FIRST AID FOR THE®

USMLE STEP 1 2014

TAO LE, MD, MHS
Associate Clinical Professor
Chief, Section of Allergy and Immunology
Department of Medicine
University of Louisville

VIKAS BHUSHAN, MD
Diagnostic Radiologist
Los Angeles

MATTHEW SOCHAT, MD
Intern, Department of Medicine
Alpert Medical School of Brown University

MAX PETERSEN
Medical Scientist Training Program
Yale School of Medicine

GORAN MICEVIC
Medical Scientist Training Program
Yale School of Medicine

KIMBERLY KALLIANOS, MD
Resident, Department of Radiology and Biomedical Imaging
University of California, San Francisco

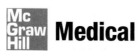 **Medical**

New York / Chicago / San Francisco / Lisbon / London / Madrid / Mexico City
Milan / New Delhi / San Juan / Seoul / Singapore / Sydney / Toronto

First Aid for the® USMLE Step 1 2014: A Student-to-Student Guide

Previous editions copyright © 1991 through 2013 by Vikas Bhushan and Tao Le. First edition copyright © 1990, 1989 by Vikas Bhushan, Jeffrey Hansen, and Edward Hon.

Photo and line art credits for this book begin on page 685 and are considered an extension of this copyright page.
Portions of this book identified with the symbol ℞ are copyright © USMLE-Rx.com (MediQ Learning, LLC).
Portions of this book identified with the symbol 🆁🆄 are copyright © Dr. Richard Usatine.
Portions of this book identified with the symbol ✷ are under license from other third parties. Please refer to page 685 for a complete list of those image source attribution notices.

First Aid for the® is a registered trademark of McGraw-Hill Education.

1 2 3 4 5 6 7 8 9 0 RMN/RMN 15 14 13

ISBN 978-0-07-183142-0
MHID 0-07-183142-8
ISSN 1532-6020

Notice

Medicine is an ever-changing science. As new research and clinical experience broaden our knowledge, changes in treatment and drug therapy are required. The authors and the publisher of this work have checked with sources believed to be reliable in their efforts to provide information that is complete and generally in accord with the standards accepted at the time of publication. However, in view of the possibility of human error or changes in medical sciences, neither the authors nor the publisher nor any other party who has been involved in the preparation or publication of this work warrants that the information contained herein is in every respect accurate or complete, and they disclaim all responsibility for any errors or omissions or for the results obtained from use of the information contained in this work. Readers are encouraged to confirm the information contained herein with other sources. For example and in particular, readers are advised to check the product information sheet included in the package of each drug they plan to administer to be certain that the information contained in this work is accurate and that changes have not been made in the recommended dose or in the contraindications for administration. This recommendation is of particular importance in connection with new or infrequently used drugs.

This book was set in Electra LH by Rainbow Graphics.
The editors were Catherine A. Johnson and Peter J. Boyle.
Project management was provided by Rainbow Graphics.
The production supervisor was Jeffrey Herzich.
RR Donnelley was printer and binder.

This book is printed on acid-free paper.

McGraw-Hill Education books are available at special quantity discounts to use as premiums and sales promotions, or for use in corporate training programs. To contact a representative please visit the Contact Us pages at www.mhprofessional.com.

Dedication

To the contributors to this and past editions, who took time to share
their knowledge, insight, and humor for the benefit of students.

Contents

▶ SECTION I   GUIDE TO EFFICIENT EXAM PREPARATION   1

▶ SECTION I SUPPLEMENT   SPECIAL SITUATIONS   25

▶ SECTION II   HIGH-YIELD GENERAL PRINCIPLES   45

Contributing Authors

FADY AKLADIOS
Medical University of the Americas
Class of 2013

RAHUL S. DALAL
Alpert Medical School of Brown University
Class of 2015

MATTHEW FOGLIA
MD/PhD Candidate
Duke University School of Medicine

ASHWANI GORE
St. George's University School of Medicine
Class of 2015

ELIZABETH L. MARSHALL
Alpert Medical School of Brown University
Class of 2015

ANDREW MARTELLA
Duke University School of Medicine
Class of 2014

MICHAEL DEAN MEHLMAN
MD/PhD Candidate
University of Queensland, Australia School of Medicine

KENNY PETTERSEN
University of California, San Francisco School of Medicine
Class of 2015

PATRICK SYLVESTER
The Ohio State University College of Medicine
Class of 2015

Image and Illustration Team

WHITNEY GREEN, MD
Resident, Department of Pathology
Johns Hopkins Hospital

PRAMOD THEETHA KARIYANNA, MBBS
Research Scholar, Division of Cardiovascular Medicine
University of Michigan Medical School

KACHIU C. LEE, MD, MPH
Resident, Department of Dermatology
Alpert Medical School of Brown University

JERRY T. LOO, MD
Resident, Department of Diagnostic Radiology
University of Southern California Keck School of Medicine

Associate Authors

DAVID H. BALLARD
Louisiana State University Health Shreveport School of Medicine
Class of 2015

ASHLEIGH C. BOUCHELION
MD/PhD Candidate
Howard University College of Medicine

JAMES M. GRAY
University College Dublin School of Medicine and Medical Science
Class of 2014

JOUZIF IBRAHIM
Medical University of the Americas
Class of 2014

EMILY LI
Alpert Medical School of Brown University
Class of 2015

M. SCOTT MOORE
Midwestern University Arizona College of Osteopathic Medicine
Class of 2014

RAZA MUSHTAQ
St. George's University School of Medicine
Class of 2015

SATYAJIT REDDY
Alpert Medical School of Brown University
Class of 2015

SASMIT SARANGI, MBBS
Research Scholar, Division of Hematology/Oncology
Massachusetts General Hospital

GRETEL TERRERO
Alpert Medical School of Brown University
Class of 2015

OLIVIER P. VAN HOUTTE
Alpert Medical School of Brown University
Class of 2015

STEPHANIE J. WONG
Boston University School of Medicine
Class of 2015

IMAGE AND ILLUSTRATION TEAM

UTKARSH ACHARYA, DO
Fellow, Department of Hematology-Oncology
University of Arizona Cancer Center

SEAN AARON LISSE
University of Michigan Medical School
Class of 2014

MICHAEL B. NATTER
Jefferson Medical College
Class of 2017

PATRICK SYLVESTER
The Ohio State University College of Medicine
Class of 2015

Faculty Reviewers

MARIA ANTONELLI, MD
Rheumatology Fellow, Department of Medicine
Metrohealth Medical Center/Case Western Reserve University

LINDA AWDISHU, PHARMD, MAS
Assistant Clinical Professor of Pharmacy
UCSD Skaggs School of Pharmacy and Pharmaceutical Sciences

ADITYA BARDIA, MBBS, MPH
Attending Physician, Massachusetts General Hospital
Harvard Medical School

LINDA S. COSTANZO, PhD
Professor of Physiology & Biophysics
Virginia Commonwealth University School of Medicine

CHARLES S. DELA CRUZ, MD, PhD
Assistant Professor, Department of Pulmonary and Critical Care Medicine
Yale School of Medicine

CONRAD FISCHER, MD
Residency Program Director, Brookdale University Hospital
Brooklyn, New York
Associate Professor of Medicine, Physiology, and Pharmacology
Touro College of Medicine

STUART D. FLYNN, MD
Dean, College of Medicine
University of Arizona College of Medicine, Phoenix

MATTHEW GARABEDIAN, MD, MPH
Department of Obstetrics and Gynecology
Santa Clara Valley Medical Center

RYAN C. W. HALL, MD
Assistant Professor, Department of Psychiatry
University of South Florida

JEFFREY W. HOFMANN
The Warren Alpert Medical School of Brown University
MD/PhD Candidate

DEEPALI JAIN, MD
Assistant Professor, Department of Pathology
All India Institute of Medical Sciences

BRIAN C. JENSEN, MD
Assistant Professor of Medicine and Pharmacology
University of North Carolina School of Medicine

KURT E. JOHNSON, PhD
Professor of Anatomy & Regenerative Biology
George Washington University School of Medicine and Health Sciences

GERALD LEE, MD
Assistant Professor, Department of Pediatrics
University of Louisville School of Medicine

ALAN I. LEIBOWITZ, MD
Professor of Medicine, Banner Good Samaritan Medical Center
University of Arizona College of Medicine, Phoenix

WARREN LEVINSON, MD, PhD
Professor, Department of Microbiology & Immunology
University of California, San Francisco School of Medicine

NICHOLAS MAHONEY, MD
Assistant Professor of Ophthalmology
Wilmer Eye Institute/Johns Hopkins Hospital

PETER MARKS, MD, PhD
Associate Professor, Department of Internal Medicine
Yale School of Medicine

MICHAEL S. RAFII, MD, PhD
Assistant Professor of Neurosciences
University of California, San Diego Health System

DANIEL J. RUBIN, MD, MSC
Assistant Professor of Medicine, Division of Endocrinology
Temple University School of Medicine

JOSEPH L. SCHINDLER, MD
Assistant Professor of Neurology and Neurosurgery
Yale School of Medicine

NATHAN W. SKELLEY, MD

Resident, Department of Orthopaedic Surgery
Barnes-Jewish Hospital/Washington University in St. Louis

VISHNU SREENIVAS, MD

Adjunct Professor of Biostatistics
All India Institute of Medical Sciences

HOWARD M. STEINMAN, PhD

Assistant Dean of Biomedical Science Education
Professor, Department of Biochemistry
Albert Einstein College of Medicine

ANDREA PROCTOR SUBHAWONG, MD

Associate Pathologist, Pathology Associates of South Miami

STEPHEN F. THUNG, MD

Associate Professor, Department of Obstetrics and Gynecology
Ohio State University College of Medicine

RICHARD P. USATINE, MD

Professor, Dermatology and Cutaneous Surgery
Professor, Family and Community Medicine
University of Texas Health Science Center San Antonio

HILARY J. VERNON, MD, PhD

Assistant Professor, McKusick Nathans Institute of Genetic Medicine
Johns Hopkins University

ADAM WEINSTEIN, MD

Assistant Professor, Section of Pediatric Nephrology
Geisel School of Medicine at Dartmonth

Preface

With this edition of *First Aid for the USMLE Step 1*, we continue our commitment to providing students with the most useful and up-to-date preparation guide for the USMLE Step 1. This edition represents an unprecedented revision to the text and illustrations, including:

- Over 50 entirely new facts and over 500 major fact updates based on the largest student survey in *First Aid* history.

- Extensive text revisions, new mnemonics, clarifications, and corrections curated by a team of 30 student authors who excelled on their Step 1 examinations. Revisions were based on over 3,000 suggestions received, and nearly 100,000 votes cast, and then verified by an expanded team of expert faculty reviewers.

- Updated with more than 350 full-color images to help visualize various disorders, descriptive findings, and basic science concepts. Labeled and captioned photographs were selected to aid retention by engaging visual memory in a manner complementary to mnemonics.

- Updated with 100+ new or revised diagrams. In partnership with USMLE-Rx.com (MedIQ Learning, LLC), we have begun introducing enhanced illustrations with improved information design to help students integrate pathophysiology, therapeutics, and diseases into memorable frameworks for annotation and personalization.

- A revised exam preparation guide with updated data from the NBME and NRMP. It also features updated USMLE advice for international medical graduates and osteopathic and podiatric students.

- An updated guide to recommended USMLE Step 1 review resources, based on a nationwide survey of randomly selected third-year medical students.

- Real-time Step 1 updates and corrections can be found exclusively on our blog at **www.firstaidteam.com**.

We invite students and faculty to continue sharing their thoughts and ideas to help us continually improve *First Aid for the USMLE Step 1* through our blog and collaborative editorial platform. (See How to Contribute, p. xvii.)

Louisville	Tao Le
Los Angeles	Vikas Bhushan
Providence	Matthew Sochat
New Haven	Goran Micevic
New Haven	Max Petersen
San Francisco	Kimberly Kallianos

Special Acknowledgments

This has been a collaborative project from the start. We gratefully acknowledge the thousands of thoughtful comments, corrections, and advice of the many medical students, international medical graduates, and faculty who have supported the authors in our continuing development of *First Aid for the USMLE Step 1*.

We provide special acknowledgment and thanks to the following students who made exemplary contributions to this edition through our voting, proofreading, and crowdsourcing platform: Daniel Aaronson, Kashif Badar, Amanda Bowers, Alice Chuang, Andrew Crisologo, Francis Deng, Joseph Farahany, Jared Gans, Alejandro Gener, Nathaniel Greenbaum, Baker Hillawy, M. Ho, Jennifer Hou, Ann Hua, Jack Hua, Hehua Huang, Mangala Iyengar, Sakshi Jain, Shana Kalaria, Tamer Khashab, Yedda Li, Ninad Maniar, Sean Martin, Xiaoliang Qiu, Nini Anastasia Sikharulidze, Justin Sysol, Charles Vu, and Jinyu Zhang.

For help on the Web, thanks to Walter F. Wiggins, Molly Lewis, Sean Martin, Luke Murray, Sarah-Grace Wesley, and Rebecca Stigall. For on-the-spot faculty review, we would like to thank Drs. Peter Chin-Hong and Ty Subhawong. For support and encouragement throughout the process, we are grateful to Thao Pham and Jonathan Kirsch, Esq. Thanks to Selina Franklin, Louise Petersen, and Trinity Kerr for organizing and supporting the project. Thanks to our publisher, McGraw-Hill, for the valuable assistance of its staff, including Midge Haramis, Jeffrey Herzich, and John Williams. For enthusiasm, support, and commitment for this ongoing and ever-challenging project, thanks to our editor, Catherine Johnson.

We are also very grateful to Dr. Fred Howell and Dr. Robert Cannon of Textensor Ltd for providing us extensive customization and support for their powerful *A.nnotate* collaborative editing platform, which allows us to efficiently manage thousands of contributions. Many thanks to Dr. Richard Usatine for his outstanding dermatologic and clinical image contributions. Thanks also to Jean-Christophe Fournet (*www.humpath.com*), Dr. Ed Uthman, and Dr. Frank Gaillard (*www.radiopaedia.org*) for generously allowing us to access some of their striking photographs.

For exceptional editorial support, enormous thanks to our tireless senior editor, Emma D. Underdown, and her team of editors, Linda Davoli, Janene Matragrano, and Isabel Nogueira. Special thanks to Jan Bednarczuk for a greatly improved index. We are also grateful to our medical illustrators, Andrea Charest, Justin Klein, Diana Kryski, Karina Metcalf, and Hans Neuhart, for their creative work on the new and updated illustrations. Lastly, tremendous thanks to Rainbow Graphics, especially David Hommel and Tina Castle, for remarkable ongoing editorial and production support under time pressure.

Louisville	Tao Le
Los Angeles	Vikas Bhushan
Providence	Matthew Sochat
New Haven	Goran Micevic
New Haven	Max Petersen
San Francisco	Kimberly Kallianos

Acknowledgments for Online Contributors

This year we were fortunate to receive the input of thousands of medical students and graduates who provided new material, clarifications, and potential corrections through our Web site and our new collaborative editing platform. This has been a tremendous help in clarifying difficult concepts, correcting errata from the previous edition, and minimizing new errata during the revision of the current edition. This reflects our long-standing vision of a true student-to-student publication. We have done our best to thank each person individually below, but we recognize that errors and omissions are likely. Therefore, we will post an updated list of acknowledgments at our Web site, **www.firstaidteam.com**. We will gladly make corrections if they are brought to our attention.

For submitting contributions and corrections, many thanks to Grant Aakre, Hasan Abbas, Khalid Abdelgadir, Yazan Abou-Ismail, Joseph Abraham, Amin Abu Khatir, Gustavo Acosta, Courtney Adams, Lance Adams, Adefunke Adedipe, Mishuka Adhikary, Jamie Adler, Gustavo Adolfo Acosta Hernandez, Abhi Aggarwal, Namita Agrawal, Nupur Agrawal, Mirza Nayyar Ahmad, Kamran Ahmed, Anosh Ahmed, Bilal Ahmed, Navid Ahmed, Umain Ahmed, Zaka Ahmed, Joanne Ahn, Hina Akbar, Arvin Akhavan, Bob Akhavan, Shola Akinshemoyin, Vivian Akoh, Anil Akoon, Ali Alagely, Ridwaan Albeiruti, Brian Alexander, Veronica Alexander, Nouman Ali, Jasim Alidina, Aness Al-Khateeb, Franz Allerberger, Netanel Alper, Katherine Altman, Aileen Alviar, Mohamed Aly Ahmed, Javier Amigon, Raj Amin, Roma Amin, Ruchi Amin, Reinaldo Amor, John Amoroso, Leonel Ampie, Zhibo An, Kapil Anand, Eric Anderson, Kristen Anderson, Ryan Anderson, Tom Anderson, Will Anderson, Kevin Andres, David Andrews, Iffat Anindo, Mohammad Ansari, Saba Ansari, Ranae Antoine, Edgar Antonio Lopez Granados, Danielle Antosh, Elizabeth Aradine, Dillon Arango, John Arcilla, Alejandro Arenas, Atif Arif, Mark Arnold, Fray Martin Arroyo-Mercado, Amir Arsalan, Hosam Asal, Aubrey Ashie, Hasan Ashkanani, Syed Ashraf, Ali Asim, Junaid Aslam, Zishan Aslam, Mwa Asplund, Roshan Asrani, Ricardo Aulet, Allen Avedian, Gabriel Axelrud, Dola Ayoade, Haripriya Ayyala, Farzana Azam, Vitali Azouz, Ryan Babienco, Solmaz Badar, Amir Badiei, Shervin Badkhshan, Rami Bahloul, Elias Baied, Christopher Bailey, Alexandra Baker, Maria Bakkal, Shruti Bala, Lindsay Baltzer, Sujani Bandela, Pavan Bang, Faustino Banuelos, Brandon Barnds, Joshua Barzilai, David Basta, James Bates, Priya Batta, Geoanna Bautista, Harinder K. Bawa, Austin Be, Yolido Beaton, Emily Beck, Vivek Behera, Babak Behseta, Rex Belgarde, Gretchen Bell, Jonathan Bell, Praveen Belur, Michael Benefiel, David Bennion, Bryan Benson, John Benson, Lauren Benson, David Bentz, Annie Laurie Benzie, Will Berlin, Kourosh Beroukhim, Frederic Bertino, Margaret Besler, Nuvpreet Bhandal, Ankit Bhatia, Vishal Bhuva, Alicia Bianco, Jake Bingham, Ryan Birdsall, John Black, Aaron Blackshaw, Craig Blakeney, Evan Blank, John Bliton, Adjoa Boateng, Maria Boboila, Nicole Bogdanovich, Joanne Boisvert, Valentina Bonev, Cecilia Bonilla, Sean Boone, Pietro Bortoletto, Eudy Bosley, Andrew Bosserman, Diana Botros, Tarrah Bowen, Mike Bowler, Venkatesh Brahma, Hemal Brahmbhatt, Cody Branch, Olga Brea, Kathryn Breidenbach, Seth Bricel, Rebeccah Briskin, Bryan Broach, Matthew Brooks, Cortlyn Brown, Fraser Brown, Kelly Brown, Sareena Brown, Zack Bryant, Carolyn Brydon, Jeff Burkeen, Phil Buss, Eduardo Bustamante, Kevin Campbell, Sanaa Cannella, Stephanie Cantu, Colby Cantu, Claudia Cao, Justin Capasso, Glenn Carr, Jessamyn Carter, Chris Cashman, Crystal Castaneda, Michael Castillo, Endri Ceka, Brian Cervoni, Phalguna Chada, Jason Chandrapal, Arjun Chandrasekaran, Kris Chang, Linda Chao, David Charles, Zeno Charles-Marcel, Marie Chase, Kiran Chatha, Shujahat Chaudhry, Yash Chavda, Peiwen Chen, Tan Chen, Wendy Chen, Zhi Cheng, Jennifer Cheung, David Chibututu Nwobu, Shideh Chinichian, David Chitty, Annie Chiu, Yu M. Chiu, Daniel Cho, Minkyung Choe, Ujval Choksi, Neesh Chop, Aneesha Chopra, Sourab Chopra, Rohit Choudhary, Amad Choudhry, Mohsin Chowdhury, Athena Christakos, Taylor Christensen, Yun Chu, George Cibulas, Dave Ciufo, Samuel Clark, Robert Clasen, Jessica Clemons, Katherine Cockerill, Steve Cohen, Laura Cohen, Alexander Cole, Jason Colip, Cristina Colon, Kelsey Conley, Brent Core, Oanea Core, Sarah Cormie, Amarilis Cornejo, Matthew Cossack, Anouchka Coste, Elliott Courter, Rachel Courtney, Steven Cox, François-Xavier Crahay, Chad Crigger, Halley Crissman, Kevin Cronin, Blake Cross, Sal Crusco, Cliff Csizmar, Ilton Cubero, Cory Cummings, Quinn Cummings, John Cummins, Wesley Cunningham, Khomthorn Cunvong, Erin Curcio, Joseph Curcio, James Dagenhart, Lekhaj Daggubati, Sarah Daigle, Bilal Dar, Alvin Das, Shayna Dattani, Chelsea Dawn Unruh, Solomon Dawson, Kevin Day, Bheesham Dayal, David Dayanim, Charles De Jesus, Sarah De los Santos, James Banks Deal Jr, Joanne Dekis, Christopher Del Prete, Kristine DeMaio, Kathryn Demitruk, Jacqueline Denysiak, Henry Derbes III, Michael

Derrick, Matthew DeSalvo, Nastassia DeSouza, Jill Desquitado, Brian Dessify, Yashu Dhamija, Asela Dharmadasa, Natasha Dhawan, Sapna Dhawan, Jennifer Diaz, August Dietrich, Peter Dietrich, Thomas Difato, Laura Diffenderfer, Om Parkash Dinani, Alex Dinh, W. James Dittmar, David DiTullio, James Doan, Isaac Dodd, John Donkersloot, Benjamin Dorfman, Andy Dornan, Elijah Douglass, Catherine Downs, Jess Dreicer, Milap Dubal, Bryce Duchman, Brandi Ducote, David Duncan, Brian Dye, Taylor Easley, Michael Eastman, Ranjitha Easwaradeva, Ryan Eaton, Christian Eccles, Sam Eccles, Jon Edgington, Jack Egbuji, Nathan Eickstaedt, Shane Eizember, Ehren Ekhause, Salem Elkhayat, Austin Ellis, Ahmed Elmetwally, Rito Escareno, Daniel Eskander, Aldo Espinoza, Michelle Estrada, Khalil Exekiel, Vaughn Eyvazian, Giselle Falconi, Mohammad Fallahzadeh, Abdelaziz Farhat, Zehra Farzal, Rebecca Fega, Benjamin Fegale, Frances Fei, Patrick Felton, Henry Feng, Dan Fer, Stuti Fernandes, Valerie Fernandez, Jaime Fineman, Emma Fink, Tucker Fischbeck, Corinne Fischer, Daniel Fischer, Sean Fischer, Juliya Fisher, Michael Flamm, Alex Flammel, Robert Flick, Manveer Victor Flora, Mario Flores, Eleanor Floyd, Megan Flynn, Julia Fong, Lindsay Forbes, Alex Fortenko, Emily Foster, Forrest Foster, Brandon Fox, Daniel Freedman, Zachary Freeland, Brian Fricke, Jonathan Fricke, Diana Fridlyand, Jessica Friedman, Gianfranco Frojo, Wendy Fujioka, William Fung, Molly Ga, James Gabriel, Mohamed Gad, Sree Gaiyahthiri Zeleznick, James Gallagher, Eva Galvane, Oliver Gantz, Elizabeth Garay, Norberto Garcia, Pablo Garcia, Nuria Garcia-Ruiz, Megha Garg, Kevin Gauvey-Kern, Josh Geleris, Colby Genrich, Nicholas George, Ryan Geosling, Trevor Gerson, Kamyar Ghabili, Laila Gharzai, Farid Gholitabar, Will Gibson, Kat Gilbert, Brian Gilberti, Simarjeet Gill, Alana Gilman, Andrew Gilman, Daniella Ginsburg, Stephanie Glass, Stephanie Gleicher, Chad Glisch, Marnie Gluck, Mustafa Goksel, Mustafa G"ksel, Daniel Goldish, Michael Goldstein, Zachary Goldstein, Edwin Golikov, Ulysses Gomez, Dibson Gondim, Andres Gonzalez, Jazmin Gonzalez, Miguel Gonzalez Velez, Joel Goodman, Farzam Gorouhi, Pishoy Gouda, Jeffrey Gould, Zain Gowani, Daniel Grabell, Kelly Grannan, Jan Grauman, Aoife Green, Ellery Greenberg, Allison Greene, Chad Greene, Alexander Greenstein, Patrick Greenwell, Michael J. E. Greff, Aaron Grober, Britt Groseclose, Joshua Gross, Andrea Grosz, Tyler Groves, Everett Gu, Lisa Gual-Bonilla, Fernando Guarderas, Angad Guliani, Jalaja Gundrathi, Xiaoyue Guo, Shabnam Gupta, Nirmal Guragai, Christie Gutierrez, Sara Hadi, Kevin Hageman, Laura Hahn, Michael Hakim, Mo Halabi, Devin Halleran, David Hamilton, Jacob Hamm, Raina Hammel, George Hanania, Bing Handler, Brittney Hanerhoff, Anna Hang, Gregory James Hanson Jr., William Harjes, Suzanna Harmouche, Jonathan Harounian, Katelyn Harris, Rebecca Hartog, Muhammad Hassan, John Hassani, Naomi Hasselblad, Katie Hateley, Nadine Haykal, Hyun Hee Kim, Christopher Heisey, Alex Helfand, Justin Hellman, Pouya Hemmati, Krista Hemmesch, Julia Heneghan, Reynold Henry, Amber Henson, Eduardo Hernandez Verge, Joseph Herron, Miriam Herschman, Ashley Hesson, Lincoln Hiatt, Ashley Higashi, Georgia Hill, Susanna Hill, Peter Hinckley, Adam Hines, Matthew Hnatow, Abby Ho, Alexander Ho, Marjorie Ho, Peter Hoang, Daniel Hoces, Aaron Hodes, Natalie Hoeting, Elizabeth Holcomb, Richard Holman, Elizabeth Horn, Noreen Hossain, Hannah Howard, Tsung Hsien Lin, Jen Hsu, Lina Hu, Jing Hua, Kevin Huang, Richard Huang, Jeff Hughes, Jenny Huo, Sook Hwang, Amr Idris, Shaz Iqbal, James Isom, Yehuda Isseroff, Rita Iyer, Yasmeen Jaber, Corbin Jacobs, Ryan Jahn, Shawn Jaikaran, Nima Jalali, Evan James, Hannah Janeway, Karl Janich, Michael Javid, Oliver Jawitz, Timothy Jay, Sarah Jenkins, Jason Jerome, Krishan Jethwa, Neil Jikaria, Damico Johnson, Ireal Johnson, Christine Johnstone, Larissa Jones, Jason Joseph, Priya Joshi, Fahad Juboori, Michael Robert Juhasz, Danielle Kacen, Zuhal Kadhim, Emily Kaditz, Michael Kagan, Alison Kahn, Sanjay Kaji, Mehboob Kalani, Jalil Kalantari, Mariya Kalashnikova, Sia Kam, Abdulrahman Kambal, Varinder Kambo, Hubert Kamecki, Jessica Kang, Angie Kao, Sushant Kapoor, David Kapp, Jerry Karp, Pallavi Karunakaran, David Karwacki, Kartikeya Kashyap, Meghana Kashyap, Lauren Kasmar, Ari Katz, Bruce Kaufman, Daniel Kaufman, Rubal Kaur, Rupinder Kaur, Stephen Kearney, Elizabeth Keiser, Billy Kennedy, Ray Kennedy, Phue Khaing, Mahmoud Khairy, Ali Khan, Khurram Khan, Mazen Khan, Simba Khan, Abhinav Khanna, Priya Khatri, Risha Khatri, Nida Khawaja, Ali Khiabani, Arshia Khorasani-Zadeh, Mani Khorsand, Mahdi Khoshchehreh, Mohammad Khoshnevisan, Shafeek Kiblawi, El Kim, Ellen Kim, Jae Kim, Jane Kim, Michael Kim, Song Kim, Youngwu Kim, Joanna Kimball, Dan Kimura, Ali Kimyaghalam, Elizabeth King, Nikhar Kinger, Mariah Kirsch, Kevin Kirschman, David Kish, Ahoy Knight, Michelle Knoll, Kevin Kolahi, Hannah Kooperkamp, Yelen Korotkaya, Maria Korte, Sujit Kotapati, Chris Kovach, David Kraft, Marat Kribis, Kaila Krishnamoorthy, Srikanth Krishnan, Emily Kronberg, Josh Kropko, Hinda Krumbein, Ryan Kuhnlein, Kaitlyn Kulesus, Anirudh Kumar, Anupam Kumar, Keerthana Kumar, Siva Kumar Aitha, Frank Kuo, David Kuppermann, Monika Kusuma-Pringle, Carmen Kut, Emmanuel Kuyinu, Daniel Kwon, Kevin Kyle, Anatalia Labilloy, Jessica Lacey, Isabella Lai, Ishan Lalani, Matthew Lam, Ragina Lancaster, Richard Lane, April Lao, Mujahed Laswi, Eric Lau, Nicholas Laucis, Dimitri Laurent, Jensen Law, Ashli Lawson, Janique Lawson, Alex Lazo, Quoc Le, Danielle Lee, David Lee, Edward Lee, Hannah Lee, Janice Amabel Lee, Janice C. Lee, Jennifer Lee, Kachiu Lee, Matthew Lee, Paul Lee, Chieng Lee Onn, Kyle Leggott, Jennifer Lehmberg, Elizabeth Lehto, Dawn Lei, Erin Leidlein, Benjamin Leist, Madelyn Lenhard, Seth Leopold, Dov Lerman-Sinkoff, Robert Leung, Maxwell Levy, Charles Li, Luming Li, Mark Liao, Huat Chye Lim, Benjamin Lin, Jonathan Lin, Peter Lin, Shawn Lin, Tsung Hsien Lin, Jason Lipof, Tyson Lippe, Matthew Lippmann, David Liu, James Liu, Junjie Liu, Mingyang Liu, Laura Llabre, Jay Llaniguez, Ahiela Logi, Stephanie Logterman, Christine Lomiguen, Zachary Lonjers, Melissa Lopez, Antonio Lopez, Laura Lopez-Roca, Dean Loporchio, Brendan Lovasik, Anna Loyal, Jing Lu, Jake Lucas, Raulee Lucero, Brooke Luo, Jeffrey Lurie, Jacob Luty, Princeton Ly, Robert Maciel, James MacKenzie, Layne Madden, Jillian Mador, Paula Magee, Lauren Mahale, Herman Mai, Leann Mainis, Ahmad Malik, Armin Malkhasian, Gopalakrishnan Manikumar, Mandip Mann, Mohamed B. Mansour, Chelsea Marion, Kent Martin, Karl Martineau, Pablo Martinez, Colton Marucci, Elham Alsadat Masoudi, Ryan Massoud, Daiva Mattis, Sergio Mauri, Ian Maya, Doug Mayeux,

Daniel Mays, Sandy Mazzoni, Patrick McAdams, Ashley McClary, Sean McGill, Andrew McGinniss, Kyle McIver, Caileigh McKenna, Travis McKevitt, Kevin McVeigh, Kevin Means, Samuel Mease, Melissa Meghpara, Hina Mehta, Dillon Meier, Chris Meinzen, Kasey Mekonnen, Ray Mendez, Joshua Mendoza-Elias, John Scott Mense, Ryan Meral, Jordan Merz, Lauren Metterle, Adam Meziani, Moeena Mian, Morgan Micheletti, Patrick Michelier, Eli Miller, Sebastien Millette, Jeff Minard, Tyler Mingo, Dennis Miraglia, Kazuya Mishima, Stuart Mitchell, Takudzwa Mkorombindo, Ahmed R. Mohsen, Hassan Reyad Mohsen, Dr. Leslie Molina, Brandon Money, Ambrose Monye, Kendall Moore, Marina Morie, Sohrab Mosaddad, Shawn Moshrefi, Geoff Motz, Rosalena Muckle, Leila Muhieddine, Dustin Mullens, Marlon Munian, Assma Murad, Daniel Murphy, Sarah Myer, Brian Myers, Rachita Navara, Nirmala Nagothu, Vijay Nagpal, Phillips Nagsuk, Edward Nahabet, Rishi Naik, Dany Nasani, Ryan Nasani, Brenton Nash, Noorul Nasir, Mohamad Nasri, Ashley Naughton, Rachita Navara, Neelima Navuluri, Nijas Nazar, Lindsey Negrete, Edward Nelson, Joseph Nelson, Jos, Nelsçn, Bryan Nevil, Neil Newman, Jason Ngo, Suzanne Ngo, Julius Ngu, Bao Nguyen, Hieu Nguyen, Kim Nguyen, Madeline Nguyen, Mai Nguyen, Michael Nguyentat, Quan Nhu, Kurt Nibelheim, Joseph Nicolazzi, Eric Niespodzany, Dhimitri Nikolla, Yifat Nir, Carolina Nocetti, Yeon-Kyeong (Caroline) Noh, Veronika Novgorodova, Yvonne Nsiah, Michael Oanea, Vanessa Obas, Nora O'Byrne, Anderson Okafor, Deborah Olmstead, Edgardo Olvera, Shi Wei Ong, Ifeanyi Onyekwe, Andrew Orr, Olusegun Osigbesan, Erik Stensj, Ben Otopalik, Giulia M. Ottaviani, Emily Oxford, Sigmund Paczkowski, Preetinder Padda, Bryce Pakso, Jon-Davy (JD) Palmer, Jason Pan, Taylor Pancoast, Mark Panetta, Kavin Panneerselvam, James Pao, Anthony Parendo, Abhishek Parikh, Pratik Parikh, Amanda Park, Jong Park, Rahul Paryani, Vanessa Pascoe, Bryce Pasko, Mike Pat, Akash Patel, Hiten Patel, Ishan Patel, Jignesh Patel, Kevin Patel, Keyur Patel, Mamta Patel, Maulin Patel, Mike Patel, Milind Patel, Nima Patel, Niraj Patel, Nisha Patel, Niti Patel, Parimal Patel, Parth Patel, Pratik Patel, Rajen Patel, Ricky Patel, Ronak Patel, Samir M. Patel, Anish Pattisapu, Jordan Patton, Michael Pelster, Rodrigo Pe¤a, Bo Peng, Lincy Bo Peng, Xuyang Peng, William Penny, Romual Perard, Rafael Perez, Abraham Peringarappillil, Alissa Petrites, Krystle Pew, Todd Pezzi, Andrew Pham, Betty Pham, Lisa Phuong, Ingrid Piat, Casey Pickett, Stephie Pierre-Louis, Emily Pinto Taylor, Crystal Piper, Collette Placek, Max Plitt, Britt Pluijmers, Alex Podolsky, Lauren K. Poindexter, Alexar Pol, Jonathan Polak, Scott Poland, Maxim Polansky, Mahesh Polavarapu, Justin Poon, Jeremy Porter, Megan Potts, Ingrid Poueriet, Kamyar Pournazari, Cee Pow, Andrew Powers, Elias Pratt, Jason Preissig, Chris Prze, Kayleigh Pung, David Purger, Anthony Purgianto, Raghuveer Puttagunta, Lucas Puttock, Eros Qamar, Zuhab Qamar, Ayman Qasrawi, Abdul Qazi, Ann Qiu, Xiaoliang Qiu, Faith Quenzer, Ann Qui, Javier A. Quintero Betancourt, Owais Qureshi, Jason Rabie, Vanessa Rackauskas, Muhammad Hamza Rafique, Preethi Raghu, Colton Ragsdale, David Rahimian, Abid Rahman, Michael Rains, Asima Raja, Thivisa Rajagopal, Vinaya Rajan, Archana Rajareddy, Ilya Rakitin, Muthukumar Ramanathan, Priya Ramaswamy, Minakshi Ramchand, Josean Ramos, Ana Maria Rams, Geoffrey Ramsdell, Gabriel Randall, Katherine Ransohoff, Robert Rash, Ali Rashid, Asheen Rauf, Misael Ravelo, Paul Ravi, Hunter Ray, Adnan Raza, Michael Reaume, Jesus Recio, Shashank Reddy, Vennela Reddy, Vibhav Reddy, Connie Redic, Sarah Reeb, Daniel Refoua, Felicia Reinitz, Michael Reopelle, David Retamar, Lindsey Retterath, Hassan Reyad Mohsen, Jose Andres Reyes, Mahsa Rezaei, Elizabeth Rhinesmith, Jamie Rhodes, Fady Riad, Jason Ricciuti, Cameron Rice, Andrew Richardson, Valery Rivas, Semnic Robert, Moshe Roberts, Dwight Robertson, Evan Robinson, Tyler Robinson, Rosa E. Rodriguez, Timmy Rogers, Pooyan Rohani, Brooke Rosen, Aaron Rosenthal, Zachary Rottmann, Ian Roy, Shubha Deep Roy, Marie Roy Babbitt, Mattan Rozenek, David Rubins, Claudia Ruiz, Danielle Rush, Christopher Russell, Jeff Ryckman, Zach Ryder, Mustafa Saad, Karl Saardi, Nouman Safdar Ali, Suparna Saha, Ryan Sahni, Peter Saikali, Glorimar Salcedo, Ahmed Salem, Yoni Samocha, Johnny Sanabria, Nilofar Sanaiha, Lakhvir Sandhar, Amanda Sandoval, Ashley Santiago, Joseph Sarcona, Anam Sarfaraz, Joyatee Sarker, Shravan Sarvepalli, Cina Sasannejad, Milan Satcher, Emma Satlof-Bedrick, Drew Satterfield, Joseph Savarese, Courtney Saw, Jeffrey Schachter, Nathan Schandevel, Matthew Schear, Nick Schiavoni, Sarah Schimansky, Sara Schlotterbeck, Joseph Schmidhofer, Andrew Schmiesing, Jonathan Schneider, Maggie Schneider, Brian Schneiderman, Lori Schoenbrun, Eran Schreter, David Schrock, Dana Scott, Paul Scott, Eric Seachrist, Meredith Sellers, Robert Semnic, Alejandro Serralvo Fuentes, Kiran Sethi, Noah Seymore, Syed Shabbir, hoda shabpiray, Raju Shah, Darshan Shah, Furqan Shah, Jarna Shah, Mihir Shah, Rutvik Shah, Sagar Shah, Tejal Shah, Ujas Shah, Elizabeth Shaheen, Rozana Shahidullah, Saate Shakil, Jonathan J. Shammaa, Shirley Shao, Zan Shareef, Kevin Sharghi, Dolly Sharma, Avijit Sharma, Sandeep Sharma, Vinny Sharma, Declan Sharp, Jonathan Sharrett, Brian Shayota, Abdul Haseeb Shehzad, Calvin Sheng, Yue Shi, Otto Shill, Jason Shimiaie, Layla Shirkhoda, Obaib Shoaib, Katoh Shoiuchi, Sara Sholar, Margo Short, Mahmud Shurafa, Adam Shurbaji, Sana Siddiqui, Zeeshan Siddiqui, Harpreet Sidhu, Peter Silverman, Anthony Simone, Brittany Simpson, Hinna Singh, Paramveer Singh, Puneet Singh, Rahul Singh, Vikal Singh, Yash Sinha, Vincent Skovira, Alex Slade, Eliza Slama, Samantha Smith, Taylor Smith, Michal Smyla, Great Snow, Andrew Snyder, Adnan Solaiman, Huijuan Song, Weihua Song, Pranay Soni, Sufian Sorathia, OsCiriah Sostan, Wilfredo Soto-Fuentes, Blake Sparks, Jeannie Sparks, Chris Spearman, Luxman Srikantha, Nandita Sriram, Marissa Srour, Amelia St. Ange, Giuseppe Staltari, Joel Stanek, Laura Stanko, Stephanie Stanley, Martin Steiner, Jonathan Sterman, Michael Stern, Evan Stevens, Nigel Stippa, Keegan Stombaugh, Jordan Stone, Melissa Stone, Erin Straight, Michelle Stram, Claudia Suarez-Makotsi, Alisha Subervi-Vazquez, Daniel Sufficool, Rebecca Suflas, Patrick Sullivan, Anitra Sumbry, Haozhe Sun, Suganja Sundaralingam, Ryan Sutherland, Thomas Sutton, Richard Swearingen, Sujan Swearingen, Lyvie-Sara Sylvestre, Peter Szpakowski, Bryan T. Young, Nathan Taillac, Rushi Talati, Wasif Talpur, Derek Tam, Jimmy Tam Huy Pham, Chung Tan, Tanya Tan, Sapna Tandon, Jessica Tanenbaum, Jackie Tanios, Maura E. Tappen, Christine Tat, Luis Taveras, Matthew Taylor, Miguel Teixeira, Alexander Teng,

Justin Teng, Zheyi Teoh, Nicholas Theodosakis, Shruthi Thiagarajasubramanian, Jordan Thiesen, Brandon Thomas, Clifford Thomas, Joshua Thomas, Emily Thompson, Rebecca Thomson, Jasmine Thum, Adam Tiagonce, Ritik Tiwari, Bridget Tobin, Misael Tollen Irizarry, Katherine Toma, Jimmy Ton, Gabriel Tonkin, Snigdha Toodi, Jen Townsend, Jake Trahan III, Michael Tran, Patrick Tran, Rebecca Tran, Daniel Treister, Jennifer Trinh, Adrian Tripp, Kent Truong, Val Tsang, Kelly Tse, Kevin Tse, Michael Tu, Michael Tuczynski, Amanda Tullos, Amity Tung, Alex Turin, Grant Turner, Victoria Tuttle, Krishna Upadhyaya, Jonathan Vacek, Neil Vadhar, Paniz Vafaei, Kimaya Vaidya, Jason Valadao, Michelle Vargas-Loaiza, Matthew Varner, Tejaswini Vasamsetty, Ashley Vaughn, Pedro-Juan V zquez Bragan, Zahra Vegdani, Meghana Vellanki, Vincent Venincasa, Bianca Verma, David Vermette, Daniel Verna, Katie Veron, Jose Villa-Uribe, Amit Vira, Suril Vithalani, Bryon Vogt, Eleftherios Vouyoukas, Jonathan Vu, Peter Vu, Jason Vuong, Nikki Vyas, Christianne Wa, Shaan Wadhawan, Michael Wallace, Amber Wallack, Joanna Wang, John Wang, Lexie Wang, Yuqi Wang, Eric Wannamaker, Muhammad Waqas, Omar Waqhar, Whitney Ward, Shane Watson, Jennifer Weinberg, Robert Weir, Sarah Weiss, David Weltman, Curt Wengel, Brian Wentworth, James West, Wells Weymouth, Raymond Whitham, Jessica Wickes, Shira Wieder, Brianna Wierz, Renee Wierz, Reid Wilkening, Dan Wilkinson, Jarrett Williams, Jason Williams, Sarah Williams, Justin Willingham, Zachary Wilseck, Suzy Wilson, Tyler Winders, Rob Winningham, Erich Wittmer, Andrew Wong, Brinton Woods, Zachary Woodward, Eric Worrall, Jason Wright, Monica Wright, Marta Wronska, James Wrubel, Edward Wu, Wayland Wu, Rong Xia, Nanfang Xu, Steven Yale, Casey Yang, Joseph Yang, Shirley Yang, Phil Yao, Niloo Yari, Daniel Yee, Jared Yee, Richard Yi, Kathleen Yip, Michael Yip, Gihee Yoon, Jane Yoon, Rachel Yoon, Albert Young, Charles Young, Christopher Young, Ibbad Yousuf, Charles Yu, Sherry Yu, Alex Yue, Sonia Yuen, Chrstine Yun, Fahd Yunus, Omer Zaman, Wayel Zanjir, Katherine Zappia, Howard Zee, Brian Zeidan, Rafik Zemokhol, Steven Zerilli, Thomas Zervos, Henry Zhan, Eddie Zhang, Jessica Zhang, Louis Zhang, Qiang Zhang, Carrie Zhao, Diana Zhong, Tianzan Zhou, Vicki Zhu Jun Bing, Audra Zimmer, Patrick Zito, Michael Zobel, Dmitri Zouev, and Sam Zuber.

For submitting book reviews, thanks to Amanda Abuaf, Ritesh Agnihothri, Gabrielle Ahlzadeh, Annie Allen, Claudia Alvarez, Nick Alvey, Jenna Anderson, Hou Andrew, Robert Apland, Zakaria Aqel, Samuel Ayo, Shruti Bala, Raksha Bangalore, Ari Berlin, Brandan Blackwell, Alexander Blair, Brittney Brown, Diondra Burney, Meisje Burton, Chris Byers, Anthony Canete, Yuan Cao, Carlos Casillas, Angad Chadha, Angela Chan, Karen Chang, Jenny Chen, Reesa Child , Kenneth Chin, Pinal Chokshi, Meir Cohen, Jared Cooke, Dan Dang, RaShonda Dennis, Charyse Diaz, Joseph Diaz, Stephanie Diebold, Brian Dinerman, Allison Dobry, Omar Dughly, Jacob Eby, Dean Ehrlich, Rachel Eliason, Pouya Entezami, Uwagbae Eweka, Christine Feigal, Shaun Fernandes, Dana Ferrari, Raul Ferrer, David Finkelstein, Caroline Fischer, Aaron Fisher, Jayson Fitter, Michael Foulks, Pavan Ganapathiraju, Himali Gandhi, Anita Garg, Merissa Garvey, Christi Gerald, Simarjeet Gill, Fatima Giron, Augustine Gnalian, Priyanka Gokhale, Maria Gomez, Preeya Goyal, Casey Graziani, Joshua Greenstein, Ashley Grief, Paula Griffith, Xiaoxiao Guo, Daniel Gutierrez, Yasmin Guzman, Anna Hang, Rebekah Harding, Erica Harple, Nadine Haykal, John Heathcote, Désmond Henry, Joyce Ho, Jessica Holley, Marianne Hom, Lindsay Hoogenboom, Safina Hossain, Kevin Hou, Meng Hsieh, Callie Hurtt, Ali Imran, Laura Irastorza, Jaspreet Jaura, Samaa Kamal, Navdeep Kang, Mohsin Khan, Neil Khanna, Amy Killeen, Alexandra Knoppel, Vanessa Kreger, Jeremy Kruger, Monika Kusuma-Pringle, Stephen Kwak, Isabella Lai, Gopal Lalchandani, Kim Tuyen Lam, Matthew Lam, Alyssa Lampe, Bradley Lander, Ji Eun Lee, Lauren Lee, David Levine, Jack Levy, Jason Lipof, Anna Loyal, Lina Lu, Andrea Lui, Elisa Lund, Alexander Ly, Paul Malczak, Lauren Maselli, Vineetha Mathew, Rica Mauricio, Daniel Mays, Caitriona McGovern, Jaine McKenzie, Chelsea McKirnan, Adam Meziani, Sebastien Millette, Nathan Mills, Michael Mitakidis, Emilie Mitten, Carmel Moazez, Norhan Mohammed, Joy Morgan, Gillian Morris, Amanda Murray, Sunny Narang, Azadeh Nasrazadani, Navin Natarajan, Anna Nguyen, Bao Nguyen, Myles Nickolich, Sarah Nickolich, James Nitti, Beatrix Ohienmhen, Blessy Oommen, Samia Osman, Navasard Ovasapians, Brent Ozaki, Aditya Paliwal, Aubrey Palmer, Karna Patel, Ruby Patel, Samir Patel, Steven Pearson, Jonathan Pelletier, Joshua Pendl, Jason Pia, Lidianny Polanco, Alex Power-Hays, Rachel Pughsley, Vinaya Rajan, Arvind Ravinutala, Sabrina Reed, Ria Richardson, Crystal Romero, Andre Rosario, Ulysses Rosas, J. S. Rowe, Alexandra Roybal, Soshian Sarrafpour, Jessica Schultz, Stacia Semple, Darshan Shah, Sonal Shah, Ahmad Shamia, Alejandro Shepard, Stephen Sheridan, Harpreet Sidhu, Molly Siegel, Megan Simon Thomas, Anna Jo Smith, Jason Solway, Haresh Soorma, Meghan Soulvie, Shravan Sridhar, Jess St. Laurent, Amelia St. Ange, Dustin Staloch, Maricarmen Stout, Ann Symonds, Vikrant Tambe, Denise Teh, Miguel Teixeira, Zheyi Teoh, David Torres, Brian Trinh, Jacob Triplet, Sandy Truong, Malcolm Vandrevala, Ruchi Vikas, Laura Villavicencio, Whitney Von Voigt, Ross Vyhmeister, Joshua Waitzman Waitzman, Shari Wallace, Marissa Watson, Rebecca Wendt, William West, Jeffrey Whitman, Jarrett Williams, Deborah Witkin, Luccie Wo, Raymond Wong, Brinton Woods, Darah Wright, Matthew Young, and Michael Zobel.

How to Contribute

This version of *First Aid for the USMLE Step 1* incorporates hundreds of contributions and improvements suggested by student and faculty reviewers. We invite you to participate in this process. Please send us your suggestions for:

- Study and test-taking strategies for the USMLE Step 1

- New facts, mnemonics, diagrams, and clinical images

- High-yield topics that may appear on future Step 1 exams

- Personal ratings and comments on review books, question banks, apps, videos, and courses

For each new entry incorporated into the next edition, you will receive up to a **$20 Amazon.com gift card** as well as personal acknowledgment in the next edition. Significant contributions will be compensated at the discretion of the authors. Also, let us know about material in this edition that you feel is low yield and should be deleted.

All submissions including potential errata should ideally be supported with hyperlinks to two current references:

- A dynamically updated Web resource such as *Wikipedia*, *eMedicine*, or *UpToDate*; and

- A link to an authoritative specialty textbook (search the "topic + *Inkling*" in Google and link to the courtesy pages available from a wide variety of major medical textbooks)

We welcome potential errata on grammar and style if the change improves readability. Please note that *First Aid* style is somewhat unique; for example, we have in this edition fully adopted the AMA *Manual of Style* recommendations on eponyms: "We recommend that the possessive form be omitted in eponymous terms."

The preferred way to submit new entries, clarifications, mnemonics, or potential corrections with a valid, authoritative reference is via our Web site: **www.firstaidteam.com**.

This Web site will be continuously updated with validated errata, new high-yield content, and a new online platform to contribute suggestions, mnemonics, diagrams, clinical images, and potential errata.

Alternatively, you can email us at: **firstaidteam@yahoo.com**.

Contributions submitted by **June 15, 2014**, receive priority consideration for the 2015 edition of *First Aid for the USMLE Step 1*. We thank you for taking the time to share your experience and apologize in advance that we cannot individually respond to all contributors as we receive thousands of contributions each year.

▶ NOTE TO CONTRIBUTORS

All contributions become property of the authors and are subject to editing and reviewing. Please verify all data and spellings carefully. Contributions should be supported by at least two high-quality references.

Please include supporting hyperlinks on all content and errata suggestions. Check our Web site first to avoid duplicate submissions. In the event that similar or duplicate entries are received, only the first complete entry received with a valid, authoritative reference will be credited. Please follow the style, punctuation, and format of this edition as much as possible.

▶ JOIN THE FIRST AID TEAM

The *First Aid* author team is pleased to offer part-time and full-time paid internships in medical education and publishing to motivated medical students and physicians. Internships range from a few months (e.g., a summer) up to a full year. Participants will have an opportunity to author, edit, and earn academic credit on a wide variety of projects, including the popular *First Aid* series.

In 2014, we are actively seeking passionate medical students and graduates with a specific interest in improving our medical illustrations and expanding our database of medical photographs. We welcome people with prior experience and talent in this area. Relevant skills include clinical imaging, digital photography, digital asset management, information design, medical illustration, and graphic design.

Please email us at **firstaidteam@yahoo.com** with a CV and summary of your interest or sample work.

How to Use This Book

Medical students who have used previous editions of this guide have given us feedback on how best to make use of the book.

START EARLY: Use this book as early as possible while learning the basic medical sciences. The first semester of your first year is not too early! Devise a study plan by reading Section I: Guide to Efficient Exam Preparation, and make an early decision on resources to use by reading Section IV: Top-Rated Review Resources.

LET FIRST AID BE YOUR GUIDE: Annotate material from other resources such as class notes or comprehensive textbooks into your copy of *First Aid*. Use it as a framework for distinguishing between high-yield and low-yield material. Note that *First Aid* is neither a textbook nor a comprehensive review book, and it is not a panacea for inadequate preparation during the first two years of medical school. We strongly recommend that you invest in the latest edition of at least one or two top-rated review resources on each subject to ensure that you learn the material thoroughly.

CONSOLIDATE THE MATERIAL: As you study new material, use the corresponding high-yield facts in *First Aid for the USMLE Step 1* as a means of consolidating knowledge. Make high-yield connections between different organ systems and general principles and focus on material that is most likely to be tested.

INTEGRATE STUDY WITH CASES AND QUESTIONS: To broaden your learning strategy, consider integrating your *First Aid* study with case-based reviews (e.g., *First Aid Cases for the USMLE Step 1*) and practice questions (e.g., *First Aid Q&A for the USMLE Step 1* or the USMLE-Rx Qmax Step 1 question bank). After reviewing a discipline or organ system chapter within *First Aid*, review cases on the same topics and test your knowledge with relevant practice questions. Maintain access to more comprehensive resources (e.g., *First Aid for the Basic Sciences: General Principles* and *Organ Systems*, *First Aid Express* and the *Ultimate* video courses) for deeper review as needed.

PRIME YOUR MEMORY: Return to your annotated Sections II and III several days before taking the USMLE Step 1. The book can serve as a useful way of retaining key associations and keeping high-yield facts fresh in your memory just prior to the exam. The Rapid Review section includes high-yield topics to help guide your studying.

CONTRIBUTE TO FIRST AID: Reviewing the book immediately after your exam can help us improve the next edition. Decide what was truly high and low yield and send us your comments. Feel free to send us scanned images from your annotated *First Aid* book as additional support. Of course, always remember that all examinees are under agreement with the USMLE to not disclose the specific details of copyrighted test material.

Common USMLE Laboratory Values

* = Included in the Biochemical Profile (SMA-12)

Blood, Plasma, Serum	Reference Range	SI Reference Intervals
*Alanine aminotransferase (ALT, GPT at 30°C)	8–20 U/L	8–20 U/L
Amylase, serum	25–125 U/L	25–125 U/L
*Aspartate aminotransferase (AST, GOT at 30°C)	8–20 U/L	8–20 U/L
Bilirubin, serum (adult)		
Total // Direct	0.1–1.0 mg/dL // 0.0–0.3 mg/dL	2–17 µmol/L // 0–5 µmol/L
*Calcium, serum (Total)	8.4–10.2 mg/dL	2.1–2.8 mmol/L
*Cholesterol, serum (Total)	140–200 mg/dL	3.6–6.5 mmol/L
*Creatinine, serum (Total)	0.6–1.2 mg/dL	53–106 µmol/L
Electrolytes, serum		
Sodium	135–147 mEq/L	135–147 mmol/L
Chloride	95–105 mEq/L	95–105 mmol/L
* Potassium	3.5–5.0 mEq/L	3.5–5.0 mmol/L
Bicarbonate	22–28 mEq/L	22–28 mmol/L
Gases, arterial blood (room air)		
P_{O_2}	75–105 mmHg	10.0–14.0 kPa
P_{CO_2}	33–44 mmHg	4.4–5.9 kPa
pH	7.35–7.45	[H$^+$] 36–44 nmol/L
*Glucose, serum	Fasting: 70–110 mg/dL	3.8–6.1 mmol/L
	2-h postprandial: < 120 mg/dL	< 6.6 mmol/L
Growth hormone – arginine stimulation	Fasting: < 5 ng/mL	< 5 µg/L
	provocative stimuli: > 7 ng/mL	> 7 µg/L
Osmolality, serum	275–295 mOsm/kg	275–295 mOsm/kg
*Phosphatase (alkaline), serum (p-NPP at 30°C)	20–70 U/L	20–70 U/L
*Phosphorus (inorganic), serum	3.0–4.5 mg/dL	1.0–1.5 mmol/L
*Proteins, serum		
Total (recumbent)	6.0–7.8 g/dL	60–78 g/L
Albumin	3.5–5.5 g/dL	35–55 g/L
Globulins	2.3–3.5 g/dL	23–35 g/L
*Urea nitrogen, serum (BUN)	7–18 mg/dL	1.2–3.0 mmol/L
*Uric acid, serum	3.0–8.2 mg/dL	0.18–0.48 mmol/L
Cerebrospinal Fluid		
Glucose	40–70 mg/dL	2.2–3.9 mmol/L

(continues)

Hematologic

Erythrocyte count	Male: 4.3–5.9 million/mm^3	$4.3–5.9 \times 10^{12}$/L
	Female: 3.5–5.5 million/mm^3	$3.5–5.5 \times 10^{12}$/L
Hematocrit	Male: 41–53%	0.41–0.53
	Female: 36–46%	0.36–0.46
Hemoglobin, blood	Male: 13.5–17.5 g/dL	2.09–2.71 mmol/L
	Female: 12.0–16.0 g/dL	1.86–2.48 mmol/L
Reticulocyte count	0.5–1.5% of red cells	0.005–0.015
Hemoglobin, plasma	1–4 mg/dL	0.16–0.62 µmol/L
Leukocyte count and differential		
Leukocyte count	4500–11,000/mm^3	$4.5–11.0 \times 10^9$/L
Segmented neutrophils	54–62%	0.54–0.62
Band forms	3–5%	0.03–0.05
Eosinophils	1–3%	0.01–0.03
Basophils	0–0.75%	0–0.0075
Lymphocytes	25–33%	0.25–0.33
Monocytes	3–7%	0.03–0.07
Mean corpuscular hemoglobin	25.4–34.6 pg/cell	0.39–0.54 fmol/cell
Mean corpuscular volume	80–100 µm^3	80–100 fL
Platelet count	150,000–400,000/mm^3	$150–400 \times 10^9$/L
Prothrombin time	11–15 seconds	11–15 seconds
Activated partial thromboplastin time	25–40 seconds	25–40 seconds
Sedimentation rate, erythrocyte (Westergren)	Male: 0–15 mm/h	0–15 mm/h
	Female: 0–20 mm/h	0–20 mm/h
Proteins in urine, total	< 150 mg/24 h	< 0.15 g/24 h

First Aid Checklist for the USMLE Step 1

This is an example of how you might use the information in Section I to prepare for the USMLE Step 1. Refer to corresponding topics in Section I for more details.

Years Prior
☐ Select top-rated review books as study guides for first-year medical school courses.
☐ Ask for advice from those who have recently taken the USMLE Step 1.

Months Prior
☐ Review computer test format and registration information.
☐ Register six months in advance. Carefully verify name and address printed on scheduling permit. Call Prometric or go online for test date ASAP.
☐ Define goals for the USMLE Step 1 (e.g., comfortably pass, beat the mean, ace the test).
☐ Set up a realistic timeline for study. Cover less crammable subjects first. Review subject-by-subject emphasis and clinical vignette format.
☐ Simulate the USMLE Step 1 to pinpoint strengths and weaknesses in knowledge and test-taking skills.
☐ Evaluate and choose study methods and materials (e.g., review books, practice tests, software).

Weeks Prior
☐ Simulate the USMLE Step 1 again. Assess how close you are to your goal.
☐ Pinpoint remaining weaknesses. Stay healthy (exercise, sleep).
☐ Verify information on admission ticket (e.g., location, date).

One Week Prior
☐ Remember comfort measures (loose clothing, earplugs, etc.).
☐ Work out test site logistics such as location, transportation, parking, and lunch.
☐ Call Prometric and confirm your exam appointment.

One Day Prior
☐ Relax.
☐ Lightly review short-term material if necessary. Skim high-yield facts.
☐ Get a good night's sleep.
☐ Make sure the name printed on your photo ID appears EXACTLY the same as the name printed on your scheduling permit.

Day of Exam
☐ Relax. Eat breakfast. Minimize bathroom breaks during the exam by avoiding excessive morning caffeine.
☐ Analyze and make adjustments in test-taking technique. You are allowed to review notes/study material during breaks on exam day.

After the Exam
☐ Celebrate, regardless.
☐ Send feedback to us on our Web site at **www.firstaidteam.com.**

Guide to Efficient Exam Preparation

"A mind of moderate capacity which closely pursues one study must infallibly arrive at great proficiency in that study."

—Mary Shelley, *Frankenstein*

"Finally, from so little sleeping and so much reading, his brain dried up and he went completely out of his mind."

—Miguel de Cervantes Saavedra, *Don Quixote*

▶ INTRODUCTION

Relax.

This section is intended to make your exam preparation easier, not harder. Our goal is to reduce your level of anxiety and help you make the most of your efforts by helping you understand more about the United States Medical Licensing Examination, Step 1 (USMLE Step 1). As a medical student, you are no doubt familiar with taking standardized examinations and quickly absorbing large amounts of material. When you first confront the USMLE Step 1, however, you may find it all too easy to become sidetracked from your goal of studying with maximal effectiveness. Common mistakes that students make when studying for Step 1 include the following:

- Not understanding how scoring is performed or what the score means
- Starting to study (including *First Aid*) too late
- Starting to study intensely too early and burning out
- Using inefficient or inappropriate study methods
- Buying the wrong books or buying more books than you can ever use
- Buying only one publisher's review series for all subjects
- Not using practice examinations to maximum benefit
- Not using review books along with your classes
- Not analyzing and improving your test-taking strategies
- Getting bogged down by reviewing difficult topics excessively
- Studying material that is rarely tested on the USMLE Step 1
- Failing to master certain high-yield subjects owing to overconfidence
- Using *First Aid* as your sole study resource
- Trying to do it all alone

In this section, we offer advice to help you avoid these pitfalls and be more productive in your studies.

> ▶ *The test at a glance:*
> - *8-hour exam*
> - *Total of 322 multiple choice items*
> - *7 test blocks (60 min/block)*
> - *46 test items per block*
> - *45 minutes of break time, plus another 15 if you skip the tutorial*

▶ USMLE STEP 1—THE BASICS

The USMLE Step 1 is the first of three examinations that you must pass in order to become a licensed physician in the United States. The USMLE is a joint endeavor of the National Board of Medical Examiners (NBME) and the Federation of State Medical Boards (FSMB). The USMLE serves as the single examination system for U.S. medical students and international medical graduates (IMGs) seeking medical licensure in the United States.

The Step 1 exam includes test items drawn from the following content areas:

- Anatomy
- Behavioral sciences
- Biochemistry
- Microbiology and immunology
- Pathology

- Pharmacology
- Physiology
- Interdisciplinary topics such as biostatistics, nutrition, genetics, and aging

How Is the Computer-Based Test (CBT) Structured?

The CBT Step 1 exam consists of one "optional" tutorial/simulation block and seven "real" question blocks of 46 questions each (see Figure 1) for a total of 322 questions, timed at 60 minutes per block. A short 11-question survey follows the last question block. The computer begins the survey with a prompt to proceed to the next block of questions.

Once an examinee finishes a particular question block on the CBT, he or she must click on a screen icon to continue to the next block. Examinees **cannot** go back and change their answers to questions from any previously completed block. However, changing answers is allowed **within** a block of questions as long as the block has not been ended and if time permits—**unless** the questions are part of a sequential item test set (see p. 4).

What Is the CBT Like?

Given the unique environment of the CBT, it's important that you become familiar ahead of time with what your test-day conditions will be like. In fact, you can easily add 15 minutes to your break time! This is because the 15-minute tutorial offered on exam day may be skipped if you are already familiar with the exam procedures and the testing interface. The 15 minutes is then added to your allotted break time of 45 minutes for a total of 1 hour of potential break time. You can download the tutorial from the USMLE Web site and do it before test day. This tutorial is the exact same interface you will use in the exam; learn it now and you can skip taking it during the exam, giving you 15 extra minutes of break time. You can also gain experience with the CBT format by taking the 150 practice questions available online or by

> ▶ *If you know the format, you can skip the tutorial and add 15 minutes to your break time!*

FIGURE 1. Schematic of CBT Exam.

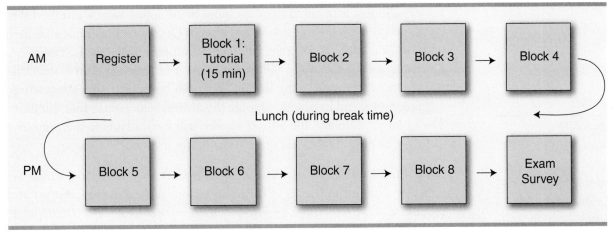

signing up for a practice session at a test center (for details, see What Does the CBT Format Mean to Me?).

For security reasons, examinees are not allowed to bring any personal electronic equipment into the testing area. This includes both digital and analog watches, iPods, tablets, calculators, cellular telephones, and electronic paging devices. Examinees are also prohibited from carrying in their books, notes, pens/pencils, and scratch paper. Food and beverages are also prohibited in the testing area. The testing centers are monitored by audio and video surveillance equipment. However, most testing centers allot each examinee a small locker outside the testing area in which he or she can store snacks, beverages, and personal items.

The typical question screen in the CBT consists of a question followed by a number of choices on which an examinee can click, together with several navigational buttons on the top of the screen. There is a countdown timer on the lower left-hand corner of the screen as well. There is also a button that allows the examinee to mark a question for review. If a given question happens to be longer than the screen (which occurs very rarely), a scroll bar will appear on the right, allowing the examinee to see the rest of the question. Regardless of whether the examinee clicks on an answer choice or leaves it blank, he or she must click the "Next" button to advance to the next question.

The USMLE features a small number of media clips in the form of audio and/or video. There may even be a question with a multimedia heart sound simulation. In these questions, a digital image of a torso appears on the screen, and the examinee directs a digital stethoscope to various auscultation points to listen for heart and breath sounds. The USMLE orientation materials include several practice questions in these formats. During the exam tutorial, examinees are given an opportunity to ensure that both the audio headphones and the volume are functioning properly. If you are already familiar with the tutorial and planning on skipping it, first skip ahead to the section where you can test your headphones. After you are sure the headphones are working properly, proceed to the exam.

A few years ago the USMLE introduced a sequential item test format for some questions. Sequential item questions are grouped together in the list of questions on the left-hand side of the screen. Questions in a sequential item set must be completed in order. After an examinee answers the first question, he or she will be given the option to proceed to the next item but will be warned that the answer to the first question will be locked. **After proceeding, examinees will not be able to change the answer selected for that question.** The question stem and the answer chosen will be available to the examinee as he or she answers the next question(s) in the sequence.

Some Step 1 questions may also contain figures or illustrations. These are typically situated to the right of the question. Although the contrast and brightness of the screen can be adjusted, there are no other ways to manipulate the picture (e.g., there is no zooming or panning).

▶ Keyboard shortcuts:

- A, B, etc.–letter choices
- Enter or spacebar–move to next question
- Esc–exit pop-up Lab and Exhibit windows
- Alt-T–countdown timers for current session and overall test

---

▶ Heart sounds are tested via media questions. Make sure you know how different heart diseases sound on auscultation.

▶ Test illustrations include:

- Gross photos
- Histology slides
- Radiographs
- Electron micrographs
- Line drawings

The examinee can call up a window displaying normal laboratory values. In order to do so, he or she must click the "Lab" icon on the top part of the screen. Afterward, the examinee will have the option to choose between "Blood," "Cerebrospinal," "Hematologic," or "Sweat and Urine." The normal-values screen may obscure the question if it is expanded. The examinee may have to scroll down to search for the needed lab values. You might want to memorize some common lab values so you spend less time on questions that require you to analyze these.

▶ *Familiarize yourself with the commonly tested lab values.*

The CBT interface provides a running list of questions on the left part of the screen at all times. The software also permits examinees to highlight or cross out information by using their mouse. Finally, there is a "Notes" icon on the top part of the screen that allows students to write notes to themselves for review at a later time. Being familiar with these features can save time and may help you better organize the information you need to answer a question.

▶ *Ctrl-Alt-Delete are the keys of death during the exam. Don't touch them!*

What Does the CBT Format Mean to Me?

The significance of the CBT to you depends on the requirements of your school and your level of computer knowledge. If you are a Mac user, you might want to spend some time using a Windows-based system and pointing and clicking icons or buttons with a mouse.

For those who feel they might benefit, the USMLE offers an opportunity to take a simulated test, or "CBT Practice Session at a Prometric center." Students are eligible to register for this three-and-one-half-hour practice session after they have received their scheduling permit.

The same USMLE Step 1 sample test items (150 questions) available on the USMLE Web site, www.usmle.org, are used at these sessions. **No new items will be presented.** The session is divided into a short tutorial and three 1-hour blocks of 50 test items each at a cost of about $75, if your testing region is in the United States or Canada. Students receive a printed percent-correct score after completing the session. **No explanations of questions are provided.**

▶ *You can take a shortened CBT practice test at a Prometric center.*

You may register for a practice session online at www.usmle.org. A separate scheduling permit is issued for the practice session. Students should allow two weeks for receipt of this permit.

How Do I Register to Take the Exam?

Prometric test centers offer Step 1 on a year-round basis, except for the first two weeks in January and major holidays. The exam is given every day except Sunday at most centers. Some schools administer the exam on their own campuses. Check with the test center you want to use before making your exam plans.

▶ *The Prometric Web site will display a calendar with open test dates.*

U.S. students can apply to take Step 1 at the NBME Web site. This application allows you to select one of 12 overlapping three-month blocks in which to be tested (e.g., April–May–June, June–July–August). Choose your three-month eligibility period wisely. If you need to reschedule outside your initial three-month period, you can request a one-time extension of eligibility for the next contiguous three-month period, and pay a rescheduling fee. The application also includes a photo ID form that must be certified by an official at your medical school to verify your enrollment. After the NBME processes your application, it will send you a scheduling permit.

The scheduling permit you receive from the NBME will contain your USMLE identification number, the eligibility period in which you may take the exam, and two additional numbers. The first of these is known as your "scheduling number." You must have this number in order to make your exam appointment with Prometric. The second number is known as the "candidate identification number," or CIN. Examinees must enter their CINs at the Prometric workstation in order to access their exams. Prometric has no access to the codes. **Do not lose your permit!** You will not be allowed to take the exam unless you present this permit along with an unexpired, government-issued photo ID that includes your signature (such as a driver's license or passport). Make sure the name on your photo ID exactly matches the name that appears on your scheduling permit.

▸ *The confirmation emails that Prometric and NBME send are not the same as the scheduling permit.*

Once you receive your scheduling permit, you may access the Prometric Web site or call Prometric's toll-free number to arrange a time to take the exam. You may contact Prometric two weeks before the test date if you want to confirm identification requirements. Although requests for taking the exam may be completed more than six months before the test date, examinees will not receive their scheduling permits earlier than six months before the eligibility period. The eligibility period is the three-month period you have chosen to take the exam. Most medical students choose the April–June or June–August period. Because exams are scheduled on a "first-come, first-served" basis, it is recommended that you contact Prometric as soon as you receive your permit. After you've scheduled your exam, it's a good idea to confirm your exam appointment with Prometric at least one week before your test date. Prometric will provide appointment confirmation on a print-out and by email. Be sure to read the *2014 USMLE Bulletin of Information* for further details.

▸ *Test scheduling is done on a "first-come, first-served" basis. It's important to call and schedule an exam date as soon as you receive your scheduling permit.*

What If I Need to Reschedule the Exam?

You can change your test date and/or center by contacting Prometric at 1-800-MED-EXAM (1-800-633-3926) or www.prometric.com. Make sure to have your CIN when rescheduling. If you are rescheduling by phone, you must speak with a Prometric representative; leaving a voice-mail message will not suffice. To avoid a rescheduling fee, you will need to request a change at least 31 calendar days before your appointment. Please note that your rescheduled test date must fall within your assigned three-month eligibility period.

When Should I Register for the Exam?

Although there are no deadlines for registering for Step 1, you should plan to register at least six months ahead of your desired test date. This will guarantee that you will get either your test center of choice or one within a 50-mile radius of your first choice. For most U.S. medical students, the desired testing window is in June, since most medical school curricula for the second year end in May or June. Thus, U.S. medical students should plan to register before January in anticipation of a June test date. The timing of the exam is more flexible for IMGs, as it is related only to when they finish exam preparation. Talk with upperclassmen who have already taken the test so you have real-life experience from students who went through a similar curriculum, then formulate your own strategy.

▶ *Register six months in advance for seating and scheduling preference.*

Where Can I Take the Exam?

Your testing location is arranged with Prometric when you call for your test date (after you receive your scheduling permit). For a list of Prometric locations nearest you, visit www.prometric.com.

How Long Will I Have to Wait Before I Get My Scores?

The USMLE reports scores in three to four weeks, unless there are delays in score processing. Examinees will be notified via email when their scores are available. By following the online instructions, examinees will be able to view, download, and print their score report. Additional information about score timetables and accessibility is available on the official USMLE Web site.

What About Time?

Time is of special interest on the CBT exam. Here's a breakdown of the exam schedule:

▶ *Gain extra break time by skipping the tutorial or finishing a block early.*

15 minutes	Tutorial (skip if familiar with test format and features)
7 hours	Seven 60-minute question blocks
45 minutes	Break time (includes time for lunch)

The computer will keep track of how much time has elapsed on the exam. However, the computer will show you only how much time you have remaining in a given block. Therefore, it is up to you to determine if you are pacing yourself properly (at a rate of approximately one question per 78 seconds).

The computer will not warn you if you are spending more than your allotted time for a break. You should therefore budget your time so that you can take a short break when you need one and have time to eat. You must be especially careful not to spend too much time in between blocks (you should keep track of how much time elapses from the time you finish a block of questions to the time you start the next block). After you finish one question block, you'll need to click on a button to proceed to the next block of questions. If you do not click to proceed to the next question block, you will automatically be entered into a break period.

Forty-five minutes is the minimum break time for the day, but you are not required to use all of it, nor are you required to use any of it. You can gain extra break time (but not time for the question blocks) by skipping the tutorial or by finishing a block ahead of the allotted time. Any time remaining on the clock when you finish a block gets added to your remaining break time. Once a new question block has been started, you may not take a break until you have reached the end of that block. If you do so, this will be recorded as an "unauthorized break" and will be reported on your final score report.

Finally, be aware that it may take a few minutes of your break time to "check out" of the secure resting room and then "check in" again to resume testing, so plan accordingly. The "check-in" process may include fingerprints and pocket checks. Some students recommend pocketless clothing on exam day to streamline the process.

> ▶ Be careful to watch the clock on your break time.

If I Freak Out and Leave, What Happens to My Score?

Your scheduling permit shows a CIN that you will enter onto your computer screen to start your exam. Entering the CIN is the same as breaking the seal on a test book, and you are considered to have started the exam when you do so. However, no score will be reported if you do not complete the exam. In fact, if you leave at any time from the start of the test to the last block, no score will be reported. The fact that you started but did not complete the exam, however, will appear on your USMLE score transcript. Even though a score is not posted for incomplete tests, examinees may still get an option to request that their scores be calculated and reported if they desire; unanswered questions will be scored as incorrect.

The exam ends when all question blocks have been completed or when their time has expired. As you leave the testing center, you will receive a printed test-completion notice to document your completion of the exam. To receive an official score, you must finish the entire exam.

What Types of Questions Are Asked?

> ▶ Nearly three fourths of Step 1 questions begin with a description of a patient.

One-best-answer multiple choice items (either singly or as part of a sequential item set) are the only question type on the exam. Most questions consist of a clinical scenario or a direct question followed by a list of five or more options. You are required to select the single best answer among the options given.

There are no "except," "not," or matching questions on the exam. A number of options may be partially correct, in which case you must select the option that best answers the question or completes the statement. Additionally, keep in mind that experimental questions may appear on the exam, which do not affect your score (see Difficult Questions, p. 20).

How Is the Test Scored?

Each Step 1 examinee receives an electronic score report that includes the examinee's pass/fail status, a three-digit test score, and a graphic depiction of the examinee's performance by discipline and organ system or subject area. The actual organ system profiles reported may depend on the statistical characteristics of a given administration of the examination.

The NBME provides a three-digit test score based on the total number of items answered correctly on the examination (see Figure 2). The score is reported as a scaled score in which the mean is 227 and the standard deviation is approximately 22.

> ▸ The mean Step 1 score for U.S. medical students continues to rise, from 200 in 1991 to 227 in 2012.

A score of 188 or higher is required to pass Step 1. The NBME does not report the minimum number of correct responses needed to pass, but estimates that it is roughly 60–70%. The NBME may adjust the minimum passing score in the future, so please check the USMLE Web site or www.firstaidteam.com for updates.

According to the USMLE, medical schools receive a listing of total scores and pass/fail results plus group summaries by discipline and organ system. Students can withhold their scores from their medical school if they wish. Official USMLE transcripts, which can be sent on request to residency programs, include only total scores, not performance profiles.

Consult the USMLE Web site or your medical school for the most current and accurate information regarding the examination.

FIGURE 2. Scoring Scale for the USMLE Step 1.

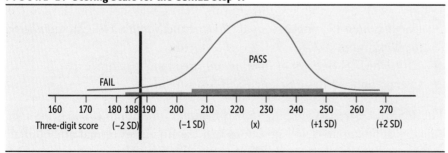

TABLE 1. Passing Rates for the 2011–2012 USMLE Step 1.

	2011		2012	
	No. Tested	**% Passing**	**No. Tested**	**% Passing**
Allopathic 1st takers	18,312	94%	18,723	96%
Repeaters	1,498	70%	1,133	68%
Allopathic total	19,810	93%	19,856	94%
Osteopathic 1st takers	2,145	89%	2,496	92%
Repeaters	66	65%	68	68%
Osteopathic total	2,211	88%	2,564	91%
Total U.S./Canadian	22,021	92%	22,420	94%
IMG 1st takers	14,855	73%	14,201	76%
Repeaters	4,621	36%	4,261	40%
IMG total	19,476	64%	18,462	68%
Total Step 1 examinees	41,497	79%	40,882	82%

What Does My Score Mean?

The most important point with the Step 1 score is passing versus failing. Passing essentially means, "Hey, you're on your way to becoming a fully licensed doc." As Table 1 shows, the majority of students pass the exam, so remember, we told you to relax.

Beyond that, the main point of having a quantitative score is to give you a sense of how well you've done on the exam and to help schools and residencies rank their students and applicants, respectively.

Official NBME/USMLE Resources

We strongly encourage students to use the materials provided by the testing agencies (see p. 23) and to study in detail the following NBME resources, all of which are available at the USMLE Web site, www.usmle.org:

- *USMLE Step 1 Computer-based Content and Sample Test Questions* (free to all examinees)
- *2014 USMLE Bulletin of Information* (free to all examinees)
- Comprehensive Basic Science Self-Assessment

> ▶ *Practice questions may be easier than the actual exam.*

The *USMLE Step 1 Computer-based Content and Sample Test Questions* contains approximately 150 questions that are similar in format and content to the questions on the actual USMLE Step 1 exam. This practice test offers one of the best means of assessing your test-taking skills. However, it does not contain enough questions to simulate the full length of the examination, and its content represents a limited sampling of the basic science material that may be covered on Step 1. Moreover, most students felt that the questions on the actual 2013 exam were more challenging than those contained in that year's sample questions. Interestingly, some students reported that they had encountered a few near-duplicates of these sample questions on the actual Step 1 exam. Presumably, these are "experimental" questions, but who knows? So the bottom line is, know these questions!

The extremely detailed *Step 1 Content Outline* provided by the USMLE has not proved useful for students studying for the exam. The USMLE even states that ". . . the content outline is not intended as a curriculum development or study guide."[1] We concur with this assessment.

The *2014 USMLE Bulletin of Information* contains detailed procedural and policy information regarding the CBT, including descriptions of all three Steps, scoring of the exams, reporting of scores to medical schools and residency programs, procedures for score rechecks and other inquiries, policies for irregular behavior, and test dates.

The NBME also offers the Comprehensive Basic Science Self-Assessment (CBSSA), which tests users on topics covered during basic science courses in a format similar to that of the USMLE Step 1 examination. Students who prepared for the examination using this Web-based tool reported that they found the format and content highly indicative of questions tested on the Step 1 examination. In addition, the CBSSA is a fair predictor of USMLE performance (see Table 2).

The CBSSA exists in two forms: a standard-paced and a self-paced format, both of which consist of four sections of 50 questions each (for a total of 200 multiple choice items). The standard-paced format allows the user up to one hour to complete each section, reflecting the time limits of the actual exam. By contrast, the self-paced format places a four-hour time limit on answering the multiple choice questions. Keep in mind that this bank of questions is available only on the Web. The NBME requires that users log on, register, and start the test within 30 days of registration. Once the assessment has begun, users are required to complete the sections within 20 days. Following completion of the questions, the CBSSA will provide a performance profile indicating each user's relative strengths and weaknesses, much like the report profile for the USMLE Step 1 exam. It is scaled with an average score of 500 and a standard deviation of 100. Please note that CBSSAs do not provide correct answers to the questions at the end of the session. However, some forms can be purchased with an extended feedback option; these tests show you which questions you answered incorrectly, but do not show you the correct answer or explain why your choice was wrong. Feedback from the self-assessment takes the form of a performance profile and nothing more. The NBME charges $50 for assessments without feedback and $60 for assessments with feedback. The fees are payable by credit card or money order. For more information regarding the CBSSA, please visit the NBME's Web site at www.nbme.org and click on the link labeled "NBME Self-Assessment Services."

TABLE 2. CBSSA to USMLE Score Prediction.

CBSSA Score	Approximate USMLE Step 1 Score
200	151
250	163
300	175
350	186
400	198
450	210
500	221
550	233
600	245
650	257
700	268
750	280
800	292

▶ DEFINING YOUR GOAL

▶ *Fourth-year medical students have the best feel for how Step 1 scores factor into the residency application process.*

It is useful to define your own personal performance goal when approaching the USMLE Step 1. Your style and intensity of preparation can then be matched to your goal. Furthermore, your goal may depend on your school's requirements, your specialty choice, your grades to date, and your personal assessment of the test's importance. Do your best to define your goals early so that you can prepare accordingly.

Certain highly competitive residency programs, such as those in plastic surgery and orthopedic surgery, have acknowledged their use of Step 1 scores in the selection process. In such residency programs, greater emphasis may be placed on attaining a high score, so students who seek to enter these programs may wish to consider aiming for a very high score on the Step 1 exam (see Figure 3). At the same time, your Step 1 score is only one of a number of factors that are assessed when you apply for residency. In fact, many residency programs value other criteria such as letters of recommendation, third-year clerkship grades, honors, and research experience more than a high score on Step 1. Fourth-year medical students who have recently completed the residency application process can be a valuable resource in this regard.

▶ *Some competitive residency programs place more weight on Step 1 scores in their selection process.*

▶ TIMELINE FOR STUDY

Before Starting

Your preparation for the USMLE Step 1 starts with entering medical school. Organize your studying so that when the time comes to prepare for the USMLE, you will be ready with a strong background.

FIGURE 3. **Median USMLE Step 1 Score by Specialty for Matched U.S. Seniors.[a]**

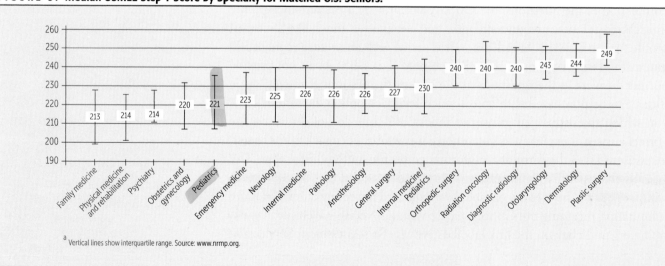

[a] Vertical lines show interquartile range. Source: www.nrmp.org.

Make a Schedule

After you have defined your goals, map out a study schedule that is consistent with your objectives, your vacation time, the difficulty of your ongoing coursework, and your family and social commitments (see Figure 4). Determine whether you want to spread out your study time or concentrate it into 14-hour study days in the final weeks. Then factor in your own history in preparing for standardized examinations (e.g., SAT, MCAT). Talk to students at your school who have recently taken Step 1. Ask them for their study schedules, especially those who have study habits and goals similar to yours.

Typically, U.S. medical students allot between five and seven weeks for dedicated preparation for Step 1. The time you dedicate to exam preparation will depend on your target score as well as your success in preparing yourself during the first two years of medical school. Some students reserve about a week at the end of their study period for final review; others save just a few days. When you have scheduled your exam date, do your best to adhere to it. Studies show that a later testing date does not translate into a higher score, so avoid pushing back your test date without good reason.[2]

▶ *Customize your schedule. Tackle your weakest section first.*

Another important consideration is when you will study each subject. Some subjects lend themselves to cramming, whereas others demand a substantial long-term commitment. The "crammable" subjects for Step 1 are those for which concise yet relatively complete review books are available. (See

FIGURE 4. Typical Timeline for the USMLE Step 1.

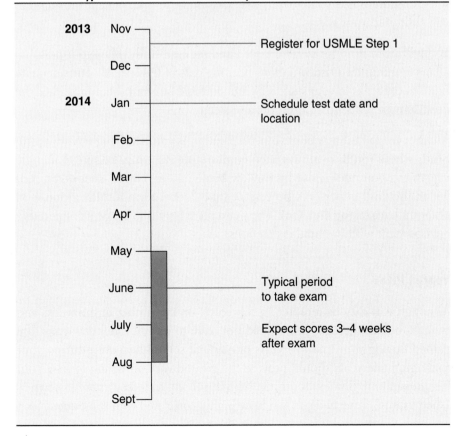

Section IV for highly rated review and sample examination materials.) Behavioral science and physiology are two subjects with concise review books. Three subjects with longer but quite comprehensive review books are microbiology, pharmacology, and biochemistry. Thus, these subjects could be covered toward the end of your schedule, whereas other subjects (anatomy and pathology) require a longer time commitment and could be studied earlier. Many students prefer using a "systems-based" approach (e.g., GI, renal, cardiovascular) to integrate the material across basic science subjects. See Section III to study embryology, anatomy, pathology, physiology, and pharmacology facts by organ system. Each subject may make up a different percentage of the test. For example, although anatomy may require a longer time commitment to review, you may encounter fewer anatomy questions on the test than questions on pharmacology. You can find more details of the breakdown of the test at the NBME's Web site.

> ▶ "Crammable" subjects should be covered later and less crammable subjects earlier.

c regards to which questions on the exam are composed of bigger sections on certain topics.

Make your schedule realistic, and set achievable goals. Many students make the mistake of studying at a level of detail that requires too much time for a comprehensive review—reading *Gray's Anatomy* in a couple of days is not a realistic goal! Have at least two catch-up days in your schedule. No matter how well you stick to your schedule, unexpected events happen. But don't let yourself procrastinate because you have catch-up days; stick to your schedule as closely as possible and revise it regularly on the basis of your actual progress. Be careful not to lose focus. Beware of feelings of inadequacy when comparing study schedules and progress with your peers. **Avoid others who stress you out.** Focus on a few top-rated resources that suit your learning style—not on some obscure books your friends may pass down to you. Accept the fact that you cannot learn it all.

You will need time for uninterrupted and focused study. Plan your personal affairs to minimize crisis situations near the date of the test. Allot an adequate number of breaks in your study schedule to avoid burnout. Maintain a healthy lifestyle with proper diet, exercise, and sleep.

> ▶ Avoid burnout. Maintain proper diet, exercise, and sleep habits.

Another important aspect of your preparation is your studying environment. **Study where you have always been comfortable studying.** Be sure to include everything you need close by (review books, notes, coffee, snacks, etc.). If you're the kind of person who cannot study alone, form a study group with other students taking the exam. The main point here is to create a comfortable environment with minimal distractions.

Year(s) Prior

Although you may be tempted to rely solely on cramming in the weeks and months before the test, you should not have to do so. The knowledge you gained during your first two years of medical school and even during your undergraduate years should provide the groundwork on which to base your test preparation. Student scores on NBME subject tests (commonly known as "shelf exams") have been shown to be highly correlated with subsequent Step

1 scores.[3] Moreover, undergraduate science GPAs as well as MCAT scores are strong predictors of performance on the Step 1 exam.[4]

We also recommend that you buy highly rated review books early in your first year of medical school and use them as you study throughout the two years. When Step 1 comes along, these books will be familiar and personalized to the way in which you learn. It is risky and intimidating to use unfamiliar review books in the final two or three weeks preceding the exam. Some students find it helpful to personalize and annotate *First Aid* throughout the curriculum.

> ▸ *Buy review books early (first year) and use while studying for courses.*

Months Prior

Review test dates and the application procedure. Testing for the USMLE Step 1 is done on a year-round basis. If you have any disabilities or "special circumstances," contact the NBME as early as possible to discuss test accommodations (see p. 43, First Aid for the Student with a Disability).

Before you begin to study earnestly, **simulate the USMLE Step 1 under "real" conditions** to pinpoint strengths and weaknesses in your knowledge, test endurance, and test-taking skills. Be sure that you are well informed about the examination and that you have planned your strategy for studying. Consider what study methods you will use, the study materials you will need, and how you will obtain your materials. Plan ahead. Do a lot of practice questions. Get advice from third- and fourth-year medical students who have recently taken the USMLE Step 1. There might be strengths and weaknesses in your school's curriculum that you should take into account in deciding where to focus your efforts. You might also choose to share books, notes, and study hints with classmates. That is how this book began.

> ▸ *Simulate the USMLE Step 1 under "real" conditions before beginning your studies.*

Three Weeks Prior

Two to four weeks before the examination is a good time to resimulate the USMLE Step 1. You may want to do this earlier depending on the progress of your review, but be sure not to do it later, when there will be little time to remedy gaps in your knowledge or test-taking skills. Make use of any remaining good-quality sample USMLE test questions, and try to simulate the computerized test conditions so that you can adequately assess your test performance. One way to simulate a full-length exam is doing a full, timed NBME CBSSA followed by three 46-question blocks from your question bank or the free 150 questions from the USMLE Web site. Recognize, too, that time pressure is increasing as more and more questions are framed as clinical vignettes. Most sample exam questions are shorter than the real thing. Focus on reviewing the high-yield facts, your own notes, clinical images, and very short review books. Do not fall into the trap of reviewing your strengths repeatedly; spend time on your weaknesses.

> ▸ *In the final two weeks, focus on review, practice questions, and endurance. Stay confident!*

One Week Prior

Make sure you have your CIN (found on your scheduling permit) as well as other items necessary for the day of the examination, including a current driver's license or another form of photo ID with your signature (make sure the name on your **ID exactly** matches that on your scheduling permit). Confirm the Prometric testing center location and test time. Work out how you will get to the testing center and what parking and traffic problems you might encounter. If possible, visit the testing site to get a better idea of the testing conditions you will face. Determine what you will do for lunch. Make sure you have everything you need to ensure that you will be comfortable and alert at the test site. It may be beneficial to adjust your schedule to start waking up at the same time that you will on your test day. And of course, make sure to maintain a healthy lifestyle and get enough sleep.

> ▶ One week before the test:
> ▪ Sleep according to the same schedule you'll use on test day
> ▪ Review the CBT tutorial one last time
> ▪ Call Prometric to confirm test date and time

One Day Prior

Try your best to relax and rest the night before the test. Double-check your admissions and test-taking materials as well as the comfort measures discussed earlier so that you will not have to deal with such details on the morning of the exam. At this point it will be more effective to review short-term memory material that you're already familiar with than to try to learn new material. The Rapid Review section at the end of this book is high yield for last-minute studying. Remember that regardless of how hard you have studied, you cannot know everything. There will be things on the exam that you have never even seen before, so do not panic. Do not underestimate your abilities.

Many students report difficulty sleeping the night prior to the exam. This is often exacerbated by going to bed much earlier than usual. Do whatever it takes to ensure a good night's sleep (e.g., massage, exercise, warm milk, no back-lit screens at night). Do not change your daily routine prior to the exam. Exam day is not the day for a caffeine-withdrawal headache.

> ▶ No notes, books, calculators, pagers, cell phones, recording devices, or watches of any kind are allowed in the testing area, but they are allowed in lockers.

Morning of the Exam

On the morning of the Step 1 exam, wake up at your regular time and eat a normal breakfast. If you think it will help you, have a close friend or family member check to make sure you get out of bed. Make sure you have your scheduling permit admission ticket, test-taking materials, and comfort measures as discussed earlier. Wear loose, comfortable clothing. Plan for a variable temperature in the testing center. Arrive at the test site 30 minutes before the time designated on the admission ticket; however, do not come too early, as doing so may intensify your anxiety. When you arrive at the test site, the proctor should give you a USMLE information sheet that will explain critical factors such as the proper use of break time. The USMLE uses the Biometric Identity Management System (BIMS) at some test center locations. BIMS converts a fingerprint, taken on test day, to a digital image used for identification of examinees during the testing process. Seating may be assigned, but ask to be reseated if necessary; you need to be seated in an area that will allow you to remain comfortable and to concentrate. Get to know your testing station, especially if you have never been in a Prometric testing center before. Listen to your proctors regarding any changes in instructions or testing procedures that may apply to your test site.

Finally, remember that it is natural (and even beneficial) to be a little nervous. Focus on being mentally clear and alert. Avoid panic. Avoid panic. Avoid panic. When you are asked to begin the exam, take a deep breath, focus on the screen, and then begin. Keep an eye on the timer. Take advantage of breaks between blocks to stretch, maybe do some jumping jacks, and relax for a moment with deep breathing or stretching.

> ▶ Arrive at the testing center 30 minutes before your scheduled exam time. If you arrive more than half an hour late, you will not be allowed to take the test.

After the Test

After you have completed the exam, be sure to have fun and relax regardless of how you may feel. Taking the test is an achievement in itself. Remember, you are much more likely to have passed than not. Enjoy the free time you have before your clerkships. Expect to experience some "reentry" phenomena as you try to regain a real life. Once you have recovered sufficiently from the test (or from partying), we invite you to send us your feedback, corrections, and suggestions for entries, facts, mnemonics, strategies, resource ratings, and the like (see p. xvii, How to Contribute). Sharing your experience will benefit fellow medical students and IMGs.

▶ STUDY MATERIALS

Quality and Cost Considerations

Although an ever-increasing number of review books and software are now available on the market, the quality of such material is highly variable. Some common problems are as follows:

- Certain review books are too detailed to allow for review in a reasonable amount of time or cover subtopics that are not emphasized on the exam.
- Many sample question books were originally written years ago and have not been adequately updated to reflect recent trends.
- Many sample question books use poorly written questions or contain factual errors in their explanations.
- Explanations for sample questions vary in quality.

Basic Science Review Books

> ▶ If a given review book is not working for you, stop using it no matter how highly rated it may be or how much it costs.

In selecting review books, be sure to weigh different opinions against each other, read the reviews and ratings in Section IV of this guide, examine the books closely in the bookstore, and choose carefully. You are investing not only money but also your limited study time. Do not worry about finding the "perfect" book, as many subjects simply do not have one, and different students prefer different formats. Supplement your chosen books with personal notes from other sources, including what you learn from question banks.

There are two types of review books: those that are stand-alone titles and those that are part of a series. Books in a series generally have the same style, and you must decide if that style works for you. However, a given style is not optimal for every subject.

You should also find out which books are up to date. Some recent editions reflect major improvements, whereas others contain only cursory changes. Take into consideration how a book reflects the format of the USMLE Step 1.

Practice Tests

Taking practice tests provides valuable information about potential strengths and weaknesses in your fund of knowledge and test-taking skills. Some students use practice examinations simply as a means of breaking up the monotony of studying and adding variety to their study schedule, whereas other students rely almost solely on practice tests. Your best preview of the computerized exam can be found in the practice exams on the USMLE Web site as well as CBSSA. You should also subscribe to one or more high-quality question banks. In addition, students report that many current practice-exam books have questions that are, on average, shorter and less clinically oriented than those on the current USMLE Step 1.

After taking a practice test, try to identify concepts and areas of weakness, not just the facts that you missed. Do not panic if you miss a lot of questions on a practice examination; instead, use the experience you have gained to motivate your study and prioritize those areas in which you need the most work. Use quality practice examinations to improve your test-taking skills. Analyze your ability to pace yourself.

Clinical Review Books

Keep your eye out for more clinically oriented review books; purchase them early and begin to use them. A number of students are turning to Step 2 CK books, pathophysiology books, and case-based reviews to prepare for the clinical vignettes. Examples of such books include:

- *First Aid Cases for the USMLE Step 1* (McGraw-Hill)
- *First Aid for the Wards* (McGraw-Hill)
- *First Aid Clerkship* series (McGraw-Hill)
- *Blueprints* clinical series (Lippincott Williams & Wilkins)
- *PreTest Physical Diagnosis* (McGraw-Hill)
- *Washington Manual* (Lippincott Williams & Wilkins)

▶ Charts and diagrams may be the best approach for physiology and biochemistry, whereas tables and outlines may be preferable for microbiology.

▶ Most practice exams are shorter and less clinical than the real thing.

▶ Use practice tests to identify concepts and areas of weakness, not just facts that you missed.

Texts, Syllabi, and Notes

Limit your use of textbooks and course syllabi for Step 1 review. Many textbooks are too detailed for high-yield review and include material that is generally not tested on the USMLE Step 1 (e.g., drug dosages, complex chemical structures). Syllabi, although familiar, are inconsistent across medical schools and frequently reflect the emphasis of individual faculty, which often does not correspond to that of the USMLE Step 1. Syllabi also tend to be less organized than top-rated books and generally contain fewer diagrams and study questions.

▶ TEST-TAKING STRATEGIES

Your test performance will be influenced by both your knowledge and your test-taking skills. You can strengthen your performance by considering each of these factors. Test-taking skills and strategies should be developed and perfected well in advance of the test date so that you can concentrate on the test itself. We suggest that you try the following strategies to see if they might work for you.

> ▶ *Practice and perfect test-taking skills and strategies well before the test date.*

Pacing

You have seven hours to complete 322 questions. Note that each one-hour block contains 46 questions. This works out to about 78 seconds per question. If you find yourself spending too much time on a question, mark the question, make an educated guess, and move on. If time permits, come back to the question later. In the past, pacing errors have been detrimental to the performance of even highly prepared examinees. The bottom line is to keep one eye on the clock at all times!

> ▶ *Time management is an important skill for exam success.*

Dealing with Each Question

There are several established techniques for efficiently approaching multiple choice questions; find what works for you. One technique begins with identifying each question as easy, workable, or impossible. Your goal should be to answer all easy questions, resolve all workable questions in a reasonable amount of time, and make quick and intelligent guesses on all impossible questions. Most students read the stem, think of the answer, and turn immediately to the choices. A second technique is to first skim the answer choices and the **last sentence of the question** and then read through the passage quickly, extracting only relevant information to answer the question. Try a variety of techniques on practice exams and see what works best for you.

Difficult Questions

Because of the exam's clinical emphasis, you may find that many of the questions on the Step 1 exam appear workable but take more time than is available to you. It can be tempting to dwell on such questions because you feel you are on the verge of "figuring it out," but resist this temptation and budget your time. Answer difficult questions with your best guess, mark them for review, and come back to them only if you have time after you have completed the rest of the questions in the block. This will keep you from inadvertently leaving any questions blank in your efforts to "beat the clock." Another reason for not dwelling too long on any one question is that certain questions may be **experimental**. These questions are typically not scored.

> ▶ *Do not dwell excessively on questions that you are on the verge of "figuring out." Make*
>
> ▶ *Remember that some questions may be experimental.*

Guessing

There is **no penalty** for wrong answers. Thus, **no test block should be left with unanswered questions.** A hunch is probably better than a random guess. If you have to guess, we suggest selecting an answer you recognize over one with which you are totally unfamiliar.

Changing Your Answer

The conventional wisdom is not to change answers that you have already marked unless there is a convincing and logical reason to do so—in other words, go with your "first hunch." However, studies show that if you change your answer, you are twice as likely to change it from an incorrect answer to a correct one than vice versa. So if you have a strong "second hunch," go for it!

> ▶ *Your first hunch is not always correct.*

Fourth-Quarter Effect (Avoiding Burnout)

Pacing and endurance are important. Practice helps develop both. Fewer and fewer examinees are leaving the examination session early. Use any extra time you might have at the end of each block to return to marked questions or to recheck your answers; you cannot add the extra time to any remaining blocks of questions. Do not be too casual in your review or you may overlook serious mistakes. Remember your goals, and keep in mind the effort you have devoted to studying compared with the small additional effort you will need to maintain focus and concentration throughout the examination. **Never give up.** If you begin to feel frustrated, try taking a 30-second breather.

> ▶ *Do not terminate a question block too early. Carefully review your answers if possible.*

▶ CLINICAL VIGNETTE STRATEGIES

In recent years, the USMLE Step 1 has become increasingly clinically oriented. This change mirrors the trend in medical education toward introducing students to clinical problem solving during the basic science years. The increasing clinical emphasis on Step 1 may be challenging to those students who attend schools with a more traditional curriculum.

▶ *Be prepared to read fast and think on your feet!*

What Is a Clinical Vignette?

A clinical vignette is a short (usually paragraph-long) description of a patient, including demographics, presenting symptoms, signs, and other information concerning the patient. Sometimes this paragraph is followed by a brief listing of important physical findings and/or laboratory results. The task of assimilating all this information and answering the associated question in the span of one minute can be intimidating. So be prepared to read quickly and think on your feet. Remember that the question is often indirectly asking something you already know.

▶ *Practice questions that include case histories or descriptive vignettes are critical for Step 1 preparation.*

Strategy

Remember that Step 1 vignettes usually describe diseases or disorders in their most classic presentation. So look for cardinal signs (e.g., malar rash for SLE or nuchal rigidity for meningitis) in the narrative history. Be aware that the question will contain classic signs and symptoms instead of buzzwords. Sometimes the data from labs and the physical exam will help you confirm or reject possible diagnoses, thereby helping you rule answer choices in or out. In some cases, they will be a dead giveaway for the diagnosis.

▶ *Step 1 vignettes usually describe diseases or disorders in their most classic presentation.*

Making a diagnosis from the history and data is often not the final answer. Not infrequently, the diagnosis is divulged at the end of the vignette, after you have just struggled through the narrative to come up with a diagnosis of your own. The question might then ask about a related aspect of the diagnosed disease.

▶ *Sometimes making a diagnosis is not necessary at all.*

One strategy that many students suggest is to skim the questions and answer choices before reading a vignette, especially if the vignette is lengthy. This focuses your attention on the relevant information and reduces the time spent on that vignette. Sometimes you may not need much of the information in the vignette to answer the question. However, be careful with skimming the answer choices; going too fast may warp your perception of what the vignette is asking.

▶ IF YOU THINK YOU FAILED

After the test, many examinees feel that they have failed, and most are at the very least unsure of their pass/fail status. There are several sensible steps you can take to plan for the future in the event that you do not achieve a passing score. First, save and organize all your study materials, including review books, practice tests, and notes. Familiarize yourself with the reapplication procedures for Step 1, including application deadlines and upcoming test dates.

▶ *If you pass Step 1, you are not allowed to retake the exam.*

Make sure you know your school's and the NBME's policies regarding retakes. The NBME allows a maximum of six attempts to pass each Step examination.[5] If the examinee has not taken any Step exam (including incompletes) before January 1, 2012, then he or she may take the same exam no more than three times in a 12-month period. Fourth and subsequent attempts must be at least 12 months after the first attempt, and at least 6 months after the most recent attempt.

The performance profiles on the back of the USMLE Step 1 score report provide valuable feedback concerning your relative strengths and weaknesses. Study these profiles closely. Set up a study timeline to strengthen gaps in your knowledge as well as to maintain and improve what you already know. Do not neglect high-yield subjects. It is normal to feel somewhat anxious about retaking the test, but if anxiety becomes a problem, seek appropriate counseling.

▶ IF YOU FAILED

Even if you came out of the exam room feeling that you failed, seeing that failing grade can be traumatic, and it is natural to feel upset. Different people react in different ways: For some it is a stimulus to buckle down and study harder; for others it may "take the wind out of their sails" for a few days; and it may even lead to a reassessment of individual goals and abilities. In some instances, however, failure may trigger weeks or months of sadness, feelings of hopelessness, social withdrawal, and inability to concentrate—in other words, true clinical depression. If you think you are depressed, please seek help.

▶ TESTING AGENCIES

- **National Board of Medical Examiners (NBME)**
  Department of Licensing Examination Services
  3750 Market Street
  Philadelphia, PA 19104-3102
  (215) 590-9500
  Fax: (215) 590-9457
  Email: webmail@nbme.org
  www.nbme.org

- **Educational Commission for Foreign Medical Graduates (ECFMG)**
  3624 Market Street
  Philadelphia, PA 19104-2685
  (215) 386-5900
  Fax: (215) 386-9196
  Email: info@ecfmg.org
  www.ecfmg.org

- **Federation of State Medical Boards (FSMB)**
  400 Fuller Wiser Road, Suite 300
  Euless, TX 76039-3856
  (817) 868-4041
  Fax: (817) 868-4098
  Email: usmle@fsmb.org
  www.fsmb.org

- **USMLE Secretariat**
  3750 Market Street
  Philadelphia, PA 19104-3102
  (215) 590-9700
  Fax: (215) 590-9457
  Email: webmail@nbme.org
  www.usmle.org

▶ REFERENCES

1. United States Medical Licensing Examination. Step 1 Content Description Online. Available at: http://www.usmle.org/pdfs/step-1/2013content_step1.pdf. Accessed October 10, 2013.
2. Pohl, Charles A., Robeson, Mary R., Hojat, Mohammadreza, and Veloski, J. Jon, "Sooner or Later? USMLE Step 1 Performance and Test Administration Date at the End of the Second Year," *Academic Medicine*, 2002, Vol. 77, No. 10, pp. S17–S19.
3. Holtman, Matthew C., Swanson, David B., Ripkey, Douglas R., and Case, Susan M., "Using Basic Science Subject Tests to Identify Students at Risk for Failing Step 1," *Academic Medicine*, 2001, Vol. 76, No. 10, pp. S48–S51.

4. Basco, William T., Jr., Way, David P., Gilbert, Gregory E., and Hudson, Andy, "Undergraduate Institutional MCAT Scores as Predictors of USMLE Step 1 Performance," *Academic Medicine*, 2002, Vol. 77, No. 10, pp. S13–S16.

5. United States Medical Licensing Examination. 2014 USMLE Bulletin: Eligibility. Available at: http://www.usmle.org/bulletin/eligibility. Accessed October 10, 2013.

Special Situations

▶ FIRST AID FOR THE INTERNATIONAL MEDICAL GRADUATE

"International medical graduate" (IMG) is the accepted term now used to describe any student or graduate of a non-U.S., non-Canadian, non–Puerto Rican medical school, regardless of whether he or she is a U.S. citizen or resident. Technically the term IMG encompasses FMGs (foreign medical graduates; i.e., medical graduates from medical schools outside the United States who are not residents of the United States—that is, U.S. citizens or green-card holders), although the terms IMG and FMG are often used interchangeably.

IMG's Steps to Licensure in the United States

To be eligible to take the USMLE Steps, you (the applicant) must be officially enrolled in a medical school located outside the United States and Canada that is listed in the International Medical Education Directory (IMED; http://www.faimer.org/resources/imed.html), both at the time you apply for examination and on your test day. In addition, your "Graduation Year" must be listed as "Current" at the time you apply and on your test day.

If you are an IMG, you must go through the following steps (not necessarily in this order) to apply for residency programs and become licensed to practice in the United States. You must complete these steps even if you are already a practicing physician and have completed a residency program in your own country.

- Pass USMLE Step 1, Step 2 CK, and Step 2 CS, as well as obtain a medical school diploma (not necessarily in this order). All three exams can be taken during medical school. If you have already graduated prior to taking any of the Steps, then you will need to verify your academic credentials (confirmation of enrollment and medical degree) prior to applying for any Step exam.
- You will be certified electronically by the Educational Commission for Foreign Medical Graduates (ECFMG) after above steps are successfully completed. You should receive your formal ECFMG certificate in the mail within the next 1–2 weeks. The ECFMG will not issue a certificate (even if all the USMLE scores are submitted) until it verifies your medical diploma with your medical school.
- You must have a valid ECFMG certificate before entering an accredited residency program in the United States, although you can begin the Electronic Residency Application Service (ERAS) application and interviews before you receive the certificate. However, many programs prefer to interview IMGs who have an ECFMG certificate, so obtaining it by the time you submit your ERAS application is ideal.
- Apply for residency positions in your fields of interest, either directly or through the ERAS and the National Residency Matching Program (NRMP), otherwise known as "the Match." To be entered into the Match, you need to have passed all the examinations necessary for ECFMG

▶ IMGs make up approximately 25% of the U.S. physician population.

▶ More detailed information can be found in the ECFMG Information Booklet, available at www.ecfmg.org/pubshome.html.

▶ Applicants may apply online for USMLE Step 1, Step 2 CK, or Step 2 CS at www.ecfmg.org.

certification (i.e., Step 1, Step 2 CK, and Step 2 CS) by the rank order list deadline (usually in late February before the Match). If you do not pass these exams by the deadline, you will be withdrawn from the Match.

■ If you are not a U.S. citizen or green-card holder (permanent resident), obtain a visa that will allow you to enter and work in the United States.

■ Sign up to receive the ECFMG and ERAS email newsletter to keep up to date with their most current policies and deadlines.

■ If required by the state in which your residency program is located, obtain an educational/training/limited medical license. Your residency program may assist you with this application. Note that medical licensing is the prerogative of each individual state, not of the federal government, and that states vary with respect to their laws about licensing.

■ Once you have the ECFMG certification, take the USMLE Step 3 during your residency, and then obtain a full medical license. Once you have a state-issued license, you are permitted to practice in federal institutions such as Veterans Affairs (VA) hospitals and Indian Health Service facilities in any state. This can open the door to "moonlighting" opportunities and possibilities for an H1B visa application if relevant. For details on individual state rules, write to the licensing board in the state in question or contact the Federation of State Medical Boards (FSMB). If you need to apply for an H1B visa for starting residency, you will need to take and pass the USMLE Step 3 exam, preferably before you Match.

■ Complete your residency and then take the appropriate specialty board exams if you wish to become board certified (e.g., in internal medicine or surgery). If you already have a specialty certification in another country, some specialty boards may grant you six months' or one year's credit toward your total residency time.

■ Currently, most residency programs are accepting applications through ERAS. For more information, see *First Aid for the Match* or contact:

> **ECFMG/ERAS Program**
> 3624 Market Street
> Philadelphia, PA 19104-2685 USA
> (215) 386-5900
> Email: eras-support@ecfmg.org
> www.ecfmg.org/eras

■ For detailed information on the USMLE Steps, visit the USMLE Web site at http://www.usmle.org.

The USMLE and the IMG

The USMLE is a series of standardized exams that give IMGs and U.S. medical graduates a level playing field. The passing marks for IMGs for Step 1, Step 2 CK, and Step 2 CS are determined by a statistical distribution that is based on the scores of U.S. medical school students. For example, to pass Step 1, you will probably have to score higher than the bottom 8–10% of U.S. and Canadian graduates.

▶ *IMGs have a maximum of six attempts to pass any USMLE Step, and must pass the USMLE Steps required for ECFMG certification within a seven-year period.*

Under USMLE program rules, a maximum of six attempts will be permitted to pass any USMLE Step or component exam. There is a limit of three attempts within a 12-month period for any of the USMLE Steps.

Timing of the USMLE

For an IMG, the timing of a complete application is critical. It is extremely important that you send in your application early if you are to obtain the maximum number of interviews. Complete all exam requirements by August of the year in which you wish to apply. Check the ECFMG Web site for deadlines to take and pass the various Step exams to be eligible for the NRMP Match.

IMG applicants must pass the USMLE Steps required for ECFMG certification within a seven-year period. The USMLE program recommends, although not all jurisdictions impose, a seven-year limit for completion of the three-step USMLE program.

▶ *If your clinical experience is recent, consider taking the Step 2 CK first, followed by the Step 1.*

In terms of USMLE exam order, arguments can be made for taking the Step 1 or the Step 2 CK exam first. For example, you may consider taking the Step 2 CK exam first if you have just graduated from medical school and the clinical topics are still fresh in your mind. However, keep in mind that there is substantial overlap between Step 1 and Step 2 CK topics in areas such as pharmacology, pathophysiology, and biostatistics. You might therefore consider taking the Step 1 and Step 2 CK exams close together to take advantage of this overlap in your test preparation.

USMLE Step 1 and the IMG

Significance of the Test. Step 1 is one of the three exams required for the ECFMG certification. Since most U.S. graduates apply to residency with their Step 1 scores only, it may be the only objective tool available with which to compare IMGs with U.S. graduates.

Eligibility Period. A three-month period of your choice.

Fee. The fee for Step 1 is $820 plus an international test delivery surcharge (if you choose a testing region other than the United States or Canada).

Statistics. In 2012–2013, 76% of IMG examinees passed Step 1 on their first attempt, compared with 96% of those from the United States and Canada.

▶ *A higher Step 1 score will improve your chances of getting into a highly competitive specialty.*

Tips. Although few if any students feel totally prepared to take Step 1, IMGs in particular require serious study and preparation in order to reach their full potential on this exam. It is also imperative that IMGs do their best on Step 1, as a poor score on Step 1 is a distinct disadvantage in applying for most residencies. Remember that if you pass Step 1, you cannot retake it in an attempt to improve your score. Your goal should thus be to beat the mean, because you can then assert with confidence that you have done better than average for U.S. students. Higher Step 1 scores will also lend credibility to your residency application and help you get into highly competitive specialties such as radiology, orthopedics, and dermatology.

Commercial Review Courses. Do commercial review courses help improve your scores? Reports vary, and such courses can be expensive. For some students these programs can provide a more structured learning environment with professional support. However, review courses consume a significant chunk of time away from independent study. Many IMGs decide to prepare for Step 1 on their own and then consider a review course only if they fail. (For more information on review courses, see Section IV.)

USMLE Step 2 CK and the IMG

What Is the Step 2 CK? It is a computerized test of the clinical sciences consisting of up to 355 multiple-choice questions divided into eight blocks. It can be taken at Prometric centers in the United States and several other countries.

Content. The Step 2 CK includes test items in the following content areas:

- Internal medicine
- Obstetrics and gynecology
- Pediatrics
- Preventive medicine
- Psychiatry
- Surgery
- Other areas relevant to the provision of care under supervision

> ▶ *The areas tested on the Step 2 CK relate to the clerkships provided at U.S. medical schools.*

Significance of the Test. The Step 2 CK is required for the ECFMG certificate. It reflects the level of clinical knowledge of the applicant. It tests clinical subjects, primarily internal medicine. Other areas that are tested are surgery, obstetrics and gynecology, pediatrics, orthopedics, psychiatry, ENT, ophthalmology, and medical ethics.

Eligibility. Students and graduates from medical schools that are listed in IMED are eligible to take the Step 2 CK. Students must have completed at least two years of medical school. This means that students must have completed the basic medical science component of the medical school curriculum by the beginning of the eligibility period selected.

Eligibility Period. A three-month period of your choice.

Fee. The fee for the Step 2 CK is $820 plus an international test delivery surcharge (if you choose a testing region other than the United States or Canada).

Statistics. In 2012–2013, 85% of ECFMG candidates passed the Step 2 CK on their first attempt, compared with 98% of U.S. and Canadian candidates.

▶ Be familiar with topics that are heavily emphasized in U.S. medicine, such as cholesterol screening.

Tips. It's better to take the Step 2 CK after your internal medicine rotation because most of the questions on the exam give clinical scenarios and ask you to make medical diagnoses and clinical decisions. In addition, because this is a clinical sciences exam, cultural and geographic considerations play a greater role than is the case with Step 1. For example, if your medical education gave you ample exposure to malaria, brucellosis, and malnutrition but little to alcohol withdrawal, child abuse, and cholesterol screening, you must work to familiarize yourself with topics that are more heavily emphasized in U.S. medicine. You must also have a basic understanding of the legal and social aspects of U.S. medicine, because you will be asked questions about communicating with and advising patients.

USMLE Step 2 CS and the IMG

What Is the Step 2 CS? The Step 2 CS is a test of clinical and communication skills administered as a one-day, eight-hour exam. It includes 10 to 12 encounters with standardized patients (15 minutes each, with 10 minutes to write a note after each encounter).

Content. The Step 2 CS tests the ability to communicate in English as well as interpersonal skills, data-gathering skills, the ability to perform a physical exam, and the ability to formulate a brief note, a differential diagnosis, and a list of diagnostic tests. The areas that are covered in the exam are as follows:

- Internal medicine
- Surgery
- Obstetrics and gynecology
- Pediatrics
- Psychiatry
- Family medicine

▶ The Step 2 CS is graded as pass/fail.

Unlike the USMLE Step 1, Step 2 CK, or Step 3, **there are no numerical grades for the Step 2 CS**—it's simply either a "pass" or a "fail." To pass, a candidate must attain a passing performance in **each** of the following three components:

- Integrated Clinical Encounter (ICE): includes Data Gathering, Physical Exam, and the Patient Note
- Spoken English Proficiency (SEP)
- Communication and Interpersonal Skills (CIS)

According to the NBME, the most commonly failed component for IMGs is the CIS.

Significance of the Test. The Step 2 CS assesses spoken English language proficiency and is required for the ECFMG certificate. The Test of English as a Foreign Language (TOEFL) is no longer required.

Eligibility. Students must have completed at least two years of medical school in order to take the test. That means students must have completed the basic medical science component of the medical school curriculum at the time they apply for the exam.

Fee. The fee for the Step 2 CS is $1440.

Scheduling. You must schedule the Step 2 CS within **four months** of the date indicated on your notification of registration. You must take the exam within 12 months of the date indicated on your notification of registration. It is generally advisable to take the Step 2 CS as soon as possible in the year before your Match, as often the results either come in late or arrive too late to allow you to retake the test and pass it before the Match.

> ▶ *Try to take the Step 2 CS the year before you plan to Match.*

Test Site Locations. The Step 2 CS is currently administered at the following five locations:

- Philadelphia, PA
- Atlanta, GA
- Los Angeles, CA
- Chicago, IL
- Houston, TX

For more information about the Step 2 CS exam, please refer to *First Aid for the Step 2 CS*.

USMLE Step 3 and the IMG

What Is the USMLE Step 3? It is a two-day computerized test in clinical medicine consisting of 480 multiple-choice questions and 12 computer-based case simulations (CCS). The exam aims at testing your knowledge and its application to patient care and clinical decision making (i.e., this exam tests if you can safely practice medicine independently and without supervision).

Significance of the Test. Taking Step 3 before residency is critical for IMGs seeking an H1B visa and is also a bonus that can be added to the residency application. Step 3 is also required to obtain a full medical license in the United States and can be taken during residency for this purpose.

> ▶ *Complete the Step 3 exam before you apply for an H1B visa.*

Fee. The fee for Step 3 is $800 in all states except Iowa ($850), South Dakota ($950), and Vermont ($835).

Eligibility. Most states require that applicants have completed one, two, or three years of postgraduate training (residency) before they apply for Step 3 and permanent state licensure. The exceptions are the 13 states mentioned below, which allow IMGs to take Step 3 at the beginning of or even before residency. So if you don't fulfill the prerequisites to taking Step 3 in your state of choice, simply use the name of one of the 13 states in your Step 3 application. You can take the exam in any state you choose regardless of the state that you mentioned on your application. Once you pass Step 3, it will be recognized by all states. Basic eligibility requirements for the USMLE Step 3 are as follows:

- Obtaining an MD or DO degree (or its equivalent) by the application deadline.
- Obtaining an ECFMG certificate if you are a graduate of a foreign medical school or are successfully completing a "fifth pathway" program (at a date no later than the application deadline).
- Meeting the requirements imposed by the individual state licensing authority to which you are applying to take Step 3. Please refer to www.fsmb.org for more information.

The following states do not have postgraduate training as an eligibility requirement to apply for Step 3:

- Arkansas
- California
- Connecticut
- Florida
- Louisiana
- Maryland
- Nebraska[a]
- New York
- South Dakota
- Texas
- Utah[a]
- Washington
- West Virginia

[a] Requires that IMGs obtain a "valid indefinite" ECFMG certificate.

The Step 3 exam is not available outside the United States. Applications can be found online at www.fsmb.org and must be submitted to the FSMB.

In 2012–2013, 83% of IMG candidates passed the Step 3 on their first attempt, compared with 96% of U.S. and Canadian candidates.

Residencies and the IMG

In the Match, the number of U.S.-citizen IMG applications has grown over the past few years, while the percentage accepted has remained constant (see Table 4). More information about residency programs can be obtained at www.ama-assn.org.

The Match and the IMG

Given the growing number of IMG candidates with strong applications, you should bear in mind that good USMLE scores are not the only way to gain a competitive edge. However, USMLE Step 1 and Step 2 CK scores continue to be used as the initial screening mechanism when candidates are being considered for interviews.

TABLE 4. IMGs in the Match.

Applicants	2011	2012	2013
U.S.-citizen IMGs	3,769	4,279	5,095
% U.S.-citizen IMGs accepted	50	49	53
Non-U.S.-citizen IMGs	6,659	6,828	7,568
% non-U.S.-citizen IMGs accepted	41	41	48
U.S. seniors (non-IMGs)	16,559	16,527	17,487
% U.S. seniors accepted	94	95	94

Source: www.nrmp.org.

Based on accumulated IMG Match experiences over recent years, here are a few pointers to help IMGs maximize their chances for a residency interview:

- **Apply early.** Programs offer a limited number of interviews and often select candidates on a first-come, first-served basis. Because of this, you should aim to complete the entire process of applying for the ERAS token, registering with the Association of American Medical Colleges (AAMC), mailing necessary documents to ERAS, and completing the ERAS application by mid-September (see Figure 5). Community programs usually send out interview offers earlier than do university and university-affiliated programs.

- **U.S. clinical experience helps.** Externships and observerships in a U.S. hospital setting have emerged as an important credential on an IMG application. Externships are like short-term medical school internships and offer hands-on clinical experience. Observerships, also called "shadowing," involve following a physician and observing how he or she manages patients. Some programs require students to have participated in an externship or observership before applying. It is best to gain such an experience before or at the time you apply to various programs so that you can mention it on your ERAS application. If such an experience or opportunity comes up after you apply, be sure to inform the programs accordingly.

  > ▶ *Most U.S. hospitals allow externship only when the applicant is actively enrolled in a medical school, so plan ahead.*

- **Clinical research helps.** University programs are attracted to candidates who show a strong interest in clinical research and academics. They may even relax their application criteria for individuals with unique backgrounds and strong research experience. Publications in well-known journals are an added bonus.

- **Time the Step 2 CS well.** ECFMG has published the new Step 2 CS score-reporting schedule for 2013–2014 at http://www.ecfmg.org. Most program directors would like to see a passing score on the Step 1, Step 2 CK, and Step 2 CS exams before they rank an IMG on their rank order list in mid-February. There have been many instances in which candidates have lost a potential Match—either because of delayed CS results or because they have been unable to retake the exam on time following a

FIGURE 5. IMG Timeline for Application.

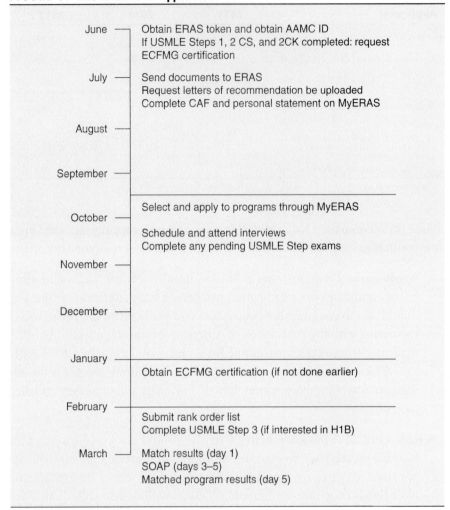

failure. It is difficult to predict a result on the Step 2 CS, since the grading process is not very transparent. Therefore, it is advisable to take the Step 2 CS as early as possible in the application year.

- **U.S. letters of recommendation help.** Letters of recommendation from clinicians practicing in the United States carry more weight than recommendations from home countries.

- **Step up the Step 3.** If H1B visa sponsorship is desired, aim to have Step 3 results by January of the Match year. In addition to the visa advantage you will gain, an early and good Step 3 score may benefit IMGs who have been away from clinical medicine for a while as well as those who have low scores on Step 1 and the Step 2 CK.

- **Verify medical credentials in a timely manner.** Do not overlook the medical school credential verification process. The ECFMG certificate arrives only after credentials have been verified and after you have passed

▶ *A good score on the Step 3 may help offset poorer scores on the Step 1 or 2 CK exams.*

Step 1, the Step 2 CK, and the Step 2 CS, so you should keep track of the process and check with the ECFMG from time to time about your status.

- **Don't count on a pre-Match.** Of note, as of the 2013 Match, programs participating in NRMP Match can no longer offer a pre-Match.

What if You Do Not Match?

For applicants who do not Match into a residency program, there's SOAP (Supplemental Offer and Acceptance Program). Under SOAP, unmatched applicants will have access to the list of unfilled programs at noon Eastern time on the Monday of Match week. The unfilled programs electing to participate in SOAP will offer positions to unmatched applicants through the Registration, Ranking, and Results (R3) system. A series of "rounds" will begin at noon Eastern time on Wednesday of Match week until 5:00 P.M. Eastern time on Friday of Match week. Detailed information about SOAP can be found at the NRMP Web site at http://www.nrmp.org.

> ▶ *The Scramble has been replaced by SOAP (Supplemental Offer and Acceptance Program).*

Resources for the IMG

- **ECFMG**
  3624 Market Street
  Philadelphia, PA 19104-2685
  (215) 386-5900
  Fax: (215) 386-9196
  www.ecfmg.org

  The ECFMG telephone number is answered only between 9:00 A.M.– 5:00 P.M. Monday through Friday EST. The ECFMG often takes a long time to answer the phone, which is frequently busy at peak times of the year, and then gives you a long voice-mail message—so it is better to write or fax early than to rely on a last-minute phone call. Do not contact the NBME, as all IMG exam matters are conducted by the ECFMG. The ECFMG also publishes an information booklet on ECFMG certification and the USMLE program, which gives details on the dates and locations of forthcoming Step tests for IMGs together with application forms. It is free of charge and is also available from the public affairs offices of U.S. embassies and consulates worldwide as well as from Overseas Educational Advisory Centers. You may order single copies of the handbook by calling (215) 386-5900, preferably on weekends or between 6 P.M. and 6 A.M. Eastern time, or by faxing to (215) 386-9196. Requests for multiple copies must be made by fax or mail on organizational letterhead. The full text of the booklet is also available on the ECFMG's Web site at www.ecfmg.org.

- **FSMB**
  400 Fuller Wiser Road, Suite 300
  Euless, TX 76039
  (817) 868-4041
  Fax: (817) 868-4098
  Email: usmle@fsmb.org
  www.fsmb.org

The FSMB has a number of publications available, including free policy documents. To obtain these publications, print and mail the order form on the Web site listed above. Alternatively, write to Federation Publications at the above address. All orders must be prepaid with a personal check drawn on a U.S. bank, a cashier's check, or a money order payable to the FSMB. Foreign orders must be accompanied by an international money order or the equivalent, payable in U.S. dollars through a U.S. bank or a U.S. affiliate of a foreign bank. For Step 3 inquiries, the telephone number is (817) 868-4041.

The AMA has dedicated a portion of its Web site to information on IMG demographics, residencies, immigration, and the like. This information can be found at www.ama-assn.org.

Other resources that may be useful and of interest to IMGs include the following:

- *The International Medical Graduate's Guide to US Medicine and Residency Training*, by Patrick C. Alquire, Gerald P. Whelan, and Vijay Rajput (2009; ISBN 9781934465080).
- *The International Medical Graduate's Best Hope*, by Franck Belibi and Suzanne Belibi (2009; ISBN 9780979877308).

▶ FIRST AID FOR THE OSTEOPATHIC MEDICAL STUDENT

What Is the COMLEX-USA Level 1?

The National Board of Osteopathic Medical Examiners (NBOME) administers the Comprehensive Osteopathic Medical Licensing Examination, or COMLEX-USA. Like the USMLE, the COMLEX-USA is administered over three levels.

The COMLEX-USA series assesses osteopathic medical knowledge and clinical skills using clinical presentations and physician tasks. A description of the COMLEX-USA Written Examination Blueprints for each level, which outline the various clinical presentations and physician tasks that examinees will encounter, is given on the NBOME Web site. Another stated goal of the COMLEX-USA Level 1 is to create a more primary care–oriented exam that integrates osteopathic principles into clinical situations.

To be eligible to take the COMLEX-USA Level 1, you must have satisfactorily completed your first year in an American Osteopathic Association (AOA)–approved medical school. The office of the dean at each school informs the NBOME that a student has completed his or her first year of school and is in good standing. At this point, the NBOME sends out an email with detailed instructions on how to register for the exam.

For all three levels of the COMLEX-USA, raw scores are converted to a percentile score and a score ranging from 5 to 800. For Levels 1 and 2, a score of 400 is required to pass; for Level 3, a score of 350 is needed. COMLEX-USA scores are posted at the NBOME Web site 4–6 weeks after the test and usually mailed within 8 weeks after the test. The mean score is always 500.

If you pass a COMLEX-USA examination, you are not allowed to retake it to improve your grade. If you fail, there is no specific limit to the number of times you can retake it in order to pass. However, a student may not take the exam more than four times in one year. Levels 2 and 3 exams must be passed in sequential order within seven years of passing Level 1.

Note that effective July 1, 2016, candidates taking COMLEX-USA examinations will be limited to a total of six attempts for each examination.

What Is the Structure of the COMLEX-USA Level 1?

The COMLEX-USA Level 1 is a computer-based examination consisting of 400 questions over an eight-hour period in a single day (nine hours if you count breaks). Most of the questions are in one-best-answer format, but a small number are matching-type questions. Some one-best-answer questions are bundled together around a common question stem that usually takes the form of a clinical scenario. Every section of the COMLEX-USA Level 1 ends with either matching questions, multiple questions around a single stem, or both. New question formats may gradually be introduced, but candidates will be notified if this occurs. In 2012, the NBOME introduced multimedia questions and have stated that multimedia questions will continue to be a larger part of the exam.

Questions are grouped into eight sections of 50 questions each in a manner similar to the USMLE. Reviewing and changing answers may be done only in the current section. A "review page" is presented for each block in order to advise test takers of questions completed, questions marked for further review, and incomplete questions for which no answer has been given.

Breaks are even more structured with COMLEX-USA than they are with the USMLE. Students are allowed to take a 10-minute break at the end of the second and sixth sections. Students who do not take these 10-minute breaks can apply the time toward their test time. After section 4, students are given a 40-minute lunch break. These are the only times a student is permitted a break. More information about the computer-based COMLEX-USA examinations can be obtained from www.nbome.org.

What Is the Difference Between the USMLE and the COMLEX-USA?

According to the NBOME, the COMLEX-USA Level 1 focuses broadly on the following categories, with osteopathic principles and practices integrated into each section:

- Health promotion and disease prevention
- The history and physical
- Diagnostic technologies
- Management
- Scientific understanding of mechanisms
- Health care delivery

▶ The test interface for the COMLEX-USA Level 1 is not the same as the USMLE Step 1 interface.

Although the COMLEX-USA and the USMLE are similar in scope, content, and emphasis, some differences are worth noting. For example, the interface is different; you cannot search for lab values. The expectation is that you can make a diagnosis without having performed testing. Fewer details are given about a patient's condition, so a savvy student needs to know how to differentiate between similar pathologies. Also, age, gender, and race are key factors for diagnosis on the COMLEX-USA. Images are embedded in the question stem and the examinee has to click an attachment button to see the image. If you don't read the question carefully, the attachment buttons are very easy to miss.

COMLEX-USA Level 1 tests osteopathic principles in addition to basic science materials but does not emphasize lab techniques. Although both exams often require that you apply and integrate knowledge over several areas of basic science to answer a given question, many students who took both tests reported that the questions differed somewhat in style. Students reported, for example, that USMLE questions generally required that the test taker reason and draw from the information given (often a two-step process), whereas those on the COMLEX-USA exam tended to be more straightforward. Furthermore, USMLE questions were on average found to be considerably longer than those on the COMLEX-USA.

COMLEX-USA test takers can expect to have only a few questions on biochemistry, molecular biology, or lab technique. On the other hand, microbiology is very heavily tested by clinical presentation and by lab identification. Another main difference is that the COMLEX-USA exam stresses osteopathic manipulative medicine. Therefore, question banks specific to the USMLE will not be adequate, and supplementation with a question bank specific to the COMLEX-USA is highly recommended.

Students also commented that the COMLEX-USA utilized "buzzwords," although limited in their use (e.g., "rose spots" in typhoid fever), whereas the USMLE avoided buzzwords in favor of descriptions of clinical findings or symptoms (e.g., rose-colored papules on the abdomen rather than rose spots). Finally, USMLE appeared to have more photographs than did the COMLEX-USA. In general, the overall impression was that the USMLE was a more "thought-provoking" exam, while the COMLEX-USA was more of a "knowledge-based" exam.

Who Should Take Both the USMLE and the COMLEX-USA?

Aside from facing the COMLEX-USA Level 1, you must decide if you will also take the USMLE Step 1. We recommend that you consider taking both the USMLE and the COMLEX-USA under the following circumstances:

- **If you are applying to allopathic residencies.** Although there is growing acceptance of COMLEX-USA certification on the part of allopathic residencies, some allopathic programs prefer or even require passage of the USMLE Step 1. These include many academic programs, programs in competitive specialties (e.g., orthopedics, ophthalmology, or dermatology), and programs in competitive geographic areas (e.g., Vermont, Utah, and California). Fourth-year doctor of osteopathy (DO) students who have already Matched may be a good source of information about which programs and specialties look for USMLE scores. It is also a good idea to contact program directors at the institutions you are interested in to ask about their policy regarding the COMLEX-USA versus the USMLE.

- **If you are unsure about your postgraduate training plans.** Successful passage of both the COMLEX-USA Level 1 and the USMLE Step 1 is certain to provide you with the greatest possible range of options when you are applying for internship and residency training.

> ▶ *If you're not sure whether you need to take either the COMLEX-USA Level 1 or the USMLE Step 1, consider taking both to keep your Match options open.*

In addition, the COMLEX-USA Level 1 has in recent years placed increasing emphasis on questions related to primary care medicine and prevention. Having a strong background in family or primary care medicine can help test takers when they face questions on prevention.

How Do I Prepare for the COMLEX-USA Level 1?

Student experience suggests that you should start studying for the COMLEX-USA four to six months before the test is given, as an early start will allow you to spend up to a month on each subject. The recommendations made in Section I regarding study and testing methods, strategies, and resources, as well as the books suggested in Section IV for the USMLE Step 1, hold true for the COMLEX-USA as well.

Another important source of information is in the *Examination Guidelines and Sample Exam*, a booklet that discusses the breakdown of each subject while also providing sample questions and corresponding answers. Many students, however, felt that this breakdown provided only a general guideline and was not representative of the level of difficulty of the actual COMLEX-USA. The sample questions did not provide examples of clinical vignettes, which made up approximately 25% of the exam. You will receive this publication with registration materials for the COMLEX-USA Level 1, but you can also receive a copy and additional information by writing:

NBOME
8765 W. Higgins Road, Suite 200
Chicago, IL 60631-4174
(773) 714-0622
Fax: (773) 714-0631
www.nbome.org

The NBOME developed the Comprehensive Osteopathic Medical Self-Assessment Examination (COMSAE) series to fill the need for self-assessment on the part of osteopathic medical students. Many students take the COMSAE exam before the COMLEX-USA in addition to using test-bank questions and board review books. Students can purchase a copy of this exam at www.nbome.org/comsae.asp.

In recent years, students have reported an emphasis in certain areas. For example:

- There was an increased emphasis on upper limb anatomy/brachial plexus.
- Specific topics were repeatedly tested on the exam. These included cardiovascular physiology and pathology, acid-base physiology, diabetes, benign prostatic hyperplasia, sexually transmitted diseases, measles, and rubella. Thyroid and adrenal function, neurology (head injury), specific drug treatments for bacterial infection, migraines/cluster headaches, and drug mechanisms also received heavy emphasis.
- Behavioral science questions were based on psychiatry.
- High-yield osteopathic manipulative technique (OMT) topics included an emphasis on the sympathetic and parasympathetic innervations of viscera and nerve roots, rib mechanics/diagnosis, and basic craniosacral theory. Students who spend time reviewing basic anatomy, studying nerve and dermatome innervations, and understanding how to perform basic OMT techniques (e.g., muscle energy or counterstrain) can improve their scores.

> ▶ *You must know the Chapman reflex points and the obscure names of physical exam signs.*

The COMLEX-USA Level 1 also includes multimedia-based questions. Such questions test the student's ability to perform a good physical exam and to elicit various physical diagnostic signs (e.g., Murphy sign).

Since topics that were repeatedly tested appeared in all four booklets, students found it useful to review them in between the two test days. It is important to understand that the topics emphasized on the current exam may not be stressed on future exams. However, some topics are heavily tested each year, so it may be beneficial to have a solid foundation in the above-mentioned topics.

▶ FIRST AID FOR THE PODIATRIC MEDICAL STUDENT

The National Board of Podiatric Medical Examiners (NBPME) offers the American Podiatric Medical Licensing Examinations (APMLE), which are designed to assess whether a candidate possesses the knowledge required to practice as a minimally competent entry-level podiatrist. The APMLE is used as part of the licensing process governing the practice of podiatric medicine. The APMLE is recognized by all 50 states and the District of Columbia, the U.S. Army, the U.S. Navy, and the Canadian provinces of Alberta, British Columbia, and Ontario. Individual states use the examination scores differently; therefore, doctor of podiatric medicine (DPM) candidates should refer to the *APMLE Bulletin of Information: 2013 Examinations.*

The APMLE Part I is generally taken after the completion of the second year of podiatric medical education. Unlike the USMLE Step 1, there is no behavioral science section, nor is biomechanics tested. The exam samples seven basic science disciplines: general anatomy (13%); lower extremity anatomy (25%); biochemistry (7%); physiology (13%); microbiology and immunology (15%); pathology (12%); and pharmacology (15%). A detailed outline of topics and subtopics covered on the exam can be found in the *APMLE Bulletin of Information*, available at www.apmle.org.

▶ *Areas tested on the NBPME Part I:*
- *General anatomy*
- *Lower extremity anatomy*
- *Biochemistry*
- *Physiology*
- *Medical microbiology & immunology*
- *Pathology*
- *Pharmacology*

Your APMLE Appointment

In early spring, your college registrar will have you fill out an application for the APMLE Part I. The exam will be offered at an independent Prometric testing facility in each city with a podiatric medical school (New York, Philadelphia, Miami, Cleveland, Chicago, Des Moines, Phoenix, Pomona, and San Francisco), along with any other city Prometric deems necessary. Please contact Prometric for a full list of testing sites or visit www.prometric.com/NBPME. You may take the exam at any of these locations regardless of which school you attend. However, you must designate on your application which testing location you desire. Specific instructions about exam dates and registration deadlines can be found in the *APMLE Bulletin.*

Exam Format

The APMLE Part I is a written exam consisting of 205 questions. The test consists of multiple choice questions that have one best answer or multiple "select all that apply" answers, as well as a drag-and-drop section. Examinees have four hours in which to take the exam and are given scratch paper and a calculator, both of which must be turned in at the end of the exam. Some questions on the exam will be "trial questions." These questions are evaluated as future board questions but are not counted in your score.

Interpreting Your Score

Three to four weeks following the exam date, the dean's office at the student's respective school will receive scores. APMLE scores are reported as pass/fail, with a scaled score of at least 75 needed to pass. Historically, 85% of first-time test takers pass the APMLE Part I. Failing candidates receive a report with a score between 55 and 74 in addition to diagnostic messages intended to help identify strengths or weaknesses in specific content areas. If you fail the APMLE Part I, you must retake the entire examination at a later date. There is no limit to the number of times you can retake the exam.

Preparation for the APMLE Part I

Students suggest that you begin studying for the APMLE Part I at least three months prior to the test date. The suggestions made in Section I regarding study and testing methods for the USMLE Step 1 can be applied to the APMLE as well. This book should, however, be used as a supplement and not as the sole source of information. Keep in mind that you need only a passing score. Neither you nor your school or future residency will ever see your actual passing numerical score. Competing with colleagues should not be an issue, and study groups are beneficial to many.

▶ *Know the anatomy of the lower extremity!*

A potential study method that helps many students is to copy the outline of the material to be tested from the *APMLE Bulletin*. Check off each topic during your study, because doing so will ensure that you have engaged each topic. If you are pressed for time, prioritize subjects on the basis of their weight on the exam. Approximately 22% of the APMLE Part I focuses on lower extremity anatomy. In this area, students should rely on the notes and material that they received from their class. Remember, lower extremity anatomy is the podiatric physician's specialty—so everything about it is important. Do not forget to study osteology. Keep your old tests and look through old lower extremity class exams, since each of the podiatric colleges submits questions from its own faculty. This strategy will give you an understanding of the types of questions that may be asked. On the APMLE Part I, you will see some of the same classic lower extremity anatomy questions you were tested on in school.

The APMLE, like the USMLE, requires that you apply and integrate knowledge over several areas of basic science in order to answer exam questions. Students report that many questions emphasize clinical presentations; however, the facts in this book are very useful in helping students recall the various diseases and organisms. DPM candidates should expand on the high-yield pharmacology section and study antifungal drugs and treatments for *Pseudomonas*, methicillin-resistant *S. aureus*, candidiasis, and erythrasma. The high-yield section focusing on pathology is very useful; however, additional emphasis on diabetes mellitus and all its secondary manifestations, particularly peripheral neuropathy, should not be overlooked. Students should also focus on renal physiology and drug elimination, the biochemistry of gout, and neurophysiology, all of which have been noted to be important topics on the APMLE Part I exam.

A sample set of questions is found on the APMLE website www.apmle.org. These samples are somewhat similar in difficulty to actual board questions. If you have any questions regarding registration, fees, test centers, authorization forms, or score reports, please contact your college registrar or:

Prometric
Phone: 877-302-8952
Fax: 800-813-6670
Email: nbpmeinquiry@prometric.com
www.prometric.com

▶ FIRST AID FOR THE STUDENT WITH A DISABILITY

The USMLE provides accommodations for students with documented disabilities. The basis for such accommodations is the Americans with Disabilities Act (ADA) of 1990. The ADA defines a disability as "a significant limitation in one or more major life activities." This includes both "observable/ physical" disabilities (e.g., blindness, hearing loss, narcolepsy) and "hidden/ mental disabilities" (e.g., attention-deficit hyperactivity disorder, chronic fatigue syndrome, learning disabilities).

To provide appropriate support, the administrators of the USMLE must be informed of both the nature and the severity of an examinee's disability. Such documentation is required for an examinee to receive testing accommodations. Accommodations include extra time on tests, low-stimulation environments, extra or extended breaks, and zoom text.

> ▶ U.S. students seeking ADA-compliant accommodations must contact the NBME directly; IMGs, contact the ECFMG.

Who Can Apply for Accommodations?

Students or graduates of a school in the United States or Canada that is accredited by the Liaison Committee on Medical Education (LCME) or the AOA may apply for test accommodations directly from the NBME. Requests are granted only if they meet the ADA definition of a disability. If you are a disabled student or a disabled graduate of a foreign medical school, you must contact the ECFMG (see the following page).

Who Is Not Eligible for Accommodations?

Individuals who do not meet the ADA definition of disabled are not eligible for test accommodations. Difficulties not eligible for test accommodations include test anxiety, slow reading without an identified underlying cognitive deficit, English as a second language, and learning difficulties that have not been diagnosed as a medically recognized disability.

Understanding the Need for Documentation

Although most learning-disabled medical students are all too familiar with the often exhausting process of providing documentation of their disability, you should realize that **applying for USMLE accommodation is different from these previous experiences.** This is because the NBME determines whether an individual is disabled solely on the basis of the guidelines set by the ADA. **Previous accommodation does not in itself justify provision of an accommodation for the USMLE,** so be sure to review the NBME guidelines carefully.

Getting the Information

The first step in applying for USMLE special accommodations is to contact the NBME and obtain a guidelines and questionnaire booklet. For the Step 1, Step 2 CK, and Step 2 CS exams, this can be obtained by calling or writing to:

Disability Services
National Board of Medical Examiners
3750 Market Street
Philadelphia, PA 19104-3102
(215) 590-9509
Fax: (215) 590-9457
Email: disabilityservices@nbme.org
www.usmle.org/test-accommodations

Internet access to this information is also available at www.nbme.org. This information is also relevant for IMGs, since the information is the same as that sent by the ECFMG.

Foreign graduates should contact the ECFMG to obtain information on special accommodations by calling or writing to:

ECFMG
3624 Market Street
Philadelphia, PA 19104-2685
(215) 386-5900
www.ecfmg.org

When you get this information, take some time to read it carefully. The guidelines are clear and explicit about what you need to do to obtain accommodations.

SECTION II

High-Yield
General Principles

"There comes a time when for every addition of knowledge you forget something that you knew before. It is of the highest importance, therefore, not to have useless facts elbowing out the useful ones."
—Sir Arthur Conan Doyle, A *Study in Scarlet*

"Never regard study as a duty, but as the enviable opportunity to learn."
—Albert Einstein

"Live as if you were to die tomorrow. Learn as if you were to live forever."
—Gandhi

▶ HOW TO USE THE DATABASE

The 2014 edition of *First Aid for the USMLE Step 1* contains a revised and expanded database of basic science material that students, student authors, and faculty authors and faculty have identified as high yield for board review. The information is presented in a partially organ-based format. Hence, Section II is devoted to pathology and the foundational principles of behavioral science, biochemistry, microbiology, immunology, and pharmacology. Section III focuses on organ systems, with subsections covering the embryology, anatomy and histology, physiology, pathology, and pharmacology relevant to each. Each subsection is then divided into smaller topic areas containing related facts. Individual facts are generally presented in a three-column format, with the **Title** of the fact in the first column, the **Description** of the fact in the second column, and the **Mnemonic** or **Special Note** in the third column. Some facts do not have a mnemonic and are presented in a two-column format. Others are presented in list or tabular form in order to emphasize key associations.

The database structure used in Sections II and III is useful for reviewing material already learned. These sections are **not** ideal for learning complex or highly conceptual material for the first time.

The database of high-yield facts is not comprehensive. Use it to complement your core study material and not as your primary study source. The facts and notes have been condensed and edited to emphasize the essential material, and as a result, each entry is "incomplete" and arguably "over-simplified." Often the more you research a topic, the more complex it gets, and certain topics resist simplification. Work with the material, add your own notes and mnemonics, and recognize that not all memory techniques work for all students.

We update the database of high-yield facts annually to keep current with new trends in boards emphasis, including clinical relevance. However, we must note that inevitably many other high-yield topics are not yet included in our database.

We actively encourage medical students and faculty to submit high-yield topics, well-written entries, diagrams, clinical images, and useful mnemonics so that we may enhance the database for future students. We also solicit recommendations of alternate tools for study that may be useful in preparing for the examination, such as charts, flashcards, apps, and online resources (see How to Contribute, p. xvii).

Image Acknowledgments

All images and diagrams marked with ℞ are © USMLE-Rx.com (MedIQ Learning, LLC) and reproduced here by special permission. All images marked with ᴿᵁ are © Dr. Richard P. Usatine and the *Color Atlas of Family Medicine* and are reproduced here by special permission (www. usatinemedia.com). Images marked with ✳ are adapted or reproduced with permission of other sources as listed on page 685.

Disclaimer

The entries in this section reflect student opinions of what is high yield. Because of the diverse sources of material, no attempt has been made to trace or reference the origins of entries individually. We have regarded mnemonics as essentially in the public domain. Errata, errors of attribution, and important omissions will gladly be corrected if brought to the attention of the authors, either through our online errata submission form at www.firstaidteam.com or directly by email to firstaidteam@yahoo.com.

Behavioral Science

"It is a mathematical fact that fifty percent of all doctors graduate in the bottom half of their class."

—Author Unknown

"It's psychosomatic. You need a lobotomy. I'll get a saw."
—Calvin, "Calvin & Hobbes"

"There are two kinds of statistics: the kind you look up and the kind you make up."

—Rex Stout

"On a long enough time line, the survival rate for everyone drops to zero."
—Chuck Palahniuk

A heterogeneous mix of epidemiology, biostatistics, ethics, psychology, sociology, and more falls under the heading of behavioral science. Many medical students do not diligently study this discipline because the material is felt to be easy or a matter of common sense. In our opinion, this is a missed opportunity.

Behavioral science questions may seem less concrete than questions from other disciplines, requiring an awareness of the social aspects of medicine. For example, if a patient does or says something, what should you do or say in response? These so-called quote questions now constitute much of the behavioral science section. Medical ethics and medical law are also appearing with increasing frequency. In addition, the key aspects of the doctor-patient relationship (e.g., communication skills, open-ended questions, facilitation, silence) are high yield, as are biostatistics and epidemiology. Make sure you can apply biostatistical concepts such as sensitivity, specificity, and predictive values in a problem-solving format.

▸ BEHAVIORAL SCIENCE–EPIDEMIOLOGY/BIOSTATISTICS

Types of studies

STUDY TYPE	DESIGN	MEASURES/EXAMPLE
Cross-sectional study Observational	Collects data from a group of people to assess frequency of disease (and related risk factors) at a particular point in time. Asks, "What is happening?"	Disease prevalence. Can show risk factor association with disease, but does not establish causality.
Case-control study Observational and retrospective	Compares a group of people with disease to a group without disease. Looks for prior exposure or risk factor. Asks, "What happened?"	Odds ratio (OR). "Patients with COPD had higher odds of a history of smoking than those without COPD had."
Cohort study Observational and prospective or retrospective	Compares a group with a given exposure or risk factor to a group without such exposure. Looks to see if exposure ↑ the likelihood of disease. Can be prospective (asks, "Who will develop disease?") or retrospective (asks, "Who developed the disease [exposed vs. nonexposed]?").	Relative risk (RR). "Smokers had a higher risk of developing COPD than nonsmokers had."
Twin concordance study	Compares the frequency with which both monozygotic twins or both dizygotic twins develop same disease.	Measures heritability and influence of environmental factors ("nature vs. nurture").
Adoption study	Compares siblings raised by biological vs. adoptive parents.	Measures heritability and influence of environmental factors.

| **Clinical trial** | Experimental study involving humans. Compares therapeutic benefits of 2 or more treatments, or of treatment and placebo. Study quality improves when study is randomized, controlled, and double-blinded (i.e., neither patient nor doctor knows whether the patient is in the treatment or control group). Triple-blind refers to the additional blinding of the researchers analyzing the data. | |

DRUG TRIALS	TYPICAL STUDY SAMPLE	PURPOSE
Phase I	Small number of healthy volunteers.	"Is it safe?" Assesses safety, toxicity, and pharmacokinetics.
Phase II	Small number of patients with disease of interest.	"Does it work?" Assesses treatment efficacy, optimal dosing, and adverse effects.
Phase III	Large number of patients randomly assigned either to the treatment under investigation or to the best available treatment (or placebo).	"Is it as good or better?" Compares the new treatment to the current standard of care.
Phase IV	Postmarketing surveillance trial of patients after approval.	"Can it stay?" Detects rare or long-term adverse effects. Can result in a drug being withdrawn from market.

Evaluation of diagnostic tests	Uses 2 × 2 table comparing test results with the actual presence of disease. TP = true positive; FP = false positive; TN = true negative; FN = false negative. Sensitivity and specificity are fixed properties of a test (vs. PPV and NPV).	
Sensitivity (true-positive rate)	Proportion of all people with disease who test positive, or the probability that a test detects disease when disease is present. Value approaching 100% is desirable for **ruling out** disease and indicates a **low false-negative rate**. High sensitivity test used for screening in diseases with low prevalence.	$= TP / (TP + FN)$ $= 1 -$ false-negative rate **SN-N-OUT** = highly **SeN**sitive test, when Negative, rules **OUT** disease If sensitivity is 100%, $TP / (TP + FN) = 1$, FN = 0, and all negatives must be TNs
Specificity (true-negative rate)	Proportion of all people without disease who test negative, or the probability that a test indicates non-disease when disease is absent. Value approaching 100% is desirable for **ruling in** disease and indicates a **low false-positive rate**. High specificity test used for confirmation after a positive screening test.	$= TN / (TN + FP)$ $= 1 -$ false-positive rate **SP-P-IN** = highly **SP**ecific test, when Positive, rules **IN** disease If specificity is 100%, $TN / (TN + FP) = 1$, FP = 0, and all positives must be TPs
Positive predictive value (PPV)	Proportion of positive test results that are true positive. Probability that person actually has the disease given a positive test result.	$= TP / (TP + FP)$ PPV varies directly with prevalence or pretest probability: high pretest probability → high PPV
Negative predictive value (NPV)	Proportion of negative test results that are true negative. Probability that person actually is disease free given a negative test result.	$= TN / (FN + TN)$ NPV varies inversely with prevalence or pretest probability: high pretest probability → low NPV

POSSIBLE CUTOFF VALUES
A = 100% sensitivity cutoff value
B = practical compromise between specificity and sensitivity
C = 100% specificity cutoff value

Incidence vs. prevalence

$$\text{Incidence rate} = \frac{\substack{\text{\# of new cases} \\ \text{in a specified time period}}}{\substack{\text{Population at risk during} \\ \text{same time period}}}$$

Incidence looks at new cases (**incidents**).

$$\text{Prevalence} = \frac{\text{\# of existing cases}}{\text{Population at risk}}$$

Prevalence looks at **all** current cases.

Prevalence ≈ incidence rate × average disease duration.

Prevalence > incidence for chronic diseases (e.g., diabetes).

Incidence and prevalence for common cold are very similar since disease duration is short.

Quantifying risk

Odds ratio (OR)	Typically used in case-control studies. Odds that the group with the disease (cases) was exposed to a risk factor (a/c) divided by the odds that the group without the disease (controls) was exposed (b/d).	$OR = \dfrac{a/c}{b/d} = \dfrac{ad}{bc}$
Relative risk (RR)	Typically used in cohort studies. Risk of developing disease in the exposed group divided by risk in the unexposed group (e.g., if 21% of smokers develop lung cancer vs. 1% of nonsmokers, RR = 21/1 = 21). If prevalence is low, RR ≈ OR.	$RR = \dfrac{a/(a+b)}{c/(c+d)}$
Relative risk reduction (RRR)	The proportion of risk reduction attributable to the intervention as compared to a control. RRR = 1 – RR (e.g., if 2% of patients who receive a flu shot develop flu, while 8% of unvaccinated patients develop the flu, then RR = 2/8 = 0.25, and RRR = 1 – RR = 0.75).	
Attributable risk (AR)	The difference in risk between exposed and unexposed groups, or the proportion of disease occurrences that are attributable to the exposure (e.g., if risk of lung cancer in smokers is 21% and risk in nonsmokers is 1%, then 20% (or .20) of the 21% risk of lung cancer in smokers is attributable to smoking).	$AR = \dfrac{a}{a+b} - \dfrac{c}{c+d}$
Absolute risk reduction (ARR)	The difference in risk (not the proportion) attributable to the intervention as compared to a control (e.g., if 8% of people who receive a placebo vaccine develop flu vs. 2% of people who receive a flu vaccine, then ARR = 8% – 2% = 6% = .06).	
Number needed to treat	Number of patients who need to be treated for 1 patient to benefit. Calculated as 1/ARR.	
Number needed to harm	Number of patients who need to be exposed to a risk factor for 1 patient to be harmed. Calculated as 1/AR.	

Disease

	⊕	⊖
Risk factor ⊕	a	b
Risk factor ⊖	c	d

Precision vs. accuracy

Precision	The consistency and reproducibility of a test (reliability). The absence of random variation in a test.	Random error—reduces precision in a test. ↑ precision → ↓ standard deviation.
Accuracy	The trueness of test measurements (validity). The absence of systematic error or bias in a test.	Systematic error—reduces accuracy in a test.

Accurate, not precise   Precise, not accurate   Accurate and precise   Not accurate, not precise

Bias and study errors

TYPE	DEFINITION	EXAMPLES	STRATEGY TO REDUCE BIAS
Recruiting participants			
Selection bias	Nonrandom assignment to participate in a study group. Most commonly a sampling bias. Examples include:		Randomization Ensure the choice of the right comparison/reference group
	▪ Berkson bias	A study looking only at inpatients	
	▪ Loss to follow-up	Studying a disease with early mortality	
	▪ Healthy worker and volunteer biases	Study populations are healthier than the general population	
Performing study			
Recall bias	Awareness of disorder alters recall by subjects; common in retrospective studies.	Patients with disease recall exposure after learning of similar cases	Decrease time from exposure to follow-up
Measurement bias	Information is gathered in a way that distorts it.	Hawthorne effect — groups who know they're being studied behave differently than they would otherwise	Use of placebo control groups with blinding to reduce influence of participants and researchers on experimental procedures and interpretation of outcomes
Procedure bias	Subjects in different groups are not treated the same.	Patients in treatment group spend more time in highly specialized hospital units	
Observer-expectancy bias	Researcher's belief in the efficacy of a treatment changes the outcome of that treatment (aka Pygmalion effect; self-fulfilling prophecy).	If observer expects treatment group to show signs of recovery, then he is more likely to document positive outcomes	
Interpreting results			
Confounding bias	When a factor is related to both the exposure and outcome, but not on the causal pathway → factor distorts or confuses effect of exposure on outcome.	Pulmonary disease is more common in coal workers than the general population; however, people who work in coal mines also smoke more frequently than the general population	Multiple/repeated studies Crossover studies (subjects act as their own controls) Matching (patients with similar characteristics in both treatment and control groups)
Lead-time bias	Early detection is confused with ↑ survival; seen with improved screening techniques.	Early detection makes it seem as though survival has increased, but the natural history of the disease has not changed	Measure "back-end" survival (adjust survival according to the severity of disease at the time of diagnosis)

Statistical distribution

Measures of central tendency	Mean = (sum of values)/(total number of values). Median = middle value of a list of data sorted from least to greatest. Mode = most common value.	If there is an even number of values, the median will be the average of the middle two values.
Measures of dispersion	Standard deviation = how much variability exists from the mean in a set of values. Standard error of the mean = an estimation of how much variability exists between the sample mean and the true population mean.	σ = SD; n = sample size. SEM = $\sigma/\sqrt{n}$. SEM ↓ as n ↑.
Normal distribution	Gaussian, also called bell-shaped. Mean = median = mode.	

Nonnormal distributions

Bimodal	Suggests two different populations (e.g., metabolic polymorphism such as fast vs. slow acetylators; suicide rate by age).	
Positive skew	Typically, mean > median > mode. Asymmetry with longer tail on right.	
Negative skew	Typically, mean < median < mode. Asymmetry with longer tail on left.	

Statistical hypotheses

Null (H₀)	Hypothesis of no difference (e.g., there is no association between the disease and the risk factor in the population).	
Alternative (H₁)	Hypothesis of some difference (e.g., there is some association between the disease and the risk factor in the population).	

Outcomes of statistical hypothesis testing

Correct result	Stating that there is an effect or difference when one exists (null hypothesis rejected in favor of alternative hypothesis). Stating that there is not an effect or difference when none exists (null hypothesis not rejected).	
Incorrect result		
Type I error (α)	Stating that there is an effect or difference when none exists (null hypothesis incorrectly rejected in favor of alternative hypothesis). α is the probability of making a type I error. p is judged against a preset α level of significance (usually $< .05$). If $p < 0.05$, then there is less than a 5% chance that the data will show something that is not really there.	Also known as false-positive error. α = you saw a difference that did not exist (e.g., convicting an innocent man).

Type II error (β)	Stating that there is not an effect or difference when one exists (null hypothesis is not rejected when it is in fact false).
	β is the probability of making a type II error. β is related to statistical power $(1 - \beta)$, which is the probability of rejecting the null hypothesis when it is false.
	↑ power and ↓ β by:
	  ▪ ↑ sample size
	  ▪ ↑ expected effect size
	  ▪ ↑ precision of measurement
		Also known as false-negative error.
		
		β = you were blind to a difference that did exist (e.g., setting a guilty man free).
		If you ↑ sample size, you ↑ power. There is power in numbers.

Meta-analysis	Pools data and integrates results from several similar studies to reach an overall conclusion. ↑ statistical power.	Limited by quality of individual studies or bias in study selection.
Confidence interval	Range of values in which a specified probability of the means of repeated samples would be expected to fall. CI = range from [mean – Z(SEM)] to [mean + Z(SEM)]. The 95% CI (corresponding to $p = .05$) is often used. For the 95% CI, Z = 1.96. For the 99% CI, Z = 2.58.	If the 95% CI for a mean difference between 2 variables includes 0, then there is no significant difference and H_0 is not rejected. If the 95% CI for odds ratio or relative risk includes 1, H_0 is not rejected. If the CIs between 2 groups do not overlap → significant difference exists. If the CIs between 2 groups overlap → usually no significant difference exists.

t-test vs. ANOVA vs. χ^2

t-test	Checks differences between means of 2 groups.	Tea is meant for 2 Example: comparing the mean blood pressure between men and women.
ANOVA	Checks differences between means of 3 or more groups.	3 words: ANalysis Of VAriance Example: comparing the mean blood pressure between members of 3 different ethnic groups.
Chi-square (χ^2)	Checks difference between 2 or more percentages or proportions of categorical outcomes (not mean values).	Pronounce Chi-tegorical Example: comparing the percentage of members of 3 different ethnic groups who have essential hypertension.

Pearson correlation coefficient (*r*)	*r* is always between −1 and +1. The closer the absolute value of *r* is to 1, the stronger the linear correlation between the 2 variables. Positive *r* value → positive correlation. Negative *r* value → negative correlation. Coefficient of determination = r^2 (value that is usually reported).

Disease prevention

Primary	Prevent disease occurrence (e.g., HPV vaccination).	PST: Prevent
Secondary	Screening early for disease (e.g., Pap smear)	Screen Treat
Tertiary	Treatment to reduce disability from disease (e.g., chemotherapy)	Quaternary—identifying patients at risk of unnecessary treatment, protecting from the harm of new interventions

Medicare and Medicaid	Medicare and Medicaid—federal programs that originated from amendments to the Social Security Act. Medicare is available to patients ≥ 65 years old, < 65 with certain disabilities, and those with end-stage renal disease. Medicaid is joint federal and state health assistance for people with very low income.	MedicarE is for Elderly. MedicaiD is for Destitute.

▶ **BEHAVIORAL SCIENCE–ETHICS**

Core ethical principles

4 principles of ethics.

Respect patient autonomy	Obligation to respect patients as individuals (→ truth-telling, confidentiality), to create conditions necessary for autonomous choice (→ informed consent), and to honor their preference in accepting or not accepting medical care.
Beneficence	Physicians have a special ethical (fiduciary) duty to act in the patient's best interest. May conflict with autonomy (an informed patient has the right to decide) or what is best for society ✳ (traditionally patient interest supersedes).
Nonmaleficence	"Do no harm." Must be balanced against beneficence; if the benefits outweigh the risks, a patient may make an informed decision to proceed (most surgeries and medications fall into this category).
Justice	To treat persons fairly and equitably. This does not always imply equally (e.g., triage).

Informed consent

A process (not just a document/signature) that legally requires:

- Disclosure: discussion of pertinent information
- Understanding: ability to comprehend (assess)
- Mental capacity: unless incompetent (a legal determination)
- Voluntariness: freedom from coercion and manipulation

Patients must have an intelligent understanding of their diagnosis and the risks/benefits of proposed treatment and alternative options, including no treatment.

Patient must be informed that he or she can revoke written consent at any time, even orally.

Exceptions to informed consent:

- Patient lacks decision-making capacity or is legally incompetent
- Implied consent in an emergency
- Therapeutic privilege—withholding information when disclosure would severely harm the patient or undermine informed decision-making capacity
- Waiver—patient explicitly waives the right of informed consent

Consent for minors

A minor is generally any person < 18 years old. Parental consent laws in relation to health care vary state by state. In general, parental consent should be obtained unless minor is legally emancipated (e.g., is married, is self-supporting, or is in the military). Some states have "mature minor" laws, in which parental consent is not required; nonetheless, physicians should always encourage healthy minor-guardian communication.

Situations in which parental consent is usually not required: parents can't stop kids from getting treatment for:

- **Sex** (contraception, STDs, pregnancy)
- **Drugs** (addiction)
- **Rock and roll** (emergency/trauma)

Decision-making capacity	Physician must determine whether the patient is psychologically and legally capable of making a particular health care decision. Components: <ul><li>Patient is ≥ 18 years old or otherwise legally emancipated</li><li>Patient makes and communicates a choice</li><li>Patient is informed (knows and understands)</li><li>Decision remains stable over time</li><li>Decision is consistent with patient's values and goals, not clouded by a mood disorder</li><li>Decision is not a result of delusions or hallucinations</li></ul>

Advance directives	Instructions given by a patient in anticipation of the need for a medical decision. Details vary per state law.
Oral advance directive	Incapacitated patient's prior oral statements commonly used as guide. Problems arise from variance in interpretation. If patient was informed, directive was specific, patient made a choice, and decision was repeated over time to multiple people, the oral directive is more valid.
Living will (written advance directive)	Describes treatments the patient wishes to receive or not receive if he/she loses decision-making capacity. Usually, patient directs physician to withhold or withdraw life-sustaining treatment if he/she develops a terminal disease or enters a persistent vegetative state.
Medical power of attorney	Patient designates an agent to make medical decisions in the event that he/she loses decision-making capacity. Patient may also specify decisions in clinical situations. Can be revoked anytime patient wishes (regardless of competence). More flexible than a living will.

Surrogate decision-maker	If an incompetent patient has not prepared an advance directive, individuals (surrogates) who know the patient must determine what the patient would have done if he/she were competent. Priority of surrogates: spouse, adult children, parents, adult siblings, other relatives.

Confidentiality	Confidentiality respects patient privacy and autonomy. If patient is not present or is incapacitated, disclosing information to family and friends should be guided by professional judgment of patient's best interest. The patient may voluntarily waive the right to confidentiality (e.g., insurance company request). General principles for exceptions to confidentiality: <ul><li>Potential physical harm to others is serious and imminent</li><li>Likelihood of harm to self is great</li><li>No alternative means exists to warn or to protect those at risk</li><li>Physicians can take steps to prevent harm</li></ul>Examples of exceptions to patient confidentiality (many are state-specific) include: <ul><li>Reportable diseases (e.g., STDs, TB, hepatitis, food poisoning)—physicians may have a duty to warn public officials, who will then notify people at risk</li><li>The Tarasoff decision—California Supreme Court decision requiring physician to directly inform and protect potential victim from harm</li><li>Child and/or elder abuse</li><li>Impaired automobile drivers (e.g., epileptics)</li><li>Suicidal/homicidal patients</li></ul>

Ethical situations

SITUATION	APPROPRIATE RESPONSE
Patient is not adherent.	Attempt to identify the reason for nonadherence and determine his/her willingness to change; do not coerce the patient into adhering or refer him/her to another physician.
Patient desires an unnecessary procedure.	Attempt to understand why the patient wants the procedure and address underlying concerns. Do not refuse to see the patient or refer him/her to another physician. Avoid performing unnecessary procedures.
Patient has difficulty taking medications.	Provide written instructions; attempt to simplify treatment regimens; use teach-back method (ask patient to repeat medication regimen back to physician) to ensure patient comprehension.
Family members ask for information about patient's prognosis.	Avoid discussing issues with relatives without the permission of the patient.
A patient's family member asks you not to disclose the results of a test if the prognosis is poor because the patient will be "unable to handle it."	Attempt to identify why the family member believes such information would be detrimental to the patient's condition. Explain that as long as the patient has decision-making capacity and does not indicate otherwise, communication of information concerning his/her care will not be withheld.
A child wishes to know more about his/her illness.	Ask what the parents have told the child about his/her illness. Parents of a child decide what information can be relayed about the illness.
A 17-year-old girl is pregnant and requests an abortion.	Many states require parental notification or consent for minors for an abortion. Unless she is at medical risk, do not advise a patient to have an abortion regardless of her age or the condition of the fetus.
A 15-year-old girl is pregnant and wants to keep the child. Her parents want you to tell her to give the child up for adoption.	The patient retains the right to make decisions regarding her child, even if her parents disagree. Provide information to the teenager about the practical issues of caring for a baby. Discuss the options, if requested. Encourage discussion between the teenager and her parents to reach the best decision.
A terminally ill patient requests physician assistance in ending own life.	In the overwhelming majority of states, refuse involvement in any form of physician-assisted suicide. Physicians may, however, prescribe medically appropriate analgesics that coincidentally shorten the patient's life.
Patient is suicidal.	Assess the seriousness of the threat; if it is serious, suggest that the patient remain in the hospital voluntarily; patient can be hospitalized involuntarily if he/she refuses.
Patient states that he/she finds you attractive.	Ask direct, closed-ended questions and use a chaperone if necessary. Romantic relationships with patients are never appropriate. Never say, "There can be no relationship while you are a patient," because this implies that a relationship may be possible if the individual is no longer a patient.
A woman who had a mastectomy says she now feels "ugly."	Find out why the patient feels this way. Do not offer falsely reassuring statements (e.g., "You still look good.").
Patient is angry about the amount of time he/she spent in the waiting room.	Acknowledge the patient's anger, but do not take a patient's anger personally. Apologize for any inconvenience. Stay away from efforts to explain the delay.
Patient is upset with the way he/she was treated by another doctor.	Suggest that the patient speak directly to that physician regarding his/her concerns. If the problem is with a member of the office staff, tell the patient you will speak to that person.
A drug company offers a "referral fee" for every patient a physician enrolls in a study.	Eligible patients who may benefit from the study may be enrolled, but it is never acceptable for a physician to receive compensation from a drug company. Patients must be told about the existence of a referral fee.
A physician orders an invasive test for the wrong patient.	No matter how serious or trivial a medical error, a physician is ethically obligated to inform a patient that a mistake has been made.
A patient requires a treatment not covered by his/her insurance.	Never limit or deny care because of the expense in time or money. Discuss all treatment options with patients, even if some are not covered by their insurance companies.

▶ BEHAVIORAL SCIENCE—DEVELOPMENT

Apgar score

Assessment of newborn vital signs following labor via a 10-point scale evaluated at 1 minute and 5 minutes. Apgar score is based on Appearance, Pulse, Grimace, Activity, and Respiration (≥ 7 = good; 4–6 = assist and stimulate; < 4 = resuscitate). If Apgar score remains < 4 at later time points, there is ↑ risk that the child will develop long-term neurological damage.

Appearance = cyanosis
Grimace = cry

Low birth weight

Defined as < 2500 g. Caused by prematurity or intrauterine growth retardation (IUGR). Associated with ↑ risk of SIDS, and with ↑ overall mortality. Other problems include impaired thermoregulation and immune function, hypoglycemia, polycythemia, and impaired neurocognitive/emotional development. Complications include infections, respiratory distress syndrome, necrotizing enterocolitis, intraventricular hemorrhage, and persistent fetal circulation.

Early developmental milestones

Milestone dates are ranges that have been approximated and vary by source. Children not meeting milestones may need assessment for potential developmental delay.

AGE	MOTOR	SOCIAL	VERBAL/COGNITIVE
Infant	**Parents**	**Start**	**Observing**
0–12 mo	Primitive reflexes disappear—Moro (by 3 mo), rooting (by 4 mo), palmar (by 6 mo), Babinski (by 12 mo) – *upgoing initially.* Posture—lifts head up prone (by 1 mo), rolls and sits (by 6 mo), crawls (by 8 mo), stands (by 10 mo), walks (by 12–18 mo) Picks—passes toys hand to hand (by 6 mo), Pincer grasp (by 10 mo) Points to objects (by 12 mo)	Social smile (by 2 mo) Stranger anxiety (by 6 mo) Separation anxiety (by 9 mo)	Orients—first to voice (by 4 mo), then to name and gestures (by 9 mo) Object permanence (by 9 mo) Oratory—says "mama" and "dada" (by 10 mo)
Toddler	**Child**	**Rearing**	**Working**
12–36 mo	Climbs stairs (by 18 mo) Cubes stacked—number = age (yr) × 3 Cultured—feeds self with fork and spoon (by 20 mo) Kicks ball (by 24 mo)	Recreation—parallel play (by 12 mo) Rapprochement—moves away from and returns to mother (by 24 mo) Realization—core gender identity formed (by 36 mo)	Words—200 words by age 2 (2 zeros), 2-word sentences
Preschool	**Don't**	**Forget, they're still**	**Learning!**
3–5 yr	Drive—tricycle (3 wheels at 3 yr) Drawings—copies line or circle, stick figure (by 4 yr) Dexterity—hops on one foot (by 4 yr), uses buttons or zippers, grooms self (by 5 yr)	Freedom—comfortably spends part of day away from mother (by 3 yr) Friends—cooperative play, has imaginary friends (by 4 yr)	Language—1000 words by age 3 (3 zeroes), uses complete sentences and prepositions (by 4 yr) Legends—can tell detailed stories (by 4 yr)

see developmental milestone module.

Changes in the elderly

Sexual changes:
- Men—slower erection/ejaculation, longer refractory period
- Women—vaginal shortening, thinning, and dryness

Sleep patterns: ↓ REM and slow-wave sleep; ↑ sleep onset latency and ↑ early awakenings

↑ suicide rate (particularly white men > 85 years old)

↓ vision, hearing, immune response, bladder control

↓ renal, pulmonary, GI function

↓ muscle mass, ↑ fat

Sexual interest does not ↓.
Intelligence does not ↓.

Presbycusis--high-frequency hearing loss due to destruction of hair cells at the cochlear base (preserved low-frequency hearing at apex).

Common causes of death (U.S.) by age

	< 1 YR	1–14 YR	15–24 YR	25–34 YR	35–44 YR	45–64 YR	65+ YR
#1	Congenital malformations	Unintentional injury	Unintentional injury	Unintentional injury	Unintentional injury	Cancer	Heart disease
#2	Preterm birth	Cancer	Homicide	Suicide	Cancer	Heart disease	Cancer
#3	SIDS	Homicide	Suicide	Homicide	Heart disease	Unintentional injury	Chronic respiratory

Biochemistry

"Biochemistry is the study of carbon compounds that crawl."

—Mike Adams

"We think we have found the basic mechanism by which life comes from life."

—Francis H. C. Crick

This high-yield material includes molecular biology, genetics, cell biology, and principles of metabolism (especially vitamins, cofactors, minerals, and single-enzyme-deficiency diseases). When studying metabolic pathways, emphasize important regulatory steps and enzyme deficiencies that result in disease, as well as reactions targeted by pharmacologic interventions. For example, understanding the defect in Lesch-Nyhan syndrome and its clinical consequences is higher yield than memorizing every intermediate in the purine salvage pathway. Do not spend time on hard-core organic chemistry, mechanisms, or physical chemistry. Detailed chemical structures are infrequently tested; however, many structures have been included here to help students learn reactions and the important enzymes involved. Familiarity with the biochemical techniques that have medical relevance—such as ELISA, immunoelectrophoresis, Southern blotting, and PCR—is useful. Beware if you placed out of your medical school's biochemistry class, as the emphasis of the test differs from that of many undergraduate courses. Review the related biochemistry when studying pharmacology or genetic diseases as a way to reinforce and integrate the material.

▶ BIOCHEMISTRY–MOLECULAR

Chromatin structure	DNA exists in the condensed, chromatin form in order to fit into the nucleus. Negatively charged DNA loops twice around positively charged histone octamer to form nucleosome "**bead**." Histones are rich in the amino acids lysine and arginine. H1 binds to the nucleosome and to "linker DNA," thereby stabilizing the chromatin fiber. In mitosis, DNA condenses to form chromosomes. DNA and histone synthesis occur during S phase.	Think of "beads on a string." H1 is the only histone that is not in the nucleosome core.
Heterochromatin	Condensed, transcriptionally inactive, sterically inaccessible.	HeteroChromatin = Highly Condensed.
Euchromatin	Less condensed, transcriptionally active, sterically accessible.	*Eu* = true, "truly transcribed."
DNA methylation	Template strand cytosine and adenine are methylated in DNA replication, which allows mismatch repair enzymes to distinguish between old and new strands in prokaryotes. DNA methylation at CpG islands represses transcription.	CpG Methylation Makes DNA Mute.
Histone methylation	Usually reversibly represses DNA transcription, but can activate it in some cases.	Histone Methylation Mostly Makes DNA Mute.
Histone acetylation	Relaxes DNA coiling, allowing for transcription.	Histone Acetylation makes DNA Active.

Nucleotides	PURines (A, G)—2 rings. PYrimidines (C, T, U)—1 ring. Thymine has a methyl. Deamination of cytosine makes uracil. Uracil found in RNA; thymine in DNA. G-C bond (3 H bonds) stronger than A-T bond (2 H bonds). ↑ G-C content → ↑ melting temperature of DNA.	PURe As Gold. CUT the PY (pie). Thymine has a methyl.

GAG—Amino acids necessary for purine synthesis:
Glycine ①
Aspartate ②
Glutamine ③
NucleoSide = base + (deoxy)ribose (Sugar).
NucleoTides = base + (deoxy)ribose + phosphaTe; linked by 3′-5′ phosphodiester bond.

De novo pyrimidine and purine synthesis

Purines	Pyrimidines
	Make temporary base (orotic acid)
Start with sugar + phosphate (PRPP)	Add sugar + phosphate (PRPP)
Add base	Modify base

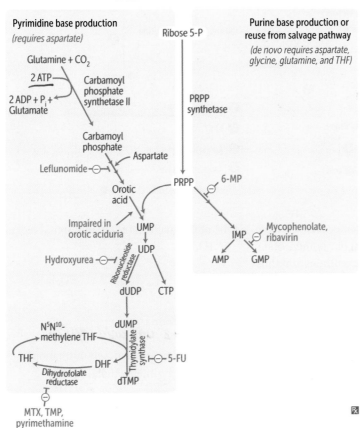

Pyrimidine base production
(requires aspartate)

Purine base production or reuse from salvage pathway
(de novo requires aspartate, glycine, glutamine, and THF)

Ribonucleotides are synthesized first and are converted to deoxyribonucleotides by ribonucleotide reductase.

Carbamoyl phosphate is involved in 2 metabolic pathways: de novo pyrimidine synthesis and the urea cycle.

Various antineoplastic and antibiotic drugs function by interfering with nucleotide synthesis:

- Leflunomide inhibits dihydroorotate dehydrogenase
- Mycophenolate and ribavirin inhibit IMP dehydrogenase
- Hydroxyurea inhibits ribonucleotide reductase
- 6-mercaptopurine (6-MP) and its prodrug azathioprine inhibit de novo purine synthesis
- 5-fluorouracil (5-FU) inhibits thymidylate synthase (↓ deoxythymidine monophosphate [dTMP])
- Methotrexate (MTX), trimethoprim (TMP), and pyrimethamine inhibit dihydrofolate reductase (↓ dTMP) in humans, bacteria, and protozoa, respectively

PRPP = phosphoribosyl pyrophosphate

THF = tetrahydrofolic acid.

Purine salvage deficiencies

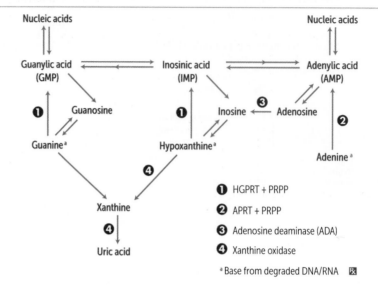

1 HGPRT + PRPP
2 APRT + PRPP
3 Adenosine deaminase (ADA)
4 Xanthine oxidase

a Base from degraded DNA/RNA

Adenosine deaminase deficiency	Excess ATP and dATP imbalances nucleotide pool via feedback inhibition of ribonucleotide reductase → prevents DNA synthesis and thus ↓ lymphocyte count.	One of the major causes of autosomal recessive SCID.
Lesch-Nyhan syndrome	Defective purine salvage due to absent HGPRT, which converts hypoxanthine to IMP and guanine to GMP. Results in excess uric acid production and de novo purine synthesis. X-linked recessive. Findings: intellectual disability, self-mutilation, aggression, hyperuricemia, gout, dystonia. Treatment: allopurinol or febuxostat (2nd line).	HGPRT: Hyperuricemia Gout → 2° uric acid crystals. Pissed off (aggression, self-mutilation) Retardation (intellectual disability) DysTonia

Genetic code features

Unambiguous	Each codon specifies only 1 amino acid.	
Degenerate/ redundant	Most amino acids are coded by multiple codons.	Exceptions: methionine and tryptophan encoded by only 1 codon (AUG and UGG, respectively).
Commaless, nonoverlapping	Read from a fixed starting point as a continuous sequence of bases.	Exceptions: some viruses.
Universal	Genetic code is conserved throughout evolution.	Exception in humans: mitochondria.

AUG = methionine
UGG = tryptophan.

DNA replication

Eukaryotic DNA replication is more complex than the prokaryotic process but uses many enzymes analogous to those listed below. In both prokaryotes and eukaryotes, DNA replication is semiconservative and involves both continuous and discontinuous (Okazaki fragment) synthesis.

A Origin of replication	Particular consensus sequence of base pairs in genome where DNA replication begins. May be single (prokaryotes) or multiple (eukaryotes).	
B Replication fork	Y-shaped region along DNA template where leading and lagging strands are synthesized.	
C Helicase	Unwinds DNA template at replication fork.	
D Single-stranded binding proteins	Prevent strands from reannealing.	
E DNA topoisomerases	Create a single- or double-stranded break in the helix to add or remove supercoils.	Fluoroquinolones—inhibit DNA gyrase (prokaryotic topoisomerase II).
F Primase	Makes an RNA primer on which DNA polymerase III can initiate replication.	
G DNA polymerase III	Prokaryotic only. Elongates leading strand by adding deoxynucleotides to the 3′ end. Elongates lagging strand until it reaches primer of preceding fragment. 3′ → 5′ exonuclease activity "proofreads" each added nucleotide.	DNA polymerase III has 5′ → 3′ synthesis and proofreads with 3′ → 5′ exonuclease.
H DNA polymerase I	Prokaryotic only. Degrades RNA primer; replaces it with DNA.	Has same functions as DNA polymerase III but also excises RNA primer with 5′ → 3′ exonuclease.
I DNA ligase	Catalyzes the formation of a phosphodiester bond within a strand of double-stranded DNA (i.e., joins Okazaki fragments).	Seals.
Telomerase	An RNA-dependent DNA polymerase that adds DNA to 3′ ends of chromosomes to avoid loss of genetic material with every duplication.	

Mutations in DNA	Severity of damage: silent << missense < nonsense < frameshift. For silent, missense, and nonsense mutations: ▪ **Transition**—purine to purine (e.g., A to G) or pyrimidine to pyrimidine (e.g., C to T). ▪ **Transversion**—purine to pyrimidine (e.g., A to T) or pyrimidine to purine (e.g., C to G).	
Silent	Nucleotide substitution but codes for same (synonymous) amino acid; often base change in 3rd position of codon (tRNA wobble).	
Missense	Nucleotide substitution resulting in changed amino acid (called conservative if new amino acid is similar in chemical structure).	Sickle cell disease
Nonsense	Nucleotide substitution resulting in early **stop** codon.	Stop the **nonsense**!
Frameshift	Deletion or insertion of a number of nucleotides not divisible by 3, resulting in misreading of all nucleotides downstream, usually resulting in a truncated, nonfunctional protein.	Duchenne muscular dystrophy

DNA repair

Single strand		
Nucleotide excision repair	Specific endonucleases release the oligonucleotide-containing damaged bases; DNA polymerase and ligase fill and reseal the gap, respectively. Repairs bulky helix-distorting lesions.	Defective in xeroderma pigmentosum, which prevents repair of pyrimidine dimers because of ultraviolet light exposure.
Base excision repair	Base-specific glycosylase recognizes altered base and creates AP site (apurinic/apyrimidinic). One or more nucleotides are removed by AP-endonuclease, which cleaves the 5′ end. Lyase cleaves the 3′ end. DNA polymerase-β fills the gap and DNA ligase seals it.	Important in repair of spontaneous/toxic deamination.
Mismatch repair	Newly synthesized strand is recognized, mismatched nucleotides are removed, and the gap is filled and resealed.	Defective in hereditary nonpolyposis colorectal cancer (HNPCC).
Double strand		
Nonhomologous end joining	Brings together 2 ends of DNA fragments to repair double-stranded breaks. No requirement for homology.	Mutated in ataxia telangiectasia.

DNA/RNA/protein synthesis direction	DNA and RNA are both synthesized 5′ → 3′. The 5′ end of the incoming nucleotide bears the triphosphate (energy source for bond). Protein synthesis is N-terminus to C-terminus.	mRNA is read 5′ to 3′. The triphosphate bond is the target of the 3′ hydroxyl attack. Drugs blocking DNA replication often have modified 3′ OH, preventing addition of the next nucleotide ("chain termination").

Start and stop codons

mRNA start codons	AUG (or rarely GUG).	AUG in**AUG**urates protein synthesis.
Eukaryotes	Codes for methionine, which may be removed before translation is completed.	
Prokaryotes	Codes for formylmethionine (f-met).	
mRNA stop codons	UGA, UAA, UAG.	UGA = U Go Away. UAA = U Are Away. UAG = U Are Gone.

Functional organization of a eukaryotic gene

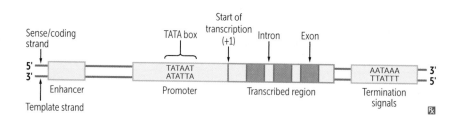

Regulation of gene expression

Promoter	Site where RNA polymerase and multiple other transcription factors bind to DNA upstream from gene locus (AT-rich upstream sequence with TATA and CAAT boxes).	Promoter mutation commonly results in dramatic ↓ in level of gene transcription.
Enhancer	Stretch of DNA that alters gene expression by binding transcription factors.	Enhancers and silencers may be located close to, far from, or even within (in an intron) the gene whose expression it regulates.
Silencer	Site where negative regulators (repressors) bind.	

RNA polymerases

Eukaryotes	RNA polymerase I makes rRNA (most numerous RNA, rampant). RNA polymerase II makes mRNA (largest RNA, massive). RNA polymerase III makes tRNA (smallest RNA, tiny). No proofreading function, but can initiate chains. RNA polymerase II opens DNA at promoter site.	I, II, and III are numbered as their products are used in protein synthesis. α-amanitin, found in *Amanita phalloides* (death cap mushrooms), inhibits RNA polymerase II. Causes severe hepatotoxicity if ingested.
Prokaryotes	1 RNA polymerase (multisubunit complex) makes all 3 kinds of RNA.	

RNA processing (eukaryotes)

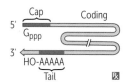

Initial transcript is called heterogeneous nuclear RNA (hnRNA). hnRNA is then modified and becomes mRNA.

The following processes occur in the nucleus following transcription:

- Capping of 5′ end (addition of 7-methylguanosine cap)
- Polyadenylation of 3′ end ($\approx$ 200 A's)
- Splicing out of introns

Capped, tailed, and spliced transcript is called mRNA.

mRNA is transported out of the nucleus into the cytosol, where it is translated.

mRNA quality control occurs at cytoplasmic P-bodies, which contain exonucleases, decapping enzymes, and microRNAs; mRNAs may be stored here for future translation.

Poly-A polymerase does not require a template.

AAUAAA = polyadenylation signal.

Splicing of pre-mRNA

❶ Primary transcript combines with small nuclear ribonucleoproteins (snRNPs) and other proteins to form spliceosome.

❷ Lariat-shaped (looped) intermediate is generated.

❸ Lariat is released to precisely remove intron and join 2 exons.

Antibodies to spliceosomal snRNPs (anti-Smith antibodies) are highly specific for SLE. Anti-U1 RNP antibodies are highly associated with mixed connective tissue disease.

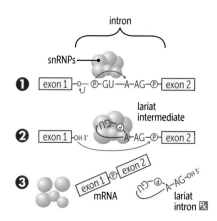

Introns vs. exons

Exons contain the actual genetic information coding for protein.

Introns are intervening noncoding segments of DNA.

Different exons are frequently combined by alternative splicing to produce a larger number of unique proteins.

Introns are intervening sequences and stay in the nucleus, whereas exons exit and are expressed.

Abnormal splicing variants are implicated in oncogenesis and many genetic disorders (e.g., β-thalassemia).

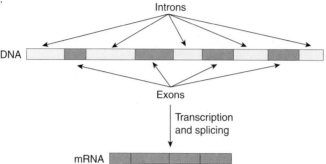

tRNA

Structure	75–90 nucleotides, 2° structure, cloverleaf form, anticodon end is opposite 3′ aminoacyl end. All tRNAs, both eukaryotic and prokaryotic, have CCA at 3′ end along with a high percentage of chemically modified bases. The amino acid is covalently bound to the 3′ end of the tRNA. **CCA Can Carry Amino acids.** T-arm: contains the TΨC (thymine, pseudouridine, cytosine) sequence necessary for tRNA-ribosome binding. D-arm: contains dihydrouracil residues necessary for tRNA recognition by the correct aminoacyl-tRNA synthetase. Acceptor stem: the 3′ CCA is the amino acid acceptor site.
Charging	Aminoacyl-tRNA synthetase (1 per amino acid; "matchmaker"; uses ATP) scrutinizes amino acid before and after it binds to tRNA. If incorrect, bond is hydrolyzed. The amino acid-tRNA bond has energy for formation of peptide bond. A mischarged tRNA reads usual codon but inserts wrong amino acid. Aminoacyl-tRNA synthetase and binding of charged tRNA to the codon are responsible for accuracy of amino acid selection.

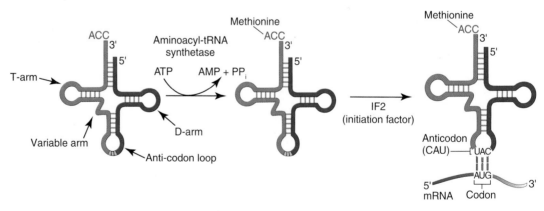

tRNA wobble Accurate base pairing is required only in the first 2 nucleotide positions of an mRNA codon, so codons differing in the 3rd "wobble" position may code for the same tRNA/amino acid (as a result of degeneracy of genetic code).

Protein synthesis

Initiation Initiated by GTP hydrolysis; initiation factors (eukaryotic IFs) help assemble the 40S ribosomal subunit with the initiator tRNA and are released when the mRNA and the ribosomal 60S subunit assemble with the complex.

Eukaryotes: 40S + 60S → 80S (Even).
PrOkaryotes: 30S + 50S → 70S (Odd).

ATP—tRNA Activation (charging).
GTP—tRNA Gripping and Going places (translocation).

Elongation
1. Aminoacyl-tRNA binds to A site (except for initiator methionine)
2. rRNA ("ribozyme") catalyzes peptide bond formation, transfers growing polypeptide to amino acid in A site
3. Ribosome advances 3 nucleotides toward 3′ end of mRNA, moving peptidyl tRNA to P site (translocation)

Think of "going APE":
A site = incoming Aminoacyl-tRNA.
P site = accommodates growing Peptide.
E site = holds Empty tRNA as it Exits.

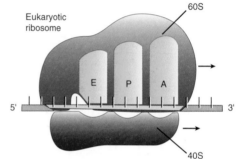

Eukaryotic ribosome

Termination Stop codon is recognized by release factor, and completed polypeptide is released from ribosome.

Posttranslational modifications

Trimming Removal of N- or C-terminal propeptides from zymogen to generate mature protein (e.g., trypsinogen to trypsin).

Covalent alterations Phosphorylation, glycosylation, hydroxylation, methylation, acetylation, and ubiquitination.

Chaperone protein Intracellular protein involved in facilitating and/or maintaining protein folding.
In yeast, some are heat shock proteins (e.g., Hsp60) that are expressed at high temperatures to prevent protein denaturing/misfolding.

▶ BIOCHEMISTRY–CELLULAR

Cell cycle phases	Checkpoints control transitions between phases of cell cycle. This process is regulated by cyclins, cyclin-dependent kinases (CDKs), and tumor suppressors. Mitosis (shortest phase of cell cycle) includes prophase, metaphase, anaphase, and telophase. G_1 and G_0 are of variable duration.	

REGULATION OF CELL CYCLE

CDKs	Constitutive and inactive.	G = Gap or Growth.
Cyclins	Regulatory proteins that control cell cycle events; phase specific; activate CDKs.	S = Synthesis.
Cyclin-CDK complexes	Must be both activated and inactivated for cell cycle to progress.	
Tumor suppressors	p53 and hypophosphorylated Rb normally inhibit G_1-to-S progression; mutations in these genes result in unrestrained cell division (e.g., Li-Fraumeni syndrome).	

CELL TYPES

Permanent	Remain in G_0, regenerate from stem cells.	Neurons, skeletal and cardiac muscle, RBCs.
Stable (quiescent)	Enter G_1 from G_0 when stimulated.	Hepatocytes, lymphocytes.
Labile	Never go to G_0, divide rapidly with a short G_1. Most affected by chemotherapy.	Bone marrow, gut epithelium, skin, hair follicles, germ cells.

Rough endoplasmic reticulum	Site of synthesis of secretory (exported) proteins and of N-linked oligosaccharide addition to many proteins. Nissl bodies (RER in neurons)—synthesize peptide neurotransmitters for secretion. Free ribosomes—unattached to any membrane; site of synthesis of cytosolic and organellar proteins.	Mucus-secreting goblet cells of the small intestine and antibody-secreting plasma cells are rich in RER.
Smooth endoplasmic reticulum	Site of steroid synthesis and detoxification of drugs and poisons. Lacks surface ribosomes.	Liver hepatocytes and steroid hormone–producing cells of the adrenal cortex and gonads are rich in SER.

Cell trafficking

Golgi is the distribution center for proteins and lipids from the ER to the vesicles and plasma membrane. Modifies N-oligosaccharides on asparagine. Adds O-oligosaccharides on serine and threonine. Adds mannose-6-phosphate to proteins for trafficking to lysosomes.

Endosomes are sorting centers for material from outside the cell or from the Golgi, sending it to lysosomes for destruction or back to the membrane/Golgi for further use.

I-cell disease (inclusion cell disease)—inherited lysosomal storage disorder; defect in phosphotransferase → failure of the Golgi to phosphorylate mannose residues (i.e., ↓ mannose-6-phosphate) on glycoproteins → proteins are secreted extracellularly rather than delivered to lysosomes. Results in coarse facial features, clouded corneas, restricted joint movement, and high plasma levels of lysosomal enzymes. Often fatal in childhood.

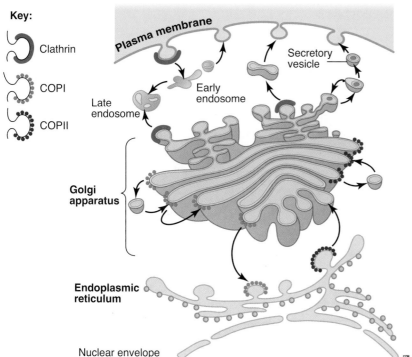

Key:
Clathrin
COPI
COPII

Plasma membrane
Secretory vesicle
Early endosome
Late endosome
Golgi apparatus
Endoplasmic reticulum
Nuclear envelope

Signal recognition particle (SRP)
Abundant, cytosolic ribonucleoprotein that traffics proteins from the ribosome to the RER. Absent or dysfunctional SRP → proteins accumulate in the cytosol.

Vesicular trafficking proteins
COPI: Golgi → Golgi (retrograde); Golgi → ER.
COPII: Golgi → Golgi (anterograde); ER → Golgi.
Clathrin: *trans*-Golgi → lysosomes; plasma membrane → endosomes (receptor-mediated endocytosis [e.g., LDL receptor activity]).

Peroxisome

Membrane-enclosed organelle involved in catabolism of very-long-chain fatty acids, branched-chain fatty acids, and amino acids.

Proteasome

Barrel-shaped protein complex that degrades damaged or ubiquitin-tagged proteins. Defects in the ubiquitin-proteasome system have been implicated in some cases of Parkinson disease.

Microtubule

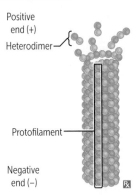

Positive end (+)

Heterodimer

Protofilament

Negative end (–)

Cylindrical structure composed of a helical array of polymerized heterodimers of α- and β-tubulin. Each dimer has 2 GTP bound. Incorporated into flagella, cilia, mitotic spindles. Grows slowly, collapses quickly. Also involved in slow axoplasmic transport in neurons.

Molecular motor proteins—transport cellular cargo toward opposite ends of microtubule tracks.
- Dynein = retrograde to microtubule (+ → –).
- Kinesin = anterograde to microtubule (– → +).

Drugs that act on microtubules (**M**icrotubules **G**et **C**onstructed **V**ery **P**oorly):
- **M**ebendazole (anti-helminthic)
- **G**riseofulvin (anti-fungal)
- **C**olchicine (anti-gout)
- **V**incristine/**V**inblastine (anti-cancer)
- **P**aclitaxel (anti-cancer)

Cilia structure

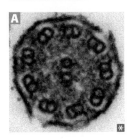

A

9 + 2 arrangement of microtubules .
Axonemal dynein—ATPase that links peripheral 9 doublets and causes bending of cilium by differential sliding of doublets.

Kartagener syndrome (1° ciliary dyskinesia)—immotile cilia due to a dynein arm defect. Results in male and female infertility due to immotile sperm and dysfunctional fallopian tube cilia, respectively; ↑ risk of ectopic pregnancy. Can cause bronchiectasis, recurrent sinusitis, and situs inversus (e.g., dextrocardia on CXR).

Cytoskeletal elements

Actin and myosin	Muscle contraction, microvilli, cytokinesis, adherens junctions. Actins are long, structural polymers. Myosins are dimeric, ATP-driven motor proteins that move along actins.
Microtubule	Movement. Cilia, flagella, mitotic spindle, axonal trafficking, centrioles.
Intermediate filaments	Structure. Vimentin, desmin, cytokeratin, lamins, glial fibrillary acid proteins (GFAP), neurofilaments.

Plasma membrane composition

Asymmetric lipid bilayer.
Contains cholesterol, phospholipids, sphingolipids, glycolipids, and proteins. Fungal membranes contain ergosterol.

Immunohistochemical stains for intermediate filaments

STAIN	CELL TYPE
Vimentin	Connective tissue
DesMin	Muscle
Cytokeratin	Epithelial cells
GFAP	NeuroGlia
Neurofilaments	Neurons

Sodium-potassium pump	Na⁺-K⁺ ATPase is located in the plasma membrane with ATP site on cytosolic side. For each ATP consumed, 3 Na⁺ go out and 2 K⁺ come in.	Ouabain inhibits by binding to K⁺ site. Cardiac glycosides (digoxin and digitoxin) directly inhibit the Na⁺-K⁺ ATPase, which leads to indirect inhibition of Na⁺/Ca²⁺ exchange → ↑ $[Ca^{2+}]_i$ → ↑ cardiac contractility.

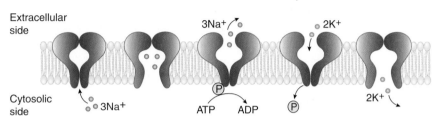

Collagen	Most abundant protein in the human body. Extensively modified by posttranslational modification. Organizes and strengthens extracellular matrix.	Be (So Totally) Cool, Read Books.
Type I	Most common (90%)—**B**one (made by osteoblasts), **S**kin, **T**endon, dentin, fascia, cornea, late wound repair.	Type I: bone. ↓ production in osteogenesis imperfecta type I.
Type II	**C**artilage (including hyaline), vitreous body, nucleus pulposus.	Type II: car**t**w**o**lage.
Type III	**R**eticulin—skin, **blood vessels**, uterus, fetal tissue, granulation tissue.	Type III: deficient in the uncommon, **vascular** type of Ehlers-Danlos syndrome (**ThreE D**).
Type IV	**B**asement membrane, basal lamina, lens.	Type IV: under the **floor** (basement membrane). Defective in Alport syndrome; targeted by autoantibodies in Goodpasture syndrome.

Collagen synthesis and structure

Inside fibroblasts	
1. Synthesis (RER)	Translation of collagen α chains (preprocollagen)—usually Gly-X-Y (X and Y are proline or lysine). Glycine content best reflects collagen synthesis (collagen is ⅓ glycine).
2. Hydroxylation (RER)	Hydroxylation of specific proline and lysine residues (requires vitamin C; deficiency → scurvy).
3. Glycosylation (RER)	Glycosylation of pro-α-chain hydroxylysine residues and formation of procollagen via hydrogen and disulfide bonds (triple helix of 3 collagen α chains). Problems forming triple helix → osteogenesis imperfecta.
4. Exocytosis	Exocytosis of procollagen into extracellular space.
Outside fibroblasts	
5. Proteolytic processing	Cleavage of disulfide-rich terminal regions of procollagen, transforming it into insoluble tropocollagen.
6. Cross-linking	Reinforcement of many staggered tropocollagen molecules by covalent lysine-hydroxylysine cross-linkage (by Cu^{2+}-containing lysyl oxidase) to make collagen fibrils. Problems with cross-linking → Ehlers-Danlos.

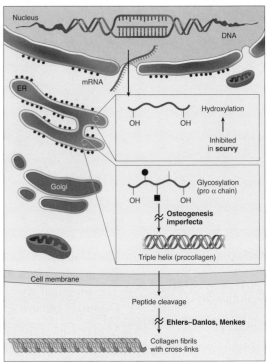

Osteogenesis imperfecta	Genetic bone disorder (brittle bone disease 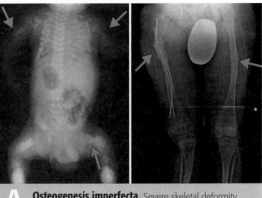) caused by a variety of gene defects.	May be confused with child abuse.

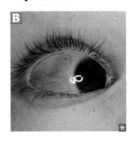

Genetic bone disorder (brittle bone disease **A**) caused by a variety of gene defects.

Most common form is autosomal dominant with ↓ production of otherwise normal type I collagen. OI manifestations can include:
- Multiple fractures with minimal trauma; may occur during the birth process
- Blue sclerae **B** due to the translucency of the connective tissue over the choroidal veins
- Hearing loss (abnormal ossicles)
- Dental imperfections due to lack of dentin

May be confused with child abuse.

A **Osteogenesis imperfecta.** Severe skeletal deformity and limb shortening due to multiple fractures in a child (left, arrows). ⚙ On the right, note bilateral proximal femur fractures (arrows); right is pinned and healing, left is healed. ⚙

Ehlers-Danlos syndrome	Faulty collagen synthesis causing hyperextensible skin, tendency to bleed (easy bruising), and hypermobile joints. 6+ types. Inheritance and severity vary. Can be autosomal dominant or recessive. May be associated with joint dislocation, berry and aortic aneurysms, organ rupture.	Hypermobility type (joint instability): most common type. Classical type (joint and skin symptoms): caused by a mutation in type V collagen. Vascular type (vascular and organ rupture): deficient type III collagen.
Menkes disease	Connective tissue disease caused by impaired copper absorption and transport. Leads to ↓ activity of lysyl oxidase (copper is a necessary cofactor). Results in brittle, "kinky" hair, growth retardation and hypotonia.	
Elastin	Stretchy protein within skin, lungs, large arteries, elastic ligaments, vocal cords, ligamenta flava (connect vertebrae → relaxed and stretched conformations). Rich in proline and glycine, nonhydroxylated forms. Tropoelastin with fibrillin scaffolding. Cross-linking takes place extracellularly and gives elastin its elastic properties. Broken down by elastase, which is normally inhibited by α_1-antitrypsin.	**Marfan syndrome**—caused by a defect in fibrillin, a glycoprotein that forms a sheath around elastin. **Emphysema**—can be caused by α_1-antitrypsin deficiency, resulting in excess elastase activity. Wrinkles of aging are due to ↓ collagen and elastin production.

▶ BIOCHEMISTRY–LABORATORY TECHNIQUES

Polymerase chain reaction	Molecular biology laboratory procedure used to amplify a desired fragment of DNA. Useful as a diagnostic tool (e.g., neonatal HIV, herpes encephalitis). Steps: 1. Denaturation—DNA is denatured by heating to generate 2 separate strands 2. Annealing—during cooling, excess premade DNA primers anneal to a specific sequence on each strand to be amplified. 3. Elongation—heat-stable DNA polymerase replicates the DNA sequence following each primer. These steps are repeated multiple times for DNA sequence amplification. Agarose gel electrophoresis—used for size separation of PCR products (smaller molecules travel further); compared against DNA ladder.

Blotting procedures

Southern blot	A DNA sample is enzymatically cleaved into smaller pieces, electrophoresed on a gel, and then transferred to a filter. The filter is then soaked in a denaturant and subsequently exposed to a radiolabeled DNA probe that recognizes and anneals to its complementary strand. The resulting double-stranded, labeled piece of DNA is visualized when the filter is exposed to film.	SNoW DRoP:
		  Southern = DNA
		  Northern = RNA
		  Western = Protein

Northern blot	Similar to Southern blot, except that an **RNA** sample is electrophoresed. Useful for studying mRNA levels, which are reflective of gene expression.	
Western blot	Sample protein is separated via gel electrophoresis and transferred to a filter. Labeled antibody is used to bind to relevant **protein.** Confirmatory test for HIV after ⊕ ELISA.	
Southwestern blot	Identifies **DNA-binding proteins** (e.g., transcription factors) using labeled oligonucleotide probes.	

Microarrays	Thousands of nucleic acid sequences are arranged in grids on glass or silicon. DNA or RNA probes are hybridized to the chip, and a scanner detects the relative amounts of complementary binding. Used to profile gene expression levels of thousands of genes simultaneously to study certain diseases and treatments. Able to detect single nucleotide polymorphisms (SNPs) and copy number variations (CNVs) for a variety of applications including genotyping, clinical genetic testing, forensic analysis, cancer mutations, and genetic linkage analysis.

Enzyme-linked immunosorbent assay	Used to detect the presence of either a specific antigen (direct) or a specific antibody (indirect) in a patient's blood sample. Patient's blood sample is probed with either: ▪ Indirect ELISA: uses a test **antigen** to see if a specific antibody is present in the patient's blood; a secondary antibody coupled to a color-generating enzyme is added to detect the first antibody. ▪ Direct ELISA: uses a test **antibody** to see if a specific antigen is present in the patient's blood; a secondary antibody coupled to a color-generating enzyme is added to detect the antigen. If the target substance is present in the sample, the test solution will have an intense color reaction, indicating a ⊕ test result.	Used in many laboratories to determine whether a particular antibody (e.g., anti-HIV) is present in a patient's blood sample. Both the sensitivity and specificity of ELISA approach 100%, but both false-positive and false-negative results occur.

Fluorescence in situ hybridization	Fluorescent DNA or RNA probe binds to specific gene site of interest on chromosomes. Used for specific localization of genes and direct visualization of anomalies (e.g., microdeletions) at molecular level (when deletion is too small to be visualized by karyotype). Fluorescence = gene is present; no fluorescence = gene has been deleted.

Cloning methods	Cloning is the production of a recombinant DNA molecule that is self perpetuating. Steps:
	1. Isolate eukaryotic mRNA (post-RNA processing steps) of interest.
	2. Expose mRNA to reverse transcriptase to produce cDNA (lacks introns).
	3. Insert cDNA fragments into bacterial plasmids containing antibiotic resistance genes.
	4. Transform recombinant plasmid into bacteria.
	5. Surviving bacteria on antibiotic medium produce cDNA.

Gene expression modifications	Transgenic strategies in mice involve: ▪ Random insertion of gene into mouse genome ▪ Targeted insertion or deletion of gene through homologous recombination with mouse gene	Knock-out = removing a gene, taking it **out**. Knock-**in** = inserting a gene.
Cre-lox system	Can inducibly manipulate genes at specific developmental points (e.g., to study a gene whose deletion causes embryonic death).	
RNA interference (RNAi)	dsRNA is synthesized that is complementary to the mRNA sequence of interest. When transfected into human cells, dsRNA separates and promotes degradation of target mRNA, "knocking down" gene expression.	

Karyotyping	A process in which metaphase chromosomes are stained, ordered, and numbered according to morphology, size, arm-length ratio, and banding pattern. Can be performed on a sample of blood, bone marrow, amniotic fluid, or placental tissue. Used to diagnose chromosomal imbalances (e.g., autosomal trisomies, sex chromosome disorders).

▶ BIOCHEMISTRY–GENETICS

Genetic terms

TERM	DEFINITION	EXAMPLE
Codominance	Both alleles contribute to the phenotype of the heterozygote.	Blood groups A, B, AB; α_1-antitrypsin deficiency.
Variable expressivity	Phenotype varies among individuals with same genotype.	2 patients with neurofibromatosis type 1 (NF1) may have varying disease severity.
Incomplete penetrance	Not all individuals with a mutant genotype show the mutant phenotype.	*BRCA1* gene mutations do not always result in breast or ovarian cancer.
Pleiotropy	One gene contributes to multiple phenotypic effects.	Untreated phenylketonuria (PKU) manifests with light skin, intellectual disability, and musty body odor.
Anticipation	Increased severity or earlier onset of disease in succeeding generations.	Trinucleotide repeat diseases (e.g., Huntington disease).
Loss of heterozygosity	If a patient inherits or develops a mutation in a tumor suppressor gene, the complementary allele must be deleted/mutated before cancer develops. This is not true of oncogenes.	Retinoblastoma and the "two-hit hypothesis."
Dominant negative mutation	Exerts a dominant effect. A heterozygote produces a nonfunctional altered protein that also prevents the normal gene product from functioning.	Mutation of a transcription factor in its allosteric site. Nonfunctioning mutant can still bind DNA, preventing wild-type transcription factor from binding.
Linkage disequilibrium	Tendency for certain alleles at 2 linked loci to occur together more often than expected by chance. Measured in a population, not in a family, and often varies in different populations.	
Mosaicism	Presence of genetically distinct cell lines in the same individual. Arises from mitotic errors after fertilization. Somatic mosaicism—mutation propagates through multiple tissues or organs. Gonadal mosaicism—mutation only in egg or sperm cells.	McCune-Albright syndrome is lethal if the mutation is somatic, but survivable if mosaic.
Locus heterogeneity	Mutations at different loci can produce a similar phenotype.	Albinism.
Allelic heterogeneity	Different mutations in the same locus produce the same phenotype.	β-thalassemia.
Heteroplasmy	Presence of both normal and mutated mtDNA, resulting in variable expression in mitochondrial inherited disease.	

Genetic terms *(continued)*

TERM	DEFINITION	EXAMPLE
Uniparental disomy	Offspring receives 2 copies of a chromosome from 1 parent and no copies from the other parent. Heterodisomy (heterozygous) indicates a meiosis I error. Isodisomy (homozygous) indicates a meiosis II error or postzygotic chromosomal duplication of one of a pair of chromosomes, and loss of the other of the original pair.	Uniparental is eUploid (correct number of chromosomes), not aneuploid. Most occurrences of UPD → normal phenotype. Consider UPD in an individual manifesting a recessive disorder when only one parent is a carrier.
Hardy-Weinberg population genetics	If a population is in Hardy-Weinberg equilibrium and if p and q are the frequencies of separate alleles, then: $p^2 + 2pq + q^2 = 1$ and $p + q = 1$, which implies that: p^2 = frequency of homozygosity for allele p q^2 = frequency of homozygosity for allele q $2pq$ = frequency of heterozygosity (carrier frequency, if an autosomal recessive disease). The frequency of an X-linked recessive disease in males = q and in females = q^2.	Hardy-Weinberg law assumptions include: ▪ No mutation occurring at the locus ▪ Natural selection is not occurring ▪ Completely random mating ▪ No net migration

		pA	qa
pA		AA $p \times p = p^2$	Aa $p \times q$
qa		Aa $p \times q$	aa $q \times q = q^2$

Genetic terms *(continued)*

TERM	DEFINITION	EXAMPLE
Imprinting	At some loci, only one allele is active; the other is inactive (imprinted/inactivated by methylation). With one allele inactivated, deletion of the active allele → disease.	Both Prader-Willi and Angelman syndromes are due to mutation or deletion of genes on chromosome 15. Can also occur as a result of uniparental disomy.
Prader-Willi syndrome	Maternal imprinting: gene from mom is normally silent and **P**aternal gene is deleted/mutated. Results in hyperphagia, obesity, intellectual disability, hypogonadism, and hypotonia.	25% of cases due to maternal uniparental disomy (two maternally imprinted genes are received; no paternal gene received).
AngelMan syndrome	Paternal imprinting: gene from dad is normally silent and **M**aternal gene is deleted/mutated. Results in inappropriate laughter ("happy puppet"), seizures, ataxia, and severe intellectual disability.	5% of cases due to paternal uniparental disomy (two paternally imprinted genes are received; no maternal gene received).

Modes of inheritance

Autosomal dominant 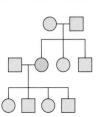	Often due to defects in structural genes. Many generations, both male and female, affected.	Often pleiotropic. Family history crucial to diagnosis.
Autosomal recessive 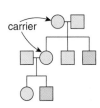	25% of offspring from 2 carrier parents are affected. Often due to enzyme deficiencies. Usually seen in only 1 generation.	Commonly more severe than dominant disorders; patients often present in childhood. ↑ risk in consanguineous families.
X-linked recessive 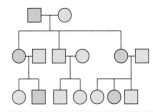	Sons of heterozygous mothers have a 50% chance of being affected. No male-to-male transmission.	Commonly more severe in males. Females usually must be homozygous to be affected.
X-linked dominant 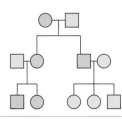	Transmitted through both parents. Mothers transmit to 50% of daughters and sons; fathers transmit to all daughters but no sons.	**Hypophosphatemic rickets**—formerly known as vitamin D–resistant rickets. Inherited disorder resulting in ↑ phosphate wasting at proximal tubule. Results in rickets-like presentation.
Mitochondrial inheritance	Transmitted only through the mother. All offspring of affected females may show signs of disease.	Variable expression in a population or even within a family due to heteroplasmy. **Mitochondrial myopathies**—rare disorders; often present with myopathy, lactic acidosis and CNS disease. 2° to failure in oxidative phosphorylation. Muscle biopsy often shows "ragged red fibers."

carrier

□ = unaffected male; ■ = affected male; ○ = unaffected female; ● = affected female.

Autosomal dominant diseases

Autosomal dominant polycystic kidney disease (ADPKD)	Formerly known as adult polycystic kidney disease. Always bilateral, massive enlargement of kidneys due to multiple large cysts. 85% of cases are due to mutation in *PKD1* (chromosome 16; 16 letters in "polycystic kidney"); remainder due to mutation in *PKD2* (chromosome 4).
Familial adenomatous polyposis	Colon becomes covered with adenomatous polyps after puberty. Progresses to colon cancer unless colon is resected. Mutations on chromosome 5 (*APC* gene); 5 letters in "polyp."
Familial hypercholesterolemia	Elevated LDL due to defective or absent LDL receptor. Leads to severe atherosclerotic disease early in life, and tendon xanthomas (classically in the Achilles tendon).
Hereditary hemorrhagic telangiectasia	Inherited disorder of blood vessels. Findings: telangiectasia, recurrent epistaxis, skin discolorations, arteriovenous malformations (AVMs), GI bleeding, hematuria. Also known as Osler-Weber-Rendu syndrome.
Hereditary spherocytosis	Spheroid erythrocytes due to spectrin or ankyrin defect; hemolytic anemia; ↑ MCHC. Treatment: splenectomy.
Huntington disease	Findings: depression, progressive dementia, choreiform movements, caudate atrophy, and ↓ levels of GABA and ACh in the brain. Gene on chromosome 4; trinucleotide repeat disorder: $(CAG)_n$. ↑ repeats → ↓ age of onset. "**Hunting 4** food."
Marfan syndrome	Fibrillin-1 gene mutation → connective tissue disorder affecting skeleton, heart, and eyes. Findings: tall with long extremities, pectus excavatum, hypermobile joints, and long, tapering fingers and toes (arachnodactyly); cystic medial necrosis of aorta → aortic incompetence and dissecting aortic aneurysms; floppy mitral valve. Subluxation of lenses, typically upward and temporally.
Multiple endocrine neoplasias (MEN)	Several distinct syndromes (1, 2A, 2B) characterized by familial tumors of endocrine glands, including those of the pancreas, parathyroid, pituitary, thyroid, and adrenal medulla. MEN 2A and 2B are associated with *ret* gene.
Neurofibromatosis type 1 (von Recklinghausen disease)	Neurocutaneous disorder characterized by café-au-lait spots and cutaneous neurofibromas. Autosomal dominant, 100% penetrance, variable expression. Caused by mutations in the *NF1* gene on chromosome 17; 17 letters in "von Recklinghausen."
Neurofibromatosis type 2	Findings: bilateral acoustic schwannomas, juvenile cataracts, meningiomas, and ependymomas. *NF2* gene on chromosome 22; type 2 = 22.
Tuberous sclerosis	Neurocutaneous disorder with multi-organ system involvement, characterized by numerous benign hamartomas. Incomplete penetrance, variable expression.
von Hippel-Lindau disease	Disorder characterized by development of numerous tumors, both benign and malignant. Associated with deletion of *VHL* gene (tumor suppressor) on chromosome 3 (3p). Von Hippel-Lindau = 3 words for chromosome 3.

Autosomal recessive diseases	Albinism, ARPKD (formerly known as infantile polycystic kidney disease), cystic fibrosis, glycogen storage diseases, hemochromatosis, Kartagener syndrome, mucopolysaccharidoses (except Hunter syndrome), phenylketonuria, sickle cell anemia, sphingolipidoses (except Fabry disease), thalassemias, Wilson disease.

Cystic fibrosis

GENETICS	Autosomal recessive; defect in *CFTR* gene on chromosome 7; commonly a deletion of Phe508. Most common lethal genetic disease in Caucasian population.
PATHOPHYSIOLOGY	*CFTR* encodes an ATP-gated Cl^- channel that secretes Cl^- in lungs and GI tract, and reabsorbs Cl^- in sweat glands. Mutations → misfolded protein → protein retained in RER and not transported to cell membrane, causing ↓ Cl^- (and H_2O) secretion; ↑ intracellular Cl^- results in compensatory ↑ Na^+ reabsorption via epithelial Na^+ channels → ↑ H_2O reabsorption → abnormally thick mucus secreted into lungs and GI tract. ↑ Na^+ reabsorption also causes more negative transepithelial potential difference.
DIAGNOSIS	↑ Cl^- concentration (>60 mEq/L) in sweat is diagnostic. Can present with contraction alkalosis and hypokalemia (ECF effects analogous to a patient taking a loop diuretic) because of ECF H_2O/Na^+ losses and concomitant renal K^+/H^+ wasting.
COMPLICATIONS	Recurrent pulmonary infections (e.g., *Pseudomonas*), chronic bronchitis and bronchiectasis → reticulonodular pattern on CXR, pancreatic insufficiency, malabsorption and steatorrhea, nasal polyps, and meconium ileus in newborns. Infertility in males (absence of vas deferens, absent sperm). Fat-soluble vitamin deficiencies (A, D, E, K).
TREATMENT	N-acetylcysteine to loosen mucus plugs (cleaves disulfide bonds within mucus glycoproteins), dornase alfa (DNAse) to clear leukocytic debris.

X-linked recessive disorders	Bruton agammaglobulinemia, Wiskott-Aldrich syndrome, Fabry disease, G6PD deficiency, Ocular albinism, Lesch-Nyhan syndrome, Duchenne (and Becker) muscular dystrophy, Hunter Syndrome, Hemophilia A and B, Ornithine transcarbamylase deficiency. Female carriers can be variably affected depending on the percentage inactivation of the X chromosome carrying the mutant vs. normal gene.	Be Wise, Fool's GOLD Heeds Silly HOpe.

Muscular dystrophies

Duchenne	X-linked **frameshift** mutation → truncated dystrophin protein → accelerated muscle breakdown. Weakness begins in pelvic girdle muscles and progresses superiorly. Pseudohypertrophy of calf muscles due to fibrofatty replacement of muscle [A]. Gower maneuver—patients use upper extremity to help them stand up. Onset before 5 years of age. Dilated cardiomyopathy is common cause of death.	Duchenne = deleted dystrophin. Dystrophin gene (*DMD*) has the longest coding region of any human gene → ↑ chance of spontaneous mutation. Dystrophin helps anchor muscle fibers, primarily in skeletal and cardiac muscle. It connects the intracellular cytoskeleton (actin) to the transmembrane proteins α- and β-dystroglycan, which are connected to the extracellular matrix (ECM). Loss of dystrophin results in myonecrosis. ↑ CPK and aldolase are seen; Western blot and muscle biopsy confirm diagnosis.
Becker	Usually, X-linked **point** mutation in dystrophin gene (no frameshift). Less severe than Duchenne. Onset in adolescence or early adulthood.	Deletions can cause both Duchenne and Becker.
Myotonic type 1	CTG trinucleotide repeat expansion in the *DMPK* gene → abnormal expression of myotonin protein kinase → myotonia, muscle wasting, frontal balding, cataracts, testicular atrophy, and arrhythmia.	

Muscle fiber

Fragile X syndrome	X-linked defect affecting the methylation and expression of the *FMR1* gene. The 2nd most common cause of genetic intellectual disability (after Down syndrome). Findings: post-pubertal macroorchidism (enlarged testes), long face with a large jaw, large everted ears, autism, mitral valve prolapse.	Trinucleotide repeat disorder $(CGG)_n$. Fragile **X** = e**X**tra large testes, jaw, ears.
Trinucleotide repeat expansion diseases	Huntington disease, myotonic dystrophy, Friedreich ataxia, fragile **X** syndrome. Fragile **X** syndrome = $(CGG)_n$. Friedreich ataxia = $(GAA)_n$. Huntington disease = $(CAG)_n$. Myotonic dystrophy = $(CTG)_n$.	Try (trinucleotide) **hunting** for my fried eggs (X). **X**-Girlfriend's **F**irst **A**id **H**elped **A**ce **M**y **T**est. May show genetic anticipation (disease severity ↑ and age of onset ↓ in successive generations).

Autosomal trisomies

Down syndrome (trisomy 21), 1:700	Findings: intellectual disability, flat facies, prominent epicanthal folds, single palmar crease, gap between 1st 2 toes, duodenal atresia, Hirschsprung disease, congenital heart disease (most commonly ostium primum-type atrial septal defect [ASD]), Brushfield spots. Associated with ↑ risk of ALL, AML, and Alzheimer disease (> 35 years old). 95% of cases due to meiotic nondisjunction of homologous chromosomes (associated with advanced maternal age; from 1:1500 in women < 20 to 1:25 in women > 45 years old). 4% of cases due to Robertsonian translocation. 1% of cases due to mosaicism (no maternal association; post-fertilization mitotic error).	Drinking age (21). Most common viable chromosomal disorder and most common cause of genetic intellectual disability. First-trimester ultrasound commonly shows: ↑ nuchal translucency and hypoplastic nasal bone; serum PAPP-A is ↓, free β-hCG is ↑. Second-trimester quad screen shows: ↓ α-fetoprotein, ↑ β-hCG, ↓ estriol, ↑ inhibin A.
Edwards syndrome (trisomy 18), 1:8000	Findings: severe intellectual disability, rocker-bottom feet, micrognathia (small jaw), low-set Ears, clenched hands, prominent occiput, congenital heart disease. Death usually occurs within 1 year of birth.	Election age (18). Most common trisomy resulting in live birth after Down syndrome. PAPP-A and free β-hCG are ↓ in first trimester. Quad screen shows: ↓ α-fetoprotein, ↓ β-hCG, ↓ estriol, ↓ or normal inhibin A.
Patau syndrome (trisomy 13), 1:15,000	Findings: severe intellectual disability, rocker-bottom feet, microphthalmia, microcephaly, cleft liP/Palate, holoProsencephaly, Polydactyly, congenital heart disease. Death usually occurs within 1 year of birth.	Puberty (13). First-trimester pregnancy screen shows: ↓ free β-hCG, ↓ PAPP-A, and ↑ nuchal translucency.

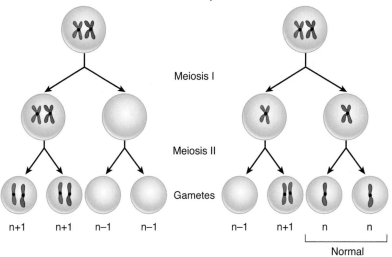

Meiotic nondisjunction

Meiosis I

Meiosis II

Gametes

n+1   n+1   n–1   n–1   n–1   n+1   n   n

Normal

Nondisjunction in meiosis I   Nondisjunction in meiosis II

Robertsonian translocation	Nonreciprocal chromosomal translocation that commonly involves chromosome pairs 13, 14, 15, 21, and 22. One of the most common types of translocation. Occurs when the long arms of 2 acrocentric chromosomes (chromosomes with centromeres near their ends) fuse at the centromere and the 2 short arms are lost. Balanced translocations normally do not cause any abnormal phenotype. Unbalanced translocations can result in miscarriage, stillbirth, and chromosomal imbalance (e.g., Down syndrome, Patau syndrome).	
Cri-du-chat syndrome	Congenital microdeletion of short arm of chromosome 5 (46,XX or XY, 5p–). Findings: microcephaly, moderate to severe intellectual disability, high-pitched crying/mewing, epicanthal folds, cardiac abnormalities (VSD).	*Cri du chat* = cry of the cat.
Williams syndrome	Congenital microdeletion of long arm of chromosome 7 (deleted region includes elastin gene). Findings: distinctive "elfin" facies, intellectual disability, hypercalcemia (↑ sensitivity to vitamin D), well-developed verbal skills, extreme friendliness with strangers, cardiovascular problems.	
22q11 deletion syndromes	Variable presentation, including Cleft palate, Abnormal facies, Thymic aplasia → T-cell deficiency, Cardiac defects, Hypocalcemia 2° to parathyroid aplasia, due to microdeletion at chromosome 22q11. DiGeorge syndrome—thymic, parathyroid, and cardiac defects. Velocardiofacial syndrome—palate, facial, and cardiac defects.	CATCH-22. Due to aberrant development of 3rd and 4th branchial pouches.

▶ BIOCHEMISTRY–NUTRITION

Vitamins: fat soluble	A, D, E, K. Absorption dependent on gut and pancreas. Toxicity more common than for water-soluble vitamins because fat-soluble vitamins accumulate in fat.	Malabsorption syndromes (steatorrhea), such as cystic fibrosis and sprue, or mineral oil intake can cause fat-soluble vitamin deficiencies.
Vitamins: water soluble	B_1 (thiamine: TPP) B_2 (riboflavin: FAD, FMN) B_3 (niacin: NAD^+) B_5 (pantothenic acid: CoA) B_6 (pyridoxine: PLP) B_7 (biotin) B_9 (folate) B_{12} (cobalamin) C (ascorbic acid)	All wash out easily from body except B_{12} and folate (stored in liver). B-complex deficiencies often result in dermatitis, glossitis, and diarrhea.

Vitamin A (retinol)

FUNCTION	Antioxidant; constituent of visual pigments (retinal); essential for normal differentiation of epithelial cells into specialized tissue (pancreatic cells, mucus-secreting cells); prevents squamous metaplasia. Used to treat measles and AML, subtype M3.	Retinol is vitamin A, so think **retin-A** (used topically for wrinkles and acne). Found in liver and leafy vegetables.
DEFICIENCY	Night blindness (nyctalopia); dry, scaly skin (xerosis cutis); alopecia; corneal degeneration (keratomalacia); immune suppression.	
EXCESS	Arthralgias, skin changes (e.g., scaliness), alopecia, cerebral edema, pseudotumor cerebri, osteoporosis, hepatic abnormalities. Teratogenic (cleft palate, cardiac abnormalities), so a ⊖ pregnancy test and reliable contraception are needed before isotretinoin is prescribed for severe acne.	

Vitamin B₁ (thiamine)

FUNCTION	In thiamine pyrophosphate (TPP), a cofactor for several dehydrogenase enzyme reactions: ▪ Pyruvate dehydrogenase (links glycolysis to TCA cycle) ▪ α-ketoglutarate dehydrogenase (TCA cycle) ▪ Transketolase (HMP shunt) ▪ Branched-chain ketoacid dehydrogenase	Think **ATP**: α-ketoglutarate dehydrogenase, Transketolase, and Pyruvate dehydrogenase. Spell beriberi as **Ber1Ber1** to remember vitamin B₁. **Wernicke-Korsakoff syndrome**—confusion, ophthalmoplegia, ataxia (classic triad) + confabulation, personality change, memory loss (permanent). Damage to medial dorsal nucleus of thalamus, mammillary bodies. **Dry beriberi**—polyneuritis, symmetrical muscle wasting. **Wet beriberi**—high-output cardiac failure (dilated cardiomyopathy), edema.
DEFICIENCY	Impaired glucose breakdown → ATP depletion worsened by glucose infusion; highly aerobic tissues (e.g., brain, heart) are affected first. Wernicke-Korsakoff syndrome and beriberi. Seen in malnutrition and alcoholism (2° to malnutrition and malabsorption). Diagnosis made by ↑ in RBC transketolase activity following vitamin B₁ administration.	

Vitamin B₂ (riboflavin)

FUNCTION	Component of flavins FAD and FMN, used as cofactors in redox reactions, e.g., the succinate dehydrogenase reaction in the TCA cycle.	FAD and FMN are derived from riboFlavin ($B_2 = 2$ ATP).
DEFICIENCY	Cheilosis (inflammation of lips, scaling and fissures at the corners of the mouth), Corneal vascularization.	The 2 C's of B_2.

Vitamin B_3 (niacin)

FUNCTION	Constituent of NAD^+, $NADP^+$ (used in redox reactions). Derived from tryptophan. Synthesis requires vitamins B_2 and B_6. Used to treat dyslipidemia; lowers levels of VLDL and raises levels of HDL.	NAD derived from Niacin (B_3 = 3 ATP).
DEFICIENCY	Glossitis. Severe deficiency leads to pellagra, which can be caused by Hartnup disease (↓ tryptophan absorption), malignant carcinoid syndrome (↑ tryptophan metabolism), and isoniazid (↓ vitamin B_6). Symptoms of pellagra: **D**iarrhea, **D**ementia (also hallucinations), **D**ermatitis (e.g., Casal necklace or hyperpigmentation of sun-exposed limbs).	The 3 D's of B_3
EXCESS	Facial flushing (induced by prostaglandin, not histamine), hyperglycemia, hyperuricemia.	

Vitamin B_5 (pantothenate)

FUNCTION	Essential component of coenzyme A (CoA, a cofactor for acyl transfers) and fatty acid synthase.	B_5 is "**pento**"thenate.
DEFICIENCY	Dermatitis, enteritis, alopecia, adrenal insufficiency.	

Vitamin B_6 (pyridoxine)

FUNCTION	Converted to pyridoxal phosphate, a cofactor used in transamination (e.g., ALT and AST), decarboxylation reactions, glycogen phosphorylase. Synthesis of cystathionine, heme, niacin, histamine, and neurotransmitters including serotonin, epinephrine, norepinephrine, dopamine, and GABA.
DEFICIENCY	Convulsions, hyperirritability, peripheral neuropathy (deficiency inducible by isoniazid and oral contraceptives), sideroblastic anemias due to impaired hemoglobin synthesis and iron excess.

Vitamin B_7 (biotin)

FUNCTION	Cofactor for carboxylation enzymes (which add a 1-carbon group): • Pyruvate carboxylase: pyruvate (3C) → oxaloacetate (4C) • Acetyl-CoA carboxylase: acetyl-CoA (2C) → malonyl-CoA (3C) • Propionyl-CoA carboxylase: propionyl-CoA (3C) → methylmalonyl-CoA (4C)	"**Avid**in in egg whites **avid**ly binds biotin."
DEFICIENCY	Relatively rare. Dermatitis, alopecia, enteritis. Caused by antibiotic use or excessive ingestion of raw egg whites.	

Vitamin B$_9$ (folic acid)

FUNCTION	Converted to tetrahydrofolate (THF), a coenzyme for 1-carbon transfer/methylation reactions. Important for the synthesis of nitrogenous bases in DNA and RNA.	Found in leafy green vegetables. Absorbed in jejunum. **Fol**ate from **fol**iage. Small reserve pool stored primarily in the liver.
DEFICIENCY	Macrocytic, megaloblastic anemia; hypersegmented polymorphonuclear cells (PMNs); glossitis; no neurologic symptoms (as opposed to vitamin B$_{12}$ deficiency). Labs: ↑ homocysteine, normal methylmalonic acid. Most common vitamin deficiency in the United States. Seen in alcoholism and pregnancy.	Deficiency can be caused by several drugs (e.g., phenytoin, sulfonamides, methotrexate). Supplemental maternal folic acid in early pregnancy decreases risk of neural tube defects.

Vitamin B$_{12}$ (cobalamin)

FUNCTION	Cofactor for homocysteine methyltransferase (transfers CH$_3$ groups as methylcobalamin) and methylmalonyl-CoA mutase.	Found in animal products. Synthesized only by microorganisms. Very large reserve pool (several years) stored primarily in the liver. Deficiency is usually caused by insufficient intake (e.g., veganism), malabsorption (e.g., sprue, enteritis, *Diphyllobothrium latum*), lack of intrinsic factor (pernicious anemia, gastric bypass surgery), or absence of terminal ileum (Crohn disease). Anti-intrinsic factor antibodies diagnostic for pernicious anemia.
DEFICIENCY	Macrocytic, megaloblastic anemia; hypersegmented PMNs; paresthesias, and subacute combined degeneration (degeneration of dorsal columns, lateral corticospinal tracts, and spinocerebellar tracts) due to abnormal myelin. Associated with ↑ serum homocysteine and methylmalonic acid levels. Prolonged deficiency → irreversible nerve damage.	

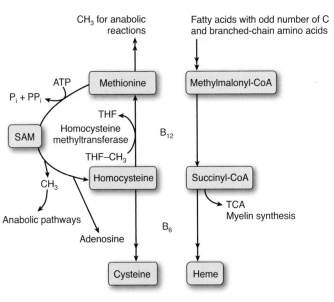

Vitamin C (ascorbic acid)

FUNCTION	Antioxidant. Also facilitates iron absorption by reducing it to Fe^{2+} state. Necessary for hydroxylation of proline and lysine in collagen synthesis. Necessary for dopamine β-hydroxylase, which converts dopamine to NE.	Found in fruits and vegetables. Pronounce "absorbic" acid. Ancillary treatment for methemoglobinemia by reducing Fe^{3+} to Fe^{2+}.
DEFICIENCY	**Scurvy**—swollen gums, bruising, hemarthrosis, anemia, poor wound healing, perifollicular and subperiosteal hemorrhages, "corkscrew" hair. Weakened immune response.	Vitamin C deficiency causes sCurvy due to a Collagen synthesis defect.
EXCESS	Nausea, vomiting, diarrhea, fatigue, calcium oxalate nephrolithiasis. Can ↑ risk of iron toxicity in predisposed individuals (e.g., those with transfusions, hereditary hemochromatosis).	

Vitamin D

Vitamin D	D_2 = ergocalciferol—ingested from plants. D_3 = cholecalciferol—consumed in milk, formed in sun-exposed skin (stratum basale). 25-OH D_3 = storage form. 1,25-$(OH)_2$ D_3 (calcitriol) = active form.	Drinking milk (fortified with vitamin D) is good for bones.
FUNCTION	↑ intestinal absorption of calcium and phosphate, ↑ bone mineralization.	
DEFICIENCY	Rickets in children (bone pain and deformity), osteomalacia in adults (bone pain and muscle weakness), hypocalcemic tetany. Breastfed infants should receive oral vitamin D. Deficiency is exacerbated by low sun exposure, pigmented skin, prematurity.	
EXCESS	Hypercalcemia, hypercalciuria, loss of appetite, stupor. Seen in sarcoidosis (↑ activation of vitamin D by epithelioid macrophages).	

A **Rickets.** X-ray of legs in toddler shows bowing of femurs (genu varum). ✴

Vitamin E (tocopherol/tocotrienol)

FUNCTION	Antioxidant (protects erythrocytes and membranes from free radical damage).	E is for Erythrocytes. Can enhance anticoagulant effects of warfarin.
DEFICIENCY	Hemolytic anemia, acanthocytosis, muscle weakness, posterior column and spinocerebellar tract demyelination.	Neurological presentation may appear similar to vitamin B_{12} deficiency, but without megaloblastic anemia, hypersegmented neutrophils, or ↑ serum methylmalonic acid levels.

Vitamin K

FUNCTION	Cofactor for the γ-carboxylation of glutamic acid residues on various proteins required for blood clotting. Synthesized by intestinal flora.	K is for Koagulation. Necessary for the activation of clotting factors II, VII, IX, X, and proteins C and S. Warfarin—vitamin K antagonist.
DEFICIENCY	Neonatal hemorrhage with ↑ PT and ↑ aPTT but normal bleeding time (neonates have sterile intestines and are unable to synthesize vitamin K). Can also occur after prolonged use of broad-spectrum antibiotics.	Not in breast milk; neonates are given vitamin K injection at birth to prevent bleeding diathesis.

Zinc

FUNCTION	Essential for the activity of 100+ enzymes. Important in the formation of zinc fingers (transcription factor motif).
DEFICIENCY	Delayed wound healing, hypogonadism, ↓ adult hair (axillary, facial, pubic), dysgeusia, anosmia, acrodermatitis enteropathica. May predispose to alcoholic cirrhosis.

Ethanol metabolism

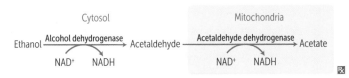

NAD⁺ is the limiting reagent.
Alcohol dehydrogenase operates via zero-order kinetics.

Ethanol metabolism ↑ NADH/NAD⁺ ratio in liver, causing:
- Pyruvate → lactate (lactic acidosis).
- Oxaloacetate → malate (prevents gluconeogenesis → fasting hypoglycemia)
- Glyceraldehyde-3-phosphate → glycerol-3-phosphate (combines with fatty acids to make triglycerides → hepatosteatosis)

End result is clinical picture seen in chronic alcoholism.
Additionally, ↑ NADH/NAD⁺ ratio disfavors TCA production of NADH → ↑ utilization of acetyl-CoA for ketogenesis (→ ketoacidosis) and lipogenesis (→ hepatosteatosis).

Fomepizole—inhibits alcohol dehydrogenase and is an antidote for methanol or ethylene glycol poisoning.
Disulfiram—inhibits acetaldehyde dehydrogenase (acetaldehyde accumulates, contributing to hangover symptoms).

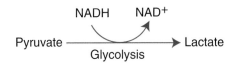

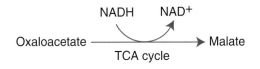

Malnutrition

Kwashiorkor	Protein malnutrition resulting in skin lesions, edema, liver malfunction (fatty change due to ↓ apolipoprotein synthesis). Clinical picture is small child with swollen belly 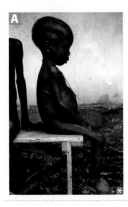.	Kwashiorkor results from a protein-deficient **MEAL**: **M**alnutrition **E**dema **A**nemia **L**iver (fatty)
Marasmus	Total calorie malnutrition resulting in tissue and muscle wasting, loss of subcutaneous fat, and variable edema.	Marasmus results in **M**uscle wasting.

▶ BIOCHEMISTRY–METABOLISM

Metabolism sites

Mitochondria	Fatty acid oxidation (β-oxidation), acetyl-CoA production, TCA cycle, oxidative phosphorylation.
Cytoplasm	Glycolysis, fatty acid synthesis, HMP shunt, protein synthesis (RER), steroid synthesis (SER), cholesterol synthesis.
Both	Heme synthesis, Urea cycle, Gluconeogenesis. **HUGs take two** (i.e., both).

Enzyme terminology	An enzyme's name often describes its function. For example, glucokinase is an enzyme that catalyzes the phosphorylation of glucose using a molecule of ATP. The following are commonly used enzyme descriptors.
Kinase	Uses ATP to add high-energy phosphate group onto substrate (e.g., phosphofructokinase).
Phosphorylase	Adds inorganic phosphate onto substrate without using ATP (e.g., glycogen phosphorylase).
Phosphatase	Removes phosphate group from substrate (e.g., fructose-1,6-bisphosphatase).
Dehydrogenase	Catalyzes oxidation-reduction reactions (e.g., pyruvate dehydrogenase).
Hydroxylase	Adds hydroxyl group (–OH) onto substrate (e.g., tyrosine hydroxylase).
Carboxylase	Transfers CO_2 groups with the help of biotin (e.g., pyruvate carboxylase).
Mutase	Relocates a functional group within a molecule (e.g., vitamin B_{12}–dependent methylmalonyl-CoA mutase).

Rate-determining enzymes of metabolic processes

PROCESS	ENZYME	REGULATORS
Glycolysis	Phosphofructokinase-1 (PFK-1)	AMP $\oplus$, fructose-2,6-bisphosphate $\oplus$ ATP $\ominus$, citrate $\ominus$
Gluconeogenesis	Fructose-1,6-bisphosphatase	ATP $\oplus$, acetyl-CoA $\oplus$ AMP $\ominus$, fructose-2,6-bisphosphate $\ominus$
TCA cycle	Isocitrate dehydrogenase	ADP $\oplus$ ATP $\ominus$, NADH $\ominus$
Glycogenesis	Glycogen synthase	Glucose-6-phosphate $\oplus$, insulin $\oplus$, cortisol $\oplus$ Epinephrine $\ominus$, glucagon $\ominus$
Glycogenolysis	Glycogen phosphorylase	Epinephrine $\oplus$, glucagon $\oplus$, AMP $\oplus$ Glucose-6-phosphate $\ominus$, insulin $\ominus$, ATP $\ominus$
HMP shunt	Glucose-6-phosphate dehydrogenase (G6PD)	NADP$^+$ $\oplus$ NADPH $\ominus$
De novo pyrimidine synthesis	Carbamoyl phosphate synthetase II	
De novo purine synthesis	Glutamine-phosphoribosylpyrophosphate (PRPP) amidotransferase	AMP $\ominus$, inosine monophosphate (IMP) $\ominus$, GMP $\ominus$
Urea cycle	Carbamoyl phosphate synthetase I	N-acetylglutamate $\oplus$
Fatty acid synthesis	Acetyl-CoA carboxylase (ACC)	Insulin $\oplus$, citrate $\oplus$ Glucagon $\ominus$, palmitoyl-CoA $\ominus$
Fatty acid oxidation	Carnitine acyltransferase I	Malonyl-CoA $\ominus$
Ketogenesis	HMG-CoA synthase	
Cholesterol synthesis	HMG-CoA reductase	Insulin $\oplus$, thyroxine $\oplus$ Glucagon $\ominus$, cholesterol $\ominus$

Summary of pathways

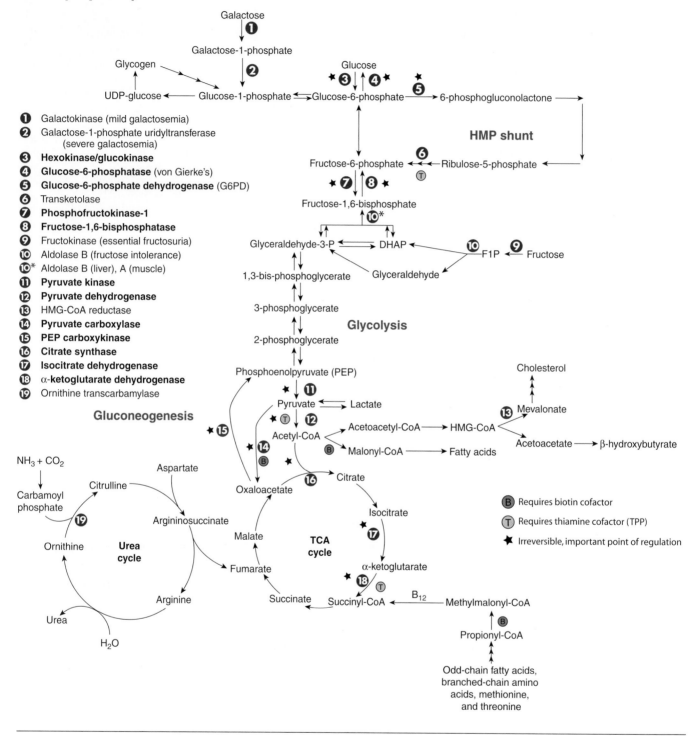

❶ Galactokinase (mild galactosemia)
❷ Galactose-1-phosphate uridyltransferase
      (severe galactosemia)
❸ **Hexokinase/glucokinase**
❹ **Glucose-6-phosphatase** (von Gierke's)
❺ **Glucose-6-phosphate dehydrogenase** (G6PD)
❻ Transketolase
❼ **Phosphofructokinase-1**
❽ **Fructose-1,6-bisphosphatase**
❾ Fructokinase (essential fructosuria)
❿ Aldolase B (fructose intolerance)
❿* Aldolase B (liver), A (muscle)
⓫ **Pyruvate kinase**
⓬ **Pyruvate dehydrogenase**
⓭ HMG-CoA reductase
⓮ **Pyruvate carboxylase**
⓯ **PEP carboxykinase**
⓰ **Citrate synthase**
⓱ **Isocitrate dehydrogenase**
⓲ **α-ketoglutarate dehydrogenase**
⓳ Ornithine transcarbamylase

Ⓑ Requires biotin cofactor
Ⓣ Requires thiamine cofactor (TPP)
★ Irreversible, important point of regulation

ATP production	Aerobic metabolism of glucose produces 32 net ATP via malate-aspartate shuttle (heart and liver), 30 net ATP via glycerol-3-phosphate shuttle (muscle). Anaerobic glycolysis produces only 2 net ATP per glucose molecule. ATP hydrolysis can be coupled to energetically unfavorable reactions.	Arsenic causes glycolysis to produce zero net ATP.

Activated carriers

CARRIER MOLECULE	CARRIED IN ACTIVATED FORM
ATP	Phosphoryl groups
NADH, NADPH, $FADH_2$	Electrons
CoA, lipoamide	Acyl groups
Biotin	CO_2
Tetrahydrofolates	1-carbon units
SAM	CH_3 groups
TPP	Aldehydes

Universal electron acceptors	Nicotinamides (NAD^+ from vitamin B_3, $NADP^+$) and flavin nucleotides (FAD^+ from vitamin B_2). NAD^+ is generally used in **catabolic** processes to carry reducing equivalents away as NADH. NADPH is used in **anabolic** processes (steroid and fatty acid synthesis) as a supply of reducing equivalents.	NADPH is a product of the HMP shunt. NADPH is used in: ▪ Anabolic processes ▪ Respiratory burst ▪ Cytochrome P-450 system ▪ Glutathione reductase

Hexokinase vs. glucokinase

Phosphorylation of glucose to yield glucose-6-P serves as the 1st step of glycolysis (also serves as the 1st step of glycogen synthesis in the liver). Reaction is catalyzed by either hexokinase or glucokinase, depending on the tissue. At low glucose concentrations, hexokinase sequesters glucose in the tissue. At high glucose concentrations, excess glucose is stored in the liver.

	Hexokinase	Glucokinase
Location	Most tissues, but not liver nor β cells of pancreas	Liver, β cells of pancreas
K_m	Lower (↑ affinity)	Higher (↓ affinity)
V_{max}	Lower (↓ capacity)	Higher (↑ capacity)
Induced by insulin	No	Yes
Feedback-inhibited by glucose-6-P	Yes	No
Gene mutation associated with maturity-onset diabetes of the young (MODY)	No	Yes

Glycolysis regulation, key enzymes	Net glycolysis (cytoplasm): Glucose + 2 P_i + 2 ADP + 2 NAD^+ → 2 pyruvate + 2 ATP + 2 NADH + 2 H^+ + 2 H_2O. Equation not balanced chemically, and exact balanced equation depends on ionization state of reactants and products.

REQUIRE ATP	Glucose ──────────→ Glucose-6-phosphate Hexokinase/glucokinase[a] Fructose-6-P ──────────→ Fructose-1,6-BP Phosphofructokinase-1 (rate-limiting step) [a]Glucokinase in liver and β cells of pancreas; hexokinase in all other tissues.	Glucose-6-P ⊖ hexokinase. Fructose-6-P ⊖ glucokinase. ATP ⊖, AMP ⊕, citrate ⊖, fructose-2,6-BP ⊕.
PRODUCE ATP	1,3-BPG ⇄──────── 3-PG Phosphoglycerate kinase Phosphoenolpyruvate ──────────→ Pyruvate Pyruvate kinase	ATP ⊖, alanine ⊖, fructose-1,6-BP ⊕.

Regulation by F2,6BP	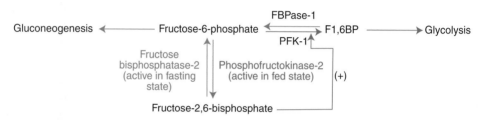

FBPase-2 and PFK-2 are the same bifunctional enzyme whose function is reversed by phosphorylation by protein kinase A.

Fasting state: ↑ glucagon → ↑ cAMP → ↑ protein kinase A → ↑ FBPase-2, ↓ PFK-2, less glycolysis, more gluconeogenesis.

Fed state: ↑ insulin → ↓ cAMP → ↓ protein kinase A → ↓ FBPase-2, ↑ PFK-2, more glycolysis, less gluconeogenesis.

Pyruvate dehydrogenase complex	Mitochondrial enzyme complex linking glycolysis and TCA cycle. Differentially regulated in fed/fasting states (active in fed state). Reaction: pyruvate + NAD^+ + CoA → acetyl-CoA + CO_2 + NADH. The complex contains 3 enzymes that require 5 cofactors: 　1. Pyrophosphate (B_1, thiamine; TPP) 　2. FAD (B_2, riboflavin) 　3. NAD (B_3, niacin) 　4. CoA (B_5, pantothenate) 　5. Lipoic acid Activated by exercise, which: 　↑ NAD^+/NADH ratio 　↑ ADP 　↑ Ca^{2+}	The complex is similar to the α-ketoglutarate dehydrogenase complex (same cofactors, similar substrate and action), which converts α-ketoglutarate → succinyl-CoA (TCA cycle). Arsenic inhibits lipoic acid. Findings: vomiting, rice-water stools, garlic breath.

Pyruvate dehydrogenase complex deficiency	Causes a buildup of pyruvate that gets shunted to lactate (via LDH) and alanine (via ALT).	Lysine and Leucine—the onLy pureLy ketogenic amino acids.
FINDINGS	Neurologic defects, lactic acidosis, ↑ serum alanine starting in infancy.	
TREATMENT	↑ intake of ketogenic nutrients (e.g., high fat content or ↑ lysine and leucine).	

Pyruvate metabolism

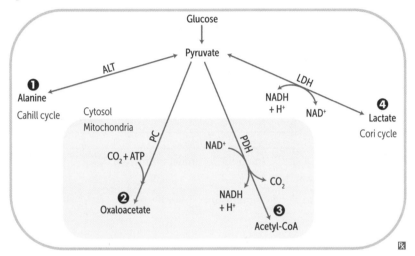

Functions of different pyruvate metabolic pathways (and their associated cofactors):

❶ Alanine aminotransferase (B_6): alanine carries amino groups to the liver from muscle

❷ Pyruvate carboxylase (biotin): oxaloacetate can replenish TCA cycle or be used in gluconeogenesis

❸ Pyruvate dehydrogenase (B_1, B_2, B_3, B_5, lipoic acid): transition from glycolysis to the TCA cycle

❹ Lactic acid dehydrogenase (B_3): end of anaerobic glycolysis (major pathway in RBCs, leukocytes, kidney medulla, lens, testes, and cornea)

TCA cycle (Krebs cycle)

Pyruvate → acetyl-CoA produces 1 NADH, 1 CO_2.

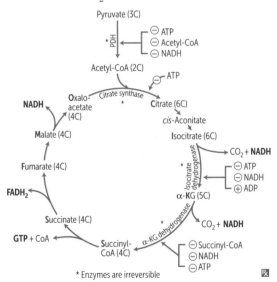

The TCA cycle produces 3 NADH, 1 $FADH_2$, 2 CO_2, 1 GTP per acetyl-CoA = 10 ATP/ acetyl-CoA (2× everything per glucose). TCA cycle reactions occur in the mitochondria.

α-ketoglutarate dehydrogenase complex requires the same cofactors as the pyruvate dehydrogenase complex (B_1, B_2, B_3, B_5, lipoic acid).

Citrate Is Krebs' Starting Substrate For Making Oxaloacetate.

Electron transport chain and oxidative phosphorylation

NADH electrons from glycolysis enter mitochondria via the malate-aspartate or glycerol-3-phosphate shuttle. FADH$_2$ electrons are transferred to complex II (at a lower energy level than NADH). The passage of electrons results in the formation of a proton gradient that, coupled to oxidative phosphorylation, drives the production of ATP.

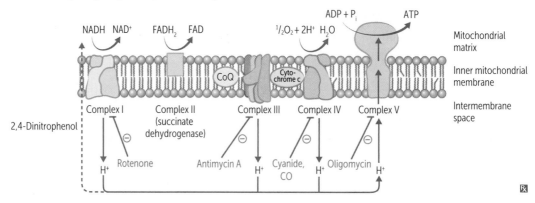

ATP PRODUCED VIA ATP SYNTHASE		
	1 NADH → 2.5 ATP; 1 FADH$_2$ → 1.5 ATP.	

OXIDATIVE PHOSPHORYLATION POISONS		
Electron transport inhibitors	Directly inhibit electron transport, causing a ↓ proton gradient and block of ATP synthesis.	Rotenone, cyanide, antimycin A, CO.
ATP synthase inhibitors	Directly inhibit mitochondrial ATP synthase, causing an ↑ proton gradient. No ATP is produced because electron transport stops.	Oligomycin.
Uncoupling agents	↑ permeability of membrane, causing a ↓ proton gradient and ↑ O$_2$ consumption. ATP synthesis stops, but electron transport continues. Produces heat.	2,4-Dinitrophenol (used illicitly for weight loss), aspirin (fevers often occur after aspirin overdose), thermogenin in brown fat.

Gluconeogenesis, irreversible enzymes

Pathway **P**roduces **F**resh **G**lucose.

Pyruvate carboxylase	In mitochondria. Pyruvate → oxaloacetate.	Requires biotin, ATP. Activated by acetyl-CoA.
Phosphoenolpyruvate carboxykinase	In cytosol. Oxaloacetate → phosphoenolpyruvate.	Requires GTP.
Fructose-1,6-bisphosphatase	In cytosol. Fructose-1,6-BP → fructose-6-P.	Citrate ⊕, fructose 2,6-bisphosphate ⊖.
Glucose-6-phosphatase	In ER. Glucose-6-P → glucose.	

Occurs primarily in liver; serves to maintain euglycemia during fasting. Enzymes also found in kidney, intestinal epithelium. Deficiency of the key gluconeogenic enzymes causes hypoglycemia. (Muscle cannot participate in gluconeogenesis because it lacks glucose-6-phosphatase).

Odd-chain fatty acids yield 1 propionyl-CoA during metabolism, which can enter the TCA cycle (as succinyl-CoA), undergo gluconeogenesis, and serve as a glucose source. Even-chain fatty acids cannot produce new glucose, since they yield only acetyl-CoA equivalents.

HMP shunt (pentose phosphate pathway)

Provides a source of NADPH from abundantly available glucose-6-P (NADPH is required for reductive reactions, e.g., glutathione reduction inside RBCs, fatty acid and cholesterol biosynthesis). Additionally, this pathway yields ribose for nucleotide synthesis and glycolytic intermediates. 2 distinct phases (oxidative and nonoxidative), both of which occur in the cytoplasm. No ATP is used or produced.

Sites: lactating mammary glands, liver, adrenal cortex (sites of fatty acid or steroid synthesis), RBCs.

REACTIONS	KEY ENZYMES	PRODUCTS
Oxidative (irreversible)	Glucose-6-P$_i$ → **Glucose-6-P dehydrogenase** (NADP⁺ → NADPH) Rate-limiting step	CO_2 2 NADPH Ribulose-5-P$_i$
Nonoxidative (reversible)	Ribulose-5-P$_i$ ← **Phosphopentose isomerase, transketolases** (Requires B$_1$)	Ribose-5-P$_i$ G3P F6P

Respiratory burst (oxidative burst)

Involves the activation of the phagocyte NADPH oxidase complex (e.g., in neutrophils, monocytes), which utilizes O_2 as a substrate. Plays an important role in the immune response → rapid release of reactive oxygen species (ROS). Note that NADPH plays a role in both the creation and neutralization of ROS. Myeloperoxidase is a blue-green heme-containing pigment that gives sputum its color.

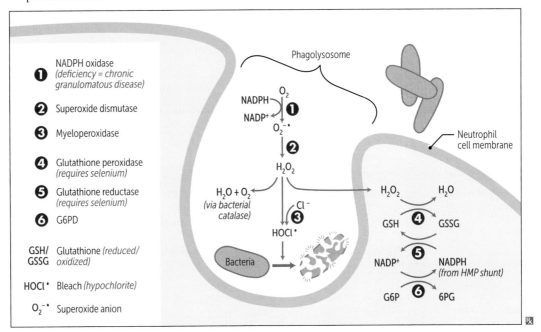

Phagocytes of patients with CGD can utilize H_2O_2 generated by invading organisms and convert it to ROS. Patients are at ↑ risk for infection by catalase ⊕ species (e.g., S. *aureus*, *Aspergillus*) capable of neutralizing their own H_2O_2, leaving phagocytes without ROS for fighting infections. Pyocyanin of *P. aeruginosa* functions to generate ROS to kill competing microbes. Lactoferrin is a protein found in secretory fluids and neutrophils that inhibits microbial growth via iron chelation.

Glucose-6-phosphate dehydrogenase deficiency

NADPH is necessary to keep glutathione reduced, which in turn detoxifies free radicals and peroxides. ↓ NADPH in RBCs leads to hemolytic anemia due to poor RBC defense against oxidizing agents (e.g., fava beans, sulfonamides, primaquine, antituberculosis drugs). Infection can also precipitate hemolysis (free radicals generated via inflammatory response can diffuse into RBCs and cause oxidative damage).

X-linked recessive disorder; most common human enzyme deficiency; more prevalent among blacks. ↑ malarial resistance.
Heinz bodies—oxidized Hemoglobin precipitated within RBCs.
Bite cells—result from the phagocytic removal of Heinz bodies by splenic macrophages. Think, "Bite into some Heinz ketchup."

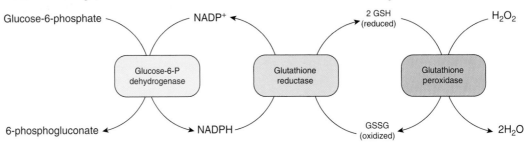

Disorders of fructose metabolism

Essential fructosuria	Involves a defect in **fructokinase.** Autosomal recessive. A benign, asymptomatic condition, since fructose is not trapped in cells. Symptoms: fructose appears in blood and urine. Disorders of fructose metabolism cause milder symptoms than analogous disorders of galactose metabolism.
Fructose intolerance	Hereditary deficiency of **aldolase B.** Autosomal recessive. Fructose-1-P accumulates, causing a ↓ in available phosphate, which results in inhibition of glycogenolysis and gluconeogenesis. Symptoms present following consumption of fruit, juice, or honey. Urine dipstick will be ⊖ (tests for glucose only); reducing sugar can be detected in the urine (nonspecific test for inborn errors of carbohydrate metabolism). Symptoms: hypoglycemia, jaundice, cirrhosis, vomiting. Treatment: ↓ intake of both fructose and sucrose (glucose + fructose).

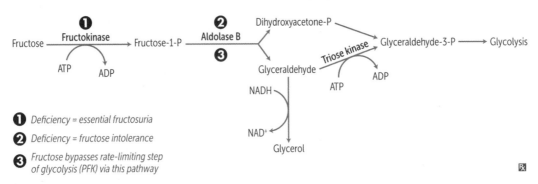

Fructose metabolism (liver)

❶ Deficiency = essential fructosuria
❷ Deficiency = fructose intolerance
❸ Fructose bypasses rate-limiting step of glycolysis (PFK) via this pathway

Disorders of galactose metabolism

Galactokinase deficiency	Hereditary deficiency of **galactokinase.** Galactitol accumulates if galactose is present in diet. Relatively mild condition. Autosomal recessive. Symptoms: galactose appears in blood and urine, infantile cataracts. May initially present as failure to track objects or to develop a social smile.
Classic galactosemia	Absence of **galactose-1-phosphate uridyltransferase.** Autosomal recessive. Damage is caused by accumulation of toxic substances (including galactitol, which accumulates in the lens of the eye). Symptoms: failure to thrive, jaundice, hepatomegaly, infantile cataracts, intellectual disability. Treatment: exclude galactose and lactose (galactose + glucose) from diet.

Galactose metabolism

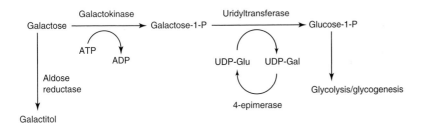

Fructose is to Aldolase B as Galactose is to UridylTransferase (**FAB GUT**).
The more serious defects lead to PO_4^{3-} depletion.
Classic galactosemia can lead to *E. coli* sepsis in neonates.

Sorbitol	An alternative method of trapping glucose in the cell is to convert it to its alcohol counterpart, called sorbitol, via aldose reductase. Some tissues then convert sorbitol to fructose using sorbitol dehydrogenase; tissues with an insufficient amount of this enzyme are at risk for intracellular sorbitol accumulation, causing osmotic damage (e.g., cataracts, retinopathy, and peripheral neuropathy seen with chronic hyperglycemia in diabetes). High blood levels of galactose also result in conversion to the osmotically active galactitol via aldose reductase.

Liver, ovaries, and seminal vesicles have both enzymes.

$$\text{Glucose} \xrightarrow[\text{NADPH}]{\textbf{Aldose reductase}} \text{Sorbitol} \xrightarrow[\text{NAD}^+]{\textbf{Sorbitol dehydrogenase}} \text{Fructose}$$

Schwann cells, retina, and kidneys have only aldose reductase. Lens has primarily aldose reductase.

$$\text{Glucose} \xrightarrow[\text{NADPH}]{\textbf{Aldose reductase}} \text{Sorbitol}$$

Lactase deficiency	Insufficient lactase enzyme → dietary lactose intolerance. Lactase functions on the brush border to digest lactose (in human and cow milk) into glucose and galactose. Primary: age-dependent decline after childhood (absence of lactase-persistent allele), common in people of Asian, African, or Native American descent. Secondary: loss of brush border due to gastroenteritis (e.g., rotavirus), autoimmune disease, etc. Congenital lactase deficiency: rare, due to defective gene. Stool demonstrates ↓ pH and breath shows ↑ hydrogen content with lactose tolerance test. Intestinal biopsy reveals normal mucosa in patients with hereditary lactose intolerance.
FINDINGS	Bloating, cramps, flatulence, osmotic diarrhea.
TREATMENT	Avoid dairy products or add lactase pills to diet; lactose-free milk.

Amino acids	Only L-form amino acids are found in proteins.	
Essential	Glucogenic: methionine (Met), valine (Val), histidine (His). Glucogenic/ketogenic: isoleucine (Ile), phenylalanine (Phe), threonine (Thr), tryptophan (Trp). Ketogenic: leucine (Leu), lysine (Lys).	All essential amino acids need to be supplied in the diet.
Acidic	Aspartic acid (Asp) and glutamic acid (Glu). Negatively charged at body pH.	
Basic	Arginine (Arg), lysine (Lys), histidine (His). Arg is most basic. His has no charge at body pH.	Arg and His are required during periods of growth. Arg and Lys are ↑ in histones, which bind negatively charged DNA.

| **Urea cycle** | Amino acid catabolism results in the formation of common metabolites (e.g., pyruvate, acetyl-CoA), which serve as metabolic fuels. Excess nitrogen (NH_3) generated by this process is converted to urea and excreted by the kidneys. | **O**rdinarily, **C**areless **C**rappers **A**re **A**lso **F**rivolous **A**bout **U**rination. |

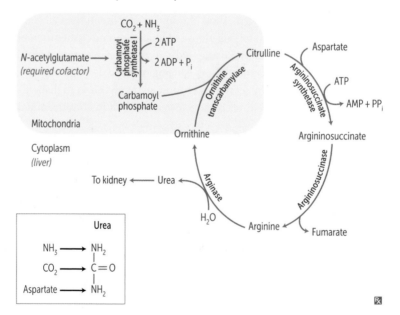

Transport of ammonia by alanine and glutamate

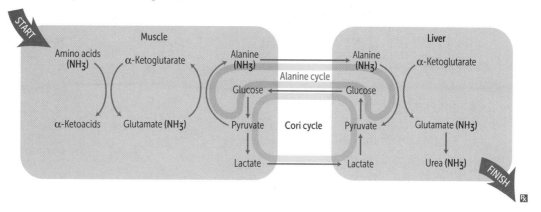

Hyperammonemia	Can be acquired (e.g., liver disease) or hereditary (e.g., urea cycle enzyme deficiencies). Results in excess NH_4^+, which depletes α-ketoglutarate, leading to inhibition of TCA cycle. Treatment: limit protein in diet. Benzoate or phenylbutyrate (both of which bind amino acid and lead to excretion) may be given to ↓ ammonia levels. Lactulose to acidify the GI tract and trap NH_4^+ for excretion.	Ammonia intoxication—tremor (asterixis), slurring of speech, somnolence, vomiting, cerebral edema, blurring of vision.

N-acetylglutamate deficiency	Required cofactor for carbamoyl phosphate synthetase I. Absence of N-acetylglutamate → hyperammonemia. Presentation is identical to carbamoyl phosphate synthetase I deficiency. However, ↑ ornithine with normal urea cycle enzymes suggests hereditary N-acetylglutamate deficiency.

Ornithine transcarbamylase deficiency	Most common urea cycle disorder. X-linked recessive (vs. other urea cycle enzyme deficiencies, which are autosomal recessive). Interferes with the body's ability to eliminate ammonia. Often evident in the first few days of life, but may present with late onset. Excess carbamoyl phosphate is converted to orotic acid (part of the pyrimidine synthesis pathway). Findings: ↑ orotic acid in blood and urine, ↓ BUN, symptoms of hyperammonemia. No megaloblastic anemia (vs. orotic aciduria).

Amino acid derivatives

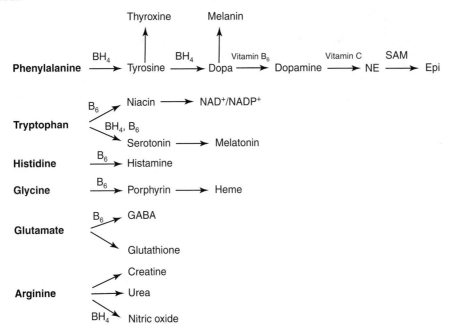

Catecholamine synthesis/tyrosine catabolism

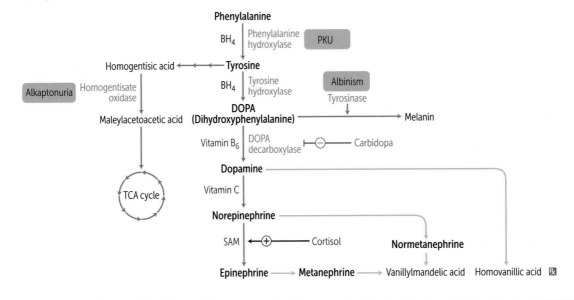

Phenylketonuria

Due to ↓ phenylalanine hydroxylase or ↓ tetrahydrobiopterin cofactor (malignant PKU). Tyrosine becomes essential. ↑ phenylalanine leads to excess phenylketones in urine.

Findings: intellectual disability, growth retardation, seizures, fair skin, eczema, musty body odor.

Treatment: ↓ phenylalanine and ↑ tyrosine in diet.

Maternal PKU—lack of proper dietary therapy during pregnancy. Findings in infant: microcephaly, intellectual disability, growth retardation, congenital heart defects.

Autosomal recessive. Incidence ≈ 1:10,000.

Screened for 2–3 days after birth (normal at birth because of maternal enzyme during fetal life).

Phenylketones—phenylacetate, phenyllactate, and phenylpyruvate.

Disorder of **aromatic** amino acid metabolism → musty body **odor**.

PKU patients must avoid the artificial sweetener aspartame, which contains phenylalanine.

Alkaptonuria (ochronosis)

Congenital deficiency of homogentisate oxidase in the degradative pathway of tyrosine to fumarate. Autosomal recessive. Benign disease.

Findings: dark connective tissue, brown pigmented sclerae, urine turns black on prolonged exposure to air. May have debilitating arthralgias (homogentisic acid toxic to cartilage).

Homocystinuria

Types (all autosomal recessive):
- Cystathionine synthase deficiency (treatment: ↓ methionine, ↑ cysteine, ↑ B_{12} and folate in diet)
- ↓ affinity of cystathionine synthase for pyridoxal phosphate (treatment: ↑↑ B_6 and ↑ cysteine in diet)
- Homocysteine methyltransferase (methionine synthase) deficiency (treatment: ↑ methionine in diet)

All forms result in excess homocysteine.

Findings: ↑↑ homocysteine in urine, intellectual disability, osteoporosis, tall stature, kyphosis, lens subluxation (downward and inward), thrombosis, and atherosclerosis (stroke and MI).

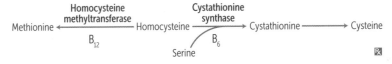

Methionine ←[Homocysteine methyltransferase / B_{12}]— Homocysteine —[Serine / Cystathionine synthase / B_6]→ Cystathionine ——→ Cysteine ℞

Cystinuria

Hereditary defect of renal PCT and intestinal amino acid transporter for **C**ysteine, **O**rnithine, **L**ysine, and **A**rginine (**COLA**).

Excess cystine in the urine can lead to precipitation of hexagonal cystine stones.

Autosomal recessive. Common (1:7000).

Urinary cyanide-nitroprusside test is diagnostic.

Treatment: urinary alkalinization (e.g., potassium citrate, acetazolamide) and chelating agents ↑ solubility of cystine stones; good hydration.

Cystine is made of 2 cysteines connected by a disulfide bond.

Maple syrup urine disease	Blocked degradation of **branched** amino acids (**I**soleucine, **L**eucine, **V**aline) due to ↓ α-ketoacid dehydrogenase (B₁). Causes ↑ α-ketoacids in the blood, especially those of leucine. Causes severe CNS defects, intellectual disability, and death.	Autosomal recessive. Urine smells like maple syrup/burnt sugar. **I L**ove **V**ermont **maple syrup** from maple trees (with **branches**). Treatment: restriction of leucine, isoleucine, and valine in diet, and thiamine supplementation.

Glycogen regulation by insulin and glucagon/epinephrine

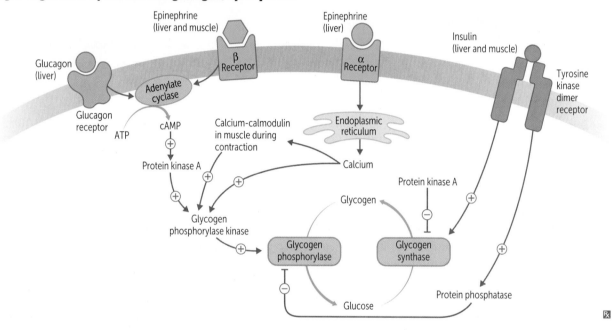

Glycogen	Branches have α-(1,6) bonds; linkages have α-(1,4) bonds.
Skeletal muscle	Glycogen undergoes glycogenolysis → glucose-1-phosphate → glucose-6-P, which is rapidly metabolized during exercise.
Hepatocytes	Glycogen is stored and undergoes glycogenolysis to maintain blood sugar at appropriate levels. Glycogen phosphorylase cleaves glucose-1-P residues off branched glycogen until four remain before a branch point. Then 4-α-D-glucanotransferase (debranching enzyme ❺) moves three glucose-1-Ps from the branch to the linkage. Then α-1,6-glucosidase (debranching enzyme ❻) cleaves off the last glucose-1-P on the branch. "Limit dextrin" refers to the one to four residues remaining on a branch after glycogen phosphorylase has already shortened it.

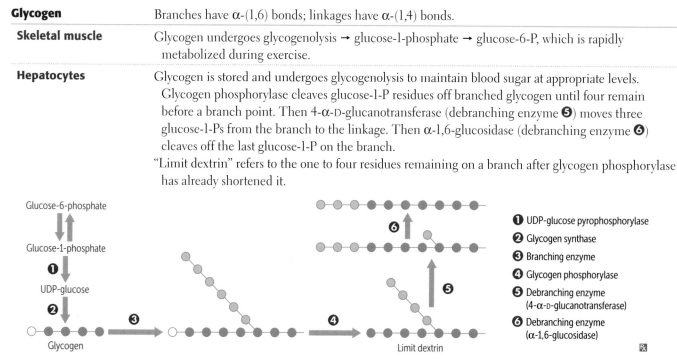

Note: A small amount of glycogen is degraded in lysosomes by α-1,4-glucosidase (acid maltase).

Glycogen storage diseases	12 types, all resulting in abnormal glycogen metabolism and an accumulation of glycogen within cells.	**V**ery **P**oor **C**arbohydrate **M**etabolism.

DISEASE	FINDINGS	DEFICIENT ENZYME	COMMENTS
Von Gierke disease (type I)	Severe fasting hypoglycemia, ↑↑ glycogen in liver, ↑ blood lactate, hepatomegaly	Glucose-6-phosphatase	Autosomal recessive. Treatment: frequent oral glucose/cornstarch; avoidance of fructose and galactose.
Pompe disease (type II)	Cardiomyopathy and systemic findings leading to early death	Lysosomal α-1,4-glucosidase (acid maltase)	Autosomal recessive. **Pompe** trashes the **Pump** (heart, liver, and muscle).
Cori disease (type III)	Milder form of type I with normal blood lactate levels	Debranching enzyme (α-1,6-glucosidase)	Autosomal recessive. Gluconeogenesis is intact.
McArdle disease (type V)	↑ glycogen in muscle, but cannot break it down, leading to painful muscle cramps, myoglobinuria (red urine) with strenuous exercise, and arrhythmia from electrolyte abnormalities.	Skeletal muscle glycogen phosphorylase (myophosphorylase)	Autosomal recessive. **McArdle** = **M**uscle.

Lysosomal storage diseases

Each is caused by a deficiency in one of the many lysosomal enzymes. Results in an accumulation of abnormal metabolic products.

DISEASE	FINDINGS	DEFICIENT ENZYME	ACCUMULATED SUBSTRATE	INHERITANCE
Sphingolipidoses				
Fabry disease	Peripheral neuropathy of hands/feet, angiokeratomas, cardiovascular/renal disease	α-galactosidase A	Ceramide trihexoside	XR
Gaucher disease 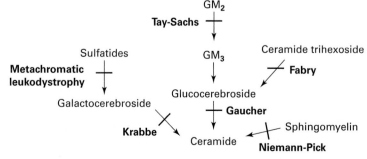	Most common. Hepatosplenomegaly, pancytopenia, aseptic necrosis of femur, bone crises, Gaucher cells **A** (lipid-laden macrophages resembling crumpled tissue paper); treatment is recombinant glucocerebrosidase.	Glucocerebrosidase (β-glucosidase)	Glucocerebroside	AR
Niemann-Pick disease	Progressive neurodegeneration, hepatosplenomegaly, "cherry-red" spot on macula, foam cells (lipid-laden macrophages) **B**	Sphingomyelinase	Sphingomyelin	AR
Tay-Sachs disease	Progressive neurodegeneration, developmental delay, "cherry-red" spot on macula **C**, lysosomes with onion skin, no hepatosplenomegaly (vs. Niemann-Pick)	Hexosaminidase A	GM$_2$ ganglioside	AR
Krabbe disease	Peripheral neuropathy, developmental delay, optic atrophy, globoid cells	Galactocerebrosidase	Galactocerebroside, psychosine	AR
Metachromatic leukodystrophy	Central and peripheral demyelination with ataxia, dementia	Arylsulfatase A	Cerebroside sulfate	AR
Mucopolysaccharidoses				
Hurler syndrome	Developmental delay, gargoylism, airway obstruction, corneal clouding, hepatosplenomegaly	α-L-iduronidase	Heparan sulfate, dermatan sulfate	AR
Hunter syndrome	Mild Hurler + aggressive behavior, no corneal clouding	Iduronate sulfatase	Heparan sulfate, dermatan sulfate	XR

No man picks (Niemann-Pick) his nose with his sphinger (sphingomyelinase).

Tay-Sa**X** lacks he**X**osaminidase.

Hunters see clearly (no corneal clouding) and aggressively aim for the **X** (**X**-linked recessive).

↑ incidence of Tay-Sachs, Niemann-Pick, and some forms of Gaucher disease in Ashkenazi Jews.

Fatty acid metabolism

Long-chain fatty acid degradation requires carnitine-dependent transport into the mitochondrial matrix.

Carnitine deficiency: inability to transport LCFAs into the mitochondria, resulting in toxic accumulation. Causes weakness, hypotonia, and hypoketotic hypoglycemia.

Acyl-CoA dehydrogenase deficiency:
↑ dicarboxylic acids, ↓ glucose and ketones. Acetyl-CoA is a ⊕ allosteric regulator of pyruvate carboxylase in gluconeogenesis. ↓ acetyl-CoA → ↓ fasting glucose.

"**SY**trate" = **SY**nthesis.
CARnitine = **CAR**nage of fatty acids.

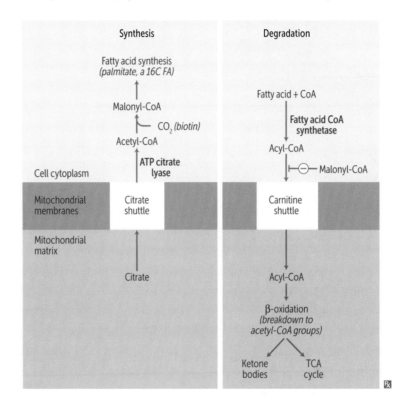

Ketone bodies

In the liver, fatty acids and amino acids are metabolized to acetoacetate and β-hydroxybutyrate (to be used in muscle and brain).

In prolonged starvation and diabetic ketoacidosis, oxaloacetate is depleted for gluconeogenesis. In alcoholism, excess NADH shunts oxaloacetate to malate. Both processes cause a buildup of acetyl-CoA, which shunts glucose and FFA toward the production of ketone bodies.

Breath smells like acetone (fruity odor). Urine test for ketones does not detect β-hydroxybutyrate.

Metabolic fuel use

Exercise

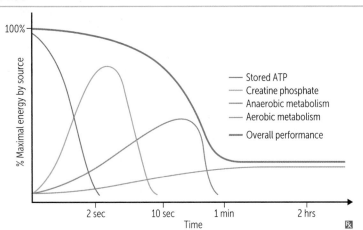

1 g protein or carbohydrate = 4 kcal.
1 g fat = 9 kcal.
1 g alcohol = 7 kcal.

Fasting and starvation	Priorities are to supply sufficient glucose to the brain and RBCs and to preserve protein.	
Fed state (after a meal)	Glycolysis and aerobic respiration.	Insulin stimulates storage of lipids, proteins, glycogen.
Fasting (between meals)	Hepatic glycogenolysis (major); hepatic gluconeogenesis, adipose release of FFA (minor).	Glucagon, adrenaline stimulate use of fuel reserves.
Starvation days 1–3	Blood glucose levels maintained by: ▪ Hepatic glycogenolysis ▪ Adipose release of FFA ▪ Muscle and liver, which shift fuel use from glucose to FFA ▪ Hepatic gluconeogenesis from peripheral tissue lactate and alanine, and from adipose tissue glycerol and propionyl-CoA (from odd-chain FFA—the only triacylglycerol components that contribute to gluconeogenesis)	Glycogen reserves depleted after day 1. RBCs lack mitochondria and so cannot use ketones.
Starvation after day 3	Adipose stores (ketone bodies become the main source of energy for the brain). After these are depleted, vital protein degradation accelerates, leading to organ failure and death. Amount of excess stores determines survival time.	

Cholesterol synthesis

Rate-limiting step is catalyzed by HMG-CoA reductase (induced by insulin), which converts HMG-CoA to mevalonate. ⅔ of plasma cholesterol is esterified by lecithin-cholesterol acyltransferase (LCAT).

Statins (e.g., lovastatin) competitively and reversibly inhibit HMG-CoA reductase.

Lipid transport, key enzymes

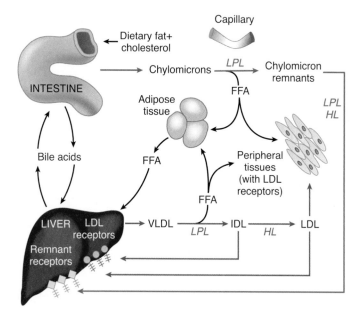

Pancreatic lipase—degradation of dietary triglycerides (TG) in small intestine.
Lipoprotein lipase (LPL)—degradation of TG circulating in chylomicrons and VLDLs. Found on vascular endothelial surface.
Hepatic TG lipase (HL)—degradation of TG remaining in IDL.
Hormone-sensitive lipase—degradation of TG stored in adipocytes.

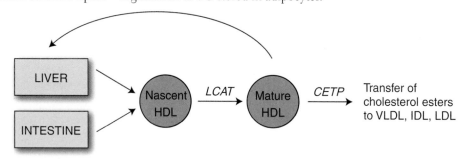

LCAT—catalyzes esterification of cholesterol.
Cholesterol ester transfer protein (CETP)—mediates transfer of cholesterol esters to other lipoprotein particles.

Major apolipoproteins

Apolipoprotein	Function	Chylomicron	Chylomicron remnant	VLDL	IDL	LDL	HDL
E	Mediates remnant uptake	✓	✓	✓	✓		✓
A-I	Activates LCAT	✓					✓
C-II	Lipoprotein lipase cofactor	✓		✓			✓
B-48	Mediates chylomicron secretion	✓	✓				
B-100	Binds LDL receptor			✓	✓	✓	

Lipoprotein functions

Lipoproteins are composed of varying proportions of cholesterol, TGs, and phospholipids. LDL and HDL carry most cholesterol.

LDL transports cholesterol from liver to tissues.

LDL is Lousy.

HDL transports cholesterol from periphery to liver.

HDL is Healthy.

Chylomicron

Delivers dietary TGs to peripheral tissue. Delivers cholesterol to liver in the form of chylomicron remnants, which are mostly depleted of their triacylglycerols. Secreted by intestinal epithelial cells.

VLDL

Delivers hepatic TGs to peripheral tissue. Secreted by liver.

IDL

Formed in the degradation of VLDL. Delivers TGs and cholesterol to liver.

LDL

Delivers hepatic cholesterol to peripheral tissues. Formed by hepatic lipase modification of IDL in the peripheral tissue. Taken up by target cells via receptor-mediated endocytosis.

HDL

Mediates reverse cholesterol transport from periphery to liver. Acts as a repository for apoC and apoE (which are needed for chylomicron and VLDL metabolism). Secreted from both liver and intestine. Alcohol ↑ synthesis.

Familial dyslipidemias

TYPE	INCREASED BLOOD LEVEL	PATHOPHYSIOLOGY
I—hyper-chylomicronemia	Chylomicrons, TG, cholesterol	Autosomal recessive. Lipoprotein lipase deficiency or altered apolipoprotein C-II. Causes pancreatitis, hepatosplenomegaly, and eruptive/pruritic xanthomas (no ↑ risk for atherosclerosis).
IIa—familial hyper-cholesterolemia	LDL, cholesterol	Autosomal dominant. Absent or defective LDL receptors. Heterozygotes (1:500) have cholesterol ≈ 300 mg/dL; homozygotes (very rare) have cholesterol ≈ 700+ mg/dL. Causes accelerated atherosclerosis (may have MI before age 20), tendon (Achilles) xanthomas, and corneal arcus.
IV—hyper-triglyceridemia	VLDL, TG	Autosomal dominant. Hepatic overproduction of VLDL. Causes pancreatitis.

Microbiology

"*Support bacteria. They're the only culture some people have.*"

—Anonymous

"*What lies behind us and what lies ahead of us are tiny matters compared to what lies within us.*"

—Oliver Wendell Holmes

This high-yield material covers the basic concepts of microbiology. The emphasis in previous examinations has been approximately 40% bacteriology (20% basic, 20% quasi-clinical), 25% immunology, 25% virology (10% basic, 15% quasi-clinical), 5% parasitology, and 5% mycology.

Microbiology questions on the Step 1 exam often require two (or more) steps: Given a certain clinical presentation, you will first need to identify the most likely causative organism, and you will then need to provide an answer regarding some feature of that organism. For example, a description of a child with fever and a petechial rash will be followed by a question that reads, "From what site does the responsible organism usually enter the blood?"

This section therefore presents organisms in two major ways: in individual microbial "profiles" and in the context of the systems they infect and the clinical presentations they produce. You should become familiar with both formats. When reviewing the systems approach, remind yourself of the features of each microbe by returning to the individual profiles. Also be sure to memorize the laboratory characteristics that allow you to identify microbes.

Additional tables that organize infectious diseases and syndromes according to the most commonly affected hosts and the most likely microbes are available on the First Aid Team blog at www. firstaidteam.com.

▶ MICROBIOLOGY–BASIC BACTERIOLOGY

Bacterial structures

STRUCTURE	FUNCTION	CHEMICAL COMPOSITION
Peptidoglycan	Gives rigid support, protects against osmotic pressure.	Sugar backbone with peptide side chains cross-linked by transpeptidase.
Cell wall/cell membrane (gram positives)	Major surface antigen.	Peptidoglycan for support. Lipoteichoic acid induces TNF and IL-1.
Outer membrane (gram negatives)	Site of endotoxin (lipopolysaccharide [LPS]); major surface antigen.	Lipid A induces TNF and IL-1; O polysaccharide is the antigen.
Plasma membrane	Site of oxidative and transport enzymes.	Phospholipid bilayer.
Ribosome	Protein synthesis.	50S and 30S subunits.
Periplasm	Space between the cytoplasmic membrane and outer membrane in gram-negative bacteria.	Contains many hydrolytic enzymes, including β-lactamases.
Capsule	Protects against phagocytosis.	Polysaccharide (except *Bacillus anthracis*, which contains D-glutamate).
Pilus/fimbria	Mediate adherence of bacteria to cell surface; sex pilus forms attachment between 2 bacteria during conjugation.	Glycoprotein.
Flagellum	Motility.	Protein.
Spore	Resistant to dehydration, heat, and chemicals.	Keratin-like coat; dipicolinic acid; peptidoglycan.
Plasmid	Contains a variety of genes for antibiotic resistance, enzymes, and toxins.	DNA.
Glycocalyx	Mediates adherence to surfaces, especially foreign surfaces (e.g., indwelling catheters).	Polysaccharide.

Cell walls

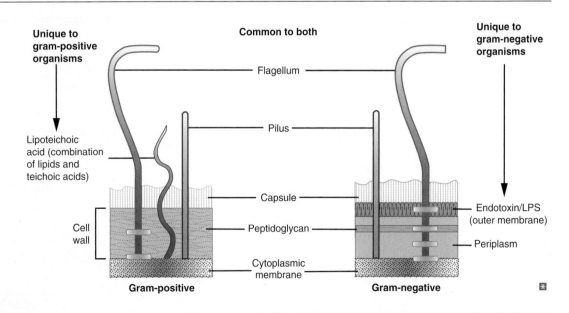

Bacterial taxonomy

MORPHOLOGY	**Gram-positive examples**	**Gram-negative examples**
Circular (coccus)	*Staphylococcus* *Streptococcus*	*Neisseria*
Rod (bacillus)	*Clostridium* *Corynebacterium* *Bacillus* *Listeria* *Mycobacterium* (acid fast) *Gardnerella* (gram variable)	Enterics: ▪ *E. coli* ▪ *Shigella* ▪ *Salmonella* ▪ *Yersinia* ▪ *Klebsiella* ▪ *Proteus* ▪ *Enterobacter* ▪ *Serratia* ▪ *Vibrio* ▪ *Campylobacter* ▪ *Helicobacter* ▪ *Pseudomonas* ▪ *Bacteroides* Respiratory: ▪ *Haemophilus* (pleomorphic) ▪ *Legionella* (silver) ▪ *Bordetella* Zoonotic: ▪ *Francisella* ▪ *Brucella* ▪ *Pasteurella* ▪ *Bartonella*
Branching filamentous	*Actinomyces* *Nocardia* (weakly acid fast)	
Pleomorphic		Rickettsiae (Giemsa) Chlamydiae (Giemsa)
Spiral		Spirochetes: ▪ *Borrelia* (Giemsa) ▪ *Leptospira* ▪ *Treponema*
No cell wall	*Mycoplasma* (does not Gram stain)	

Bacteria with unusual cell membranes/walls

Mycoplasma	Contain sterols and have no cell wall.
Mycobacteria	Contain mycolic acid. High lipid content.

Gram stain limitations	These bugs do not Gram stain well:	These Microbes May Lack Real Color.
	Treponema (too thin to be visualized).	Treponemes—dark-field microscopy and fluorescent antibody staining.
	Mycobacteria (high lipid content in cell wall detected by carbolfuchsin in acid-fast stain).	
	Mycoplasma (no cell wall).	
	Legionella pneumophila (primarily intracellular).	*Legionella*—silver stain.
	Rickettsia (intracellular parasite).	
	Chlamydia (intracellular parasite; lacks muramic acid in cell wall).	

Stains

Giemsa	*Chlamydia*, *Borrelia*, Rickettsiae, Trypanosomes, *Plasmodium*.	Certain Bugs Really Try my Patience.
PAS (periodic acid–Schiff)	Stains glycogen, mucopolysaccharides; used to diagnose Whipple disease (*Tropheryma whipplei*).	PASs the sugar.
Ziehl-Neelsen (carbol fuchsin)	Acid-fast organisms (*Nocardia*, *Mycobacterium*).	
India ink	*Cryptococcus neoformans* (mucicarmine can also be used to stain thick polysaccharide capsule red).	
Silver stain	Fungi (e.g., *Pneumocystis*), *Legionella*, *Helicobacter pylori*.	

Special culture requirements

BUG	MEDIA USED FOR ISOLATION
H. influenzae	Chocolate agar with factors V (NAD$^+$) and X (hematin)
N. gonorrhoeae, N. meningitidis	Thayer-Martin (or VPN) media—Vancomycin (inhibits gram-positive organisms), Polymyxin (inhibits gram-negative organisms except *Neisseria*), and Nystatin (inhibits fungi); "to connect to *Neisseria*, please use your **VPN** client"
B. pertussis	Bordet-Gengou (potato) agar (**Bordet** for **Bordetella**)
C. diphtheriae	Tellurite agar, Löffler medium
M. tuberculosis	Löwenstein-Jensen agar
M. pneumoniae	Eaton agar, requires cholesterol
Lactose-fermenting enterics	Pink colonies on MacConkey agar (fermentation produces acid, turning colony pink); *E. coli* is also grown on eosin–methylene blue (EMB) agar as colonies with green metallic sheen
Legionella	Charcoal yeast extract agar buffered with cysteine and iron
Fungi	Sabouraud agar. "Sab's a **fun guy**!"

Obligate aerobes	Use an O_2-dependent system to generate ATP. Examples include *Nocardia*, *Pseudomonas aeruginosa*, and *MycoBacterium tuberculosis*. Reactivation of *M. tuberculosis* (e.g., after immune compromise or TNF-α inhibitor use) has a predilection for the apices of the lung, which have the highest P_{O_2}.	Nagging Pests Must Breathe. *P. aeruginosa* is an aerobe seen in burn wounds, complications of diabetes, nosocomial pneumonia, and pneumonias in cystic fibrosis patients.
Obligate anaerobes	Examples include *Clostridium*, *Bacteroides*, and *Actinomyces*. They lack catalase and/or superoxide dismutase and are thus susceptible to oxidative damage. Generally foul smelling (short-chain fatty acids), are difficult to culture, and produce gas in tissue (CO_2 and H_2).	Anaerobes Can't Breathe Air. Anaerobes are normal flora in GI tract, pathogenic elsewhere. $AminO_2glycosides$ are ineffective against anaerobes because these antibiotics require O_2 to enter into bacterial cell.

Intracellular bugs

Obligate intracellular	*Rickettsia*, *Chlamydia*. Can't make own ATP.	Stay inside (cells) when it is Really Cold.
Facultative intracellular	*Salmonella*, *Neisseria*, *Brucella*, *Mycobacterium*, *Listeria*, *Francisella*, *Legionella*, *Yersinia pestis*.	Some Nasty Bugs May Live FacultativeLY.

Encapsulated bacteria	Examples are *Streptococcus pneumoniae*, *Haemophilus influenzae* type B, *Neisseria meningitidis*, *Escherichia coli*, *Salmonella*, *Klebsiella pneumoniae*, and group B Strep. Their capsules serve as an antiphagocytic virulence factor. Capsule + protein conjugate serves as an antigen in vaccines.	SHiNE SKiS. Are opsonized, and then cleared by spleen. Asplenics have ↓ opsonizing ability and are at risk for severe infections. Give *S. pneumoniae*, *H. influenzae*, *N. meningitidis* vaccines.
Catalase-positive organisms	Catalase degrades H_2O_2 before it can be converted to microbicidal products by the enzyme myeloperoxidase. People with chronic granulomatous disease (NADPH oxidase deficiency) have recurrent infections with catalase ⊕ organisms. Examples: *Pseudomonas*, *Listeria*, *Aspergillus*, *Candida*, *E. coli*, *S. aureus*, *Serratia*.	You need **PLACESS** for your cats.

Encapsulated bacteria vaccines	Some vaccines containing polysaccharide capsule antigens are conjugated to a carrier protein, enhancing immunogenicity by promoting T-cell activation and subsequent class switching. A polysaccharide antigen alone cannot be presented to T cells.	Pneumococcal vaccine: PCV (pneumococcal conjugate vaccine, i.e., Prevnar); PPSV (pneumococcal polysaccharide vaccine with no conjugated protein, i.e., Pneumovax) *H. influenzae* type B (conjugate vaccine) Meningococcal vaccine (conjugate vaccine)
Urease-positive bugs	*Cryptococcus, H. pylori, Proteus, Ureaplasma, Nocardia, Klebsiella, S. epidermidis, S. saprophyticus.*	**CH**uck Norris hates **PUNKSS**.
Pigment-producing bacteria	*Actinomyces israelii*—yellow "sulfur" granules, which are composed of filaments of bacteria.	Israel has yellow sand.
	S. aureus—yellow pigment.	*aureus* (Latin) = gold.
	Pseudomonas aeruginosa—blue-green pigment.	Aerugula is green.
	Serratia marcescens—red pigment.	*Serratia marcescens*—think red maraschino cherries.
Bacterial virulence factors	These promote evasion of host immune response.	
Protein A	Binds Fc region of IgG. Prevents opsonization and phagocytosis. Expressed by *S. aureus*.	
IgA protease	Enzyme that cleaves IgA. Secreted by *S. pneumoniae, H. influenzae* type B, and *Neisseria* (**SHiN**) in order to colonize respiratory mucosa.	
M protein	Helps prevent phagocytosis. Expressed by group A streptococci.	

Main features of exotoxins and endotoxins

PROPERTY	Exotoxin	Endotoxin
SOURCE	Certain species of some gram-positive and gram-negative bacteria	Outer cell membrane of most gram-negative bacteria
SECRETED FROM CELL	Yes	No
CHEMISTRY	Polypeptide	Lipopolysaccharide (structural part of bacteria; released when lysed)
LOCATION OF GENES	Plasmid or bacteriophage	Bacterial chromosome
TOXICITY	High (fatal dose on the order of 1 μg)	Low (fatal dose on the order of hundreds of micrograms)
CLINICAL EFFECTS	Various effects (see following pages)	Fever, shock (hypotension), DIC
MODE OF ACTION	Various modes (see following pages)	Induces TNF, IL-1, and IL-6
ANTIGENICITY	Induces high-titer antibodies called antitoxins	Poorly antigenic
VACCINES	Toxoids used as vaccines	No toxoids formed and no vaccine available
HEAT STABILITY	Destroyed rapidly at 60°C (except staphylococcal enterotoxin)	Stable at 100°C for 1 hr
TYPICAL DISEASES	Tetanus, botulism, diphtheria	Meningococcemia; sepsis by gram-negative rods

Bugs with exotoxins

BACTERIA	TOXIN	MECHANISM	MANIFESTATION
Inhibit protein synthesis			
Corynebacterium diphtheriae	Diphtheria toxin[a]	Inactivate elongation factor (EF-2)	Pharyngitis with pseudomembranes in throat and severe lymphadenopathy (bull neck)
Pseudomonas aeruginosa	Exotoxin A[a]		Host cell death
Shigella spp.	Shiga toxin (ST)[a]	Inactivate 60S ribosome by removing adenine from rRNA	GI mucosal damage → dysentery; ST also enhances cytokine release, causing hemolytic-uremic syndrome (HUS)
Enterohemorrhagic *E. coli* (EHEC), including O157:H7 strain	Shiga-like toxin (SLT)[a]		SLT enhances cytokine release, causing HUS; unlike *Shigella*, EHEC does not invade host cells
Increase fluid secretion			
Enterotoxigenic *E. coli* (ETEC)	Heat-labile toxin (LT)[a]	Overactivates adenylate cyclase ($\uparrow$ cAMP) → $\uparrow$ Cl$^-$ secretion in gut and H$_2$O efflux	Watery diarrhea: **labile** in the Air (Adenylate cyclase), **stable** on the Ground (Guanylate cyclase)
	Heat-**stable** toxin (ST)	Overactivates guanylate cyclase ($\uparrow$ cGMP) → $\downarrow$ resorption of NaCl and H$_2$O in gut	
Bacillus anthracis	Edema factor	Mimics the adenylate cyclase enzyme ($\uparrow$ cAMP)	Likely responsible for characteristic edematous borders of black eschar in cutaneous anthrax
Vibrio cholerae	Cholera toxin[a]	Overactivates adenylate cyclase ($\uparrow$ cAMP) by permanently activating G$_s$ → $\uparrow$ Cl$^-$ secretion in gut and H$_2$O efflux	Voluminous "rice-water" diarrhea
Inhibit phagocytic ability			
Bordetella pertussis	Pertussis toxin[a]	Overactivates adenylate cyclase ($\uparrow$ cAMP) by disabling G$_i$, impairing phagocytosis to permit survival of microbe	**Whooping cough**: child coughs on expiration and "whoops" on inspiration (toxin may not actually be a cause of cough; can cause "100-day cough" in adults)
Inhibit release of neurotransmitter			
Clostridium tetani	Tetanospasmin	Both are proteases that cleave SNARE proteins required for neurotransmitter release	Spasticity, risus sardonicus, and "lockjaw"; toxin prevents release of **inhibitory** (GABA and glycine) neurotransmitters from Renshaw cells in spinal cord
Clostridium botulinum	Botulinum toxin		Flaccid paralysis, floppy baby; toxin prevents release of **stimulatory** (ACh) signals at neuromuscular junctions → flaccid paralysis

[a]Toxin is an ADP ribosylating A-B toxin: B (binding) component binds to host cell surface receptor, enabling endocytosis; A (active) component attaches ADP-ribosyl to disrupt host cell proteins.

Bugs with exotoxins (continued)

BACTERIA	TOXIN	MECHANISM	MANIFESTATION
Lyse cell membranes			
Clostridium perfringens	Alpha toxin	Phospholipase (lecithinase) that degrades tissue and cell membranes	Degradation of phospholipids → myonecrosis ("gas gangrene") and hemolysis ("double zone" of hemolysis on blood agar)
Streptococcus pyogenes	Streptolysin O	Protein that degrades cell membrane	Lyses RBCs; contributes to β-hemolysis; host antibodies against toxin (ASO) used to diagnose rheumatic fever (do not confuse with immune complexes of poststreptococcal glomerulonephritis)
Superantigens causing shock			
Staphylococcus aureus	Toxic shock syndrome toxin (TSST-1)	Bring MHC II and TCR in proximity to outside of antigen binding site to cause overwhelming release of IFN-γ and IL-2 → shock	Toxic shock syndrome: fever, rash, shock; other toxins cause scalded skin syndrome (exfoliative toxin) and food poisoning (enterotoxin)
Streptococcus pyogenes	Exotoxin A		Toxic shock syndrome: fever, rash, shock

Endotoxin

An LPS found in outer membrane of gram-negative bacteria (both cocci and rods).

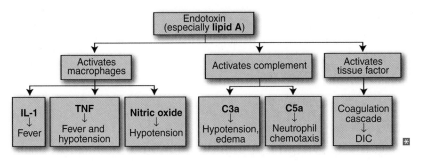

ENDOTOXIN:
Edema
Nitric oxide
DIC/Death
Outer membrane
TNF-α
O-antigen
eXtremely heat stable
IL-1
Neutrophil chemotaxis

Bacterial genetics

Transformation	Ability to take up naked DNA (i.e., from cell lysis) from environment (also known as "competence"). A feature of many bacteria, especially *S. pneumoniae*, *H. influenzae* type B, and *Neisseria* (**SHiN**). Any DNA can be used. Adding deoxyribonuclease to environment will degrade naked DNA in medium → no transformation seen.
Conjugation	
F⁺ × F⁻	F⁺ plasmid contains genes required for sex pilus and conjugation. Bacteria without this plasmid are termed F⁻. Plasmid (dsDNA) is replicated and transferred through pilus from F⁺ cell. No transfer of chromosomal genes.
Hfr × F⁻	F⁺ plasmid can become incorporated into bacterial chromosomal DNA, termed high-frequency recombination (Hfr) cell. Replication of incorporated plasmid DNA may include some flanking chromosomal DNA. Transfer of plasmid and chromosomal genes.
Transposition	Segment of DNA (e.g., transposon) that can "jump" (excision and reintegration) from one location to another, can transfer genes from plasmid to chromosome and vice versa. When excision occurs, may include some flanking chromosomal DNA, which can be incorporated into a plasmid and transferred to another bacterium. Examples include antibiotic resistance genes on R plasmid.
Transduction	
Generalized	A "packaging" event. Lytic phage infects bacterium, leading to cleavage of bacterial DNA. Parts of bacterial chromosomal DNA may become packaged in viral capsid. Phage infects another bacterium, transferring these genes.
Specialized	An "excision" event. Lysogenic phage infects bacterium; viral DNA incorporates into bacterial chromosome. When phage DNA is excised, flanking bacterial genes may be excised with it. DNA is packaged into phage viral capsid and can infect another bacterium. Genes for the following 5 bacterial toxins are encoded in a lysogenic phage (**ABCDE**): ▪ Shig**A**-like toxin ▪ **B**otulinum toxin (certain strains) ▪ **C**holera toxin ▪ **D**iphtheria toxin ▪ **E**rythrogenic toxin of *Streptococcus pyogenes*

Gram-positive lab algorithm

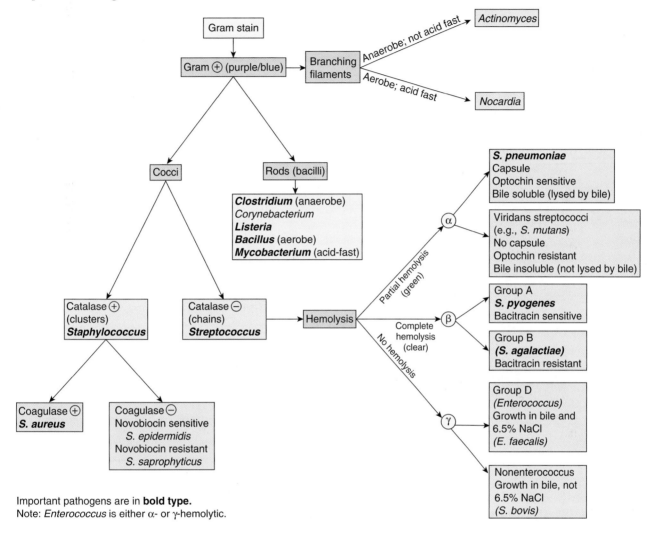

Important pathogens are in **bold type.**
Note: *Enterococcus* is either α- or γ-hemolytic.

Identification of gram-positive cocci

Staphylococci	NOvobiocin—*Saprophyticus* is Resistant; *Epidermidis* is Sensitive.	On the office's "staph" retreat, there was NO StRESs.
Streptococci	Optochin—*Viridans* is Resistant; *Pneumoniae* is Sensitive.	OVRPS (overpass).
	Bacitracin—group B strep are Resistant; group A strep are Sensitive.	B-BRAS.

α-hemolytic bacteria	Form green ring around colonies on blood agar. Include the following organisms:
	▪ *Streptococcus pneumoniae* (catalase ⊖ and optochin sensitive)
	▪ Viridans streptococci (catalase ⊖ and optochin resistant)

β-hemolytic bacteria	Form clear area of hemolysis on blood agar. Include the following organisms:
	▪ *Staphylococcus aureus* (catalase and coagulase ⊕)
	▪ *Streptococcus pyogenes*—group A strep (catalase ⊖ and bacitracin sensitive)
	▪ *Streptococcus agalactiae*—group B strep (catalase ⊖ and bacitracin resistant)
	▪ *Listeria monocytogenes* (tumbling motility, meningitis in newborns, unpasteurized milk)

Staphylococcus aureus

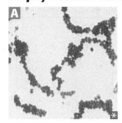

Gram-positive cocci in clusters **A**. Protein A (virulence factor) binds Fc-IgG, inhibiting complement activation and phagocytosis. Commonly colonizes the nose.

Causes:
- Inflammatory disease—skin infections, organ abscesses, pneumonia (often after influenza virus infection), endocarditis, and osteomyelitis
- Toxin-mediated disease—toxic shock syndrome (TSST-1), scalded skin syndrome (exfoliative toxin), rapid-onset food poisoning (enterotoxins)
- MRSA (methicillin-resistant S. *aureus*) infection—important cause of serious nosocomial and community-acquired infections; resistant to methicillin and nafcillin because of altered penicillin-binding protein

TSST is a superantigen that binds to MHC II and T-cell receptor, resulting in polyclonal T-cell activation. Presents as fever, vomiting, rash, desquamation, shock, end-organ failure. Use of vaginal or nasal tampons predisposes to toxic shock syndrome.

S. *aureus* food poisoning due to ingestion of preformed toxin → short incubation period (2–6 hr). Enterotoxin is heat stable → not destroyed by cooking.

Staph make catalase because they have more "**staff**." Bad staph (*aureus*) make coagulase and toxins. Forms fibrin clot around self → abscess.

Staphylococcus epidermidis

Infects prosthetic devices and intravenous catheters by producing adherent biofilms. Component of normal skin flora; contaminates blood cultures. Novobiocin sensitive.

Staphylococcus saprophyticus

Second most common cause of uncomplicated UTI in young women (first is E. *coli*). Novobiocin resistant.

Streptococcus pneumoniae

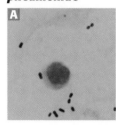

Most common cause of:
- Meningitis
- Otitis media (in children)
- Pneumonia
- Sinusitis

Lancet-shaped, gram-positive diplococci **A**. Encapsulated. IgA protease.

S. *pneumoniae* MOPS are Most OPtochin Sensitive.

Pneumococcus is associated with "rusty" sputum, sepsis in sickle cell anemia and splenectomy.

No virulence without capsule.

Viridans group streptococci	Viridans streptococci are α-hemolytic. They are normal flora of the oropharynx and cause dental caries (*Streptococcus mutans*) and subacute bacterial endocarditis at damaged valves (*S. sanguinis*). Resistant to optochin, differentiating them from *S. pneumoniae*, which is α-hemolytic but is optochin sensitive.	*Sanguis* = blood. There is lots of blood in the heart (endocarditis). *S. sanguinis* makes dextrans, which bind to fibrin-platelet aggregates on damaged heart valves. Viridans group strep live in the mouth because they are not afraid of-the-chin (op-to-chin resistant).
Streptococcus pyogenes (group A streptococci)	Causes: ■ Pyogenic—pharyngitis, cellulitis, impetigo ■ Toxigenic—scarlet fever, toxic shock–like syndrome, necrotizing fasciitis ■ Immunologic—rheumatic fever, acute glomerulonephritis Bacitracin sensitive. Antibodies to M protein enhance host defenses against *S. pyogenes* but can give rise to rheumatic fever. ASO titer detects recent *S. pyogenes* infection.	J♥NES criteria for rheumatic fever: Joints—polyarthritis ♥—carditis Nodules (subcutaneous) Erythema marginatum Sydenham chorea **Pharyngitis** can result in rheumatic "**phever**" and glomerulone**phritis**. Impetigo more commonly precedes glomerulonephritis than pharyngitis. **Scarlet fever:** scarlet rash with sandpaper-like texture, strawberry tongue, circumoral pallor.
Streptococcus agalactiae (group B streptococci)	Bacitracin resistant, β-hemolytic, colonizes vagina; causes pneumonia, meningitis, and sepsis, mainly in **babies**. Produces CAMP factor, which enlarges the area of hemolysis formed by *S. aureus*. (Note: CAMP stands for the authors of the test, not cyclic AMP.) Hippurate test ⊕. Screen pregnant women at 35–37 weeks. Patients with ⊕ culture receive intrapartum penicillin prophylaxis.	Group **B** for **B**abies!
Enterococci (group D streptococci) 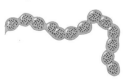	Enterococci (*Enterococcus faecalis* and *E. faecium*) are normal colonic flora that are penicillin G resistant and cause UTI, biliary tract infections, and subacute endocarditis (following GI/GU procedures). Lancefield group D includes the enterococci and the nonenterococcal group D streptococci. Lancefield grouping is based on differences in the C carbohydrate on the bacterial cell wall. Variable hemolysis. VRE (vancomycin-resistant enterococci) are an important cause of nosocomial infection.	Enterococci, hardier than nonenterococcal group D, can grow in 6.5% NaCl and bile (lab test). *Entero* = intestine, *faecalis* = feces, *strepto* = twisted (chains), *coccus* = berry.

Streptococcus bovis (group D streptococci)	Colonizes the gut. Can cause bacteremia and subacute endocarditis in colon cancer patients.	Bovis in the blood = cancer in the colon.
Corynebacterium diphtheriae 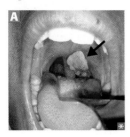	Causes diphtheria via exotoxin encoded by β-prophage. Potent exotoxin inhibits protein synthesis via ADP-ribosylation of EF-2. Symptoms include pseudomembranous pharyngitis (grayish-white membrane **A**) with lymphadenopathy, myocarditis, and arrhythmias. Lab diagnosis based on gram-positive rods with metachromatic (blue and red) granules and Elek test for toxin. Toxoid vaccine prevents diphtheria.	*Coryne* = club shaped. Black colonies on cystine-tellurite agar. **ABCDEFG:** ADP-ribosylation Beta-prophage *Corynebacterium* *Diphtheriae* Elongation Factor 2 Granules
Spores: bacterial	Some bacteria can form spores at the end of the stationary phase when nutrients are limited. Spores are highly resistant to heat and chemicals. Have dipicolinic acid in their core. Have no metabolic activity. Must autoclave to kill spores (as is done to surgical equipment) by steaming at 121°C for 15 minutes.	Spore-forming gram-positive bacteria found in soil: *Bacillus anthracis, Clostridium perfringens, C. tetani.* Other spore formers include *B. cereus, C. botulinum, Coxiella burnetii.*
Clostridia (with exotoxins)	Gram-positive, spore-forming, obligate anaerobic bacilli.	
C. tetani	Produces tetanospasmin, an exotoxin causing tetanus. Tetanus toxin (and botulinum toxin) are proteases that cleave releasing proteins for neurotransmitters.	Tetanus is tetanic paralysis (blocks glycine and GABA release [both are inhibitory neurotransmitters] from Renshaw cells in spinal cord). Causes spastic paralysis, trismus (lockjaw), and risus sardonicus.
C. botulinum	Produces a preformed, heat-labile toxin that inhibits ACh release at the neuromuscular junction, causing botulism. In adults, disease is caused by ingestion of preformed toxin. In babies, ingestion of spores in honey causes disease (floppy baby syndrome).	*Botulinum* is from bad bottles of food and honey (causes a flaccid paralysis).
C. perfringens	Produces α toxin ("lecithinase," a phospholipase) that can cause myonecrosis (gas gangrene) and hemolysis.	*Perfringens* perforates a gangrenous leg.
C. difficile	Produces 2 toxins. Toxin A, enterotoxin, binds to the brush border of the gut. Toxin B, cytotoxin, causes cytoskeletal disruption via actin depolymerization → pseudomembranous colitis → diarrhea. Often 2° to antibiotic use, especially clindamycin or ampicillin. Diagnosed by detection of one or both toxins in stool.	*Difficile* causes diarrhea. Treatment: metronidazole or oral vancomycin. For recurring cases, fecal transplant may prevent relapse.

Anthrax	Caused by *Bacillus anthracis*, a gram-positive, spore-forming rod (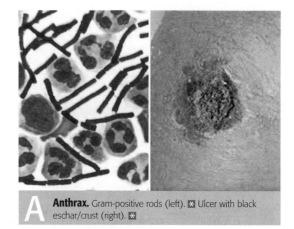, left) that produces anthrax toxin. The only bacterium with a polypeptide capsule (contains D-glutamate).	

A **Anthrax.** Gram-positive rods (left). ✸ Ulcer with black eschar/crust (right). ✸

Cutaneous anthrax	Boil-like lesion → ulcer with black eschar (**A**, right) (painless, necrotic) → uncommonly progresses to bacteremia and death.
Pulmonary anthrax	Inhalation of spores → flu-like symptoms that rapidly progress to fever, pulmonary hemorrhage, mediastinitis, and shock.	Woolsorters' disease—inhalation of spores from contaminated wool.

Bacillus cereus	Causes food poisoning. Spores survive cooking rice. Keeping rice warm results in germination of spores and enterotoxin formation. Emetic type usually seen with rice and pasta. Nausea and vomiting within 1–5 hr. Caused by cereulide, a preformed toxin. Diarrheal type causes watery, nonbloody diarrhea and GI pain within 8–18 hr.	Reheated rice syndrome.

Listeria monocytogenes	Facultative intracellular microbe; acquired by ingestion of unpasteurized dairy products and deli meats, via transplacental transmission, or by vaginal transmission during birth. Form "rocket tails" (via actin polymerization) that allow them to move through the cytoplasm and into the cell membrane, thereby avoiding antibody. Characteristic tumbling motility; is only gram-positive organism to produce LPS.
	Can cause amnionitis, septicemia, and spontaneous abortion in pregnant women; granulomatosis infantiseptica; neonatal meningitis; meningitis in immunocompromised patients; mild gastroenteritis in healthy individuals. Treatment: gastroenteritis usually self-limited; ampicillin in infants, immunocompromised patients, and the elderly in empirical treatment of meningitis.

Actinomyces vs. Nocardia

Both form long, branching filaments resembling fungi.

Actinomyces	Nocardia
Gram-positive anaerobe A	Gram-positive aerobe
Not acid fast	Acid fast (weak) B
Normal oral flora	Found in soil
Causes oral/facial abscesses that drain through sinus tracts, forms yellow "sulfur granules"	Causes pulmonary infections in immunocompromised and cutaneous infections after trauma in immunocompetent
Treat with penicillin	Treat with sulfonamides

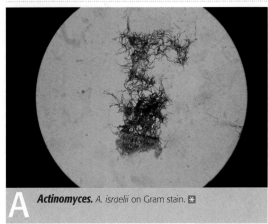

A **Actinomyces.** *A. israelii* on Gram stain. ✱

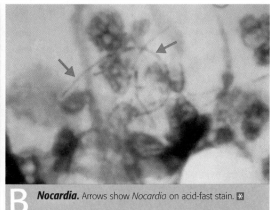

B **Nocardia.** Arrows show *Nocardia* on acid-fast stain. ✱

1° and 2° tuberculosis

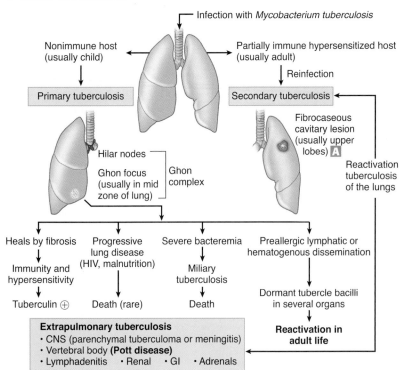

Infection with *Mycobacterium tuberculosis*

Nonimmune host (usually child) — Partially immune hypersensitized host (usually adult)

Primary tuberculosis

Reinfection

Secondary tuberculosis ← Reactivation tuberculosis of the lungs

Fibrocaseous cavitary lesion (usually upper lobes) A

Hilar nodes

Ghon focus (usually in mid zone of lung) — Ghon complex

Heals by fibrosis → Immunity and hypersensitivity → Tuberculin ⊕

Progressive lung disease (HIV, malnutrition) → Death (rare)

Severe bacteremia → Miliary tuberculosis → Death

Preallergic lymphatic or hematogenous dissemination → Dormant tubercle bacilli in several organs → **Reactivation in adult life**

Extrapulmonary tuberculosis
- CNS (parenchymal tuberculoma or meningitis)
- Vertebral body **(Pott disease)**
- Lymphadenitis　· Renal　· GI　· Adrenals

PPD⊕ if current infection, past exposure, or BCG vaccinated.

PPD⊖ if no infection or anergic (steroids, malnutrition, immunocompromise) and in sarcoidosis.

Interferon-γ release assay (IGRA) is a more specific test; has fewer false positives from BCG vaccination.

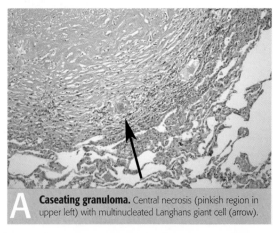

A **Caseating granuloma.** Central necrosis (pinkish region in upper left) with multinucleated Langhans giant cell (arrow).

Mycobacteria

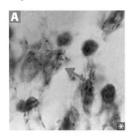

Mycobacterium tuberculosis (TB, often resistant to multiple drugs).

M. kansasii (pulmonary TB-like symptoms).

M. avium–intracellulare (causes disseminated, non-TB disease in AIDS; often resistant to multiple drugs). Prophylactic treatment with azithromycin.

All mycobacteria are acid-fast organisms 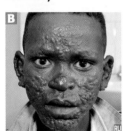.

TB symptoms include fever, night sweats, weight loss, and hemoptysis.

Cord factor in virulent strains inhibits macrophage maturation and induces release of TNF-α. Sulfatides (surface glycolipids) inhibit phagolysosomal fusion.

Leprosy (Hansen disease)

Caused by *Mycobacterium leprae*, an acid-fast bacillus that likes cool temperatures (infects skin and superficial nerves—"glove and stocking" loss of sensation) and cannot be grown in vitro. Reservoir in United States: armadillos.

Hansen disease has 2 forms:

- **Lepromatous**—presents diffusely over the skin 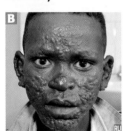, with leonine (lion-like) facies , and is communicable; characterized by low cell-mediated immunity with a humoral Th_2 response.
- **Tuberculoid**—limited to a few hypoesthetic, hairless skin plaques; characterized by high cell-mediated immunity with a largely Th_1-type immune response.

Treatment: multidrug therapy consisting of dapsone and rifampin for 6 months for tuberculoid form; and dapsone, rifampin, and clofazimine for 2–5 years for lepromatous form.

Lepromatous can be lethal.

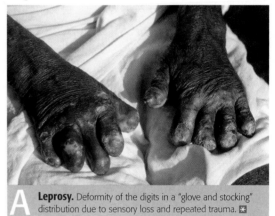

Leprosy. Deformity of the digits in a "glove and stocking" distribution due to sensory loss and repeated trauma.

Gram-negative lab algorithm

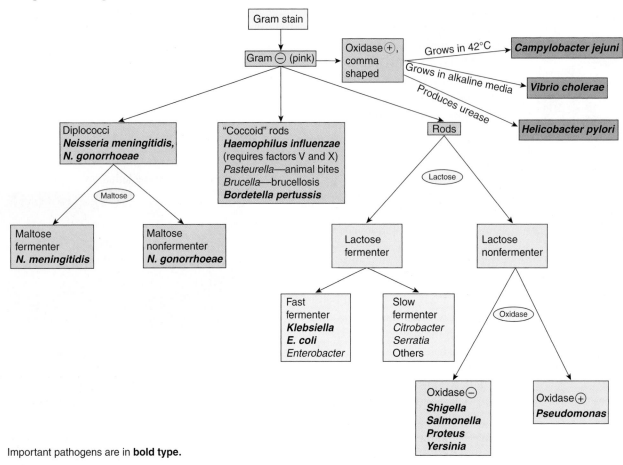

Important pathogens are in **bold type.**

Lactose-fermenting enteric bacteria	Grow pink colonies on MacConkey agar. Examples include *Citrobacter*, *Klebsiella*, *E. coli*, *Enterobacter*, and *Serratia* (weak fermenter). *E. coli* produces β-galactosidase, which breaks down lactose into glucose and galactose.	Lactose is **KEE**. Test with MacCon**KEE'S** agar. EMB agar—lactose fermenters grow as purple/black colonies. *E. coli* grows purple colonies with a green sheen.
Penicillin and gram-negative bugs	Gram-negative bacilli are resistant to penicillin G but may be susceptible to penicillin derivatives such as ampicillin and amoxicillin. The gram-negative outer membrane layer inhibits entry of penicillin G and vancomycin.	

Neisseria

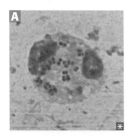

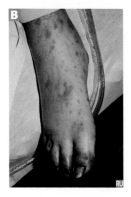

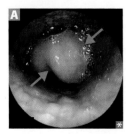

Gram-negative diplococci. Both ferment glucose and produce IgA proteases. *N. gonorrhoeae* is often intracellular (within neutrophils) **A**.

MeninGococci ferment Maltose and Glucose. Gonococci ferment Glucose.

Gonococci	Meningococci
No polysaccharide capsule	Polysaccharide capsule
No maltose fermentation	Maltose fermentation
No vaccine (due to rapid antigenic variation of pilus proteins)	Vaccine (none for type B)
Sexually transmitted	Respiratory and oral secretions
Causes gonorrhea, septic arthritis, neonatal conjunctivitis, pelvic inflammatory disease (PID), and Fitz-Hugh–Curtis syndrome	Causes meningococcemia **B** and meningitis, Waterhouse-Friderichsen syndrome
Condoms prevent sexual transmission. Erythromycin ointment prevents neonatal transmission	Rifampin, ciprofloxacin, or ceftriaxone prophylaxis in close contacts
Treatment: ceftriaxone + (azithromycin or doxycycline) for possible chlamydia coinfection	Treatment: ceftriaxone or penicillin G

Haemophilus influenzae

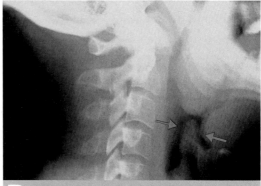

Small gram-negative (coccobacillary) rod. Aerosol transmission. Most invasive disease caused by capsular type B. Nontypeable strains cause mucosal infections (otitis media, conjunctivitis, bronchitis). Produces IgA protease. Culture on **chocolate** agar requires factors **V** (NAD⁺) and **X** (hematin) for growth; can also be grown with *S. aureus*, which provides factor V. *HaEMOPhilus* causes Epiglottitis **A B** ("cherry red" in children), Meningitis, Otitis media, and Pneumonia.

Treat mucosal infections with amoxicillin +/– clavulanate.

Treat meningitis with ceftriaxone. Rifampin prophylaxis in close contacts.

When a child has "flu," mom goes to five (**V**) and dime (**X**) store to buy some **chocolate**.

Vaccine contains type B capsular polysaccharide (polyribosylribitol phosphate) conjugated to diphtheria toxoid or other protein. Given between 2 and 18 months of age.

Does not cause the flu (influenza virus does).

B ***Haemophilus influenzae* epiglottitis.** Thickening of the epiglottis ("thumbprint sign") on lateral neck radiograph.

Legionella pneumophila	Gram-negative rod. Gram stains poorly—use silver stain. Grow on **charcoal** yeast extract culture with **iron** and **cysteine**. Detected clinically by presence of antigen in urine. Aerosol transmission from environmental water source habitat (e.g., air conditioning systems, hot water tanks). No person-to-person transmission. Treatment: macrolide or quinolone.	Labs show hyponatremia.
	Legionnaires' disease = severe pneumonia, fever, GI and CNS symptoms. **Pontiac fever** = mild flu-like syndrome.	Think of a French **legionnaire** (soldier) with his **silver** helmet, sitting around a campfire (**charcoal**) with his **iron** dagger—he is no **sissy** (cysteine).

Pseudomonas aeruginosa 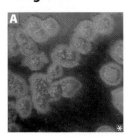	Aerobic gram-negative rod. Non-lactose fermenting, oxidase ⊕. Produces pyocyanin (blue-green pigment **A**); has a grape-like odor. Water source. Produces endotoxin (fever, shock) and exotoxin A (inactivates EF-2). **PSEUDO***monas* is associated with **w**ound and burn infections, **P**neumonia (especially in cystic fibrosis), **S**epsis, **E**xternal otitis (swimmer's ear), **U**TI, **D**rug use and **D**iabetic **O**steomyelitis, and hot tub folliculitis. Malignant otitis externa in diabetics. **Ecthyma gangrenosum**—rapidly progressive, necrotic cutaneous lesions **B** caused by *Pseudomonas* bacteremia. Typically seen in immunocompromised patients. Treatment: aminoglycoside plus extended-spectrum penicillin (e.g., piperacillin, ticarcillin, cefepime, imipenem, meropenem).	Aeruginosa—aerobic. Think water connection and blue-green pigment. Think *Pseudomonas* in burn victims. Chronic pneumonia in cystic fibrosis patients is associated with biofilm. 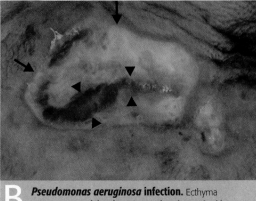 **B** ***Pseudomonas aeruginosa* infection.** Ecthyma gangrenosum of the chest. Large ulcer (arrows) with necrotic region (arrowheads). ✳

E. coli	*E. coli* virulence factors: fimbriae—cystitis and pyelonephritis; K capsule—pneumonia, neonatal meningitis; LPS endotoxin—septic shock.	
STRAIN	**TOXIN AND MECHANISM**	**PRESENTATION**
EIEC	Microbe invades intestinal mucosa and causes necrosis and inflammation. Clinical manifestations similar to *Shigella*.	Invasive; dysentery.
ETEC	Produces heat-labile and heat-stable enteroToxins. No inflammation or invasion.	Travelers' diarrhea (watery).
EPEC	No toxin produced. Adheres to apical surface, flattens villi, prevents absorption.	Diarrhea usually in children (Pediatrics).
EHEC	O157:H7 is the most common serotype. Produces Shiga-like toxin that causes Hemolytic-uremic syndrome (triad of anemia, thrombocytopenia, and acute renal failure). Also called STEC (Shiga toxin–producing *E. coli*). Microthrombi form on endothelium damaged by toxin → mechanical hemolysis (schistocytes formed) and ↓ renal blood flow; microthrombi consume platelets → thrombocytopenia.	Dysentery (toxin alone causes necrosis and inflammation). Does not ferment sorbitol (distinguishes it from other *E. coli*).

Klebsiella	An intestinal flora that causes lobar pneumonia in alcoholics and diabetics when aspirated. Very mucoid colonies caused by abundant polysaccharide capsules. Red "currant jelly" sputum. Also cause of nosocomial UTIs.	4 A's: Aspiration pneumonia Abscess in lungs and liver Alcoholics di-A-betics

Salmonella vs. Shigella	**Salmonella**	**Shigella**
	Have flagella (**salmon** swim)	No flagella
	Can disseminate hematogenously	Cell to cell transmission; no hematogenous spread
	Have many animal reservoirs	Only reservoirs are humans and primates
	Produce hydrogen sulfide	Does not produce hydrogen sulfide
	Antibiotics may prolong fecal excretion of organism	Antibiotics shorten duration of fecal excretion of organism
	Invades intestinal mucosa and causes a monocytic response	Invades intestinal mucosa and causes PMN infiltration
	Can cause bloody diarrhea	Often causes bloody diarrhea
	Does not ferment lactose	Does not ferment lactose

Salmonella typhi	Causes typhoid fever. Found only in humans. Characterized by rose spots on the abdomen, fever, headache, and diarrhea. Can remain in gallbladder and cause a carrier state.

Campylobacter jejuni

Major cause of bloody diarrhea, especially in children. Fecal-oral transmission through foods such as poultry, meat, unpasteurized milk. Comma or S-shaped, oxidase ⊕, grows at 42°C ("*Campylobacter* likes the hot **camp**fire"). Common antecedent to Guillain-Barré syndrome and reactive arthritis.

Vibrio cholerae

Produces profuse rice-water diarrhea via enterotoxin that permanently activates G_s, ↑ cAMP. Comma shaped, oxidase ⊕, grows in alkaline media. Endemic to developing countries. Prompt oral rehydration is necessary.

Yersinia enterocolitica

Usually transmitted from pet feces (e.g., puppies), contaminated milk, or pork. Causes mesenteric adenitis that can mimic Crohn disease or appendicitis.

Helicobacter pylori

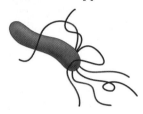

Causes gastritis and peptic ulcers (especially duodenal). Risk factor for peptic ulcer, gastric adenocarcinoma and lymphoma. Curved gram-negative rod that is catalase, oxidase, and urease ⊕ (can use urea breath test or fecal antigen test for diagnosis). Creates alkaline environment. Most common initial treatment is triple therapy: proton pump inhibitor + clarithromycin + either amoxicillin or metronidazole.

Spirochetes

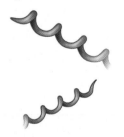

The spirochetes are spiral-shaped bacteria with axial filaments and include *Borrelia* (big size), *Leptospira*, and *Treponema*. Only *Borrelia* can be visualized using aniline dyes (Wright or Giemsa stain) in light microscopy. *Treponema* is visualized by dark-field microscopy.

BLT.
B is **B**ig.

Leptospira interrogans

Found in water contaminated with animal urine, causes leptospirosis: flu-like symptoms, jaundice, photophobia with conjunctival suffusion (erythema without exudate). Prevalent among surfers and in tropics (i.e., Hawaii).

Weil disease (icterohemorrhagic leptospirosis)—severe form with jaundice and azotemia from liver and kidney dysfunction; fever, hemorrhage, and anemia.

Lyme disease

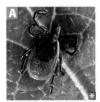

Caused by *Borrelia burgdorferi*, which is transmitted by the tick *Ixodes* 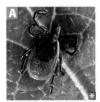 (also vector for *Babesia*). Natural reservoir is the mouse. Mice are important to tick life cycle.

Common in northeastern United States.

- Initial symptoms—erythema chronicum migrans **B**, flu-like symptoms, +/− facial nerve palsy.
- Later symptoms—monoarthritis (large joints) and migratory polyarthritis, cardiac (AV nodal block), neurologic (encephalopathy, facial nerve palsy, polyneuropathy).

Treatment: doxycycline, ceftriaxone.

FAKE a Key Lyme pie:
Facial nerve palsy (typically bilateral)
Arthritis
Kardiac block
Erythema migrans

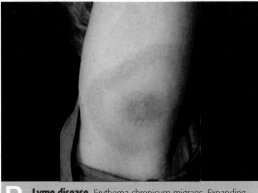

B **Lyme disease.** Erythema chronicum migrans. Expanding "bull's eye" red rash. ✱

Syphilis

Caused by spirochete *Treponema pallidum.*

Treatment: penicillin G.

1° syphilis

Localized disease presenting with **painless** chancre **A**. If available, use dark-field microscopy to visualize treponemes in fluid from chancre **B**. Serologic testing: VDRL/RPR (non-specifc), confirm diagnosis with specific test (e.g., FTA-ABS).

2° syphilis

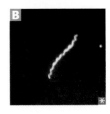

Disseminated disease with constitutional symptoms, maculopapular rash (palms and soles), condylomata lata (also confirmable with dark-field microscopy).

Serologic testing: VDRL/RPR (non-specific), confirm diagnosis with specific test (e.g., FTA-ABS).

Secondary syphilis = **S**ystemic. Latent syphilis (⊕ serology without symptoms) follows.

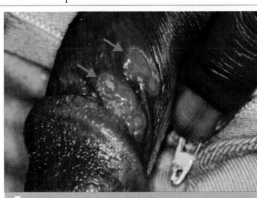

A **Painless chancre.** Painless ulcerated lesions on shaft of penis. ✱

3° syphilis

Gummas (chronic granulomas), aortitis (vasa vasorum destruction), neurosyphilis (tabes dorsalis, "general paresis"), Argyll Robertson pupil.

Signs: broad-based ataxia, ⊕ Romberg, Charcot joint, stroke without hypertension.

For neurosyphilis: test spinal fluid with VDRL or RPR.

Congenital syphilis

Saber shins, saddle nose, CN VIII deafness, Hutchinson teeth, mulberry molars.

To prevent, treat mother early in pregnancy, as placental transmission typically occurs after first trimester.

Argyll Robertson pupil	Argyll Robertson pupil constricts with accommodation but is not reactive to light. Associated with 3° syphilis.	"Prostitute pupil"—accommodates but does not react.

VDRL false positives	VDRL detects nonspecific antibody that reacts with beef cardiolipin. Inexpensive, widely available test for syphilis, quantitative, sensitive but not specific. Many false positives, including viral infection (e.g., mononucleosis [EBV], hepatitis), some drugs, and SLE.	**VDRL:** **V**iruses (mono, hepatitis) **D**rugs **R**heumatic fever **L**upus and leprosy

Jarisch-Herxheimer reaction	Flu-like syndrome after antibiotics are started—due to killed bacteria releasing pyrogens.

Zoonotic bacteria	Zoonosis: infectious disease transmitted between animals and humans.

SPECIES	DISEASE	TRANSMISSION AND SOURCE
Anaplasma spp.	Anaplasmosis	*Ixodes* ticks (live on deer and mice)
Bartonella spp.	Cat scratch disease, bacillary angiomatosis	Cat scratch
Borrelia burgdorferi	Lyme disease	*Ixodes* ticks (live on deer and mice)
Borrelia recurrentis	Relapsing fever	Louse (recurrent due to variable surface antigens)
Brucella spp.	Brucellosis/undulant fever	Unpasteurized dairy
Campylobacter	Bloody diarrhea	Puppies, livestock (fecal-oral, ingestion of undercooked meat)
Chlamydophila psittaci	Psittacosis	Parrots, other birds
Coxiella burnetii	Q fever	Aerosols of cattle/sheep amniotic fluid
Ehrlichia chaffeensis	Ehrlichiosis	Lone Star ticks
Francisella tularensis	Tularemia	Ticks, rabbits, deer fly
Leptospira spp.	Leptospirosis	Animal urine
Mycobacterium leprae	Leprosy	Humans with lepromatous leprosy; armadillo (rare)
Pasteurella multocida	Cellulitis, osteomyelitis	Animal bite, cats, dogs
Rickettsia prowazekii	Epidemic typhus	Louse
Rickettsia rickettsii	Rocky Mountain spotted fever	*Dermacentor* ticks
Rickettsia typhi	Endemic typhus	Fleas
Yersinia pestis	Plague	Fleas (rats and prairie dogs are reservoirs)

Gardnerella vaginalis

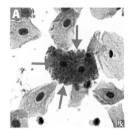

A pleomorphic, gram-variable rod that is involved in vaginosis. Presents as a gray vaginal discharge with a **fishy** smell; nonpainful (vs. vaginitis). Associated with sexual activity, but not sexually transmitted. Bacterial vaginosis is also characterized by overgrowth of certain anaerobic bacteria in vagina. **Clue** cells, or vaginal epithelial cells covered with *Gardnerella* bacteria, are visible under the microscope (arrow) **A**.

Treatment: metronidazole or (to treat anaerobic bacteria) clindamycin.

I don't have a **clue** why I smell **fish** in the **vagina garden**!

Rickettsial diseases and vector-borne illness	Treatment for all: doxycycline.	
RASH COMMON		
Rocky Mountain spotted fever	*Rickettsia rickettsii*, vector is tick. Despite its name, disease occurs primarily in the South Atlantic states, especially North Carolina. Rash typically starts at wrists and ankles and then spreads to trunk, palms, and soles 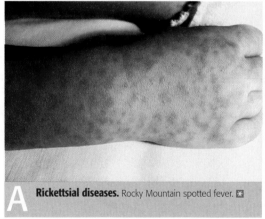. Rickettsiae are obligate intracellular organisms that need CoA and NAD⁺ because they cannot synthesize ATP.	Classic triad—headache, fever, rash (vasculitis). **Palms** and **soles** rash is seen in Coxsackievirus **A** infection (hand, foot, and mouth disease), **R**ocky Mountain spotted fever, and 2° **S**yphilis (you drive **CARS** using your **palms** and **soles**).
Typhus	Endemic (fleas)—*R. typhi*. Epidemic (human body louse)—*R. prowazekii*. Rash starts centrally and spreads out, sparing palms and soles.	*Rickettsii* on the w**R**ists, **T**yphus on the **T**runk.
RASH RARE		
Ehrlichiosis	*Ehrlichia*; vector is tick. Monocytes with morulae 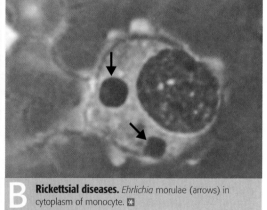 (berry-like inclusions) in cytoplasm.	
Anaplasmosis	*Anaplasma*, vector is tick. Granulocytes with morulae in cytoplasm.	
Q fever	*Coxiella burnetii*; no arthropod vector. Tick feces and cattle placenta release spores that are inhaled as aerosols. Presents as pneumonia.	**Q** fever is **Q**ueer because it has no rash or vector and its causative organism can survive outside in its endospore form. Not in the *Rickettsia* genus, but closely related.

A **Rickettsial diseases.** Rocky Mountain spotted fever. ✴

B **Rickettsial diseases.** *Ehrlichia* morulae (arrows) in cytoplasm of monocyte. ✴

Chlamydiae

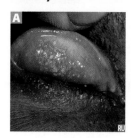

Chlamydiae cannot make their own ATP. They are obligate intracellular organisms that cause mucosal infections. 2 forms:

- Elementary body (small, dense) is "**E**nfectious" and **E**nters cell via **E**ndocytosis; transforms into reticulate body.
- Reticulate body **R**eplicates in cell by fission; reorganizes into elementary bodies.

Chlamydia trachomatis causes reactive arthritis (Reiter syndrome), follicular conjunctivitis **A**, nongonococcal urethritis, and PID.

C. pneumoniae and *C. psittaci* cause atypical pneumonia; transmitted by aerosol.

Treatment: azithromycin (favored because one-time treatment) or doxycycline.

Chlamys = cloak (intracellular).
Chlamydophila psittaci—notable for an avian reservoir.
Lab diagnosis: cytoplasmic inclusions seen on Giemsa or fluorescent antibody–stained smear.
The chlamydial cell wall is unusual in that it lacks muramic acid.

Chlamydia trachomatis serotypes

Types A, B, and C	Chronic infection, cause blindness due to follicular conjunctivitis in Africa.	ABC = Africa/Blindness/Chronic infection.
Types D–K	Urethritis/PID, ectopic pregnancy, neonatal pneumonia (staccato cough), neonatal conjunctivitis.	D–K = everything else. Neonatal disease can be acquired during passage through infected birth canal.
Types L1, L2, and L3	Lymphogranuloma venereum—small, painless ulcers on genitals → swollen, painful inguinal lymph nodes that ulcerate ("buboes"). Treat with doxycycline.	

Mycoplasma pneumoniae

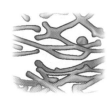

Classic cause of atypical "walking" pneumonia (insidious onset, headache, nonproductive cough, patchy or diffuse interstitial infiltrate). X-ray looks worse than patient. High titer of cold agglutinins (IgM), which can agglutinate or lyse RBCs. Grown on Eaton agar.
Treatment: macrolide, doxycycline, or fluoroquinolone (penicillin ineffective since *Mycoplasma* have no cell wall).

No cell wall. Not seen on Gram stain.
Bacterial membrane contains sterols for stability.
Mycoplasmal pneumonia is more common in patients <30 years old.
Frequent outbreaks in military recruits and prisons.

▸ **MICROBIOLOGY–MYCOLOGY**

Systemic mycoses	All of the following can cause pneumonia and can disseminate. All are caused by dimorphic fungi: cold (20°C) = mold; heat (37°C) = yeast. The only exception is coccidioidomycosis, which is a spherule (not yeast) in tissue. Treatment: fluconazole or itraconazole for **local** infection; amphotericin B for **systemic** infection. Systemic mycoses can mimic TB (granuloma formation), except, unlike TB, have no person-person transmission.

DISEASE	ENDEMIC LOCATION AND PATHOLOGIC FEATURES	NOTES
Histoplasmosis	Mississippi and Ohio River valleys. Causes pneumonia. Macrophage filled with *Histoplasma* (smaller than RBC) **A**.	Histo hides (within macrophages). Bird or bat droppings.
Blastomycosis	States east of Mississippi River and Central America. Causes inflammatory lung disease and can disseminate to skin and bone. Forms granulomatous nodules. Broad-base budding (same size as RBC) **B**.	Blasto buds broadly.
Coccidioidomycosis	Southwestern United States, California. Causes pneumonia and meningitis; can disseminate to bone and skin. Case rate ↑ after earthquakes (spores in dust are thrown up in the air and become spherules in lungs). Spherule (much larger than RBC) filled with endospores **C**.	Coccidio crowds. "(San Joaquin) Valley fever" "Desert bumps" = erythema nodosum "Desert rheumatism" = arthralgias
Paracoccidioidomycosis	Latin America. Budding yeast with "**captain's wheel**" formation (much larger than RBC) **D**.	Paracoccidio parasails with the **captain's wheel** all the way to **Latin America**.

Cutaneous mycoses

Tinea versicolor 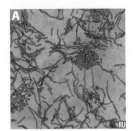	Caused by *Malassezia furfur*. Degradation of lipids produces acids that damage melanocytes and cause hypopigmented and/or hyperpigmented patches. Occurs in hot, humid weather. Treatment: topical miconazole, selenium sulfide (Selsun). "Spaghetti and meatball" appearance **A**.
Other tineae	Includes tinea pedis (foot), tinea cruris (groin), tinea corporis (ringworm, on body), tinea capitis (head, scalp), tinea unguium (onychomycosis, on fingernails). Pruritic lesions with central clearing resembling a ring, caused by dermatophytes (*Microsporum*, *Trichophyton*, and *Epidermophyton*). See mold hyphae in KOH prep, not dimorphic.

Opportunistic fungal infections

Candida albicans [A]

alba = white.

Systemic or superficial fungal infection. Oral and esophageal thrush in immunocompromised (neonates, steroids, diabetes, AIDS), vulvovaginitis (diabetes, use of antibiotics), diaper rash, endocarditis in IV drug users, disseminated candidiasis (to any organ), chronic mucocutaneous candidiasis.

Treatment: topical azole for vaginal; fluconazole or caspofungin for oral/esophageal; fluconazole, amphotericin B, or caspofungin for systemic.

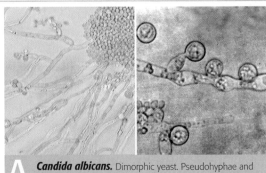

A *Candida albicans.* Dimorphic yeast. Pseudohyphae and budding yeasts at 20°C (left). ✴ Germ tubes at 37°C (right). ✴

Aspergillus fumigatus [B]

Invasive aspergillosis, especially in immunocompromised and those with chronic granulomatous disease.

Allergic bronchopulmonary aspergillosis (ABPA): associated with asthma and cystic fibrosis; may cause bronchiectasis and eosinophilia.

Aspergillomas in lung cavities, especially after TB infection.

Some species of *Aspergillus* produce aflatoxins, which are associated with hepatocellular carcinoma.

Think "A" for Acute Angles in Aspergillus. Not dimorphic.

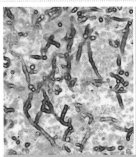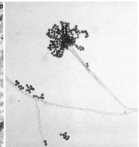

B *Aspergillus fumigatus.* Septate hyphae that branch at 45° angle (left). ✴ Conidiophore with radiating chains of spores (right). ✴

Cryptococcus neoformans [C]

Cryptococcal meningitis, cryptococcosis. Heavily encapsulated yeast. Not dimorphic. Found in soil, pigeon droppings. Acquired through inhalation with hematogenous dissemination to meninges. Culture on Sabouraud agar. Stains with India ink and mucicarmine. Latex agglutination test detects polysaccharide capsular antigen and is more specific. "Soap bubble" lesions in brain.

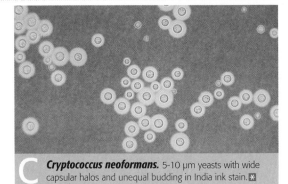

C *Cryptococcus neoformans.* 5-10 μm yeasts with wide capsular halos and unequal budding in India ink stain. ✴

Mucor [D] **and Rhizopus** spp.

Mucormycosis. Disease mostly in ketoacidotic diabetic and leukemic patients. Fungi proliferate in blood vessel walls when there is excess ketone and glucose, penetrate cribriform plate, and enter brain. Rhinocerebral, frontal lobe abscesses. Headache, facial pain, black necrotic eschar on face; may have cranial nerve involvement.

Treatment: amphotericin B.

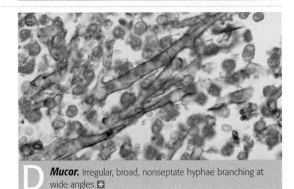

D *Mucor.* Irregular, broad, nonseptate hyphae branching at wide angles. ✴

Pneumocystis jirovecii

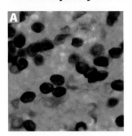

Causes *Pneumocystis* pneumonia (PCP), a diffuse interstitial pneumonia. Yeast (originally classified as protozoan). Inhaled. Most infections are asymptomatic. Immunosuppression (e.g., AIDS) predisposes to disease. Diffuse, bilateral CXR appearance. Diagnosed by lung biopsy or lavage. Disc-shaped yeast forms on methenamine silver stain of lung tissue **A**.

Treatment/prophylaxis: TMP-SMX, pentamidine, dapsone (prophylaxis only), atovaquone (prophylaxis only). Start prophylaxis when CD4 count drops < 200 cells/mm^3 in HIV patients.

Sporothrix schenckii

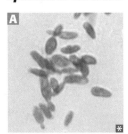

Sporotrichosis. Dimorphic, cigar-shaped budding yeast that lives on vegetation **A**. When spores are traumatically introduced into the skin, typically by a thorn ("**rose** gardener's" disease), causes local pustule or ulcer with nodules along draining lymphatics (ascending lymphangitis). Little systemic illness.

Treatment: itraconazole or **pot**assium iodide.

"Plant a **rose** in the **pot**."

▶ MICROBIOLOGY–PARASITOLOGY

Protozoa—GI infections

ORGANISM	DISEASE	TRANSMISSION	DIAGNOSIS	TREATMENT
Giardia lamblia	Giardiasis: bloating, flatulence, foul-smelling, fatty diarrhea (often seen in campers/hikers)— think fat-rich Ghirardelli chocolates for fatty stools of *Giardia*	Cysts in water	Trophozoites A or cysts B in stool	Metronidazole
Entamoeba histolytica	Amebiasis: bloody diarrhea (dysentery), liver abscess ("anchovy paste" exudate), RUQ pain (histology shows flask-shaped ulcer if submucosal abscess of colon ruptures)	Cysts in water	Serology and/or trophozoites (with RBCs in the cytoplasm) C or cysts (with up to 4 nuclei) D in stool	Metronidazole; iodoquinol for asymptomatic cyst passers
Cryptosporidium	Severe diarrhea in AIDS Mild disease (watery diarrhea) in nonimmunocompromised	Oocysts in water	Oocysts on acid-fast stain E	Prevention (by filtering city water supplies); nitazoxanide in immunocompetent hosts

Protozoa–CNS infections

ORGANISM	DISEASE	TRANSMISSION	DIAGNOSIS	TREATMENT
Toxoplasma gondii	Brain abscess in HIV (seen as ring-enhancing brain lesions on CT/MRI); congenital toxoplasmosis = "classic triad" of chorioretinitis, hydrocephalus, and intracranial calcifications	Cysts in meat or oocysts in cat feces; crosses placenta (pregnant women should avoid cats)	Serology, biopsy (tachyzoite) A	Sulfadiazine + pyrimethamine
Naegleria fowleri	Rapidly fatal meningoencephalitis	Swimming in **freshwater** lakes (think **Nalgene** bottle filled with **fresh water** containing *Naegleria*); enters via cribriform plate	Amoebas in spinal fluid B	Amphotericin B has been effective for a few survivors
Trypanosoma brucei	African sleeping sickness: enlarged lymph nodes, recurring fever (due to antigenic variation), somnolence, coma Two subspecies: *Trypanosoma brucei rhodesiense, Trypanosoma brucei gambiense*	Tsetse fly, a painful bite	Blood smear C	**Suramin** for blood-borne disease or **melarsoprol** for CNS penetration ("it **sure** is nice to go to sleep"; **melatonin** helps with sleep)

Protozoa–Hematologic infections

ORGANISM	DISEASE	TRANSMISSION	DIAGNOSIS	TREATMENT
Plasmodium **P. vivax/ovale** **P. falciparum** **P. malariae** 	Malaria: fever, headache, anemia, splenomegaly P. vivax/ovale—48-hr cycle (tertian; includes fever on first day and third day, thus fevers are actually 48 hr apart); dormant form (hypnozoite) in liver P. falciparum—severe; irregular fever patterns; parasitized RBCs occlude capillaries in brain (cerebral malaria), kidneys, lungs P. malariae—72-hr cycle (quartan)	Mosquito (Anopheles)	Blood smear, trophozoite ring form within RBC **A**, schizont containing merozoites **B** 	Begin with chloroquine, which blocks Plasmodium heme polymerase; if resistant, use mefloquine or atovaquone/proguanil If life-threatening, use intravenous quinidine (test for G6PD deficiency) Vivax/ovale—add primaquine for hypnozoite (test for G6PD deficiency)
Babesia 	Babesiosis: fever and hemolytic anemia; predominantly in northeastern United States; asplenia ↑ risk of severe disease	Ixodes tick (same as Borrelia burgdorferi of Lyme disease; may often coinfect humans)	Blood smear, ring form **C1**, "Maltese cross" **C2**; PCR	Atovaquone + azithromycin

Protozoa–Others

ORGANISM	DISEASE	TRANSMISSION	DIAGNOSIS	TREATMENT
Visceral infections				
Trypanosoma cruzi	Chagas disease: dilated cardiomyopathy, megacolon, megaesophagus; predominantly in South America	Reduviid bug ("kissing bug") feces, deposited in a painless bite (much like a kiss)	Blood smear Ⓐ	Benznidazole or nifurtimox
Leishmania donovani	Visceral leishmaniasis (kala-azar): spiking fevers, hepatosplenomegaly, pancytopenia	Sandfly	Macrophages containing amastigotes Ⓑ	Amphotericin B, sodium stibogluconate
STDs				
Trichomonas vaginalis	Vaginitis: foul-smelling, greenish discharge; itching and burning; do not confuse with *Gardnerella vaginalis*, a gram-variable bacterium associated with bacterial vaginosis	Sexual (cannot exist outside human because it cannot form cysts)	Trophozoites (motile) Ⓒ on wet mount; "strawberry cervix"	Metronidazole for patient and partner (prophylaxis)

Nematodes (roundworms)

ORGANISM	TRANSMISSION	DISEASE	TREATMENT
Intestinal			
Enterobius vermicularis (pinworm)	Fecal-oral	Intestinal infection causing anal pruritus (diagnosed via the Scotch Tape test)	Bendazoles or pyrantel pamoate (because worms are bendy)
Ascaris lumbricoides (giant roundworm)	Fecal-oral; eggs visible in feces under microscope	Intestinal infection	Bendazoles or pyrantel pamoate
Strongyloides stercoralis	Larvae in soil penetrate the skin	Intestinal infection causing vomiting, diarrhea, epigastric pain (may be peptic ulcer-like)	Ivermectin or albendazole
Ancylostoma duodenale, Necator americanus (hookworms)	Larvae penetrate skin	Intestinal infection causing anemia by sucking blood from intestinal walls	Bendazoles or pyrantel pamoate
Tissue			
Onchocerca volvulus	Female blackfly bite	Hyperpigmented skin and river blindness (**black** flies, **black** skin nodules, "**black** sight"); allergic reaction to microfilaria possible	Ivermectin (ivermectin for river blindness)
Loa loa	Deer fly, horse fly, mango fly	Swelling in skin, worm in conjunctiva	Diethylcarbamazine
Wuchereria bancrofti	Female mosquito	Blocks lymphatic vessels: elephantiasis; takes 9 mo–1 yr after bite to become symptomatic	Diethylcarbamazine
Toxocara canis	Fecal-oral	Visceral larva migrans	Albendazole or mebendazole

Nematode routes of infection	Ingested—*Enterobius, Ascaris, Toxocara* Cutaneous—*Strongyloides, Ancylostoma, Necator* Bites—*Loa loa, Onchocerca volvulus, Wuchereria bancrofti*	You'll get sick if you **EAT** these! These get into your feet from the **SAN**d. Lay **LOW** to avoid getting bitten.

Cestodes (tapeworms)

ORGANISM	TRANSMISSION	DISEASE	TREATMENT
Taenia solium	Ingestion of larvae encysted in undercooked pork	Intestinal infection	Praziquantel
	Ingestion of eggs	Cysticercosis, neurocysticercosis	Praziquantel; albendazole for neurocysticercosis
Diphyllobothrium latum	Ingestion of larvae from raw freshwater fish	Vitamin B_{12} deficiency (tapeworm competes for B_{12} in intestine) → anemia	Praziquantel
Echinococcus granulosus	Ingestion of eggs from dog feces	Hydatid cysts in liver, causing anaphylaxis if antigens released (surgeons preinject with ethanol to kill cysts before removal)	Albendazole

Trematodes (flukes)

ORGANISM	TRANSMISSION	DISEASE	TREATMENT
Schistosoma	Snails are host; cercariae penetrate skin of humans	Liver and spleen granulomas, fibrosis, and inflammation Chronic infection with *S. haematobium* can lead to squamous cell carcinoma of the bladder (painless hematuria)	Praziquantel
Clonorchis sinensis	Undercooked fish	Biliary tract inflammation → pigmented gallstones Associated with cholangiocarcinoma	Praziquantel

Parasite hints

ASSOCIATIONS	ORGANISM
Biliary tract disease, cholangiocarcinoma	*Clonorchis sinensis*
Brain cysts, seizures	*Taenia solium* (cysticercosis)
Hematuria, bladder cancer	*Schistosoma haematobium*
Liver (hydatid) cysts	*Echinococcus granulosus*
Microcytic anemia	*Ancylostoma, Necator*
Perianal pruritus	*Enterobius*
Portal hypertension	*Schistosoma mansoni, Schistosoma japonicum*
Vitamin B_{12} deficiency	*Diphyllobothrium latum*

▶ MICROBIOLOGY–VIROLOGY

Viral structure—general features

Naked virus with icosahedral capsid

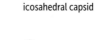
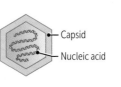

Capsid

Nucleic acid

Enveloped virus with icosahedral capsid

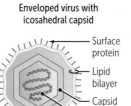

Surface protein

Lipid bilayer

Capsid

Nucleic acid

Enveloped virus with helical capsid

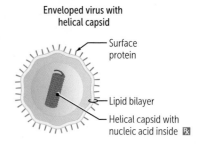

Surface protein

Lipid bilayer

Helical capsid with nucleic acid inside

Viral genetics

Recombination	Exchange of genes between 2 chromosomes by crossing over within regions of significant base sequence homology.
Reassortment	When viruses with segmented genomes (e.g., influenza virus) exchange segments. High-frequency recombination. Cause of worldwide influenza pandemics.
Complementation	When 1 of 2 viruses that infect the cell has a mutation that results in a nonfunctional protein. The nonmutated virus "complements" the mutated one by making a functional protein that serves both viruses.
Phenotypic mixing	Occurs with simultaneous infection of a cell with 2 viruses. Genome of virus A can be partially or completely coated (forming pseudovirion) with the surface proteins of virus B. Type B protein coat determines the tropism (infectivity) of the hybrid virus. However, the progeny from this infection have a type A coat that is encoded by its type A genetic material.

Viral vaccines

Live attenuated vaccines	Induce humoral and cell-mediated immunity but have reverted to virulence on rare occasions. Killed/inactivated vaccines induce only humoral immunity but are stable. Live attenuated—smallpox, yellow fever, chickenpox (VZV), Sabin polio virus, MMR, Influenza (intranasal).	No booster needed for live attenuated vaccines. Dangerous to give live vaccines to immunocompromised patients or their close contacts. "**Live!** One night only! See small yellow **chickens** get vaccinated with **Sabin** and **MMR**! It's incredible!" MMR = measles, mumps, rubella (live attenuated vaccine that can be given to HIV-positive patients who do not show signs of immunodeficiency).
Killed	Rabies, Influenza (injected), Salk Polio, and HAV vaccines.	Sal**K** = **K**illed. **RIP A**lways.
Recombinant	HBV (antigen = recombinant HBsAg), HPV (types 6, 11, 16, and 18).	

DNA viral genomes | All DNA viruses except the Parvoviridae are dsDNA.
All are linear except papilloma-, polyoma-, and hepadnaviruses (circular). | All are dsDNA (like our cells), except "part-of-a-virus" (parvovirus) is ssDNA.
Parvus = small. |

RNA viral genomes	All RNA viruses except Reoviridae are ssRNA. Positive-stranded RNA viruses: I went to a **retro** (retrovirus) **toga** (togavirus) party, where I drank **flavored** (flavivirus) **Corona** (coronavirus) and ate **hippy** (hepevirus) **California** (calicivirus) **pickles** (picornavirus).	All are ssRNA (like our mRNA), except "repeato-virus" (reovirus) is dsRNA.

Naked viral genome infectivity	Purified nucleic acids of most dsDNA (except poxviruses and HBV) and ⊕ strand ssRNA (≈ mRNA) viruses are infectious. Naked nucleic acids of ⊖ strand ssRNA and dsRNA viruses are not infectious. They require polymerases contained in the complete virion.

Viral replication

DNA viruses	All replicate in the nucleus (except poxvirus).
RNA viruses	All replicate in the cytoplasm (except influenza virus and retroviruses).

Viral envelopes	**Naked** (nonenveloped) viruses include **Papillomavirus, Adenovirus, Parvovirus, Polyomavirus, Calicivirus, Picornavirus, Reovirus,** and **Hepevirus.** Generally, enveloped viruses acquire their envelopes from plasma membrane when they exit from cell. Exceptions include herpesviruses, which acquire envelopes from nuclear membrane.	Give **PAPP** smears and **CPR** to a naked **Heppy** (hippy). DNA = **PAPP**; RNA = **CPR** and hepevirus.

DNA virus characteristics	Some general rules—all DNA viruses:

GENERAL RULE	COMMENTS
Are **HHAPPPP**y viruses	Hepadna, Herpes, Adeno, Pox, Parvo, Papilloma, Polyoma.
Are double stranded	Except parvo (single stranded).
Are linear	Except papilloma and polyoma (circular, supercoiled) and hepadna (circular, incomplete).
Are icosahedral	Except pox (complex).
Replicate in the nucleus	Except pox (carries own DNA-dependent RNA polymerase).

DNA viruses

VIRAL FAMILY	ENVELOPE	DNA STRUCTURE	MEDICAL IMPORTANCE
Herpesviruses	Yes	DS and linear	HSV-1—oral (and some genital) lesions, spontaneous temporal lobe encephalitis, keratoconjunctivitis HSV-2—genital (and some oral) lesions VZV (HHV-3)—chickenpox, zoster (shingles); vaccine available EBV (HHV-4)—mononucleosis, Burkitt lymphoma, Hodgkin lymphoma CMV (HHV-5)—infection in immunosuppressed patients (AIDS retinitis), especially transplant recipients; congenital defects ("**sight**omegalovirus") HHV-6—roseola (exanthem subitum) HHV-7—less common cause of roseola HHV-8—causes Kaposi sarcoma
Hepadnavirus	Yes	Partially DS and circular	HBV: ▪ Acute or chronic hepatitis ▪ Vaccine available—contains HBV surface antigen ▪ Not a retrovirus but has reverse transcriptase
Adenovirus	No	DS and linear	Febrile pharyngitis—sore throat Acute hemorrhagic cystitis Pneumonia Conjunctivitis—"pink eye"
Parvovirus	No	SS and linear (–) (smallest DNA virus)	B19 virus—aplastic crises in sickle cell disease, "slapped cheeks" rash in children—erythema infectiosum (fifth disease), RBC destruction in fetus leads to hydrops fetalis and death, pure RBC aplasia and rheumatoid arthritis–like symptoms in adults
Papillomavirus	No	DS and circular	HPV—warts (1, 2, 6, 11), CIN, cervical cancer (16, 18) vaccine available
Polyomavirus	No	DS and circular	JC virus—progressive multifocal leukoencephalopathy (PML) in HIV BK virus—transplant patients, commonly targets kidney (**JC**: Junky Cerebrum; **BK**: Bad Kidney)
Poxvirus	Yes	DS and linear (largest DNA virus)	Smallpox, although eradicated, could be used in germ warfare Cowpox ("milkmaid blisters") Molluscum contagiosum—flesh-colored dome lesions with central umbilicated dimple

DS, double-stranded; SS, single-stranded

Herpesviruses

HSV-1	Gingivostomatitis, keratoconjunctivitis **A**, temporal lobe encephalitis (most common cause of sporadic encephalitis in the United States), herpes labialis **B**. Latent in trigeminal ganglia. Transmitted by respiratory secretions, saliva.
HSV-2	Herpes genitalis **C**, neonatal herpes. Latent in sacral ganglia. Transmitted by sexual contact, perinatally.
VZV	Varicella-zoster (chickenpox, shingles) **D**, encephalitis, pneumonia. Latent in dorsal root or trigeminal ganglia. Most common complication of shingles is post-herpetic neuralgia. Transmitted by respiratory secretions.
EBV	Mononucleosis. Characterized by fever, hepatosplenomegaly, pharyngitis, and lymphadenopathy (especially posterior cervical nodes). Transmitted by respiratory secretions and saliva; also called "kissing disease" since commonly seen in teens, young adults. Infects B cells. Atypical lymphocytes seen on peripheral blood smear **E** are not infected B cells but rather reactive cytotoxic T cells. Detect by ⊕ Monospot test—heterophile antibodies detected by agglutination of sheep or horse RBCs. Associated with Hodgkin lymphoma, endemic Burkitt lymphoma, nasopharyngeal carcinoma.
CMV	Congenital infection, mononucleosis (⊖ Monospot), pneumonia, retinitis. Infected cells have characteristic "owl eye" inclusions **F**. Latent in mononuclear cells. Transmitted congenitally and by transfusion, sexual contact, saliva, urine, transplant.
HHV-6	Roseola: high fevers for several days that can cause seizures, followed by a diffuse macular rash **G**. Transmitted by saliva.
HHV-8	Kaposi sarcoma, a neoplasm of endothelial cells. Seen in HIV/AIDS and transplant patients. Dark/violaceous flat and nodular skin lesions **H** representing endothelial growths. Can also affect GI tract and lungs. Transmitted by sexual contact.

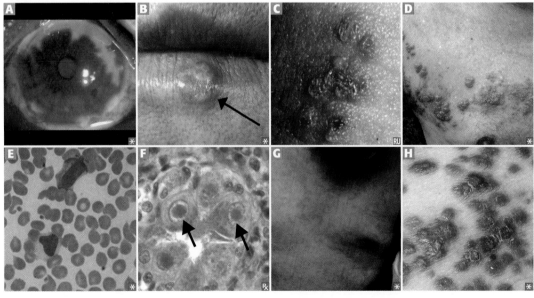

HSV identification

Viral culture for skin/genitalia.
CSF PCR for herpes encephalitis.
Tzanck test (genital herpes)—a smear of an opened skin vesicle to detect multinucleated giant cells 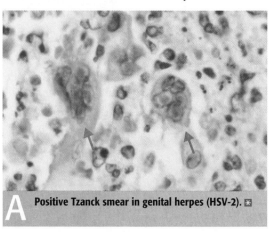.
Infected cells also have intranuclear Cowdry A inclusions.

Tzanck heavens I do not have herpes.

Positive Tzanck smear in genital herpes (HSV-2). ✷

RNA viruses

VIRAL FAMILY	ENVELOPE	RNA STRUCTURE	CAPSID SYMMETRY	MEDICAL IMPORTANCE
Reoviruses	No	DS linear 10–12 segments	Icosahedral (double)	Coltivirus[a]—Colorado tick fever Rotavirus—#1 cause of fatal diarrhea in children
Picornaviruses	No	SS ⊕ linear	Icosahedral	Poliovirus—polio-Salk/Sabin vaccines—IPV/OPV Echovirus—aseptic meningitis Rhinovirus—"common cold" Coxsackievirus—aseptic meningitis; herpangina (mouth blisters, fever); hand, foot, and mouth disease; myocarditis; pericarditis HAV—acute viral hepatitis **PERCH**
Hepevirus	No	SS ⊕ linear	Icosahedral	HEV
Caliciviruses	No	SS ⊕ linear	Icosahedral	Norovirus—viral gastroenteritis
Flaviviruses	Yes	SS ⊕ linear	Icosahedral	HCV Yellow fever[a] Dengue[a] St. Louis encephalitis[a] West Nile virus[a]
Togaviruses	Yes	SS ⊕ linear	Icosahedral	Rubella Eastern equine encephalitis[a] Western equine encephalitis[a]
Retroviruses	Yes	SS ⊕ linear	Icosahedral (HTLV), complex and conical (HIV)	Have reverse transcriptase HTLV—T-cell leukemia HIV—AIDS
Coronaviruses	Yes	SS ⊕ linear	Helical	Coronavirus—"common cold" and SARS
Orthomyxoviruses	Yes	SS ⊖ linear 8 segments	Helical	Influenza virus

Paramyxoviruses	Yes	SS ⊖ linear Nonsegmented	Helical	PaRaMyxovirus:
				     Parainfluenza—croup
				     RSV—bronchiolitis in babies; Rx—ribavirin
				     Measles, Mumps

Rhabdoviruses	Yes	SS ⊖ linear	Helical	Rabies
Filoviruses	Yes	SS ⊖ linear	Helical	Ebola/Marburg hemorrhagic fever—often fatal!
Arenaviruses	Yes	SS ⊖ circular 2 segments	Helical	LCMV—lymphocytic choriomeningitis virus Lassa fever encephalitis—spread by mice
Bunyaviruses	Yes	SS ⊖ circular 3 segments	Helical	California encephalitis[a] Sandfly/Rift Valley fevers[a] Crimean-Congo hemorrhagic fever[a] Hantavirus—hemorrhagic fever, pneumonia
Delta virus	Yes	SS ⊖ circular	Uncertain	HDV is a "defective" virus that requires HBV co-infection

SS, single-stranded; DS, double-stranded; ⊕, positive sense; ⊖, negative sense; [a]= arbovirus, transmitted by arthropods (mosquitoes, ticks).

(Adapted, with permission, from Levinson W, Jawetz E. *Medical Microbiology and Immunology: Examination and Board Review,* 6th ed. New York: McGraw-Hill, 2000: 182.)

Negative-stranded viruses	Must transcribe ⊖ strand to ⊕. Virion brings its own RNA-dependent RNA polymerase. They include Arenaviruses, Bunyaviruses, Paramyxoviruses, Orthomyxoviruses, Filoviruses, and Rhabdoviruses.	**A**lways **B**ring **P**olymerase **O**r **F**ail **R**eplication.
Segmented viruses	All are RNA viruses. They include **B**unyaviruses, **O**rthomyxoviruses (influenza viruses), **A**renaviruses, and **R**eoviruses.	**BOAR.**
Picornavirus	Includes **P**oliovirus, **E**chovirus, **R**hinovirus, **C**oxsackievirus, **H**AV. RNA is translated into 1 large polypeptide that is cleaved by proteases into functional viral proteins. Can cause aseptic (viral) meningitis (except rhinovirus and HAV). All are enteroviruses (fecal-oral spread) except rhinovirus.	**Pico**RNA**virus** = small **RNA** virus. **PERCH** on a "peak" (pico).
Rhinovirus	A picornavirus. Nonenveloped RNA virus. Cause of common cold; > 100 serologic types. Acid labile—destroyed by stomach acid; therefore, does not infect the GI tract (unlike the other picornaviruses).	**Rhino** has a runny nose.
Yellow fever virus	A flavivirus (also an arbovirus) transmitted by *Aedes* mosquitoes. Virus has a monkey or human reservoir. Symptoms: high fever, black vomitus, and jaundice.	*Flavi* = yellow, jaundice.
Rotavirus 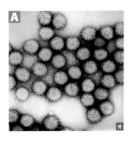	Rotavirus **A**, the most important global cause of infantile gastroenteritis, is a segmented dsRNA virus (a reovirus). Major cause of acute diarrhea in the United States during winter, especially in day-care centers, kindergartens. Villous destruction with atrophy leads to ↓ absorption of Na⁺ and loss of K⁺.	**ROTA**virus = **R**ight **O**ut **T**he **A**nus. CDC recommends routine vaccination of all infants.

Influenza viruses	Orthomyxoviruses. Enveloped, ⊖ ssRNA viruses with 8-segment genome. Contain hemagglutinin (promotes viral entry) and neuraminidase (promotes progeny virion release) antigens. Patients at risk for fatal bacterial superinfection. Rapid genetic changes.	Reformulated vaccine ("the flu shot") containing the viral strains most likely to appear during the flu season. Killed viral vaccine is most frequently used. Live, attenuated (temperature-sensitive mutant) vaccine that replicates in the nose but not in the lung, administered intranasally.
Genetic shift / antigenic shifts	Causes pandemics. Reassortment of viral genome; segments undergo high-frequency recombination, such as when human flu A virus recombines with swine flu A virus.	Sudden shift is more deadly than gradual drift.
Genetic drift	Causes epidemics. Minor (antigenic drift) changes based on random mutation.	

Rubella virus	A togavirus. Causes rubella, once known as German (3-day) measles. Fever, postauricular and other lymphadenopathy, arthralgias, and fine rash A. Causes mild disease in children but serious congenital disease (a ToRCHeS infection). Congenital rubella findings include "blueberry muffin" appearance, indicative of extramedullary hematopoiesis B.

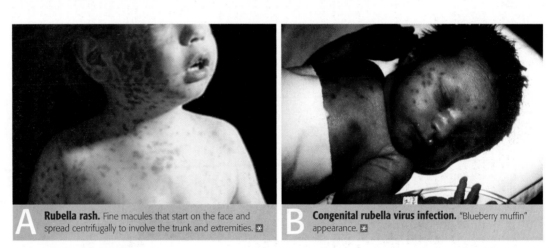

A **Rubella rash.** Fine macules that start on the face and spread centrifugally to involve the trunk and extremities. ✳

B **Congenital rubella virus infection.** "Blueberry muffin" appearance. ✳

Paramyxoviruses	Paramyxoviruses cause disease in children. They include those that cause parainfluenza (croup: seal-like barking cough), mumps, and measles as well as RSV, which causes respiratory tract infection (bronchiolitis, pneumonia) in infants. All contain surface F (fusion) protein, which causes respiratory epithelial cells to fuse and form multinucleated cells. Palivizumab (monoclonal antibody against F protein) prevents pneumonia caused by RSV infection in premature infants.

Measles virus

A paramyxovirus that causes measles. Koplik spots 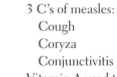 and descending maculopapular rash B are characteristic. SSPE (subacute sclerosing panencephalitis, occurring years later), encephalitis (1:2000), and giant cell pneumonia (rarely, in immunosuppressed) are possible sequelae.

3 C's of measles:
  Cough
  Coryza
  Conjunctivitis
Vitamin A used to prevent severe exfoliative dermatitis in malnourished children.

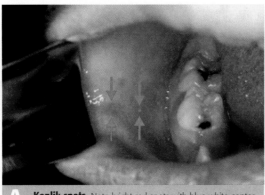

A **Koplik spots.** Note bright red spots with blue-white center on buccal mucosa (arrows) that precede the measles rash by 1–2 days. ✖

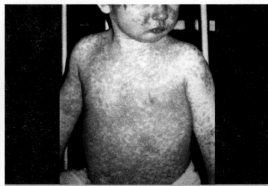

B **Rash of measles.** Discrete erythematous rash, presents late, and includes limbs (vs. rubella) as it spreads downward. ✖

Mumps virus

A paramyxovirus.
Symptoms: Parotitis **A**, Orchitis (inflammation of testes), and aseptic Meningitis. Can cause sterility (especially after puberty).

Mumps makes your parotid glands and testes as big as **POM**-poms.

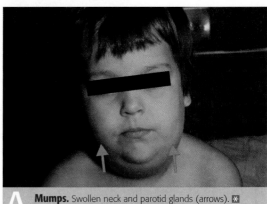

A **Mumps.** Swollen neck and parotid glands (arrows). ✖

Rabies virus

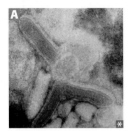

Bullet-shaped virus **A**. Negri bodies **B** commonly found in Purkinje cells of cerebellum and in hippocampal neurons. Rabies has long incubation period (weeks to months) before symptom onset. Postexposure treatment is wound cleansing and vaccination ± rabies immune globulin.

Travels to the CNS by migrating in a retrograde fashion up nerve axons.

Progression of disease: fever, malaise
→ agitation, photophobia, hydrophobia
→ paralysis, coma → death.

More commonly from bat, raccoon, and skunk bites than from dog bites in the United States.

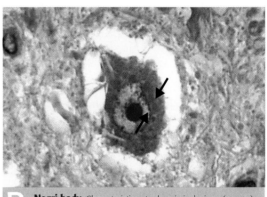

B **Negri body.** Characteristic cytoplasmic inclusions (arrows) in neurons infected by rabies virus. ✳

Hepatitis viruses

	VIRUS	TRANSMISSION	CARRIER	INCUBATION	HCC RISK	NOTES
HAV[a]	RNA picornavirus	Fecal-oral	No	Short (weeks)	No	Asymptomatic (usually), Acute, Alone (no carriers)
HBV[b]	DNA hepadnavirus	Parenteral, sexual, maternal-fetal	Yes	Long (months)	Yes: integrates into host genome, acts as oncogene	
HCV	RNA flavivirus	Primarily blood (IVDU, post-transfusion)	Yes	Long	Yes: from chronic inflammation	Chronic, Cirrhosis, Carcinoma, Carrier
HDV	RNA delta virus	Parenteral, sexual, maternal-fetal	Yes	Superinfection (HDV after HBV)—short Co-infection (HDV with HBV)—long	Yes	Defective virus Dependent on HBV; superinfection → ↓ prognosis
HEV[a]	RNA hepevirus	Fecal-oral, especially with waterborne epidemics	No	Short	No	High mortality in pregnant women; Enteric, Expectant mothers, Epidemic

Signs and symptoms of all hepatitis viruses: episodes of fever, jaundice, ↑ ALT and AST.

[a]HAV and HEV are fecal-oral: The **vowels** hit your **bowels**. Naked viruses do not rely on an envelope so they are not destroyed by the gut.

[b]In HBV, the DNA polymerase has both DNA- and RNA-dependent activities. Upon entry into the nucleus, the polymerase functions to complete the partial dsDNA. The host RNA polymerase transcribes mRNA from viral DNA to make viral proteins. The DNA polymerase then reverse transcribes viral RNA to DNA, which helps form new viral particles.

Hepatitis serologic markers

Anti-HAV (IgM)	IgM antibody to HAV; best test to detect active hepatitis A.
Anti-HAV (IgG)	IgG antibody indicates prior HAV infection and/or prior vaccination; protects against reinfection.
HBsAg	Antigen found on surface of HBV; indicates hepatitis B infection.
Anti-HBs	Antibody to HBsAg; indicates immunity to hepatitis B.
HBcAg	Antigen associated with core of HBV.
Anti-HBc	Antibody to HBcAg; IgM = acute/recent infection; IgG = prior exposure or chronic infection. Positive during window period.
HBeAg	A second, different antigenic determinant in the HBV core. HBeAg indicates active viral replication and therefore high transmissibility.
Anti-HBe	Antibody to HBeAg; indicates low transmissibility.

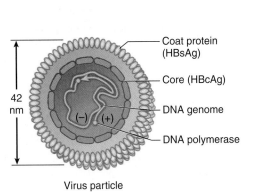

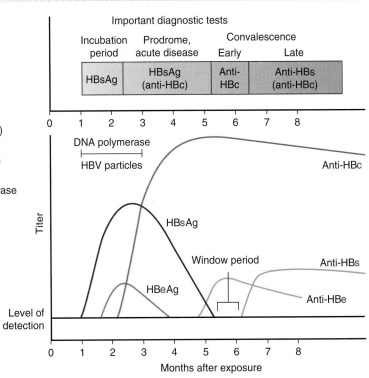

In viral hepatitis, ALT > AST.
In alcoholic hepatitis, AST > ALT.
SECES: SE are antigens, CES
are antibodies; labeled on figure
in order of appearance.

	HBsAg	Anti-HBs	HBeAg	Anti-HBe	Anti-HBc
Acute HBV	✓		✓		IgM
Window				✓	IgM
Chronic HBV (high infectivity)	✓		✓		IgG
Chronic HBV (low infectivity)	✓			✓	IgG
Recovery		✓		✓	IgG
Immunized		✓			

HIV

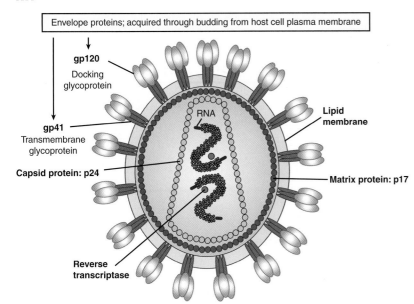

Envelope proteins; acquired through budding from host cell plasma membrane

gp120
Docking glycoprotein

gp41
Transmembrane glycoprotein

Capsid protein: p24

Reverse transcriptase

RNA

Lipid membrane

Matrix protein: p17

Diploid genome (2 molecules of RNA).
The 3 structural genes (protein coded for):
- *env* (gp120 and gp41):
  - Formed from cleavage of gp160 to form envelope glycoproteins.
  - gp120—attachment to host CD4+ T cell.
  - gp41—fusion and entry.
- *gag* (p24)—capsid protein.
- *pol*—reverse transcriptase, aspartate protease, integrase.

Reverse transcriptase synthesizes dsDNA from RNA; dsDNA integrates into host genome.
Virus binds CCR5 (early) or CXCR4 (late) co-receptor and CD4 on T cells; binds CCR5 and CD4 on macrophages.
Homozygous CCR5 mutation = immunity.
Heterozygous CCR5 mutation = slower course.

HIV diagnosis

Presumptive diagnosis made with ELISA (sensitive, high false-positive rate and low threshold, **rule out** test); ⊕ results are then confirmed with Western blot assay (specific, high false-negative rate and high threshold, **rule in** test).

HIV PCR/viral load tests determine the amount of viral RNA in the plasma. High viral load associated with poor prognosis. Also use viral load to monitor effect of drug therapy.

AIDS diagnosis ≤ 200 CD4+ cells/mm^3 (normal: 500–1500 cells/mm^3). HIV-positive with AIDS-defining condition (e.g., *Pneumocystis* pneumonia) or CD4 percentage < 14%.

ELISA/Western blot tests look for antibodies to viral proteins; these tests often are falsely negative in the first 1–2 months of HIV infection and falsely positive initially in babies born to infected mothers (anti-gp120 crosses placenta).

Time course of untreated HIV infection

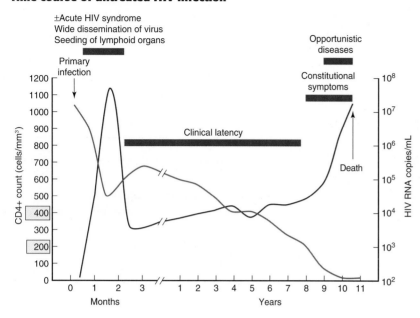

Four stages of untreated infection:
1. Flu-like (acute)
2. Feeling fine (latent)
3. Falling count
4. Final crisis

During latent phase, virus replicates in lymph nodes.

Red line = CD4+ T-lymphocyte count (cells/mm³); blue line = HIV RNA copies/mL plasma.

Blue boxes on vertical CD4+ count axis indicate moderate immunocompromise (< 400 CD4+ cells/mm³) and when AIDS-defining illnesses emerge (< 200 CD4+ cells/mm³).

Common diseases of HIV-positive adults

As CD4+ count ↓, risk of reactivation of past infections (e.g., TB, HSV, shingles), dissemination of bacterial infections and fungal infections (e.g., coccidioidomycosis), and non-Hodgkin lymphomas ↑.

CLINICAL PRESENTATION	FINDINGS/LABS	PATHOGEN
Systemic		
Low-grade fevers, cough, hepatosplenomegaly, tongue ulcer	Oval yeast cells within macrophages, CD4+ < 100 cells/mm^3	*Histoplasma capsulatum* (causes only pulmonary symptoms in immunocompetent hosts)
Dermatologic		
Fluffy white cottage-cheese lesions	Pseudohyphae, commonly oral if CD4+ < 400 cells/mm^3, esophageal if CD4+ < 100 cells/mm^3	*C. albicans* (causes oral thrush and esophagitis)
Hairy leukoplakia	Often on lateral tongue	EBV
Superficial vascular proliferation	Biopsy reveals neutrophilic inflammation	*Bartonella henselae* (causes bacillary angiomatosis)
Gastrointestinal		
Chronic, watery diarrhea	Acid-fast cysts seen in stool especially when CD4+ < 200 cells/mm^3	*Cryptosporidium* spp.
Neurologic		
Abscesses	Many ring-enhancing lesions on imaging, CD4+ < 100 cells/mm^3	*Toxoplasma gondii*
Dementia	Must differentiate from other causes	Directly associated with HIV
Encephalopathy	Due to reactivation of a latent virus; results in demyelination, CD4+ < 200 cells/mm^3	JC virus reactivation (cause of PML)
Meningitis	India ink stain reveals yeast with narrow-based budding and large capsule, CD4+ < 50 cells/mm^3	*Cryptococcus neoformans*
Retinitis	Cotton-wool spots on fundoscopic exam and may also occur with esophagitis, CD4+ < 50 cells/mm^3	CMV
Oncologic		
Non-Hodgkin lymphoma (large cell type)	Often on oropharynx (Waldeyer ring)	May be associated with EBV
Primary CNS lymphoma	Focal or multiple, differentiate from toxoplasmosis	Often associated with EBV
Squamous cell carcinoma	Often in anus (men who have sex with men) or cervix	HPV
Superficial neoplastic proliferation of vasculature	Biopsy reveals lymphocytic inflammation	HHV-8 (causes Kaposi sarcoma), do not confuse with bacillary angiomatosis caused by *B. henselae*
Respiratory		
Interstitial pneumonia	Biopsy reveals cells with intranuclear (owl eye) inclusion bodies	CMV
Invasive aspergillosis	Pleuritic pain, hemoptysis, infiltrates on imaging	*Aspergillus fumigatus*
Pneumocystis pneumonia	Especially with CD4+ < 200 cells/mm^3 Ground-glass appearance on imaging	*Pneumocystis jirovecii*
Pneumonia	Generally with CD4+ > 200 cells/mm^3	*S. pneumoniae*
Tuberculosis-like disease	Especially with CD4+ < 50 cells/mm^3	*Mycobacterium avium–intracellulare*, also known as *Mycobacterium avium* complex (MAC)

Prions

Prion diseases are caused by the conversion of a normal (predominantly α-helical) protein termed prion protein (PrP^c) to a β-pleated form (PrP^{sc}), which is transmissible. PrP^{sc} resists protease degradation and facilitates the conversion of still more PrP^c to PrP^{sc}. Accumulation of PrP^{sc} results in spongiform encephalopathy and dementia, ataxia, and death. It can be sporadic (Creutzfeldt-Jakob disease—rapidly progressive dementia), inherited (Gerstmann-Sträussler-Scheinker syndrome), or acquired (kuru).

▶ MICROBIOLOGY–SYSTEMS

Normal flora: dominant

LOCATION	MICROORGANISM
Skin	S. epidermidis
Nose	S. epidermidis; colonized by S. aureus
Oropharynx	Viridans group streptococci
Dental plaque	S. mutans
Colon	B. fragilis > E. coli
Vagina	Lactobacillus, colonized by E. coli and group B strep

Neonates delivered by C-section have no flora but are rapidly colonized after birth.

Bugs causing food poisoning

S. aureus and B. cereus food poisoning starts quickly and ends quickly.

MICROORGANISM	SOURCE OF INFECTION
B. cereus	Reheated rice. "Food poisoning from reheated rice? **Be serious!**" (**B. cereus**)
C. botulinum	Improperly canned foods (sign is bulging cans)
C. perfringens	Reheatved meat dishes
E. coli O157:H7	Undercooked meat
Salmonella	Poultry, meat, and eggs
S. aureus	Meats, mayonnaise, custard; preformed toxin
V. parahaemolyticus and V. vulnificus[a]	Contaminated seafood

[a]V. vulnificus can also cause wound infections from contact with contaminated water or shellfish.

Bugs causing diarrhea

Bloody diarrhea	
Campylobacter	Comma- or S-shaped organisms; growth at 42°C
E. histolytica	Protozoan; amebic dysentery; liver abscess
Enterohemorrhagic *E. coli*	O157:H7; can cause HUS; makes Shiga-like toxin
Enteroinvasive *E. coli*	Invades colonic mucosa
Salmonella	Lactose ⊖; flagellar motility; has animal reservoir, especially poultry and eggs
Shigella	Lactose ⊖; very low ID_{50}; produces Shiga toxin (human reservoir only); bacillary dysentery
Y. enterocolitica	Day-care outbreaks, pseudoappendicitis
Watery diarrhea	
C. difficile	Pseudomembranous colitis. Caused by antibiotics. Occasionally bloody diarrhea.
C. perfringens	Also causes gas gangrene
Enterotoxigenic *E. coli*	Travelers' diarrhea; produces heat-labile (LT) and heat-stable (ST) toxins
Protozoa	*Giardia, Cryptosporidium* (in immunocompromised)
V. cholerae	Comma-shaped organisms; rice-water diarrhea; often from infected seafood
Viruses	Rotavirus, norovirus

Common causes of pneumonia

NEONATES (< 4 WK)	CHILDREN (4 WK–18 YR)	ADULTS (18–40 YR)	ADULTS (40–65 YR)	ELDERLY
Group B streptococci *E. coli*	Viruses (**RSV**) *Mycoplasma* *C. trachomatis* (infants–3 yr) *C. pneumoniae* (school-aged children) *S. pneumoniae* Runts May Cough Chunky Sputum	*Mycoplasma* *C. pneumoniae* *S. pneumoniae*	*S. pneumoniae* *H. influenzae* Anaerobes Viruses *Mycoplasma*	*S. pneumoniae* Influenza virus Anaerobes *H. influenzae* Gram-negative rods
Special groups				
Alcoholic/IV drug user	*S. pneumoniae, Klebsiella, Staphylococcus*			
Aspiration	Anaerobes			
Atypical	*Mycoplasma, Legionella, Chlamydia*			
Cystic fibrosis	*Pseudomonas, S. aureus, S. pneumoniae*			
Immunocompromised	*Staphylococcus*, enteric gram-negative rods, fungi, viruses, *P. jirovecii* (with HIV)			
Nosocomial (hospital acquired)	*Staphylococcus, Pseudomonas*, other enteric gram-negative rods			
Postviral	*Staphylococcus, H. influenzae, S. pneumoniae*			

Common causes of meningitis

NEWBORN (0–6 MO)	CHILDREN (6 MO–6 YR)	6–60 YR	60 YR +
Group B streptococci E. coli Listeria	S. pneumoniae N. meningitidis H. influenzae type B Enteroviruses	S. pneumoniae N. meningitidis (#1 in teens) Enteroviruses HSV	S. pneumoniae Gram-negative rods Listeria

Give ceftriaxone and vancomycin empirically (add ampicillin if *Listeria* is suspected).

Viral causes of meningitis—enteroviruses (esp. coxsackievirus), HSV-2 (HSV-1 = encephalitis), HIV, West Nile virus, VZV.

In HIV—*Cryptococcus*, CMV, toxoplasmosis (brain abscess), JC virus (PML).

Note: Incidence of *H. influenzae* meningitis has ↓ greatly with introduction of the conjugate *H. influenzae* vaccine in last 10–15 years. Today, cases are usually seen in unimmunized children.

CSF findings in meningitis

	OPENING PRESSURE	CELL TYPE	PROTEIN	SUGAR
Bacterial	↑	↑ PMNs	↑	↓
Fungal/TB	↑	↑ lymphocytes	↑	↓
Viral	Normal/↑	↑ lymphocytes	Normal/↑	Normal

Osteomyelitis

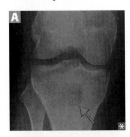
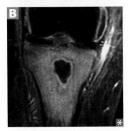

RISK FACTOR	CAUSE
Assume if no other information is available	S. aureus (most common overall)
Sexually active	Neisseria gonorrhoeae (rare), septic arthritis more common
Diabetics and IV drug users	Pseudomonas aeruginosa, Serratia
Sickle cell	Salmonella
Prosthetic joint replacement	S. aureus and S. epidermidis
Vertebral involvement	Mycobacterium tuberculosis (Pott disease)
Cat and dog bites	Pasteurella multocida

Most osteomyelitis occurs in children.

Elevated CRP and ESR observed but nonspecific.

Can be subtle on radiographs (arrow in **A**); same lesion more easily seen on MRI **B**.

Urinary tract infections

Cystitis presents with dysuria, frequency, urgency, suprapubic pain, and WBCs (but not WBC casts) in urine. Primarily caused by ascension of microbes from urethra to bladder. Males— infants with congenital defects, vesicoureteral reflux. Elderly—enlarged prostate. Ascension to kidney results in pyelonephritis, which presents with fever, chills, flank pain, costovertebral angle tenderness, hematuria, and WBC casts.

Ten times more common in women (shorter urethras colonized by fecal flora). Other predisposing factors include obstruction, kidney surgery, catheterization, GU malformation, diabetes, and pregnancy.

Diagnostic markers: leukocyte esterase test ⊕ = bacterial UTI; nitrite test ⊕ = gram-negative bacterial UTI.

UTI bugs

SPECIES	FEATURES	COMMENTS
Escherichia coli	Leading cause of UTI. Colonies show green metallic sheen on EMB agar.	Diagnostic markers:
Staphylococcus saprophyticus	2nd leading cause of UTI in sexually active women.	⊕ Leukocyte esterase = bacterial. ⊕ Nitrite test = gram-negative bugs. ⊕ Urease test = urease-producing bugs (e.g., *Proteus, Klebsiella*).
Klebsiella pneumoniae	3rd leading cause of UTI. Large mucoid capsule and viscous colonies.	⊖ Urease test = *E. coli, Enterococcus*.
Serratia marcescens	Some strains produce a red pigment; often nosocomial and drug resistant.	
Enterobacter cloacae	Often nosocomial and drug resistant.	
Proteus mirabilis	Motility causes "swarming" on agar; produces urease; associated with struvite stones.	
Pseudomonas aeruginosa	Blue-green pigment and fruity odor; usually nosocomial and drug resistant.	

Common vaginal infections

	Bacterial vaginosis	**Trichomoniasis**	***Candida* vulvovaginitis**
SIGNS AND SYMPTOMS	No inflammation Thin, white discharge with fishy odor	Inflammation Frothy, grey-green, foul-smelling discharge	Inflammation Thick, white, "cottage cheese" discharge
LAB FINDINGS	Clue cells pH > 4.5	Motile trichomonads pH > 4.5	Pseudohyphae pH normal (4.0–4.5)
TREATMENT	Metronidazole	Metronidazole Treat sexual partner	-azoles

ToRCHeS infections

Microbes that may pass from mother to fetus. Transmission is transplacental in most cases, or via delivery (especially HSV-2). Nonspecific signs common to many **ToRCHeS** infections include hepatosplenomegaly, jaundice, thrombocytopenia, and growth retardation.

Other important infectious agents include *Streptococcus agalactiae* (group B streptococci), *E. coli*, and *Listeria monocytogenes*—all causes of meningitis in neonates. Parvovirus B19 causes hydrops fetalis.

AGENT	MODE OF TRANSMISSION	MATERNAL MANIFESTATIONS	NEONATAL MANIFESTIONS
Toxoplasma gondii	Cat feces or ingestion of undercooked meat	Usually asymptomatic; lymphadenopathy (rarely)	Classic triad: chorioretinitis, hydrocephalus, and intracranial calcifications
Rubella	Respiratory droplets	Rash, lymphadenopathy, arthritis	Classic triad: PDA (or pulmonary artery hypoplasia), cataracts, and deafness ± "blueberry muffin" rash
CMV	Sexual contact, organ transplants	Usually asymptomatic; mononucleosis-like illness	Hearing loss, seizures, petechial rash, "blueberry muffin" rash
HIV	Sexual contact, needlestick	Variable presentation depending on CD4+ count	Recurrent infections, chronic diarrhea
Herpes simplex virus-2	Skin or mucous membrane contact	Usually asymptomatic; herpetic (vesicular) lesions	Encephalitis, herpetic (vesicular) lesions
Syphilis	Sexual contact	Chancre (1°) and disseminated rash (2°) are the two stages likely to result in fetal infection	Often results in stillbirth, hydrops fetalis; if child survives, presents with facial abnormalities A (notched teeth B, saddle nose, short maxilla), saber shins, CN VIII deafness

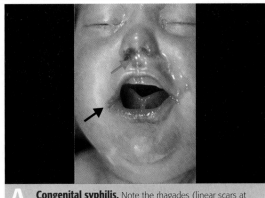

A **Congenital syphilis.** Note the rhagades (linear scars at angle of mouth, black arrow) and snuffles (nasal discharge, red arrow) full of syphilis spirochetes. ✲

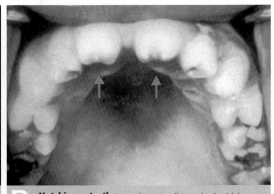

B **Hutchinson teeth.** Note the centrally notched, widely spaced central incisors (arrows). Patients may also have saddle nose and short maxilla. ✲

Red rashes of childhood

AGENT	ASSOCIATED SYNDROME/DISEASE	CLINICAL PRESENTATION
Coxsackievirus type A	Hand-foot-mouth disease	Vesicular rash on palms and soles 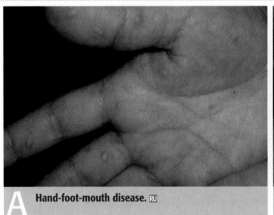; vesicles and ulcers in oral mucosa
HHV-6	Roseola	A macular rash over body appears after several days of high fever; can present with febrile seizures; usually affects infants
Measles virus	Measles (rubeola)	A paramyxovirus; beginning at head and moving down; rash is preceded by cough, coryza, conjunctivitis, and blue-white (Koplik) spots on buccal mucosa
Parvovirus B19	Erythema infectiosum (fifth disease)	"Slapped cheek" rash on face 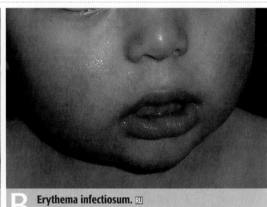 (can cause hydrops fetalis in pregnant women)
Rubella virus	Rubella	Rash begins at head and moves down; → fine truncal rash; postauricular lymphadenopathy
Streptococcus pyogenes	Scarlet fever	Erythematous, sandpaper-like rash with fever and sore throat
VZV	Chickenpox	Vesicular rash begins on trunk; spreads to face and extremities with lesions of different ages

A Hand-foot-mouth disease. RU

B Erythema infectiosum. RU

Sexually transmitted diseases

DISEASE	CLINICAL FEATURES	ORGANISM
AIDS	Opportunistic infections, Kaposi sarcoma, lymphoma	HIV
Chancroid	Painful genital ulcer, inguinal adenopathy	*Haemophilus **ducreyi*** (it's so painful, you "do cry")
Chlamydia	Urethritis, cervicitis, conjunctivitis, reactive arthritis, PID	*Chlamydia trachomatis* (D–K)
Condylomata acuminata	Genital warts, koilocytes	HPV-6 and -11
Genital herpes	Painful penile, vulvar, or cervical vesicles and ulcers; can cause systemic symptoms such as fever, headache, myalgia	HSV-2, less commonly HSV-1
Gonorrhea	Urethritis, cervicitis, PID, prostatitis, epididymitis, arthritis, creamy purulent discharge	*Neisseria gonorrhoeae*
Hepatitis B	Jaundice	HBV
Lymphogranuloma venereum	Infection of lymphatics; painless genital ulcers, painful lymphadenopathy (i.e., buboes)	*C. trachomatis* (L1–L3)
1° syphilis	Painless chancre	*Treponema pallidum*
2° syphilis	Fever, lymphadenopathy, skin rashes, condylomata lata	
3° syphilis	Gummas, tabes dorsalis, general paresis, aortitis, Argyll Robertson pupil	
Trichomoniasis	Vaginitis, strawberry cervix, motile in wet prep	*Trichomonas vaginalis*

Pelvic inflammatory disease

Top bugs—*Chlamydia trachomatis* (subacute, often undiagnosed), *Neisseria gonorrhoeae* (acute). *C. trachomatis*—the most common bacterial STD in the United States. Cervical motion tenderness (chandelier sign), purulent cervical discharge **A**. PID may include salpingitis, endometritis, hydrosalpinx, and tubo-ovarian abscess. Can lead to **Fitz-Hugh–Curtis syndrome**—infection of the liver capsule and "violin string" adhesions of peritoneum to liver **B**.

Salpingitis is a risk factor for ectopic pregnancy, infertility, chronic pelvic pain, and adhesions.

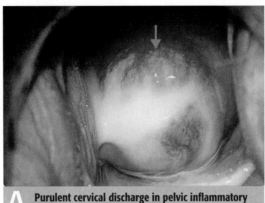

A **Purulent cervical discharge in pelvic inflammatory disease.** ✳

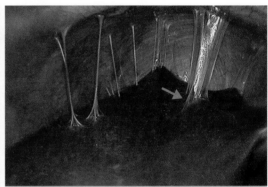

B **Adhesions in Fitz-Hugh–Curtis syndrome.** Note the adhesions (arrow) extending from the peritoneum anchored to the surface of the liver. ✳

Nosocomial infections

PATHOGEN	RISK FACTOR	NOTES
Candida albicans	Hyperalimentation	
CMV, RSV	Newborn nursery	
E. coli, Proteus mirabilis	Urinary catheterization	The 2 most common causes of nosocomial infections are *E. coli* (UTI) and *S. aureus* (wound infection).
HBV	Work in renal dialysis unit	
Legionella	Water aerosols	Think *Legionella* when water source is involved.
Pseudomonas aeruginosa	Respiratory therapy equipment	Presume *Pseudomonas "airuginosa"* when **air** or burns are involved.

Bugs affecting unimmunized children

CLINICAL PRESENTATION	FINDINGS/LABS	PATHOGEN
Dermatologic		
Rash	Beginning at head and moving down with postauricular lymphadenopathy	Rubella virus
	Beginning at head and moving down; rash preceded by cough, coryza, conjunctivitis, and blue-white (Koplik) spots on buccal mucosa	Measles virus
Neurologic		
Meningitis	Microbe colonizes nasopharynx	*H. influenzae* type B
	Can also lead to myalgia and paralysis	Poliovirus
Respiratory		
Epiglottitis	Fever with dysphagia, drooling, and difficulty breathing due to edematous "cherry red" epiglottis; "thumbprint sign" on X-ray	*H. influenzae* type B (also capable of causing epiglottitis in fully immunized children)
Pharyngitis	Grayish oropharyngeal exudate ("pseudomembranes" may obstruct airway); painful throat	*Corynebacterium diphtheriae* (elaborates toxin that causes necrosis in pharynx, cardiac, and CNS tissue)

Bug hints (if all else fails)	CHARACTERISTIC	ORGANISM
	Asplenic patient (due to surgical splenectomy or autosplenectomy, e.g., chronic sickle cell anemia)	Encapsulated microbes, especially **SHiN** (*S. pneumoniae* >> *H. influenzae* type B > *N. meningitidis*)
	Branching rods in oral infection, sulfur granules	*Actinomyces israelii*
	Chronic granulomatous disease	Catalase ⊕ microbes, especially *S. aureus*
	"Currant jelly" sputum	*Klebsiella*
	Dog or cat bite	*Pasteurella multocida*
	Facial nerve palsy	*Borrelia burgdorferi* (Lyme disease)
	Fungal infection in diabetic or immunocompromised patient	*Mucor* or *Rhizopus* spp.
	Health care provider	HBV (from needle stick)
	Neutropenic patients	*Candida albicans* (systemic), *Aspergillus*
	Organ transplant recipient	CMV
	PAS ⊕	*Tropheryma whipplei* (Whipple disease)
	Pediatric infection	*Haemophilus influenzae* (including epiglottitis)
	Pneumonia in cystic fibrosis, burn infection	*Pseudomonas aeruginosa*
	Pus, empyema, abscess	*S. aureus*
	Rash on hands and feet	Coxsackie A virus, *Treponema pallidum*, *Rickettsia rickettsii*
	Sepsis/meningitis in newborn	Group B strep
	Surgical wound	*S. aureus*
	Traumatic open wound	*Clostridium perfringens*

▶ MICROBIOLOGY–ANTIMICROBIALS

Antimicrobial therapy

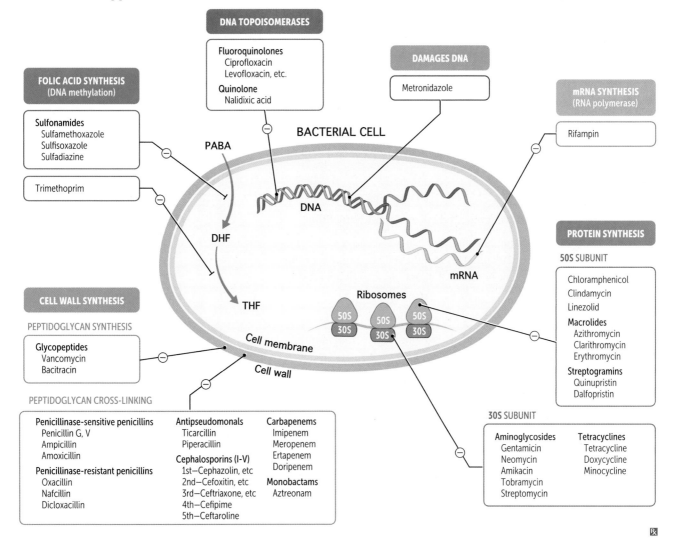

Penicillin G, V	Penicillin G (IV and IM form), penicillin V (oral). Prototype β-lactam antibiotics.
MECHANISM	Bind penicillin-binding proteins (transpeptidases). Block transpeptidase cross-linking of peptidoglycan. Activate autolytic enzymes.
CLINICAL USE	Mostly used for gram-positive organisms (*S. pneumoniae*, *S. pyogenes*, *Actinomyces*). Also used for *N. meningitidis* and *T. pallidum*. Bactericidal for gram-positive cocci, gram-positive rods, gram-negative cocci, and spirochetes. Penicillinase sensitive.
TOXICITY	Hypersensitivity reactions, hemolytic anemia.
RESISTANCE	Penicillinase in bacteria (a type of β-lactamase) cleaves β-lactam ring.

Ampicillin, amoxicillin (aminopenicillins, penicillinase-sensitive penicillins)

MECHANISM	Same as penicillin. Wider spectrum; penicillinase sensitive. Also combine with clavulanic acid to protect against β-lactamase.	AMinoPenicillins are AMPed-up penicillin. AmOxicillin has greater Oral bioavailability than ampicillin.
CLINICAL USE	Extended-spectrum penicillin—*Haemophilus influenzae*, *E. coli*, *Listeria monocytogenes*, *Proteus mirabilis*, *Salmonella*, *Shigella*, enterococci.	Coverage: ampicillin/amoxicillin **HELPSS** kill enterococci.
TOXICITY	Hypersensitivity reactions; rash; pseudomembranous colitis.	
MECHANISM OF RESISTANCE	Penicillinase in bacteria (a type of β-lactamase) cleaves β-lactam ring.	

Oxacillin, nafcillin, dicloxacillin (penicillinase-resistant penicillins)

MECHANISM	Same as penicillin. Narrow spectrum; penicillinase resistant because bulky R group blocks access of β-lactamase to β-lactam ring.	
CLINICAL USE	*S. aureus* (except MRSA; resistant because of altered penicillin-binding protein target site).	"Use **naf** (nafcillin) for **staph**."
TOXICITY	Hypersensitivity reactions, interstitial nephritis.	

Ticarcillin, piperacillin (antipseudomonals)

MECHANISM	Same as penicillin. Extended spectrum.
CLINICAL USE	*Pseudomonas* spp. and gram-negative rods; susceptible to penicillinase; use with β-lactamase inhibitors.
TOXICITY	Hypersensitivity reactions.

β-lactamase inhibitors	Include Clavulanic Acid, Sulbactam, Tazobactam. Often added to penicillin antibiotics to protect the antibiotic from destruction by β-lactamase (penicillinase).	CAST.

Cephalosporins (generations I, II, III, IV, V)

MECHANISM	β-lactam drugs that inhibit cell wall synthesis but are less susceptible to penicillinases. Bactericidal.	Organisms typically not covered by cephalosporins are **LAME**: *Listeria*, Atypicals (*Chlamydia*, *Mycoplasma*), MRSA, and Enterococci. Exception: ceftaroline covers MRSA.
CLINICAL USE	1st generation (cefazolin, cephalexin)—gram-positive cocci, *Proteus mirabilis*, *E. coli*, *Klebsiella pneumoniae*. Cefazolin used prior to surgery to prevent *S. aureus* wound infections.	1st generation—**PEcK**.
	2nd generation (cefoxitin, cefaclor, cefuroxime)—gram-positive cocci, *Haemophilus influenzae*, *Enterobacter aerogenes*, *Neisseria* spp., *Proteus mirabilis*, *E. coli*, *Klebsiella pneumoniae*, *Serratia marcescens*.	2nd generation—**HEN PEcKS**.
	3rd generation (ceftriaxone, cefotaxime, ceftazidime)—serious gram-negative infections resistant to other β-lactams.	Ceftriaxone—meningitis and gonorrhea. Ceftazidime—*Pseudomonas*.
	4th generation (cefepime)—↑ activity against *Pseudomonas* and gram-positive organisms.	
	5th generation (ceftaroline)—broad gram-positive and gram-negative organism coverage, including MRSA; does not cover *Pseudomonas*.	
TOXICITY	Hypersensitivity reactions, vitamin K deficiency. Low cross-reactivity with penicillins. ↑ nephrotoxicity of aminoglycosides.	

Aztreonam

MECHANISM	A monobactam; resistant to β-lactamases. Prevents peptidoglycan cross-linking by binding to penicillin-binding protein 3. Synergistic with aminoglycosides. No cross-allergenicity with penicillins.
CLINICAL USE	Gram-negative rods only—no activity against gram-positives or anaerobes. For penicillin-allergic patients and those with renal insufficiency who cannot tolerate aminoglycosides.
TOXICITY	Usually nontoxic; occasional GI upset.

Carbapenems	Imipenem, meropenem, ertapenem, doripenem.	
MECHANISM	Imipenem is a broad-spectrum, β-lactamase– resistant carbapenem. Always administered with cilastatin (inhibitor of renal dehydropeptidase I) to ↓ inactivation of drug in renal tubules.	With imipenem, "the kill is **lastin'** with **cilastatin**." Newer carbapenems include ertapenem (limited *Pseudomonas* coverage) and doripenem.
CLINICAL USE	Gram-positive cocci, gram-negative rods, and anaerobes. Wide spectrum, but significant side effects limit use to life-threatening infections or after other drugs have failed. Meropenem has a ↓ risk of seizures and is stable to dehydropeptidase I.	
TOXICITY	GI distress, skin rash, and CNS toxicity (seizures) at high plasma levels.	

Vancomycin	
MECHANISM	Inhibits cell wall peptidoglycan formation by binding D-ala D-ala portion of cell wall precursors. Bactericidal.
CLINICAL USE	Gram positive only—serious, multidrug-resistant organisms, including MRSA, enterococci, and *Clostridium difficile* (oral dose for pseudomembranous colitis).
TOXICITY	Well tolerated in general—but **NOT** trouble free. Nephrotoxicity, Ototoxicity, Thrombophlebitis, diffuse flushing—**red man syndrome** (can largely prevent by pretreatment with antihistamines and slow infusion rate).
MECHANISM OF RESISTANCE	Occurs in bacteria via amino acid modification of **D-ala D-ala** to D-ala D-lac. "Pay back **2 D-alas** (dollars) for **v**andalizing (**v**ancomycin)."

Protein synthesis inhibitors

Specifically target smaller bacterial ribosome (70S, made of 30S and 50S subunits), leaving human ribosome (80S) unaffected.

"Buy AT 30, CCEL (sell) at 50."

30S inhibitors

A = Aminoglycosides [bactericidal]
T = Tetracyclines [bacteriostatic]

50S inhibitors

C = Chloramphenicol, Clindamycin [bacteriostatic]
E = Erythromycin (macrolides) [bacteriostatic]
L = Linezolid [variable]

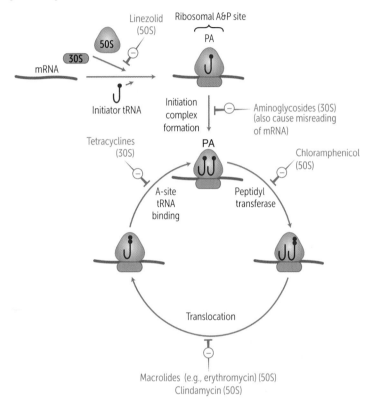

Aminoglycosides	Gentamicin, Neomycin, Amikacin, Tobramycin, Streptomycin.	"**Mean**" (aminoglycoside) GNATS caNNOT kill anaerobes.
MECHANISM	Bactericidal; inhibit formation of initiation complex and cause misreading of mRNA. Also block translocation. Require O_2 for uptake; therefore ineffective against anaerobes.	A "initiates" the Alphabet.
CLINICAL USE	Severe gram-negative rod infections. Synergistic with β-lactam antibiotics. Neomycin for bowel surgery.	
TOXICITY	Nephrotoxicity (especially when used with cephalosporins), Neuromuscular blockade, Ototoxicity (especially when used with loop diuretics). Teratogen.	
MECHANISM OF RESISTANCE	Bacterial transferase enzymes inactivate the drug by acetylation, phosphorylation, or adenylation.	

Tetracyclines	Tetracycline, doxycycline, minocycline.
MECHANISM	Bacteriostatic; bind to 30S and prevent attachment of aminoacyl-tRNA; limited CNS penetration. Doxycycline is fecally eliminated and can be used in patients with renal failure. Do not take with milk (Ca^{2+}), antacids (Ca^{2+} or Mg^{2+}), or iron-containing preparations because divalent cations inhibit its absorption in the gut.
CLINICAL USE	*Borrelia burgdorferi, M. pneumoniae*. Drug's ability to accumulate intracellularly makes it very effective against *Rickettsia* and *Chlamydia*. Also used to treat acne.
TOXICITY	GI distress, discoloration of teeth and inhibition of bone growth in children, photosensitivity. Contraindicated in pregnancy.
MECHANISM OF RESISTANCE	↓ uptake or ↑ efflux out of bacterial cells by plasmid-encoded transport pumps.

Macrolides	Azithromycin, clarithromycin, erythromycin.
MECHANISM	Inhibit protein synthesis by blocking translocation ("macroslides"); bind to the 23S rRNA of the 50S ribosomal subunit. Bacteriostatic.
CLINICAL USE	Atypical pneumonias (*Mycoplasma, Chlamydia, Legionella*), STDs (for *Chlamydia*), and gram-positive cocci (streptococcal infections in patients allergic to penicillin).
TOXICITY	MACRO: Gastrointestinal Motility issues, Arrhythmia caused by prolonged QT, acute Cholestatic hepatitis, Rash, eOsinophilia. Increases serum concentration of theophyllines, oral anticoagulants.
MECHANISM OF RESISTANCE	Methylation of 23S rRNA-binding site prevents binding of drug.

Chloramphenicol

MECHANISM	Blocks peptidyltransferase at 50S ribosomal subunit. Bacteriostatic.
CLINICAL USE	Meningitis (*Haemophilus influenzae*, *Neisseria meningitidis*, *Streptococcus pneumoniae*) and Rocky Mountain spotted fever (*Rickettsia rickettsii*). Limited use owing to toxicities but often still used in developing countries because of low cost.
TOXICITY	Anemia (dose dependent), aplastic anemia (dose independent), gray baby syndrome (in premature infants because they lack liver UDP-glucuronyl transferase).
MECHANISM OF RESISTANCE	Plasmid-encoded acetyltransferase inactivates the drug.

Clindamycin

MECHANISM	Blocks peptide transfer (translocation) at 50S ribosomal subunit. Bacteriostatic.	
CLINICAL USE	Anaerobic infections (e.g., *Bacteroides* spp., *Clostridium perfringens*) in aspiration pneumonia, lung abscesses, and oral infections. Also effective against invasive Group A streptococcal (GAS) infection.	Treats anaerobes **above** the diaphragm vs. metronidazole (anaerobic infections **below** diaphragm).
TOXICITY	Pseudomembranous colitis (*C. difficile* overgrowth), fever, diarrhea.	

Sulfonamides

Sulfamethoxazole (SMX), sulfisoxazole, sulfadiazine.

MECHANISM	Inhibit folate synthesis. *Para*-aminobenzoic acid (PABA) antimetabolites inhibit dihydropteroate synthase. Bacteriostatic.
CLINICAL USE	Gram-positive, gram-negative, *Nocardia*, *Chlamydia*. Triple sulfas or SMX for simple UTI.
TOXICITY	Hypersensitivity reactions, hemolysis if G6PD deficient, nephrotoxicity (tubulointerstitial nephritis), photosensitivity, kernicterus in infants, displace other drugs from albumin (e.g., warfarin).
MECHANISM OF RESISTANCE	Altered enzyme (bacterial dihydropteroate synthase), ↓ uptake, or ↑ PABA synthesis.

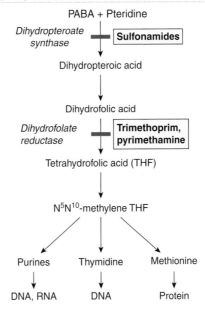

Trimethoprim

MECHANISM	Inhibits bacterial dihydrofolate reductase. Bacteriostatic.
CLINICAL USE	Used in combination with sulfonamides (trimethoprim-sulfamethoxazole [TMP-SMX]), causing sequential block of folate synthesis. Combination used for UTIs, *Shigella*, *Salmonella*, *Pneumocystis jirovecii* pneumonia treatment and prophylaxis, toxoplasmosis prophylaxis.
TOXICITY	Megaloblastic anemia, leukopenia, granulocytopenia. (May alleviate with supplemental folinic acid).

TMP: Treats Marrow Poorly.

Fluoroquinolones

Ciprofloxacin, norfloxacin, levofloxacin, ofloxacin, sparfloxacin, moxifloxacin, gemifloxacin, enoxacin (fluoroquinolones), nalidixic acid (a quinolone).

MECHANISM	Inhibit DNA gyrase (topoisomerase II) and topoisomerase IV. Bactericidal. Must not be taken with antacids.
CLINICAL USE	Gram-negative rods of urinary and GI tracts (including *Pseudomonas*), *Neisseria*, some gram-positive organisms.
TOXICITY	GI upset, superinfections, skin rashes, headache, dizziness. Less commonly, can cause tendonitis, tendon rupture, leg cramps, and myalgias. Contraindicated in pregnant women, nursing mothers, and children under 18 years old due to possible damage to cartilage. Some may cause prolonged QT interval. May cause tendon rupture in people > 60 years old and in patients taking prednisone.
MECHANISM OF RESISTANCE	Chromosome-encoded mutation in DNA gyrase, plasmid-mediated resistance, efflux pumps.

Fluoroquinolones hurt attachments to your **bones**.

Metronidazole

MECHANISM	Forms free radical toxic metabolites in the bacterial cell that damage DNA. Bactericidal, antiprotozoal.	
CLINICAL USE	Treats *Giardia*, *Entamoeba*, *Trichomonas*, *Gardnerella vaginalis*, Anaerobes (*Bacteroides*, *C. difficile*). Used with a proton pump inhibitor and clarithromycin for "triple therapy" against *H. Pylori*.	**GET GAP** on the **Metro** with metronidazole! Treats anaerobic infection **below** the diaphragm vs. clindamycin (anaerobic infections **above** diaphragm).
TOXICITY	Disulfiram-like reaction (severe flushing, tachycardia, hypotension) with alcohol; headache, metallic taste.	

Antimycobacterial drugs

BACTERIUM	PROPHYLAXIS	TREATMENT
M. tuberculosis	Isoniazid	Rifampin, Isoniazid, Pyrazinamide, Ethambutol (**RIPE** for treatment)
M. avium–intracellulare	Azithromycin, rifabutin	More drug resistant than *M. tuberculosis*. Azithromycin or clarithromycin + ethambutol. Can add rifabutin or ciprofloxacin.
M. leprae	N/A	Long-term treatment with dapsone and rifampin for tuberculoid form. Add clofazimine for lepromatous form.

Isoniazid (INH)

MECHANISM	↓ synthesis of mycolic acids. Bacterial catalase-peroxidase (encoded by KatG) needed to convert INH to active metabolite.	
CLINICAL USE	*Mycobacterium tuberculosis*. The only agent used as solo prophylaxis against TB.	Different INH half-lives in fast vs. slow acetylators.
TOXICITY	Neurotoxicity, hepatotoxicity. Pyridoxine (vitamin B_6) can prevent neurotoxicity, lupus.	**INH** Injures Neurons and Hepatocytes.

Rifamycins

Rifampin, rifabutin

MECHANISM	Inhibits DNA-dependent RNA polymerase.	Rifampin's 4 R's:
CLINICAL USE	*Mycobacterium tuberculosis*; delays resistance to dapsone when used for leprosy. Used for meningococcal prophylaxis and chemoprophylaxis in contacts of children with *Haemophilus influenzae* type B.	RNA polymerase inhibitor Ramps up microsomal cytochrome P-450 Red/orange body fluids Rapid resistance if used alone Rifampin ramps up cytochrome P-450, but rifabutin does not
TOXICITY	Minor hepatotoxicity and drug interactions (↑ P-450); orange body fluids (nonhazardous side effect). Rifabutin favored over rifampin in patients with HIV infection due to less cytochrome P-450 stimulation.	

Pyrazinamide

MECHANISM	Mechanism uncertain. Thought to acidify intracellular environment via conversion to pyrazinoic acid. Effective in acidic pH of phagolysosomes, where TB engulfed by macrophages is found.
CLINICAL USE	*Mycobacterium tuberculosis.*
TOXICITY	Hyperuricemia, hepatotoxicity.

Ethambutol

MECHANISM	↓ carbohydrate polymerization of mycobacterium cell wall by blocking arabinosyltransferase.
CLINICAL USE	*Mycobacterium tuberculosis.*
TOXICITY	Optic neuropathy (red-green color blindness).

Antimicrobial prophylaxis

CONDITION	MEDICATION
Endocarditis with surgical or dental procedures	Penicillins
Gonorrhea	Ceftriaxone
History of recurrent UTIs	TMP-SMX
Meningococcal infection	Ciprofloxacin (drug of choice), rifampin for children
Pregnant woman carrying group B strep	Ampicillin
Prevention of gonococcal or chlamydial conjunctivitis in newborn	Erythromycin ointment
Prevention of postsurgical infection due to *S. aureus*	Cefazolin
Prophylaxis of strep pharyngitis in child with prior rheumatic fever	Oral penicillin
Syphilis	Benzathine penicillin G

Prophylaxis in HIV patients

CELL COUNT	PROPHYLAXIS	INFECTION
CD4 < 200 cells/mm^3	TMP-SMX[a]	*Pneumocystis* pneumonia
CD4 < 100 cells/mm^3	TMP-SMX[a]	*Pneumocystis* pneumonia and toxoplasmosis
CD4 < 50 cells/mm^3	Azithromycin	*Mycobacterium avium* complex

[a]Aerosolized pentamidine may be used if patient is unable to tolerate TMP-SMX, but this may not prevent toxoplasmosis infection concurrently.

Treatment of highly resistant bacteria

MRSA—vancomycin, daptomycin, linezolid (can cause serotonin syndrome), tigecycline, ceftaroline.
VRE—linezolid and streptogramins (quinupristin/dalfopristin).

Antifungal therapy

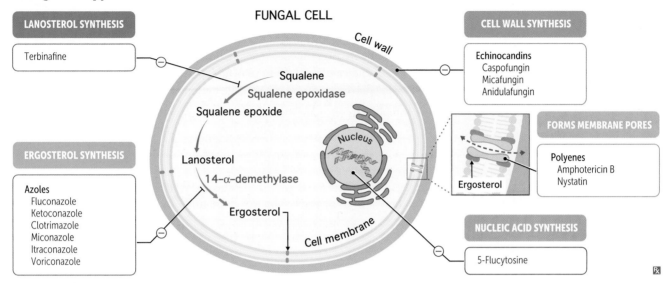

Amphotericin B

MECHANISM	Binds ergosterol (unique to fungi); forms membrane pores that allow leakage of electrolytes.	Amphotericin "**tears**" holes in the fungal membrane by forming pores.
CLINICAL USE	Serious, systemic mycoses. *Cryptococcus* (amphotericin B with/without flucytosine for cryptococcal meningitis), *Blastomyces*, *Coccidioides*, *Histoplasma*, *Candida*, *Mucor*. Intrathecally for fungal meningitis. Supplement K^+ and Mg^{2+} because of altered renal tubule permeability.	
TOXICITY	Fever/chills ("shake and bake"), hypotension, nephrotoxicity, arrhythmias, anemia, IV phlebitis ("**amphoterrible**"). Hydration ↓ nephrotoxicity. Liposomal amphotericin ↓ toxicity.	

Nystatin

MECHANISM	Same as amphotericin B. Topical form because too toxic for systemic use.
CLINICAL USE	"Swish and swallow" for oral candidiasis (thrush); topical for diaper rash or vaginal candidiasis.

Azoles	Fluconazole, ketoconazole, clotrimazole, miconazole, itraconazole, voriconazole.
MECHANISM	Inhibit fungal sterol (ergosterol) synthesis, by inhibiting the cytochrome P-450 enzyme that converts lanosterol to ergosterol.
CLINICAL USE	Local and less serious systemic mycoses. Fluconazole for chronic suppression of cryptococcal meningitis in AIDS patients and candidal infections of all types. Itraconazole for *Blastomyces*, *Coccidioides*, *Histoplasma*. Clotrimazole and miconazole for topical fungal infections.
TOXICITY	Testosterone synthesis inhibition (gynecomastia, esp. with ketoconazole), liver dysfunction (inhibits cytochrome P-450).

Flucytosine	
MECHANISM	Inhibits DNA and RNA biosynthesis by conversion to 5-fluorouracil by cytosine deaminase.
CLINICAL USE	Systemic fungal infections (esp. meningitis caused by *Cryptococcus*) in combination with amphotericin B.
TOXICITY	Bone marrow suppression.

Echinocandins	Caspofungin, micafungin, anidulafungin.
MECHANISM	Inhibits cell wall synthesis by inhibiting synthesis of β-glucan.
CLINICAL USE	Invasive aspergillosis, *Candida*.
TOXICITY	GI upset, flushing (by histamine release).

Terbinafine	
MECHANISM	Inhibits the fungal enzyme squalene epoxidase.
CLINICAL USE	Dermatophytoses (especially onychomycosis—fungal infection of finger or toe nails).
TOXICITY	GI upset, headaches, hepatotoxicity, taste disturbance.

Griseofulvin	
MECHANISM	Interferes with microtubule function; disrupts mitosis. Deposits in keratin-containing tissues (e.g., nails).
CLINICAL USE	Oral treatment of superficial infections; inhibits growth of dermatophytes (tinea, ringworm).
TOXICITY	Teratogenic, carcinogenic, confusion, headaches, ↑ P-450 and warfarin metabolism.

Antiprotozoan therapy	Pyrimethamine (toxoplasmosis), suramin and melarsoprol (*Trypanosoma brucei*), nifurtimox (*T. cruzi*), sodium stibogluconate (leishmaniasis).

Chloroquine

MECHANISM	Blocks detoxification of heme into hemozoin. Heme accumulates and is toxic to plasmodia.
CLINICAL USE	Treatment of plasmodial species other than *P. falciparum* (frequency of resistance in *P. falciparum* is too high). Resistance due to membrane pump that ↓ intracellular concentration of drug. Treat *P. falciparum* with artemether/lumefantrine or atovaquone/proguanil. For life-threatening malaria, use quinidine in U.S. (quinine elsewhere) or artesunate.
TOXICITY	Retinopathy; pruritus (especially in dark-skinned individuals).

Antihelminthic therapy

Mebendazole, pyrantel pamoate, ivermectin, diethylcarbamazine, praziquantel; immobilize helminths. Use praziquantel against flukes (trematodes) such as *Schistosoma*.

Antiviral therapy

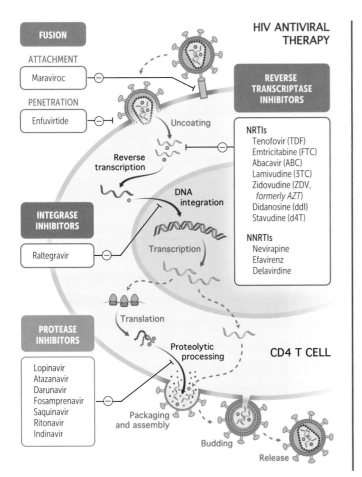

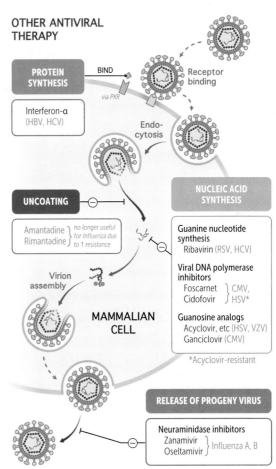

Zanamivir, oseltamivir

MECHANISM	Inhibit influenza neuraminidase → ↓ the release of progeny virus.
CLINICAL USE	Treatment and prevention of both influenza A and B.

Ribavirin

MECHANISM	Inhibits synthesis of guanine nucleotides by competitively inhibiting inosine monophosphate dehydrogenase.
CLINICAL USE	RSV, chronic hepatitis C.
TOXICITY	Hemolytic anemia. Severe teratogen.

Acyclovir, famciclovir, valacyclovir

MECHANISM	Monophosphorylated by HSV/VZV thymidine kinase and not phosphorylated in uninfected cells → few adverse effects. Guanosine analog. Triphosphate formed by cellular enzymes. Preferentially inhibits viral DNA polymerase by chain termination.
CLINICAL USE	HSV and VZV. Weak activity against EBV. No activity against CMV. Used for HSV-induced mucocutaneous and genital lesions as well as for encephalitis. Prophylaxis in immunocompromised patients. No effect on latent forms of HSV and VZV. Valacyclovir, a prodrug of acyclovir, has better oral bioavailability. For herpes zoster, use a related agent, famciclovir.
TOXICITY	Obstructive crystalline nephropathy and acute renal failure if not adequately hydrated.
MECHANISM OF RESISTANCE	Mutated viral thymidine kinase.

Ganciclovir

MECHANISM	5′-monophosphate formed by a CMV viral kinase. Guanosine analog. Triphosphate formed by cellular kinases. Preferentially inhibits viral DNA polymerase.
CLINICAL USE	CMV, especially in immunocompromised patients. Valganciclovir, a prodrug of ganciclovir, has better oral bioavailability.
TOXICITY	Leukopenia, neutropenia, thrombocytopenia, renal toxicity. More toxic to host enzymes than acyclovir.
MECHANISM OF RESISTANCE	Mutated CMV DNA polymerase or lack of viral kinase.

Foscarnet

MECHANISM	Viral DNA polymerase inhibitor that binds to the pyrophosphate-binding site of the enzyme. Does not require activation by viral kinase. **F**oscarnet = p**y**ro**f**osphate analog.
CLINICAL USE	CMV retinitis in immunocompromised patients when ganciclovir fails; acyclovir-resistant HSV.
TOXICITY	Nephrotoxicity.
MECHANISM OF RESISTANCE	Mutated DNA polymerase.

Cidofovir

MECHANISM	Preferentially inhibits viral DNA polymerase. Does not require phosphorylation by viral kinase.
CLINICAL USE	CMV retinitis in immunocompromised patients; acyclovir-resistant HSV. Long half-life.
TOXICITY	Nephrotoxicity (coadminister with probenecid and IV saline to ↓ toxicity).

HIV therapy

Highly active antiretroviral therapy (HAART): initiated when patients present with AIDS-defining illness, low CD4 cell counts (< 500 cells/mm^3), or high viral load. Regimen consists of 3 drugs to prevent resistance:

[2 nucleoside reverse transcriptase inhibitors (NRTIs)] +

[1 non-nucleoside reverse transcriptase inhibitor (NNRTI) OR 1 protease inhibitor OR 1 integrase inhibitor]

DRUG	MECHANISM	TOXICITY
Protease inhibitors		
Atazanavir Darunavir Fosamprenavir Indinavir Lopinavir Ritonavir Saquinavir	Assembly of virions depends on HIV-1 protease (*pol* gene), which cleaves the polypeptide products of HIV mRNA into their functional parts. Thus, protease inhibitors prevent maturation of new viruses. Ritonavir can "boost" other drug concentrations by inhibiting cytochrome P-450. All protease inhibitors end in -*navir*. **Navir** (never) tease a **protease**.	Hyperglycemia, GI intolerance (nausea, diarrhea), lipodystrophy. Nephropathy, hematuria (indinavir).
NRTIs		
Abacavir (ABC) Didanosine (ddl) Emtricitabine (FTC) Lamivudine (3TC) Stavudine (d4T) Tenofovir (TDF) Zidovudine (ZDV, formerly AZT)	Competitively inhibit nucleotide binding to reverse transcriptase and terminate the DNA chain (lack a 3′ OH group). Tenofovir is a nucleoTide; the others are nucleosides and need to be phosphorylated to be active. ZDV is used for general prophylaxis and during pregnancy to ↓ risk of fetal transmission. Have you dined (vudine) with my nuclear (nucleosides) family?	Bone marrow suppression (can be reversed with granulocyte colony-stimulating factor [G-CSF] and erythropoietin), peripheral neuropathy, lactic acidosis (nucleosides), rash (non-nucleosides), anemia (ZDV), pancreatitis (didanosine).
NNRTIs		
Efavirenz Nevirapine Delavirdine	Bind to reverse transcriptase at site different from NRTIs. Do not require phosphorylation to be active or compete with nucleotides.	Rash and hepatotoxicity are common to all NNRTIs. Vivid dreams and CNS symptoms are common with efavirenz. Delavirdine and efavirenz are contraindicated in pregnancy.
Integrase inhibitors		
Raltegravir	Inhibits HIV genome integration into host cell chromosome by reversibly inhibiting HIV integrase.	Hypercholesterolemia.
Fusion inhibitors		
Enfuvirtide	Binds gp41, inhibiting viral entry.	Skin reaction at injection sites.
Maraviroc	Binds CCR-5 on surface of T cells/monocytes, inhibiting interaction with gp120.	

Interferons

MECHANISM	Glycoproteins normally synthesized by virus-infected cells, exhibiting a wide range of antiviral and antitumoral properties.
CLINICAL USE	IFN-α: chronic hepatitis B and C, Kaposi sarcoma, hairy cell leukemia, condyloma acuminatum, renal cell carcinoma, malignant melanoma. IFN-β: multiple sclerosis. IFN-γ: chronic granulomatous disease.
TOXICITY	Neutropenia, myopathy.

Antibiotics to avoid in pregnancy

ANTIBIOTIC	ADVERSE EFFECT
Sulfonamides	Kernicterus
Aminoglycosides	Ototoxicity
Fluoroquinolones	Cartilage damage
Clarithromycin	Embryotoxic
Tetracyclines	Discolored teeth, inhibition of bone growth
Ribavirin (antiviral)	Teratogenic
Griseofulvin (antifungal)	Teratogenic
Chloramphenicol	"Gray baby"

SAFe **C**hildren **T**ake **R**eally **G**ood **C**are.

Immunology

"I hate to disappoint you, but my rubber lips are immune to your charms."
—Batman & Robin

"No State shall make or enforce any law which shall abridge the privileges or immunities of citizens of the United States . . ."
—The United States Constitution

The immunology content on the Step 1 exam has been expanded and reclassified into a new category called the immune system. Mastery of the basic principles and facts in this area will be useful. Cell surface markers are important to know because they are clinically useful (e.g., in identifying specific types of immune deficiency or cancer) and are functionally critical to the jobs immune cells carry out. By spending a little extra effort here, it is possible to turn a traditionally difficult subject into one that is high yield.

▸ **IMMUNOLOGY–LYMPHOID STRUCTURES**

Lymph node	A 2° lymphoid organ that has many afferents, 1 or more efferents. Encapsulated, with trabeculae. Functions are nonspecific filtration by macrophages, storage of B and T cells, and immune response activation.

Follicle Site of B-cell localization and proliferation. In outer cortex. 1° follicles are dense and dormant. 2° follicles have pale central germinal centers and are active.

Medulla Consists of medullary cords (closely packed lymphocytes and plasma cells) and medullary sinuses. Medullary sinuses communicate with efferent lymphatics and contain reticular cells and macrophages.

Paracortex Houses T cells. Region of cortex between follicles and medulla. Contains high endothelial venules through which T and B cells enter from blood. Not well developed in patients with DiGeorge syndrome.

Paracortex enlarges in an extreme cellular immune response (e.g., viral infection).

Lymph drainage

LYMPH NODE CLUSTER	AREA OF BODY DRAINED
Cervical	Head and neck
Hilar	Lungs
Mediastinal	Trachea and esophagus
Axillary	Upper limb, breast, skin above umbilicus
Celiac	Liver, stomach, spleen, pancreas, upper duodenum
Superior mesenteric	Lower duodenum, jejunum, ileum, colon to splenic flexure
Inferior mesenteric	Colon from splenic flexure to upper rectum
Internal iliac	Lower rectum to anal canal (above pectinate line), bladder, vagina (middle third), prostate
Para-aortic	Testes, ovaries, kidneys, uterus
Superficial inguinal	Anal canal (below pectinate line), skin below umbilicus (except popliteal territory)
Popliteal	Dorsolateral foot, posterior calf

Right lymphatic duct—drains right side of body above diaphragm.
Thoracic duct—drains everything else into junction of left subclavian and internal jugular veins.

Sinusoids of spleen

Long, vascular channels in red pulp with fenestrated "barrel hoop" basement membrane. Macrophages found nearby.

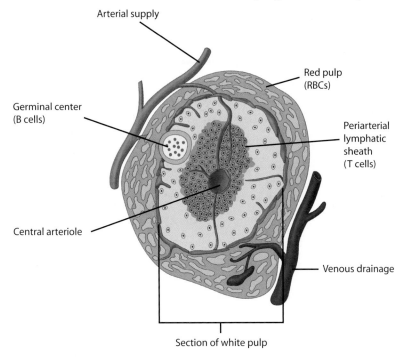

Arterial supply

Red pulp (RBCs)

Germinal center (B cells)

Periarterial lymphatic sheath (T cells)

Central arteriole

Venous drainage

Section of white pulp

T cells are found in the periarterial lymphatic sheath within the white pulp of the spleen. B cells are found in follicles within the white pulp of the spleen. The marginal zone, in between the red pulp and white pulp, contains APCs and specialized B cells, and is where APCs present blood-borne antigens.

Macrophages in the spleen remove encapsulated bacteria.

Splenic dysfunction (e.g., postsplenectomy, sickle cell disease): ↓ IgM → ↓ complement activation → ↓ C3b opsonization → ↑ susceptibility to encapsulated organisms (SHiNE SKiS):

- *Streptococcus pneumoniae*
- *Haemophilus influenzae* type B
- *Neisseria meningitidis*
- *Escherichia coli*
- *Salmonella* spp.
- *Klebsiella pneumoniae*
- Group B Streptococci

Postsplenectomy:

- Howell-Jolly bodies (nuclear remnants)
- Target cells
- Thrombocytosis

Thymus

Site of T-cell differentiation and maturation. Encapsulated. From epithelium of 3rd pharyngeal pouches. Lymphocytes of mesenchymal origin. Cortex is dense with immature T cells; medulla is pale with mature T cells and Hassall corpuscles containing epithelial reticular cells.

T cells = Thymus
B cells = Bone marrow

▶ IMMUNOLOGY–LYMPHOCYTES

Innate vs. adaptive immunity

	Innate immunity	Adaptive immunity
COMPONENTS	Neutrophils, macrophages, monocytes, dendritic cells, NK cells (lymphoid origin), complement	T cells, B cells, circulating antibodies
RESISTANCE	Germline encoded Resistance persists through generations, does not change within an organism's lifetime	Variation through V(D)J recombination during lymphocyte development Microbial resistance not heritable
RESPONSE TO PATHOGENS	Nonspecific Occurs rapidly (minutes to hours)	Highly specific, refined over time Develops over long periods; memory response is faster and more robust
PHYSICAL BARRIERS	Epithelial tight junctions, mucus	—
SECRETED PROTEINS	Lysozyme, complement, CRP, defensins	Immunoglobulins
KEY FEATURES IN PATHOGEN RECOGNITION	Toll-like receptors (TLRs): pattern recognition receptors that recognize pathogen-associated molecular patterns (PAMPs). Examples of PAMPs include LPS (gram-negative bacteria), flagellin (bacteria), ssRNA (viruses)	Memory cells: activated B and T cells; subsequent exposure to a previously encountered antigen → stronger, quicker immune response

MHC I and II

MHC encoded by HLA genes. Present antigen fragments to T cells and bind TCRs.

	MHC I	MHC II
LOCI	HLA-A, HLA-B, HLA-C	HLA-DR, HLA-DP, HLA-DQ
BINDING	TCR and CD8	TCR and CD4
EXPRESSION	Expressed on all nucleated cells Not expressed on RBCs	Expressed only on APCs
FUNCTION	Present **endogenously** synthesized **antigens** (e.g., viral) to **CD8+ cytotoxic T cells**	Present **exogenously** synthesized **proteins** (e.g., bacterial proteins, viral capsid proteins) to **T-helper cells**
ANTIGEN LOADING	Antigen peptides loaded onto MHC I in RER after delivery via TAP peptide transporter	Antigen loaded following release of invariant chain in an acidified endosome
MODE OF TRANSPORT TO CELL SURFACE	β_2-microglobulin	Unknown

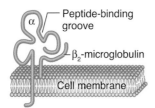

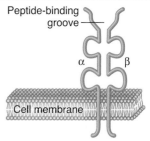

HLA subtypes associated with diseases

A3	Hemochromatosis.	
B27	Psoriatic arthritis, Ankylosing spondylitis, arthritis of Inflammatory bowel disease, Reactive arthritis (formerly Reiter syndrome).	**PAIR.** Also known as seronegative arthropathies.
DQ2/DQ8	Celiac disease.	
DR2	Multiple sclerosis, hay fever, SLE, Goodpasture syndrome.	
DR3	Diabetes mellitus type 1, SLE, Graves disease.	
DR4	Rheumatoid arthritis, diabetes mellitus type 1.	There are 4 walls in a "**rheum**" (room).
DR5	Pernicious anemia → vitamin B_{12} deficiency, Hashimoto thyroiditis.	

Natural killer cells	Use perforin and granzymes to induce apoptosis of virally infected cells and tumor cells. Only lymphocyte member of innate immune system. Activity enhanced by IL-2, IL-12, IFN-β, and IFN-α. Induced to kill when exposed to a nonspecific activation signal on target cell and/or to an absence of class I MHC on target cell surface. Also kills via antibody-dependent cell-mediated cytotoxicity (CD16 binds Fc region of bound Ig, activating the NK cell).

Major functions of B and T cells

B cell functions	Recognize antigen—undergo somatic hypermutation to optimize antigen specificity. Produce antibody—differentiate into plasma cells to secrete specific immunoglobulins. Maintain immunologic memory—memory B cells persist and accelerate future response to antigen.
T cell functions	CD4+ T cells help B cells make antibody and produce cytokines to activate other cells of immune system. CD8+ T cells kill virus-infected cells directly. Delayed cell-mediated hypersensitivity (type IV). Acute and chronic cellular organ rejection. **Rule of 8:** MHC **II** × CD4 = 8; MHC **I** × CD8 = 8.

Differentiation of T cells

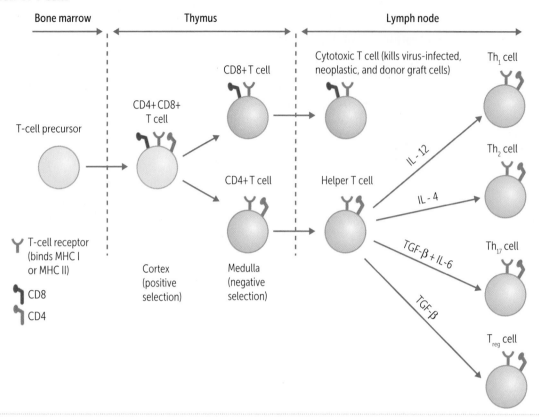

Positive selection	Thymic cortex. T cells expressing TCRs capable of binding surface self MHC molecules survive.
Negative selection	Medulla. T cells expressing TCRs with high affinity for self antigens undergo apoptosis.

T and B cell activation	Antigen-presenting cells (APCs): B cells, macrophages, dendritic cells. Two signals are required for T cell activation, B cell activation, and class switching.
Naive T cell activation	1. Foreign body is phagocytosed by dendritic cell. 2. Foreign antigen is presented on MHC II and recognized by TCR on Th (helper) cell. Antigen is presented on MHC I to Tc (cytotoxic) cells (signal 1). 3. "Costimulatory signal" is given by interaction of B7 and CD28 (signal 2). 4. Th cell activates and produces cytokines. Tc cell activates and is able to recognize and kill virus-infected cell.
B cell activation and class switching	1. Helper T cell activation as above. 2. B cell receptor-mediated endocytosis; foreign antigen is presented on MHC II and recognized by TCR on Th cell (signal 1). 3. CD40 receptor on B cell binds CD40 ligand on Th cell (signal 2). 4. Th cell secretes cytokines that determine Ig class switching of B cell. B cell activates and undergoes class switching, affinity maturation, and antibody production.

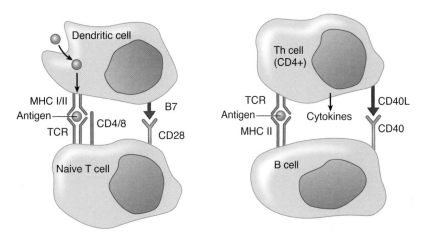

Helper T cells	**Th_1 cell**	**Th_2 cell**
	Secretes IFN-γ	Secretes IL-4, IL-5, IL-6, IL-13
	Activates macrophages and cytotoxic T lymphocytes (CTLs)	Recruits eosinophils for parasite defense and promotes IgE production by B cells
	Inhibited by IL-4 and IL-10 (from Th_2 cell)	Inhibited by IFN-γ (from Th_1 cell)

Macrophage-lymphocyte interaction—macrophages release IL-12, which stimulates T cells to differentiate into Th_1 cells. Th_1 cells release IFN-γ to stimulate macrophages.
Helper T cells have CD4, which binds to MHC II on APCs.

Cytotoxic T cells	Kill virus-infected, neoplastic, and donor graft cells by inducing apoptosis. Release cytotoxic granules containing preformed proteins (perforin—helps to deliver the content of granules into target cell; granzyme B—a serine protease, activates apoptosis inside target cell; granulysin—antimicrobial, induces apoptosis). Cytotoxic T cells have CD8, which binds to MHC I on virus-infected cells.

Regulatory T cells

Help maintain specific immune tolerance by suppressing CD4 and CD8 T-cell effector functions. Identified by expression of cell surface markers CD3, CD4, CD25 (α chain of IL-2 receptor), and transcription factor FOXP3.

Activated regulatory T cells produce anti-inflammatory cytokines like IL-10 and TGF-β.

Antibody structure and function

Variable part of L and H chains recognizes antigens. Fc portion of IgM and IgG fixes complement. Heavy chain contributes to Fc and Fab fractions. Light chain contributes only to Fab fraction.

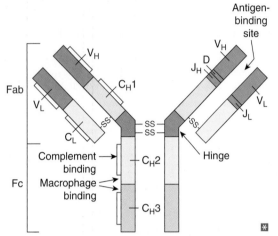

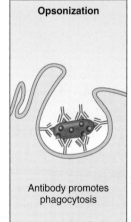 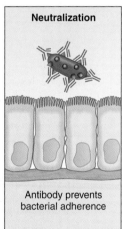 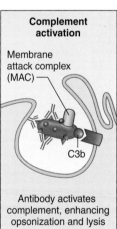

Opsonization	Neutralization	Complement activation
Antibody promotes phagocytosis	Antibody prevents bacterial adherence	Antibody activates complement, enhancing opsonization and lysis

Membrane attack complex (MAC)

C3b

Fab:
- Antigen-binding fragment
- Determines idiotype: unique antigen-binding pocket; only 1 antigenic specificity expressed per B cell

Fc:
- Constant
- Carboxy terminal
- Complement binding
- Carbohydrate side chains
- Determines isotype (IgM, IgD, etc.)

Antibody diversity is generated by:
- Random "recombination" of VJ (light-chain) or V(D)J (heavy-chain) genes
- Random combination of heavy chains with light chains
- Somatic hypermutation (following antigen stimulation)
- Addition of nucleotides to DNA during recombination (see 1st entry in this list) by terminal deoxynucleotidyl transferase

Immunoglobulin isotypes	Mature B lymphocytes express IgM and IgD on their surfaces. They may differentiate in germinal centers of lymph nodes by isotype switching (gene rearrangement; mediated by cytokines and CD40 ligand) into plasma cells that secrete IgA, IgE, or IgG.
IgG	Main antibody in 2° (**delayed**) response to an antigen. Most abundant isotype in serum. Fixes complement, crosses the placenta (provides infants with passive immunity), opsonizes bacteria, neutralizes bacterial toxins and viruses. → neutralizes
IgA	Prevents attachment of bacteria and viruses to mucous membranes; does not fix complement. Monomer (in circulation) or dimer (when secreted). Crosses epithelial cells by transcytosis. Most produced antibody overall, but released into secretions (tears, saliva, mucus) and early breast milk (known as colostrum). Picks up secretory component from epithelial cells before secretion.
IgM	Produced in the 1° (**immediate**) response to an antigen. Fixes complement but does not cross the placenta. Antigen receptor on the surface of B cells. Monomer on B cell or pentamer when secreted. Shape of pentamer allows it to efficiently trap free antigens out of tissue while humoral response evolves.
IgD	Unclear function. Found on the surface of many B cells and in serum.
IgE	Binds mast cells and basophils; cross-links when exposed to allergen, mediating immediate (type I) hypersensitivity through release of inflammatory mediators such as histamine. Mediates immunity to worms by activating eosinophils. Lowest concentration in serum.

Antigen type and memory

Thymus-independent antigens	Antigens lacking a peptide component (e.g., lipopolysaccharides from gram-negative bacteria); cannot be presented by MHC to T cells. Weakly or nonimmunogenic; vaccines often require boosters (e.g., pneumococcal polysaccharide vaccine).
Thymus-dependent antigens	Antigens containing a protein component (e.g., diphtheria vaccine). Class switching and immunologic memory occur as a result of direct contact of B cells with Th cells (CD40–CD40 ligand interaction). long term memory.

▶ IMMUNOLOGY–IMMUNE RESPONSES

Acute-phase reactants	Factors whose serum concentrations change significantly in response to inflammation; produced by the liver in both acute and chronic inflammatory states. Induced by IL-6, IL-1, TNF-α, and IFN-γ.
POSITIVE (UPREGULATED)	
Serum amyloid A	Prolonged elevation can lead to amyloidosis.
C-reactive protein	Opsonin; fixes complement and facilitates phagocytosis. Measured clinically as a sign of ongoing inflammation.
Ferritin	Binds and sequesters iron to inhibit microbial iron scavenging. microbes we inn
Fibrinogen	Coagulation factor; promotes endothelial repair; correlates with ESR. if ESR ↑ fibrinogen ↑
Hepcidin	Prevents release of iron bound by ferritin → anemia of chronic disease.
NEGATIVE (DOWNREGULATED)	
Albumin	Reduction conserves amino acids for positive reactants.
Transferrin	Internalized by macrophages to sequester iron.

Complement

Overview	System of interacting plasma proteins that play a role in innate immunity and inflammation. MAC defends against gram-negative bacteria.	
Activation	Classic pathway—IgG or IgM mediated. Alternative pathway—microbe surface molecules. Lectin pathway—mannose or other sugars on microbe surface.	GM makes classic cars.
Functions	C3b—opsonization. C3a, C4a, C5a—anaphylaxis. C5a—neutrophil chemotaxis. C5b-9—cytolysis by membrane attack complex (MAC).	C3b binds bacteria.
Opsonins	C3b and IgG are the two 1° opsonins in bacterial defense; C3b also helps clear immune complexes.	
Inhibitors	Decay-accelerating factor (DAF, aka CD55) and C1 esterase inhibitor help prevent complement activation on self cells (e.g., RBC).	

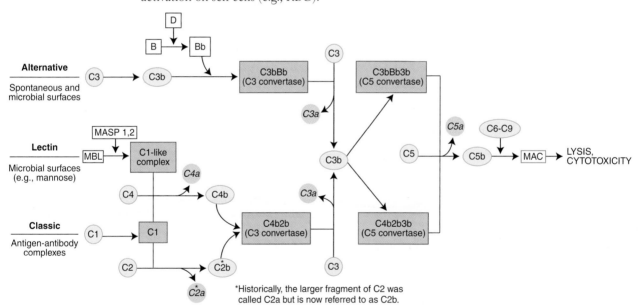

*Historically, the larger fragment of C2 was called C2a but is now referred to as C2b.

Complement disorders

C1 esterase inhibitor deficiency	Causes hereditary angioedema. ACE inhibitors are contraindicated.
C3 deficiency	Increases risk of severe, recurrent pyogenic sinus and respiratory tract infections; ↑ susceptibility to type III hypersensitivity reactions.
C5–C9 deficiencies	Increase susceptibility to recurrent *Neisseria* bacteremia.
DAF (GPI anchored enzyme) deficiency	Causes complement-mediated lysis of RBCs and paroxysmal nocturnal hemoglobinuria.

Important cytokines

SECRETED BY MACROPHAGES

IL-1	An endogenous pyrogen, also called osteoclast-activating factor. Causes fever, acute inflammation. Activates endothelium to express adhesion molecules; induces chemokine secretion to recruit leukocytes.	"Hot T-bone stEAK": IL-1: fever (hot). IL-2: stimulates T cells. IL-3: stimulates bone marrow. IL-4: stimulates IgE production. IL-5: stimulates IgA production. IL-6: stimulates aKute-phase protein production.
IL-6	An endogenous pyrogen. Also secreted by Th_2 cells. Causes fever and stimulates production of acute-phase proteins.	
IL-8	Major chemotactic factor for neutrophils.	"Clean up on aisle 8." Neutrophils are recruited by IL-8 to clear infections.
IL-12	Induces differentiation of T cells into Th_1 cells. Activates NK cells. Also secreted by B cells.	
TNF-α	Mediates septic shock. Activates endothelium. Causes leukocyte recruitment, vascular leak.	

SECRETED BY ALL T CELLS

IL-2	Stimulates growth of helper, cytotoxic, and regulatory T cells.	
IL-3	Supports the growth and differentiation of bone marrow stem cells. Functions like GM-CSF.	

FROM Th_1 CELLS

Interferon-γ	Has antiviral and antitumor properties. Activates NK cells to kill virus-infected cells, Increases MHC expression and antigen presentation in all cells.	

FROM Th_2 CELLS

IL-4	Induces differentiation into Th_2 cells. Promotes growth of B cells. Enhances class switching to IgE and IgG.	
IL-5	Promotes differentiation of B cells. Enhances class switching to IgA. Stimulates the growth and differentiation of eosinophils.	
IL-10	Modulates inflammatory response. Inhibits actions of activated T cells and Th_1. Also secreted by regulatory T cells.	TGF-β has similar actions to IL-10, because it is involved in inhibiting inflammation.

Interferon α and β	A part of innate host defense against both RNA and DNA viruses. **Interferons** are glycoproteins synthesized by viral-infected cells that act locally on uninfected cells, "priming them" for viral defense. When a virus infects "primed" cells, viral dsRNA activates: • RNAase L → degradation of viral/host mRNA. • Protein kinase → inhibition of viral/host protein synthesis. Essentially results in apoptosis, thereby interrupting viral amplification.	**Inter**feres with viruses.

Cell surface proteins	All cells except mature RBCs have MHC I.	
T cells	TCR (binds antigen-MHC complex) CD3 (associated with TCR for signal transduction) CD28 (binds B7 on APC)	
Helper T cells	CD4, CD40 ligand	
Cytotoxic T cells	CD8	
B cells	Ig (binds antigen) CD19, CD20, CD21 (receptor for EBV), CD40 MHC II, B7	You can drink **B**eer at the **Bar** when you're **21**: **B** cells, **E**pstein-**B**arr virus; CD-**21**.
Macrophages	CD14, CD40 MHC II, B7 Fc and C3b receptors (enhanced phagocytosis)	
NK cells	CD16 (binds Fc of IgG), CD56 (unique marker for NK)	

Anergy	Self-reactive T cells become nonreactive without costimulatory molecule. B cells also become anergic, but tolerance is less complete than in T cells.

Effects of bacterial toxins	Superantigens (*S. pyogenes* and *S. aureus*)—cross-link the β region of the T-cell receptor to the MHC class II on APCs. Can activate any T cell, leading to massive release of cytokines. Endotoxins/lipopolysaccharide (gram-negative bacteria)—directly stimulate macrophages by binding to endotoxin receptor CD14; Th cells are not involved.

Antigenic variation

Classic examples:
- Bacteria—*Salmonella* (2 flagellar variants), *Borrelia* (relapsing fever), *Neisseria gonorrhoeae* (pilus protein).
- Virus—influenza (major = shift, minor = drift).
- Parasites—trypanosomes (programmed rearrangement).

Some mechanisms for variation include DNA rearrangement and RNA segment reassortment (e.g., influenza major shift).

Passive vs. active immunity

	Passive	Active
MEANS OF ACQUISITION	Receiving preformed antibodies	Exposure to foreign antigens
ONSET	Rapid	Slow
DURATION	Short span of antibodies (half-life = 3 weeks)	Long-lasting protection (memory)
EXAMPLES	IgA in breast milk, maternal IgG crossing placenta, antitoxin, humanized monoclonal antibody	Natural infection, vaccines, toxoid
NOTES	After exposure to Tetanus toxin, Botulinum toxin, HBV, or Rabies virus, patients are given preformed antibodies (passive)—"To Be Healed Rapidly"	Combined passive and active immunizations can be given for hepatitis B or rabies exposure

Vaccination

Vaccines are used to induce an active immune response (humoral and/or cellular) to specific pathogens.

VACCINE TYPE	DESCRIPTION	PROS/CONS	EXAMPLES
Live attenuated vaccine	Microorganism loses its pathogenicity but retains capacity for transient growth within inoculated host. Mainly induces a **cellular response.**	Pro: induces strong, often lifelong immunity. Con: may revert to virulent form. Often contraindicated in pregnancy and immune deficiency.	Measles, mumps, rubella, polio (Sabin), influenza (intranasal), varicella, yellow fever.
Inactivated or killed vaccine	Pathogen is inactivated by heat or chemicals; maintaining epitope structure on surface antigens is important for immune response. **Humoral immunity** induced.	Pro: stable and safer than live vaccines. Con: weaker immune response; booster shots usually required.	Cholera, hepatitis A, polio (Salk), influenza (injection), rabies.

Hypersensitivity types

| **Type I** | Anaphylactic and atopic—free antigen cross-links IgE on presensitized mast cells and basophils, triggering immediate release of vasoactive amines that act at postcapillary venules (i.e., histamine). Reaction develops rapidly after antigen exposure because of preformed antibody. Delayed response follows due to production of arachidonic acid metabolites (e.g., leukotrienes). | First (type) and Fast (anaphylaxis). Types I, II, and III are all antibody mediated. Test: skin test for specific IgE. |

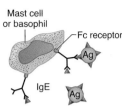

Mast cell or basophil — Fc receptor — Ag — IgE — Ag

| **Type II** | Cytotoxic (antibody mediated)—IgM, IgG bind to fixed antigen on "enemy" cell, leading to cellular destruction.
 3 mechanisms:
 ▪ Opsonization leading to phagocytosis or complement activation
 ▪ Complement-mediated lysis
 ▪ Antibody-dependent cell-mediated cytotoxicity, usually due to NK cells or macrophages | Type II is cy-2-toxic.
 Antibody and complement lead to membrane attack complex (MAC).
 Test: direct and indirect Coombs'.
 Direct: detects antibodies that **have** adhered to patient's RBCs (e.g., test an Rh ⊕ infant of an Rh ⊖ mother).
 Indirect: detects antibodies that **can** adhere to other RBCs (e.g., test an Rh ⊖ woman for Rh ⊕ antibodies). |

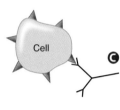

Cell Ⓒ

Ⓒ = complement

| **Type III** | Immune complex—antigen-antibody (IgG) complexes activate complement, which attracts neutrophils; neutrophils release lysosomal enzymes.

 Serum sickness—an immune complex disease (type III) in which antibodies to the foreign proteins are produced (takes 5 days). Immune complexes form and are deposited in membranes, where they fix complement (leads to tissue damage). More common than Arthus reaction.

 Arthus reaction—a local subacute antibody-mediated hypersensitivity (type III) reaction. Intradermal injection of antigen induces antibodies, which form antigen-antibody complexes in the skin. Characterized by edema, necrosis, and activation of complement. | In type III reaction, imagine an immune complex as **3** things stuck together: antigen-antibody-complement.

 Most serum sickness is now caused by drugs (not serum) acting as haptens. Fever, urticaria, arthralgias, proteinuria, lymphadenopathy 5–10 days after antigen exposure.

 Antigen-antibody complexes cause the Arthus reaction.
 Test: immunofluorescent staining. |

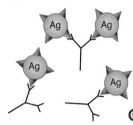

Ag Ag Ag Ag Ⓒ

| **Type IV** | Delayed (T-cell-mediated) type—sensitized T lymphocytes encounter antigen and then release lymphokines (leads to macrophage activation; no antibody involved). | 4th and last—delayed. Cell mediated; therefore, it is not transferable by serum.
 4 T's = T lymphocytes, Transplant rejections, TB skin tests, Touching (contact dermatitis).
 Test: patch test, PPD.

 ACID:
 Anaphylactic and Atopic (type I)
 Cytotoxic (antibody mediated) (type II)
 Immune complex (type III)
 Delayed (cell mediated) (type IV) |

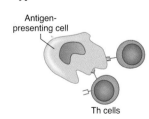

Antigen-presenting cell

Th cells

Hypersensitivity disorders

REACTION	EXAMPLES	PRESENTATION
Type I	Anaphylaxis (e.g., bee sting, some food/drug allergies) Allergic and atopic disorders (e.g., rhinitis, hay fever, eczema, hives, asthma)	Immediate, anaphylactic, atopic
Type II	Autoimmune hemolytic anemia Pernicious anemia Idiopathic thrombocytopenic purpura Erythroblastosis fetalis Acute hemolytic transfusion reactions Rheumatic fever Goodpasture syndrome Bullous pemphigoid Pemphigus vulgaris	Disease tends to be specific to tissue or site where antigen is found
Type III	SLE Polyarteritis nodosa Poststreptococcal glomerulonephritis Serum sickness Arthus reaction (e.g., swelling and inflammation following tetanus vaccine)	Can be associated with vasculitis and systemic manifestations
Type IV	Multiple sclerosis Guillain-Barré syndrome Graft-versus-host disease PPD (test for *M. tuberculosis*) Contact dermatitis (e.g., poison ivy, nickel allergy)	Response is delayed and does **not** involve antibodies (vs. types I, II, and III)

Blood transfusion reactions

TYPE	PATHOGENESIS	CLINICAL PRESENTATION
Allergic reaction	Type I hypersensitivity reaction against plasma proteins in transfused blood.	Urticaria, pruritus, wheezing, fever. Treat with antihistamines.
Anaphylactic reaction	Severe allergic reaction. IgA-deficient individuals must receive blood products that lack IgA.	Dyspnea, bronchospasm, hypotension, respiratory arrest, shock.
Febrile nonhemolytic transfusion reaction	Type II hypersensitivity reaction. Host antibodies against donor HLA antigens and leukocytes.	Fever, headaches, chills, flushing.
Acute hemolytic transfusion reaction	Type II hypersensitivity reaction. Intravascular hemolysis (ABO blood group incompatibility) or extravascular hemolysis (host antibody reaction against foreign antigen on donor RBCs).	Fever, hypotension, tachypnea, tachycardia, flank pain, hemoglobinemia (intravascular), jaundice (extravascular hemolysis).

Autoantibodies

AUTOANTIBODY	ASSOCIATED DISORDER
Anti-ACh receptor	Myasthenia gravis
Anti-basement membrane	Goodpasture syndrome
Anti-cardiolipin, lupus anticoagulant	SLE, antiphospholipid syndrome
Anticentromere	Limited scleroderma (CREST syndrome)
Anti-desmoglein	Pemphigus vulgaris
Anti-dsDNA, anti-Smith	SLE
Anti-glutamate decarboxylase	Type 1 diabetes mellitus
Anti-hemidesmosome	Bullous pemphigoid
Antihistone	Drug-induced lupus
Anti-Jo-1, anti-SRP, anti-Mi-2	Polymyositis, dermatomyositis
Antimicrosomal, antithyroglobulin	Hashimoto thyroiditis
Antimitochondrial	1° biliary cirrhosis
Antinuclear antibodies	SLE, nonspecific
Anti-Scl-70 (anti-DNA topoisomerase I)	Scleroderma (diffuse)
Anti-smooth muscle	Autoimmune hepatitis
Anti-SSA, anti-SSB (anti-Ro, anti-La)	Sjögren syndrome
Anti-TSH receptor	Graves disease
Anti-U1 RNP (ribonucleoprotein)	Mixed connective tissue disease
c-ANCA (PR3-ANCA)	Granulomatosis with polyangiitis (Wegener)
IgA antiendomysial, IgA anti-tissue transglutaminase	Celiac disease
p-ANCA (MPO-ANCA)	Microscopic polyangiitis, Churg-Strauss syndrome
Rheumatoid factor (antibody, most commonly IgM, specific to IgG Fc region), anti-CCP	Rheumatoid arthritis

Infections in immunodeficiency

PATHOGEN	NO T CELLS	NO B CELLS	NO GRANULOCYTE	NO COMPLEMENT
Bacteria	Sepsis	Encapsulated: *Streptococcus pneumoniae*, *Haemophilus influenzae* type B, *Neisseria meningitidis*, *Escherichia coli*, *Salmonella*, *Klebsiella pneumoniae*, group B Strep (SHiNE SKiS)	*Staphylococcus*, *Burkholderia cepacia*, *Serratia*, *Nocardia*	*Neisseria* (no membrane attack complex)
Virus	CMV, EBV, JCV, VZV chronic infection with respiratory/GI viruses	Enteroviral encephalitis, poliovirus (live vaccine contraindicated)	N/A	N/A
Fungi/parasites	*Candida*, PCP	GI giardiasis (no IgA)	*Candida*, *Aspergillus*	N/A

Note: B-cell deficiencies tend to produce recurrent bacterial infections, whereas T-cell deficiencies produce more fungal and viral infections.

Immune deficiencies

DISEASE	DEFECT	PRESENTATION	FINDINGS
B-cell disorders			
X-linked (Bruton) agammaglobulinemia	Defect in *BTK*, a tyrosine kinase gene → no B cell maturation. X-linked recessive (↑ in Boys).	Recurrent bacterial and enteroviral infections after 6 months (↓ maternal IgG).	Normal CD19+ B cell count, ↓ pro-B, ↓ Ig of all classes. Absent/scanty lymph nodes and tonsils.
Selective IgA deficiency	Unknown. Most common 1° immunodeficiency.	Majority Asymptomatic. Can see Airway and GI infections, Autoimmune disease, Atopy, Anaphylaxis to IgA-containing products.	IgA < 7 mg/dL with normal IgG, IgM levels.
Common variable immunodeficiency	Defect in B-cell differentiation. Many causes.	Can be acquired in 20s–30s; ↑ risk of autoimmune disease, bronchiectasis, lymphoma, sinopulmonary infections.	↓ plasma cells, ↓ immunoglobulins.
T-cell disorders			
Thymic aplasia (DiGeorge syndrome)	22q11 deletion; failure to develop 3rd and 4th pharyngeal pouches → absent thymus and parathyroids.	Tetany (hypocalcemia), recurrent viral/fungal infections (T-cell deficiency), conotruncal abnormalities (e.g., tetralogy of Fallot, truncus arteriosus).	↓ T cells, ↓ PTH, ↓ Ca^{2+}. Absent thymic shadow on CXR. 22q11 deletion detected by FISH.
IL-12 receptor deficiency	↓ Th_1 response. Autosomal recessive.	Disseminated mycobacterial and fungal infections; may present after administration of BCG vaccine.	↓ IFN-γ.
Autosomal dominant hyper-IgE syndrome (Job syndrome)	Deficiency of Th_{17} cells due to *STAT3* mutation → impaired recruitment of neutrophils to sites of infection.	FATED: coarse Facies, cold (noninflamed) staphylococcal Abscesses, retained primary Teeth, ↑ IgE, Dermatologic problems (eczema).	↑ IgE, ↓ IFN-γ.
Chronic mucocutaneous candidiasis	T-cell dysfunction. Many causes.	Noninvasive *Candida albicans* infections of skin and mucous membranes.	Absent in vitro T-cell proliferation in response to *Candida* antigens. Absent cutaneous reaction to *Candida* antigens.

Immune deficiencies (continued)

DISEASE	DEFECT	PRESENTATION	FINDINGS
B- and T-cell disorders			
Severe combined immunodeficiency (SCID)	Several types including defective IL-2R gamma chain (most common, X-linked), adenosine deaminase deficiency (autosomal recessive).	Failure to thrive, chronic diarrhea, thrush. Recurrent viral, bacterial, fungal, and protozoal infections. Treatment: bone marrow transplant (no concern for rejection).	↓ T-cell receptor excision circles (TRECs). Absence of thymic shadow (CXR), germinal centers (lymph node biopsy), and T cells (flow cytometry).
Ataxia-telangiectasia	Defects in *ATM* gene → DNA double strand breaks → cell cycle arrest.	Triad: cerebellar defects (**A**taxia), spider **A**ngiomas (telangiectasia), Ig**A** deficiency.	↑ AFP. ↓ IgA, IgG, and IgE. Lymphopenia, cerebellar atrophy.
Hyper-IgM syndrome	Most commonly due to defective CD40L on Th cells = class switching defect; X-linked recessive.	Severe pyogenic infections early in life; opportunistic infection with *Pneumocystis*, *Cryptosporidium*, CMV.	↑ IgM. ↓↓ IgG, IgA, IgE.
Wiskott-Aldrich syndrome	Mutation in *WAS* gene (X-linked recessive); T cells unable to reorganize actin cytoskeleton.	**WATER**: **W**iskott-Aldrich: **T**hrombocytopenic purpura, **E**czema, **R**ecurrent infections. ↑ risk of autoimmune disease and malignancy.	↓ to normal IgG, IgM. ↑ IgE, IgA. Fewer and smaller platelets.
Phagocyte dysfunction			
Leukocyte adhesion deficiency (type 1)	Defect in LFA-1 integrin (CD18) protein on phagocytes; impaired migration and chemotaxis; autosomal recessive.	Recurrent bacterial skin and mucosal infections, absent pus formation, impaired wound healing, delayed separation of umbilical cord (>30 days).	↑ neutrophils. Absence of neutrophils at infection sites.
Chédiak-Higashi syndrome	Defect in lysosomal trafficking regulator gene (*LYST*). Microtubule dysfunction in phagosome-lysosome fusion; autosomal recessive.	Recurrent pyogenic infections by staphylococci and streptococci, partial albinism, peripheral neuropathy, progressive neurodegeneration, infiltrative lymphohistiocytosis.	Giant granules in neutrophils and platelets. Pancytopenia. Mild coagulation defects.
Chronic granulomatous disease	Defect of NADPH oxidase →↓ reactive oxygen species (e.g., superoxide) and absent respiratory burst in neutrophils; X-linked recessive.	↑ susceptibility to catalase ⊕ organisms (**PLACESS**): *Pseudomonas*, *Listeria*, *Aspergillus*, *Candida*, *E. coli*, *S. aureus*, *Serratia*.	Abnormal dihydrorhodamine (flow cytometry) test. Nitroblue tetrazolium dye reduction test is ⊖ (test out of favor).

Grafts

Autograft	From self.
Syngeneic graft	From identical twin or clone.
Allograft	From nonidentical individual of same species.
Xenograft	From different species.

Transplant rejection

TYPE OF REJECTION	ONSET	PATHOGENESIS	FEATURES
Hyperacute	Within minutes	Pre-existing recipient antibodies react to donor antigen (type II reaction), activate complement.	Widespread thrombosis of graft vessels → ischemia/necrosis. Graft must be removed.
Acute	Weeks to months	Cellular: CTLs activated against donor MHCs. Humoral: similar to hyperacute, except antibodies develop after transplant.	Vasculitis of graft vessels with dense interstitial lymphocytic infiltrate. Prevent/reverse with immunosuppressants.
Chronic	Months to years	Recipient T cells perceive donor MHC as recipient MHC and react against donor antigens presented. Both cellular and humoral components.	Irreversible. T-cell and antibody-mediated damage. Organ specific: Heart—atherosclerosis. Lungs—bronchiolitis obliterans. Liver—vanishing bile ducts. Kidney—vascular fibrosis, glomerulopathy.
Graft-versus-host disease	Varies	Grafted immunocompetent T cells proliferate in the immunocompromised host and reject host cells with "foreign" proteins → severe organ dysfunction.	Maculopapular rash, jaundice, diarrhea, hepatosplenomegaly. Usually in bone marrow and liver transplants (rich in lymphocytes). Potentially beneficial in bone marrow transplant for leukemia (graft-versus-tumor effect).

▶ **IMMUNOLOGY–IMMUNOSUPPRESSANTS**

Immunosuppressants   Agents that block lymphocyte activation and proliferation. Reduce acute transplant rejection by suppressing cellular immunity. Frequently combined to achieve greater efficacy with ↓ toxicity. Chronic suppression ↑ risk of infection and malignancy.

DRUG	MECHANISM	USE	TOXICITY	NOTES
Cyclosporine	Calcineurin inhibitor; binds cyclophilin. Blocks T cell activation by **preventing IL-2 transcription.**	Transplant rejection prophylaxis, psoriasis, rheumatoid arthritis.	**Nephrotoxicity,** hypertension, hyperlipidemia, hyperglycemia, tremor, hirsutism, gingival hyperplasia.	Both calcineurin inhibitors are highly nephrotoxic.
Tacrolimus	Calcineurin inhibitor; binds FK506 binding protein (FKBP). Blocks T cell activation by **preventing IL-2 transcription.**	Transplant rejection prophylaxis.	Similar to cyclosporine, ↑ risk of diabetes and neurotoxicity; no gingival hyperplasia or hirsutism.	-limus drugs bind FKBP.
Sirolimus (Rapamycin)	mTOR inhibitor; binds FKBP. Blocks T cell activation and B cell differentiation by **preventing IL-2 signal transduction.**	Kidney transplant rejection prophylaxis.	Anemia, thrombocytopenia, leukopenia, insulin resistance, hyperlipidemia; **non-nephrotoxic.**	Kidney "sir-vives." Synergistic with cyclosporine. Also used in drug-eluting stents.
Basiliximab	Monoclonal antibody; blocks IL-2R.	Kidney transplant rejection prophylaxis.	Edema, hypertension, tremor.	
Azathioprine	Antimetabolite precursor of 6-mercaptopurine. Inhibits lymphocyte proliferation by blocking nucleotide synthesis.	Transplant rejection prophylaxis, rheumatoid arthritis, Crohn disease, glomerulonephritis, other autoimmune conditions.	Leukopenia, anemia, thrombocytopenia.	6-MP degraded by xanthine oxidase; toxicity ↑ by allopurinol. Pronounce "azathio-**purine.**"
Glucocorticoids	Inhibit NF-κB. Suppress both B and T cell function by ↓ transcription of many cytokines.	Transplant rejection prophylaxis (immune suppression), many autoimmune disorders, inflammation.	Hyperglycemia, osteoporosis, central obesity, muscle breakdown, psychosis, acne, hypertension, cataracts, peptic ulcers.	Can cause iatrogenic Cushing syndrome.

Immunosuppression targets

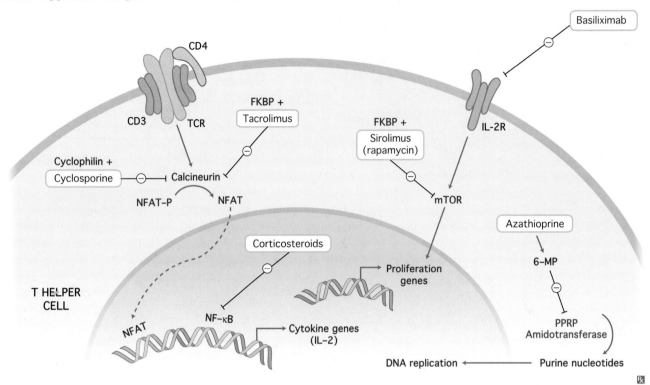

Recombinant cytokines and clinical uses

AGENT	CLINICAL USES
Epoetin alfa (erythropoietin)	Anemias (especially in renal failure)
Thrombopoietin	Thrombocytopenia
Oprelvekin (interleukin-11)	Thrombocytopenia
Filgrastim (granulocyte colony-stimulating factor)	Recovery of bone marrow
Sargramostim (granulocyte-macrophage colony-stimulating factor)	Recovery of bone marrow
Aldesleukin (interleukin-2)	Renal cell carcinoma, metastatic melanoma
IFN-α	Chronic hepatitis B and C, Kaposi sarcoma, hairy cell leukemia, condyloma acuminatum, renal cell carcinoma, malignant melanoma
IFN-β	Multiple sclerosis
IFN-γ	Chronic granulomatous disease

Therapeutic antibodies

AGENT	TARGET	CLINICAL USE	NOTES
Cancer therapy			
Alemtuzumab	CD52	CLL	"Alymtuzumab"—chronic lymphocytic leukemia
Bevacizumab	VEGF	Colorectal cancer, renal cell carcinoma	
Cetuximab	EGFR	Stage IV colorectal cancer, head and neck cancer	
Rituximab	CD20	B-cell non-Hodgkin lymphoma, rheumatoid arthritis (with MTX), ITP	
Trastuzumab	HER2/neu	Breast cancer, gastric cancer	HER2—"tras2zumab"
Autoimmune disease therapy			
Infliximab, adalimumab	TNF-α	IBD, rheumatoid arthritis, ankylosing spondylitis, psoriasis	Rheumatoid arthritis "**inflix**" pain in "**da limbs**"
Natalizumab	α4-integrin	Multiple sclerosis, Crohn disease	α4-integrin: leukocyte adhesion Risk of PML in patients with JC virus
Other			
Abciximab	Glycoprotein IIb/IIIa	Anti-platelet agent for prevention of ischemic complications in patients undergoing percutaneous coronary intervention	IIb times IIIa equals "absiximab"
Denosumab	RANKL	Osteoporosis; inhibits osteoclast maturation (mimics osteoprotegrin)	Denosumab affects osteoclasts
Digoxin immune Fab	Digoxin	Antidote for digoxin toxicity	
Omalizumab	IgE	Allergic asthma; prevents IgE binding to FcϵRI	
Palivizumab	RSV F protein	RSV prophylaxis for high-risk infants	PaliVIzumab—VIrus

▶ NOTES

Pathology

"Digressions, objections, delight in mockery, carefree mistrust are signs of health; everything unconditional belongs in pathology."

—Friedrich Nietzsche

The fundamental principles of pathology are key to understanding diseases in all organ systems. Major topics such as inflammation and neoplasia appear frequently in questions across different organ systems, and such topics are definitely high yield. For example, the concepts of cell injury and inflammation are key to understanding the inflammatory response that follows myocardial infarction, a very common subject of board questions. Similarly, a familiarity with the early cellular changes that culminate in the development of neoplasias—for example, esophageal or colon cancer—is critical. Finally, make sure you recognize the major tumor-associated genes and are comfortable with key cancer concepts such as tumor staging and metastasis.

▶ **PATHOLOGY–INFLAMMATION**

Apoptosis

Programmed cell death; ATP required. Intrinsic or extrinsic pathway; both pathways → activation of cytosolic caspases that mediate cellular breakdown.

No significant inflammation (unlike necrosis).

Characterized by deeply eosinophilic cytoplasm, cell shrinkage, nuclear shrinkage (pyknosis) and basophilia, membrane blebbing, nuclear fragmentation (karyorrhexis), and formation of apoptotic bodies, which are then phagocytosed.

DNA laddering is a sensitive indicator of apoptosis; during karyorrhexis, endonucleases cleave at internucleosomal regions, yielding 180-bp fragments. Radiation therapy causes apoptosis of tumors and surrounding tissue via free radical formation and dsDNA breakage. Rapidly dividing cells (e.g., skin, GI mucosa) are very susceptible to radiation therapy-induced apoptosis.

Intrinsic pathway

Involved in tissue remodeling in embryogenesis. Occurs when a regulating factor is withdrawn from a proliferating cell population (e.g., ↓ IL-2 after a completed immunological reaction → apoptosis of proliferating effector cells). Also occurs after exposure to injurious stimuli (e.g., radiation, toxins, hypoxia).

Changes in proportions of anti- and pro-apoptotic factors lead to ↑ mitochondrial permeability and cytochrome c release. BAX and BAK are pro-apoptotic proteins; Bcl-2 is anti-apoptotic.

Bcl-2 prevents cytochrome c release by binding to and inhibiting Apaf-1. Apaf-1 normally induces the activation of caspases. If Bcl-2 is overexpressed (e.g., follicular lymphoma), then Apaf-1 is overly inhibited, leading to ↓ caspase activation and tumorigenesis.

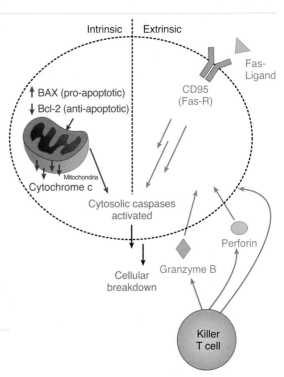

Extrinsic pathway

2 pathways:
- Ligand receptor interactions (FasL binding to Fas [CD95])
- Immune cell (cytotoxic T-cell release of perforin and granzyme B)

Fas-FasL interaction is necessary in thymic medullary negative selection. Mutations in Fas ↑ numbers of circulating self-reacting lymphocytes due to failure of clonal deletion.

After Fas crosslinks with FasL, multiple Fas molecules coalesce, forming a binding site for a death domain–containing adapter protein, FADD. FADD binds inactive caspases, activating them.

Defective Fas-FasL interaction is the basis for autoimmune disorders.

Necrosis	Enzymatic degradation and protein denaturation of a cell resulting from exogenous injury. Intracellular components leak; inflammatory process (unlike apoptosis).

Types	Characteristics
Coagulative	Heart, liver, kidney; occurs in tissues supplied by end-arteries; ↑ cytoplasmic binding of acidophilic dye. Proteins denature first, followed by enzymatic degradation.
Liquefactive	Brain, bacterial abscess; occurs in CNS due to high fat content. In contrast to coagulative necrosis, enzymatic degradation due to the release of lysosomal enzymes occurs first.
Caseous	TB, systemic fungi, *Nocardia*.
Fatty	Enzymatic (pancreatitis [saponification]) and nonenzymatic (e.g., breast trauma); calcium deposits appear dark blue on staining.
Fibrinoid	Vasculitides (e.g., Henoch-Schönlein purpura, Churg-Strauss syndrome), malignant hypertension; amorphous and pink on H&E.
Gangrenous	Dry (ischemic coagulative) and wet (infection); common in limbs and GI tract.

Cell injury	REVERSIBLE WITH O_2	IRREVERSIBLE
	ATP depletion	Nuclear pyknosis, karyorrhexis, karyolysis
	Cellular/mitochondrial swelling (↓ ATP → ↓ activity of Na^+/K^+ pumps)	Plasma membrane damage (degradation of membrane phospholipid)
	Nuclear chromatin clumping	Lysosomal rupture
	↓ glycogen	Mitochondrial permeability/vacuolization; phospholipid-containing amorphous densities within mitochondria (swelling alone is reversible)
	Fatty change	
	Ribosomal/polysomal detachment (↓ protein synthesis)	
	Membrane blebbing	

Ischemia: susceptible areas

Areas susceptible to hypoxia/ischemia and infarction:

ORGAN	LOCATION
Brain	ACA/MCA/PCA boundary areas[a,b]
Heart	Subendocardium (LV)
Kidney	Straight segment of proximal tubule (medulla) Thick ascending limb (medulla)
Liver	Area around central vein (zone III)
Colon	Splenic flexure,[a] rectum[a]

[a]Watershed areas (border zones) receive dual blood supply from most distal branches of 2 arteries, which protects these areas from single-vessel focal blockage. However, these areas are susceptible to ischemia from systemic hypoperfusion.

[b]Hypoxic ischemic encephalopathy (HIE) affects pyramidal cells of hippocampus and Purkinje cells of cerebellum.

Infarcts: red vs. pale	Reperfusion injury is due to damage by free radicals.
Red	Red (hemorrhagic) infarcts (left in **A**) occur in loose tissues with multiple blood supplies, such as liver, lungs, and intestine. Red = reperfusion.
Pale	Pale infarcts (right in **A**) occur in solid tissues with a single blood supply, such as heart, kidney, and spleen.

A **Infarcts.** Image on left shows red infarct (arrows). ℞ Image on right shows pale infarct (arrow). ✖

Shock

First sign of shock is tachycardia. Shock in the setting of DIC 2° to trauma is likely due to sepsis. Distributive shock includes septic, neurogenic, and anaphylactic shock.

Distributive	Hypovolemic/cardiogenic
High-output failure (↓ TPR, ↑ CO, ↑ venous return)	Low-output failure (↑ TPR, ↓ CO, ↓ venous return)
↓ PCWP	PCWP ↑ in cardiogenic PCWP ↓ in hypovolemic
Vasodilation (warm, dry skin)	Vasoconstriction (cold, clammy patient)
Failure to ↑ blood pressure with IV fluids	Blood pressure restored with IV fluids

---

Atrophy

Reduction in the size and/or number of cells. Causes include:
- ↓ endogenous hormones (e.g., post-menopausal ovaries)
- ↑ exogenous hormones (e.g., factitious thyrotoxicosis, steroid use)
- ↓ innervation (e.g., motor neuron damage)
- ↓ blood flow/nutrients
- ↓ metabolic demand (e.g., prolonged hospitalization, paralysis)
- ↑ pressure (e.g., nephrolithiasis)
- Occlusion of secretory ducts (e.g., cystic fibrosis)

Inflammation	Characterized by *rubor* (redness), *dolor* (pain), *calor* (heat), *tumor* (swelling), and *functio laesa* (loss of function).
Vascular component	↑ vascular permeability, vasodilation, endothelial injury.
Cellular component	Neutrophils extravasate from circulation to injured tissue to participate in inflammation through phagocytosis, degranulation, and inflammatory mediator release.
Acute	Neutrophil, eosinophil, and antibody mediated. Acute inflammation is rapid onset (seconds to minutes), lasts minutes to days. Outcomes include complete resolution, abscess formation, and progression to chronic inflammation.
Chronic	Mononuclear cell and fibroblast mediated; characterized by persistent destruction and repair. Associated with blood vessel proliferation, fibrosis. Granuloma: nodular collections of epithelioid macrophages and giant cells. Outcomes include scarring and amyloidosis.

Chromatolysis 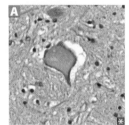	Process involving the cell body following axonal injury. Changes reflect ↑ protein synthesis in effort to repair the damaged axon. Characterized by: ▪ Round cellular swelling **A** ▪ Displacement of the nucleus to the periphery ▪ Dispersion of Nissl substance throughout cytoplasm

Types of calcification

Dystrophic calcification	Calcium deposition in tissues 2° to necrosis. Tends to be localized (e.g., on heart valves). Seen in TB (lungs and pericardium), liquefactive necrosis of chronic abscesses, fat necrosis, infarcts, thrombi, schistosomiasis, Mönckeberg arteriolosclerosis, congenital CMV + toxoplasmosis, psammoma bodies. Is not directly associated with hypercalcemia (i.e., patients are usually **normocalcemic**).
Metastatic calcification	Widespread (i.e., diffuse, metastatic) deposition of calcium in normal tissue 2° to hypercalcemia (e.g., 1° hyperparathyroidism, sarcoidosis, hypervitaminosis D) or high calcium-phosphate product (e.g., chronic renal failure + 2° hyperparathyroidism, long-term dialysis, calciphylaxis, warfarin). Calcium deposits predominantly in interstitial tissues of kidney, lungs, and gastric mucosa (these tissues lose acid quickly; ↑ pH favors deposition). Patients are usually **not normocalcemic**.

Leukocyte extravasation

Extravasation predominantly occurs at postcapillary venules.

Leukocytes exit from blood vessels at sites of tissue injury and inflammation in 4 steps:

STEP	VASCULATURE/STROMA	LEUKOCYTE
❶ Margination and rolling	E-selectin P-selectin GlyCAM-1, CD34	Sialyl-Lewis^X Sialyl-Lewis^X L-selectin
❷ Tight-binding	ICAM-1 (CD54) VCAM-1 (CD106)	CD11/18 integrins (LFA-1, Mac-1) VLA-4 integrin
❸ Diapedesis—leukocyte travels between endothelial cells and exits blood vessel	PECAM-1 (CD31)	PECAM-1 (CD31)
❹ Migration—leukocyte travels through interstitium to site of injury or infection guided by chemotactic signals	Chemotactic products released in response to bacteria: C5a, IL-8, LTB$_4$, kallikrein, platelet-activating factor	Various

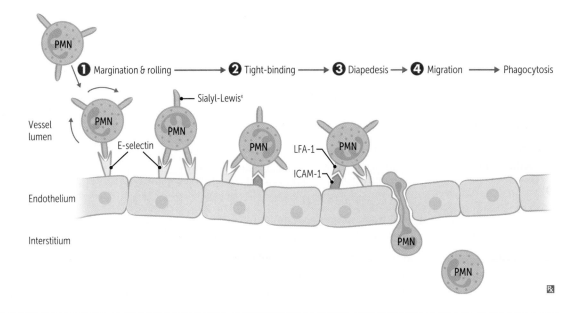

Free radical injury

Free radicals damage cells via membrane lipid peroxidation, protein modification, and DNA breakage.

Initiated via radiation exposure (e.g., cancer therapy), metabolism of drugs (phase I), redox reactions, nitric oxide, transition metals, leukocyte oxidative burst.

Free radicals can be eliminated by enzymes (e.g., catalase, superoxide dismutase, glutathione peroxidase), spontaneous decay, antioxidants (e.g., vitamins A, C, E).

Pathologies include:
- Retinopathy of prematurity
- Bronchopulmonary dysplasia
- Carbon tetrachloride, leading to liver necrosis (fatty change)
- Acetaminophen overdose (fulminant hepatitis, renal papillary necrosis)
- Iron overload (hemochromatosis)
- Reperfusion injury (e.g., superoxide), especially after thrombolytic therapy

Inhalation injury   Most common pulmonary complication after exposure to fire. Inhalation of products of combustion (e.g., carbon particles, toxic fumes) → chemical tracheobronchitis, edema, and pneumonia.

Scar formation   70–80% of tensile strength returns at 3 months following wound; little additional tensile strength will be regained. Two common pathologic types.

	Hypertrophic scars A	**Keloid scars** B
COLLAGEN SYNTHESIS	↑	↑↑↑
COLLAGEN ARRANGEMENT	Parallel	Disorganized
EXTENT	Confined to borders of original wound	Extend beyond borders of original wound
RECURRENCE	Infrequently recur following resection	Frequently recur following resection

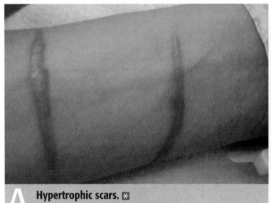

A **Hypertrophic scars.** ✷

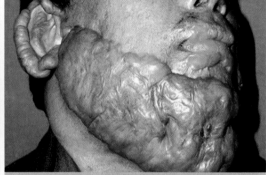

B **Keloid scar.** In a young person, with characteristic "claw-like" projections. Higher risk in African-Americans. ✷

Wound healing

Tissue mediators

MEDIATOR	ROLE
PDGF	Secreted by activated platelets and macrophages Induces vascular remodeling and smooth muscle cell migration Stimulates fibroblast growth for collagen synthesis
FGF	Stimulates all aspects of angiogenesis
EGF	Stimulates cell growth via tyrosine kinases (e.g., EGFR, as expressed by *ERBB2*)
TGF-β	Angiogenesis, fibrosis, cell cycle arrest
Metalloproteinases	Tissue remodeling

PHASE OF WOUND HEALING	MEDIATORS	CHARACTERISTICS
Inflammatory (immediate)	Platelets, neutrophils, macrophages	Clot formation, ↑ vessel permeability and neutrophil migration into tissue; macrophages clear debris 2 days later
Proliferative (2–3 days after wound)	Fibroblasts, myofibroblasts, endothelial cells, keratinocytes, macrophages	Deposition of granulation tissue and collagen, angiogenesis, epithelial cell proliferation, dissolution of clot, and wound contraction (mediated by myofibroblasts)
Remodeling (1 week after wound)	Fibroblasts	Type III collagen replaced by type I collagen, ↑ tensile strength of tissue

Granulomatous diseases

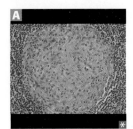

Bartonella henselae (cat scratch disease)
Berylliosis
Churg-Strauss syndrome
Crohn disease
Francisella tularensis
Fungal infections (e.g., histoplasmosis, blastomycosis)
Granulomatosis with polyangiitis (Wegener)
Listeria monocytogenes (granulomatosis infantiseptica)
M. leprae (leprosy; Hansen disease)
M. tuberculosis
Treponema pallidum (tertiary syphilis)
Sarcoidosis **A**
Schistosomiasis

Th_1 cells secrete γ-interferon, activating macrophages. TNF-α from macrophages induce and maintain granuloma formation. Anti-TNF drugs can, as a side effect, cause sequestering granulomas to breakdown, leading to disseminated disease. Always test for latent TB before starting anti-TNF therapy.

Exudate vs. transudate

Exudate ("Thick...")	Transudate ("and thin")
Cellular	Hypocellular
Protein-rich	Protein-poor
Specific gravity > 1.020	Specific gravity < 1.012
Due to: ▪ Lymphatic obstruction ▪ Inflammation/infection ▪ Malignancy	Due to: ▪ ↑ hydrostatic pressure (e.g., CHF) ▪ ↓ oncotic pressure (e.g., cirrhosis) ▪ Na^+ retention

---

Erythrocyte sedimentation rate

Products of inflammation (e.g., fibrinogen) coat RBCs and cause aggregation. When aggregated, RBCs fall at a faster rate within the test tube.

↑ ESR	↓ ESR
Most anemias Infections Inflammation (e.g., temporal arteritis) Cancer (e.g., multiple myeloma) Pregnancy Autoimmune disorders (e.g., SLE)	Sickle cell (altered shape) Polycythemia (↑ RBCs "dilute" aggregation factors) CHF (unknown)

Iron poisoning

One of the leading causes of fatality from toxicologic agents in children.

MECHANISM	Cell death due to peroxidation of membrane lipids.
SYMPTOMS	Acute—nausea, vomiting, gastric bleeding, lethargy. Chronic—metabolic acidosis, scarring leading to GI obstruction.
TREATMENT	Chelation (e.g., IV deferoxamine, oral deferasirox) and dialysis.

Amyloidosis	Abnormal aggregation of proteins (or their fragments) into β-pleated sheet structures A B → damage and apoptosis.
COMMON TYPES	**DESCRIPTION**
AL (primary)	Due to deposition of proteins from Ig Light chains. Can occur as a plasma cell disorder or associated with multiple myeloma. Often affects multiple organ systems, including renal (nephrotic syndrome), cardiac (restrictive cardiomyopathy, arrhythmia), hematologic (easy bruising), GI (hepatomegaly), and neurologic (neuropathy).
AA (secondary)	Seen with chronic conditions, such as rheumatoid arthritis, IBD, spondyloarthropathy, protracted infection. Fibrils composed of serum Amyloid A. Often multisystem like AL amyloidosis.
Dialysis-related	Fibrils composed of β_2-microglobulin in patients with ESRD and/or on long-term dialysis. May present as carpal tunnel syndrome.
Heritable	Heterogeneous group of disorders. Example is ATTR neurologic/cardiac amyloidosis due to transthyretin (TTR or prealbumin) gene mutation.
Age-related (senile) systemic	Due to deposition of normal (wild-type) TTR in myocardium and other sites. Slower progression of cardiac dysfunction relative to AL amyloidosis.
Organ-specific	Amyloid deposition localized to a single organ. Most important form is amyloidosis in Alzheimer disease due to deposition of amyloid-β protein cleaved from amyloid precursor protein (APP). Islet amyloid polypeptide (IAPP) is commonly seen in diabetes mellitus type 2 and is caused by deposition of amylin in pancreatic islets.

A **Amyloidosis.** Congo red stain shows amyloid deposits within vessel walls.

B **Amyloidosis.** Congo red stain shows apple green birefringence under polarized light.

Lipofuscin

A yellow-brown "wear and tear" pigment 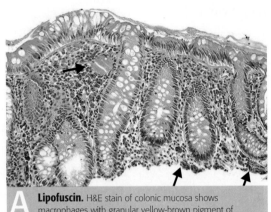 associated with normal aging.

Formed by oxidation and polymerization of autophagocytosed organellar membranes.

Autopsy of elderly person will reveal deposits in heart, liver, kidney, eye, and other organs.

A **Lipofuscin.** H&E stain of colonic mucosa shows macrophages with granular yellow-brown pigment of lipofuscin. ✱

▶ PATHOLOGY–NEOPLASIA

Neoplastic progression
Hallmarks of cancer—evasion of apoptosis, growth signal self-sufficiency, anti-growth signal insensitivity, sustained angiogenesis, limitless replicative potential, tissue invasion, and metastasis.

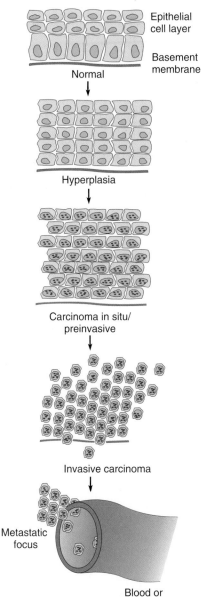

• Normal cells with basal → apical differentiation

• Cells ↑ in number—**hyperplasia**
• Abnormal proliferation of cells with loss of size, shape, and orientation—**dysplasia**

Carcinoma in situ/preinvasive
• Neoplastic cells have not invaded basement membrane
• High nuclear/cytoplasmic ratio and clumped chromatin
• Neoplastic cells encompass entire thickness

Invasive carcinoma
• Cells have invaded basement membrane using **collagenases** and **hydrolases** (metalloproteinases)
• Can metastasize if they reach a blood or lymphatic vessel

Metastasis—spread to distant organ
• Must survive immune attack
• "Seed and soil" theory of metastasis
  • Seed = tumor embolus
  • Soil = target organ—liver, lungs, bone, brain, etc.

P-glycoprotein
Also known as multidrug resistance protein 1 (MDR1). Expressed by some cancer cells (e.g., colon, liver) to pump out toxins, including chemotherapeutic agents (one mechanism of ↓ responsiveness or resistance to chemotherapy over time).

-plasia definitions

REVERSIBLE	
Hyperplasia	↑ in number of cells.
Metaplasia	One adult cell type is replaced by another. Often 2° to irritation (e.g., Barrett esophagus) and/or environmental exposure (e.g., smoking-induced tracheal/bronchial squamous metaplasia).
Dysplasia	Abnormal growth with loss of cellular orientation, shape, and size in comparison to normal tissue maturation; commonly preneoplastic.
IRREVERSIBLE	
Anaplasia	Loss of structural differentiation and function of cells, resembling primitive cells of same tissue; often equated with undifferentiated malignant neoplasms. May see "giant cells" with single large nucleus or several nuclei.
Neoplasia	A clonal proliferation of cells that is uncontrolled and excessive. Neoplasia may be benign or malignant.
Desmoplasia	Fibrous tissue formation in response to neoplasm (e.g., linitis plastica in diffuse stomach cancer).

Tumor grade vs. stage

Grade	Determined by degree of cellular differentiation and mitotic activity on histology. Usually graded 1–4; 1 = low grade, well differentiated; 4 = high grade, poorly differentiated, anaplastic.	Stage usually has more prognostic value than grade.
Stage	Degree of localization/spread based on site and size of 1° lesion, spread to regional lymph nodes, presence of metastases. Based on clinical (c) or pathology (p) findings. Example: cT3N1M0	TNM staging system (Stage = Spread): T = Tumor size N = Node involvement M = Metastases TMN each has independent prognostic value.

Tumor nomenclature

The term **carcinoma** implies epithelial origin, whereas **sarcoma** denotes mesenchymal origin. Both terms imply malignancy. Most carcinomas spread lymphatically, whereas most sarcomas spread hematogenously. Notable exceptions to carcinomas that spread lymphatically include renal cell carcinoma (often invades renal vein), hepatocellular carcinoma (often invades hepatic vein), follicular carcinoma of the thyroid, and choriocarcinoma, all of which may spread hematogenously.

CELL TYPE	BENIGN	MALIGNANT
Epithelium	Adenoma, papilloma	Adenocarcinoma, papillary carcinoma
Mesenchyme		
Blood cells		Leukemia, lymphoma
Blood vessels	Hemangioma	Angiosarcoma
Smooth muscle	Leiomyoma	Leiomyosarcoma
Striated muscle	Rhabdomyoma	Rhabdomyosarcoma
Connective tissue	Fibroma	Fibrosarcoma
Bone	Osteoma	Osteosarcoma
Fat	Lipoma	Liposarcoma

Tumor differences

Benign	Usually well differentiated, low mitotic activity, well demarcated, no metastasis, no necrosis.
Malignant	May be poorly differentiated, erratic growth, locally invasive/diffuse, may metastasize, ↓ apoptosis (upregulation of telomerase prevents chromosome shortening and cell death).

Cachexia

Weight loss, muscle atrophy, and fatigue that occur in chronic disease (e.g., cancer, AIDS, heart failure, TB). Mediated by TNF-α (nicknamed cachectin), IFN-γ, and IL-6.

Disease conditions associated with neoplasms

CONDITION	NEOPLASM
Acanthosis nigricans (hyperpigmentation and epidermal thickening)	Visceral malignancy (esp. stomach)
Actinic keratosis	Squamous cell carcinoma of skin
AIDS	Aggressive malignant lymphomas (non-Hodgkin) and Kaposi sarcoma
Autoimmune diseases (e.g., Hashimoto thyroiditis, SLE)	Lymphoma
Barrett esophagus (chronic GI reflux)	Esophageal adenocarcinoma
Chronic atrophic gastritis, pernicious anemia, postsurgical gastric remnants	Gastric adenocarcinoma
Cirrhosis	Hepatocellular carcinoma
Cushing syndrome	Small cell lung cancer
Dermatomyositis	Lung cancer
Down syndrome	**ALL** ("we **ALL** fall **Down**"), AML
Dysplastic nevus	Malignant melanoma
Hypercalcemia	Squamous cell lung cancer
Immunodeficiency states	Malignant lymphomas
Lambert-Eaton myasthenic syndrome	Small cell lung cancer
Myasthenia gravis, pure RBC aplasia	Thymoma
Paget disease of bone	2° osteosarcoma and fibrosarcoma
Plummer-Vinson syndrome (↓ iron)	Squamous cell carcinoma of esophagus
Polycythemia	Renal cell carcinoma, hepatocellular carcinoma
Radiation exposure	Leukemia, sarcoma, papillary thyroid cancer, and breast cancer
SIADH	Small cell lung cancer
Tuberous sclerosis (facial angiofibroma, seizures, intellectual disability)	Giant cell astrocytoma, renal angiomyolipoma, and cardiac rhabdomyoma
Ulcerative colitis	Colonic adenocarcinoma
Xeroderma pigmentosum, albinism	Melanoma, basal cell carcinoma, and especially squamous cell carcinomas of skin

Oncogenes Gain of function → ↑ cancer risk. Need damage to only 1 allele.

GENE	ASSOCIATED TUMOR	GENE PRODUCT
BCR-ABL	CML, ALL	Tyrosine kinase
bcl-2	Follicular and undifferentiated lymphomas	Anti-apoptotic molecule (inhibits apoptosis)
BRAF	Melanoma	Serine/threonine kinase
c-kit	Gastrointestinal stromal tumor (GIST)	Cytokine receptor (for stem cell factor)
c-myc	Burkitt lymphoma	Transcription factor
HER2/neu (c-erbB2)	Breast, ovarian, and gastric carcinomas	Tyrosine kinase
L-myc	Lung tumor	Transcription factor
N-myc	Neuroblastoma	Transcription factor
ras	Colon cancer, lung cancer, pancreatic cancer	GTPase
ret	MEN 2A and 2B	Tyrosine kinase

Tumor suppressor genes Loss of function → ↑ cancer risk; both alleles must be lost for expression of disease.

GENE	ASSOCIATED TUMOR	GENE PRODUCT
APC	Colorectal cancer (associated with FAP)	
BRCA1	Breast and ovarian cancer	DNA repair protein
BRCA2	Breast and ovarian cancer	DNA repair protein
CPD4/SMAD4	Pancreatic cancer	DPC—Deleted in Pancreatic Cancer
DCC	Colon cancer	DCC—Deleted in Colon Cancer
MEN1	MEN type I	
NF1	NeuroFibromatosis type 1	RAS GTPase activating protein (neurofibromin)
NF2	NeuroFibromatosis type 2	Merlin (schwannomin) protein
p16	Melanoma	Cyclin-dependent kinase inhibitor 2A
p53	Most human cancers, Li-Fraumeni syndrome	Transcription factor for p21, blocks G_1 → S phase
PTEN	Breast cancer, prostate cancer, endometrial cancer	
Rb	Retinoblastoma, osteosarcoma	Inhibits E2F; blocks G_1 → S phase
TSC1	Tuberous sclerosis	Hamartin protein
TSC2	Tuberous sclerosis	Tuberin protein
VHL	von Hippel-Lindau disease	Inhibits hypoxia inducible factor 1a
WT1	Wilms Tumor (nephroblastoma)	
WT2	Wilms Tumor (nephroblastoma)	

Tumor markers	Tumor markers should not be used as the 1° tool for cancer diagnosis. They may be used to monitor tumor recurrence and response to therapy, but definitive diagnosis can be made only via biopsy.	
Alkaline phosphatase	Metastases to bone, liver, Paget disease of bone, seminoma (placental ALP).	
α-fetoprotein	Normally made by fetus. Hepatocellular carcinoma, hepatoblastoma, yolk sac (endodermal sinus) tumor, testicular cancer, mixed germ cell tumor (co-secreted with β-hCG).	
β-hCG	Hydatidiform moles and Choriocarcinomas (Gestational trophoblastic disease), testicular cancer.	Commonly associated with pregnancy.
CA-15-3/CA-27-29	Breast cancer.	
CA-19-9	Pancreatic adenocarcinoma.	
CA-125	Ovarian cancer.	
Calcitonin	Medullary thyroid carcinoma.	
CEA	CarcinoEmbryonic Antigen. Very nonspecific but produced by ~ 70% of colorectal and pancreatic cancers; also produced by gastric, breast, and medullary thyroid carcinomas.	
PSA	Prostate-specific antigen. Used to follow prostate adenocarcinoma. Can also be elevated in BPH and prostatitis. Questionable risk/benefit for screening.	
S-100	Neural crest origin (e.g., melanomas, neural tumors, schwannomas, Langerhans cell histiocytosis).	
TRAP	Tartrate-Resistant Acid Phosphatase (**TRAP**). **Hairy** cell leukemia—a B-cell neoplasm.	**TRAP** the **hairy** animal. Largely replaced by flow cytometry.

Oncogenic microbes

Microbe	Associated cancer
EBV	Burkitt lymphoma, Hodgkin lymphoma, nasopharyngeal carcinoma, CNS lymphoma (in immunocompromised patients)
HBV, HCV	Hepatocellular carcinoma
HHV-8 (Kaposi sarcoma–associated herpesvirus)	Kaposi sarcoma, body cavity fluid B-cell lymphoma
HPV	Cervical and penile/anal carcinoma (16, 18), head and neck or throat cancer
H. pylori	Gastric adenocarcinoma and MALT lymphoma
HTLV-1	Adult T-cell leukemia/lymphoma
Liver fluke *(Clonorchis sinensis)*	Cholangiocarcinoma
Schistosoma haematobium	Bladder cancer (squamous cell)

Carcinogens

TOXIN	ORGAN	IMPACT
Aflatoxins (*Aspergillus*)	Liver	Hepatocellular carcinoma
Alkylating agents	Blood	Leukemia/lymphoma
Aromatic amines (e.g., benzidine, 2-naphthylamine)	Bladder	Transitional cell carcinoma
Arsenic	Liver	Angiosarcoma
	Lung	Lung cancer
	Skin	Squamous cell carcinoma
Asbestos	Lung	Bronchogenic carcinoma > mesothelioma
Carbon tetrachloride	Liver	Centrilobular necrosis, fatty change
Cigarette smoke	Bladder	Transitional cell carcinoma
	Esophagus	Squamous cell carcinoma/adenocarcinoma
	Kidney	Renal cell carcinoma
	Larynx	Squamous cell carcinoma
	Lung	Squamous cell and small cell carcinoma
	Pancreas	Pancreatic adenocarcinoma
Ethanol	Liver	Hepatocellular carcinoma
Ionizing radiation	Thyroid	Papillary thyroid carcinoma
Nitrosamines (smoked foods)	Stomach	Gastric cancer
Radon	Lung	Lung cancer (2nd leading cause after cigarette smoke)
Vinyl chloride	Liver	Angiosarcoma

Paraneoplastic syndromes

HORMONE/AGENT	EFFECT	NEOPLASM(S)
1,25-$(OH)_2$ D_3 (calcitriol)	Hypercalcemia	Hodgkin lymphoma, some non-Hodgkin lymphomas
ACTH	Cushing syndrome	Small cell lung carcinoma
ADH	SIADH	Small cell lung carcinoma and intracranial neoplasms
Antibodies against presynaptic Ca^{2+} channels at NMJ	Lambert-Eaton myasthenic syndrome (muscle weakness)	Small cell lung carcinoma
Erythropoietin	Polycythemia	Renal cell carcinoma, thymoma, hemangioblastoma, hepatocellular carcinoma, leiomyoma, pheochromocytoma
PTHrP	Hypercalcemia	Squamous cell lung carcinoma, renal cell carcinoma, breast cancer

Psammoma bodies

Laminated, concentric, calcific spherules 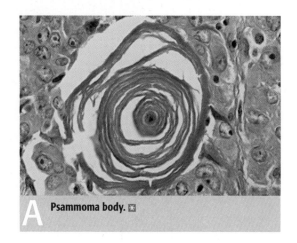, PSaMMoma bodies are seen in:
- Papillary carcinoma of thyroid
- Serous papillary cystadenocarcinoma of ovary
- Meningioma
- Malignant mesothelioma

A Psammoma body. ✴

Cancer epidemiology

	MALE	FEMALE	NOTES
Incidence	Prostate (32%) Lung (16%) Colon/rectum (12%)	Breast (32%) Lung (13%) Colon/rectum (13%)	Lung cancer incidence has dropped in men, but has not changed significantly in women.
Mortality	Lung (33%) Prostate (13%)	Lung (23%) Breast (18%)	Cancer is the 2nd leading cause of death in the United States (heart disease is 1st).

Common metastases

SITE OF METASTASIS	1° TUMOR	NOTES
Brain	Lung > breast > genitourinary > osteosarcoma > melanoma > GI.	50% of brain tumors are from metastases **A**. Commonly seen as multiple well-circumscribed tumors at gray/white matter junction.
Liver	Colon >> stomach > pancreas.	Liver **B** **C** and lung are the most common sites of metastasis after the regional lymph nodes.
Bone	Prostate, breast > lung > thyroid.	Bone metastasis **D** >> 1° bone tumors (e.g., multiple myeloma, lytic). Whole-body bone scan **E** shows tumor predilection for axial skeleton. Prostate = blastic. Breast = lytic and blastic.

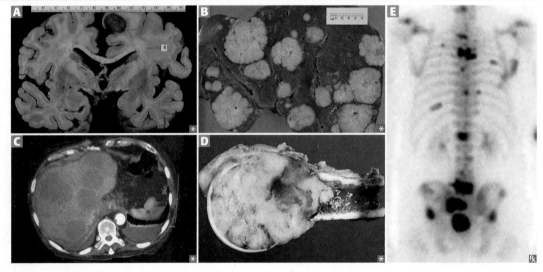

HIGH-YIELD PRINCIPLES IN

Pharmacology

"Take me, I am the drug; take me, I am hallucinogenic."

—Salvador Dali

"I was under medication when I made the decision not to burn the tapes."

—Richard Nixon

"I wondher why ye can always read a doctor's bill an' ye niver can read his purscription."

—Finley Peter Dunne

"Once you get locked into a serious drug collection, the tendency is to push it as far as you can."

—Hunter S. Thompson

Preparation for questions on pharmacology is straightforward. Memorizing all the key drugs and their characteristics (e.g., mechanisms, clinical use, and important side effects) is high yield. Focus on understanding the prototype drugs in each class. Avoid memorizing obscure derivatives. Learn the "classic" and distinguishing toxicities of the major drugs. Specific drug dosages or trade names are generally not testable. Reviewing associated biochemistry, physiology, and microbiology can be useful while studying pharmacology. There is a strong emphasis on ANS, CNS, antimicrobial, and cardiovascular agents as well as on NSAIDs. Much of the material is clinically relevant. Newer drugs on the market are also fair game.

▶ PHARMACOLOGY–PHARMACOKINETICS & PHARMACODYNAMICS

Enzyme kinetics

Michaelis-Menten kinetics	[S] = concentration of substrate; V = velocity. 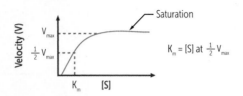	K_m is inversely related to the affinity of the enzyme for its substrate. V_{max} is directly proportional to the enzyme concentration. Most enzymatic reactions follow a hyperbolic curve (follow Michaelis-Menten kinetics); however, enzymatic reactions that exhibit a sigmoid curve usually indicate cooperative kinetics (i.e., hemoglobin).
Lineweaver-Burk plot	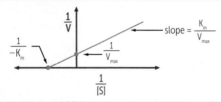	↑ y-intercept, ↓ V_{max}. The further to the right the x-intercept (i.e., closer to zero), the greater the K_m and the lower the affinity.
Enzyme inhibition	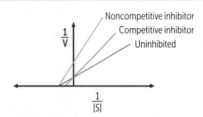	Competitive inhibitors cross each other competitively, whereas noncompetitive inhibitors do not.

	Competitive inhibitors, reversible	Competitive inhibitors, irreversible	Noncompetitive inhibitors
Resemble substrate	Yes	Yes	No
Overcome by ↑ [S]	Yes	No	No
Bind active site	Yes	Yes	No
Effect on V_{max}	Unchanged	↓	↓
Effect on K_m	↑	Unchanged	Unchanged
Pharmacodynamics	↓ potency	↓ efficacy	↓ efficacy

Pharmacokinetics vs. pharmacodynamics

Pharmacokinetics	The effects of the body on the drug.	ADME: <ul><li>Absorption</li><li>Distribution</li><li>Metabolism</li><li>Excretion</li></ul>
Pharmacodynamics	The effects of the drug on the body.	Includes concepts of receptor binding, drug efficacy, drug potency, toxicity.

Pharmacokinetics

Bioavailability (F)	Fraction of administered drug that reaches systemic circulation unchanged. For an IV dose, $F = 100\%$. Orally: F typically <100% due to incomplete absorption and first-pass metabolism.
Volume of distribution (V$_d$)	Theoretical volume occupied by the total absorbed drug amount at the plasma concentration. Apparent V_d of plasma protein–bound drugs can be altered by liver and kidney disease (↓ protein binding, ↑ V_d). Drugs may distribute in more than one compartment. $$V_d = \frac{\text{amount of drug in the body}}{\text{plasma drug concentration}}$$

V_d	COMPARTMENT	DRUG TYPES
Low	Blood (4–8 L)	Large/charged molecules; plasma protein bound
Medium	ECF	Small hydrophilic molecules
High	All tissues including fat	Small lipophilic molecules, especially if bound to tissue protein

Half-life (t$_{1/2}$)	The time required to change the amount of drug in the body by ½ during elimination (or constant infusion). Property of first-order elimination. A drug infused at a constant rate takes 4–5 half-lives to reach steady state. It takes 3.3 half-lives to reach 90% of the steady-state level. $$t_{1/2} = \frac{0.693 \times V_d}{CL}$$

# of half-lives	1	2	3	4
% remaining	50%	25%	12.5%	6.25%

Clearance (CL)	The volume of plasma cleared of drug per unit time. Clearance may be impaired with defects in cardiac, hepatic, or renal function. $$CL = \frac{\text{rate of elimination of drug}}{\text{plasma drug concentration}} = V_d \times K_e \text{ (elimination constant)}$$

Dosage calculations	$$\text{Loading dose} = \frac{C_p \times V_d}{F}$$ $$\text{Maintenance dose} = \frac{C_p \times CL \times \tau}{F}$$ C_p = target plasma concentration at steady state τ = dosage interval (time between doses), if not administered continuously	In renal or liver disease, maintenance dose ↓ and loading dose is usually unchanged. Time to steady state depends primarily on $t_{1/2}$ and is independent of dose and dosing frequency.

Elimination of drugs

Zero-order elimination	Rate of elimination is constant regardless of C_p (i.e., constant **amount** of drug eliminated per unit time). C_p ↓ linearly with time. Examples of drugs—**P**henytoin, **E**thanol, and **A**spirin (at high or toxic concentrations).	Capacity-limited elimination. **PEA.** (A pea is round, shaped like the "0" in "zero-order.")
First-order elimination	Rate of elimination is directly proportional to the drug concentration (i.e., constant **fraction** of drug eliminated per unit time). C_p ↓ exponentially with time.	Flow-dependent elimination.

Zero-order elimination

2.5 units/h elimination rate

2.5 units/h

2.5 units/h

Plasma concentration

Time (h)

First-order elimination

5 units/h elimination rate

2.5 units/h

1.25 units/h

Plasma concentration

Time (h)

Urine pH and drug elimination

Ionized species are trapped in urine and cleared quickly. Neutral forms can be reabsorbed.

Weak acids	Examples: phenobarbital, methotrexate, aspirin. Trapped in basic environments. Treat overdose with bicarbonate.

$$RCOOH \rightleftharpoons RCOO^- + H^+$$
(lipid soluble)   (trapped)

Weak bases	Example: amphetamines. Trapped in acidic environments. Treat overdose with ammonium chloride.

$$RNH_3^+ \rightleftharpoons RNH_2 + H^+$$
(trapped)   (lipid soluble)

Drug metabolism

Phase I	Reduction, oxidation, hydrolysis with cytochrome P-450 usually yield slightly polar, water-soluble metabolites (often still active).	Geriatric patients lose phase I first.
Phase II	Conjugation (**G**lucuronidation, **A**cetylation, **S**ulfation) usually yields very polar, inactive metabolites (renally excreted).	Geriatric patients have **GAS** (phase II). Patients who are slow acetylators have greater side effects from certain drugs because of ↓ rate of metabolism.

Efficacy vs. potency

Efficacy

Maximal effect a drug can produce. High-efficacy drug classes are analgesic (pain) medications, antibiotics, antihistamines, and decongestants. Partial agonists have less efficacy than full agonists.

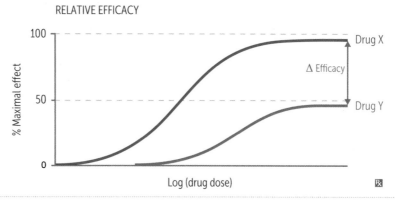

Potency

Amount of drug needed for a given effect. ↑ potency, ↑ affinity for receptor. Highly potent drug classes include chemotherapeutic (cancer) drugs, antihypertensive (blood pressure) drugs, and lipid-lowering (cholesterol) drugs.

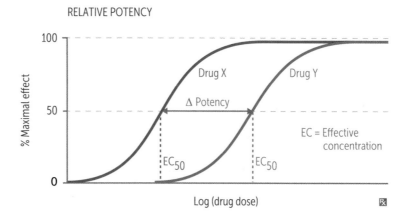

Receptor binding

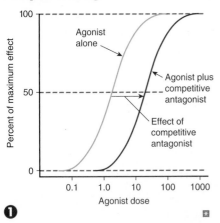

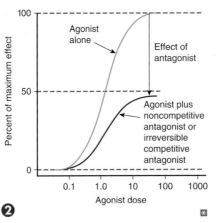

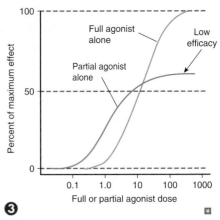

FIGURE	EFFECT	EXAMPLE
❶ Competitive antagonist	Shifts curve to right (↓ potency), no change in efficacy. Can be overcome by ↑ the concentration of agonist substrate.	Diazepam + **flumazenil** (competitive antagonist) on GABA receptor.
❷ Noncompetitive antagonist	Shifts curve down (↓ efficacy). Cannot be overcome by ↑ agonist substrate concentration.	Glutamate + **ketamine** (noncompetitive antagonist) on NMDA receptors.
Irreversible competitive antagonist		Norepinephrine + **phenoxybenzamine** (irreversible competitive antagonist) on α-receptors.
❸ Partial agonist	Acts at same site as full agonist, but with lower maximal effect (↓ efficacy). Potency is an independent variable.	Morphine vs. **buprenorphine** (partial agonist) at opioid μ-receptors.

Therapeutic index

Measurement of drug safety.

$$\frac{TD_{50}}{ED_{50}} = \frac{\text{median toxic dose}}{\text{median effective dose}}$$

Therapeutic window—measure of clinical drug effectiveness for a patient.

TITE: Therapeutic Index = TD_{50}/ED_{50}.
Safer drugs have higher TI values. Examples of drugs with low TI values include digoxin, lithium, theophylline, and warfarin.
LD_{50} (lethal median dose) often replaces TD_{50} in animal studies.

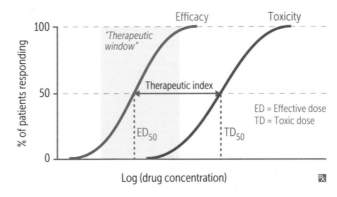

▶ PHARMACOLOGY–AUTONOMIC DRUGS

Central and peripheral nervous system

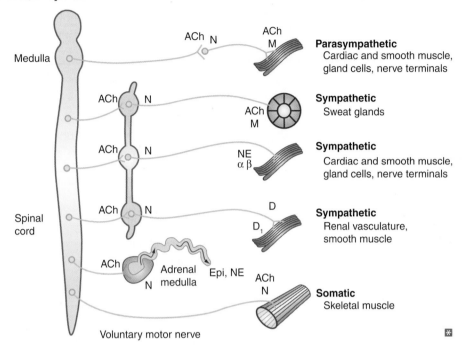

Note that the adrenal medulla and sweat glands are part of the sympathetic nervous system but are innervated by cholinergic fibers.

Botulinum toxin prevents release of neurotransmitter at all cholinergic terminals.

ACh receptors	Nicotinic ACh receptors are ligand-gated Na^+/K^+ channels; N_N (found in autonomic ganglia) and N_M (found in neuromuscular junction) subtypes.
	Muscarinic ACh receptors are G-protein–coupled receptors that usually act through 2nd messengers; 5 subtypes: M_1, M_2, M_3, M_4, and M_5.

G-protein–linked 2nd messengers

RECEPTOR	G-PROTEIN CLASS	MAJOR FUNCTIONS
Sympathetic		
α_1	q	↑ vascular smooth muscle contraction, ↑ pupillary dilator muscle contraction (mydriasis), ↑ intestinal and bladder sphincter muscle contraction
α_2	i	↓ sympathetic outflow, ↓ insulin release ↓ lipolysis, ↑ platelet aggregation
β_1	s	↑ heart rate, ↑ contractility, ↑ renin release, ↑ lipolysis
β_2	s	Vasodilation, bronchodilation, ↑ heart rate, ↑ contractility, ↑ lipolysis, ↑ insulin release, ↓ uterine tone (tocolysis), ciliary muscle relaxation, ↑ aqueous humor production
Parasympathetic		
M_1	q	CNS, enteric nervous system
M_2	i	↓ heart rate and contractility of atria
M_3	q	↑ exocrine gland secretions (e.g., lacrimal, salivary, gastric acid), ↑ gut peristalsis, ↑ bladder contraction, bronchoconstriction, ↑ pupillary sphincter muscle contraction (miosis), ciliary muscle contraction (accommodation)
Dopamine		
D_1	s	Relaxes renal vascular smooth muscle
D_2	i	Modulates transmitter release, especially in brain
Histamine		
H_1	q	↑ nasal and bronchial mucus production, ↑ vascular permeability, contraction of bronchioles, pruritus, and pain
H_2	s	↑ gastric acid secretion
Vasopressin		
V_1	q	↑ vascular smooth muscle contraction
V_2	s	↑ H_2O permeability and reabsorption in the collecting tubules of the kidney (V_2 is found in the 2 kidneys)

"**Q**iss (kiss) and **q**i**q** (kick) till you're **s**i**q** (sick) of **sqs** (super qinky sex)."

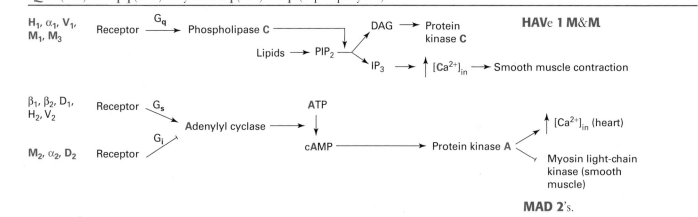

$H_1, \alpha_1, V_1,$ M_1, M_3 → Receptor —G_q→ Phospholipase **C** → DAG → Protein kinase **C**   **HAV**e **1 M&M**

Lipids → PIP_2 → IP_3 → ↑ $[Ca^{2+}]_{in}$ → Smooth muscle contraction

$\beta_1, \beta_2, D_1,$ H_2, V_2 → Receptor —G_s→ Adenylyl cyclase → ATP ↓ cAMP → Protein kinase **A** → ↑ $[Ca^{2+}]_{in}$ (heart) / Myosin light-chain kinase (smooth muscle)

M_2, α_2, D_2 → Receptor —G_i→

MAD 2's.

Autonomic drugs

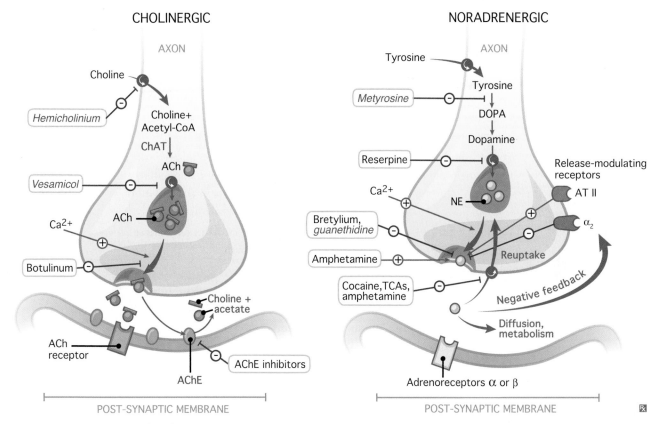

Circles with rotating arrows represent transporters. Drugs in *italics* are generally not clinically used.

Release of norepinephrine from a sympathetic nerve ending is modulated by norepinephrine itself, acting on presynaptic α_2-autoreceptors, angiotensin II, and other substances.

Cholinomimetic agents

DRUG	CLINICAL APPLICATIONS	ACTION
Direct agonists		
Bethanechol	Postoperative ileus, neurogenic ileus, and urinary retention	Activates bowel and bladder smooth muscle; resistant to AChE. "**Bethany, call** (bethanechol) me, maybe, if you want to activate your bowels and bladder."
Carbachol	Glaucoma, pupillary constriction, and relief of intraocular pressure	Carbon copy of acetylcholine.
Pilocarpine	Potent stimulator of sweat, tears, and saliva Open-angle and closed-angle glaucoma	Contracts ciliary muscle of eye (open-angle glaucoma), pupillary sphincter (closed-angle glaucoma); resistant to AChE. "You cry, drool, and sweat on your 'pilow.'"
Methacholine	Challenge test for diagnosis of asthma	Stimulates muscarinic receptors in airway when inhaled.
Indirect agonists (anticholinesterases)		
Neostigmine	Postoperative and neurogenic ileus and urinary retention, myasthenia gravis, reversal of neuromuscular junction blockade (postoperative)	↑ endogenous ACh. Neo CNS = No CNS penetration.
Pyridostigmine	Myasthenia gravis (long acting); does not penetrate CNS	↑ endogenous ACh; ↑ strength. Pyridostigmine gets rid of myasthenia gravis.
Physostigmine	Anticholinergic toxicity (crosses blood-brain barrier → CNS)	↑ endogenous ACh. Physostigmine "phyxes" atropine overdose.
Donepezil, rivastigmine, galantamine	Alzheimer disease	↑ endogenous ACh.
Edrophonium	Historically, diagnosis of myasthenia gravis (extremely short acting). Myasthenia now diagnosed by anti-AChR Ab (anti-acetylcholine receptor antibody) test.	↑ endogenous ACh.

Note: With all cholinomimetic agents, watch for exacerbation of COPD, asthma, and peptic ulcers when giving to susceptible patients.

Cholinesterase inhibitor poisoning	Often due to organophosphates, such as parathion, that **irreversibly** inhibit AChE. Causes Diarrhea, Urination, Miosis, Bronchospasm, Bradycardia, Excitation of skeletal muscle and CNS, Lacrimation, Sweating, and Salivation.	DUMBBELSS. Organophosphates are components of insecticides; poisoning usually seen in farmers. Antidote—atropine (competitive inhibitor) + pralidoxime (regenerates AChE if given early).

Muscarinic antagonists

DRUGS	ORGAN SYSTEMS	APPLICATIONS
Atropine, homatropine, tropicamide	Eye	Produce mydriasis and cycloplegia.
Benztropine	CNS	Parkinson disease—"Park my Benz."
Scopolamine	CNS	Motion sickness.
Ipratropium, tiotropium	Respiratory	COPD, asthma ("**I pray** I can breathe soon!").
Oxybutynin, darifenacin, and solifenacin	Genitourinary	Reduce urgency in mild cystitis and reduce bladder spasms. Other agents: tolterodine, fesoterodine, trospium.
Glycopyrrolate	Gastrointestinal, respiratory	Parenteral: preoperative use to reduce airway secretions. Oral: drooling, peptic ulcer.

Atropine Muscarinic antagonist. Used to treat bradycardia and for ophthalmic applications.

ORGAN SYSTEM	ACTION	NOTES
Eye	↑ pupil dilation, cycloplegia	Blocks **DUMBBeLSS**. Skeletal muscle and CNS excitation mediated by nicotinic receptors. See previous page.
Airway	↓ secretions	
Stomach	↓ acid secretion	
Gut	↓ motility	
Bladder	↓ urgency in cystitis	
TOXICITY	↑ body **temperature** (due to ↓ sweating); rapid pulse; dry mouth; **dry, flushed skin**; **cycloplegia**; constipation; **disorientation** Can cause acute angle-closure glaucoma in elderly (due to mydriasis), urinary retention in men with prostatic hyperplasia, and hyperthermia in infants	Side effects: **Hot** as a hare **Dry** as a bone **Red** as a beet **Blind** as a bat **Mad** as a hatter Jimson weed *(Datura)* → gardeners pupil (mydriasis due to plant alkaloids)

Sympathomimetics

DRUG	EFFECT	APPLICATIONS
Direct sympathomimetics		
Epinephrine	$\beta > \alpha$	Anaphylaxis, open angle glaucoma, asthma, hypotension; α effects predominate at high doses
Norepinephrine	$\alpha_1 > \alpha_2 > \beta_1$	Hypotension (but ↓ renal perfusion)
Isoproterenol	$\beta_1 = \beta_2$	Electrophysiologic evaluation of tachyarrhythmias. Can worsen ischemia.
Dopamine	$D_1 = D_2 > \beta > \alpha$	Unstable bradycardia, heart failure, shock; inotropic and chronotropic α effects predominate at high doses
Dobutamine	$\beta_1 > \beta_2, \alpha$	Heart failure (inotropic > chronotropic), cardiac stress testing
Phenylephrine	$\alpha_1 > \alpha_2$	Hypotension (vasoconstrictor), ocular procedures (mydriatic), rhinitis (decongestant)
Albuterol, salmeterol, terbutaline	$\beta_2 > \beta_1$	Albuterol for acute asthma; salmeterol for long-term asthma or COPD control; terbutaline to reduce premature uterine contractions
Indirect sympathomimetics		
Amphetamine	Indirect general agonist, reuptake inhibitor, also releases stored catecholamines	Narcolepsy, obesity, attention deficit disorder
Ephedrine	Indirect general agonist, releases stored catecholamines	Nasal decongestion, urinary incontinence, hypotension
Cocaine	Indirect general agonist, reuptake inhibitor	Causes vasoconstriction and local anesthesia; never give β-blockers if cocaine intoxication is suspected (can lead to unopposed α_1 activation and extreme hypertension)

Norepinephrine vs. isoproterenol

Norepinephrine causes ↑ in systolic and diastolic pressures as a result of α_1-mediated vasoconstriction → ↑ mean arterial pressure → bradycardia. However, isoproterenol (no longer commonly used) has little α effect but causes β_2-mediated vasodilation, resulting in ↓ mean arterial pressure and ↑ heart rate through β_1 and reflex activity.

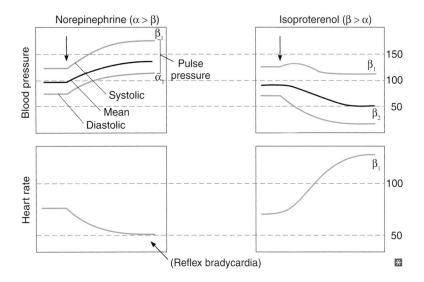

Sympatholytics (α_2-agonists)

DRUG	APPLICATIONS	TOXICITY
Clonidine	Hypertensive urgency (limited situations); does not decrease renal blood flow ADHD, severe pain, and a variety of off-label indications (e.g., ethanol and opioid withdrawal)	CNS depression, bradycardia, hypotension, respiratory depression, and small pupil size
α-methyldopa	Hypertension in pregnancy Safe in pregnancy	Direct Coombs ⊕ hemolytic anemia, SLE-like syndrome

α-blockers

DRUG	APPLICATIONS	TOXICITY
Nonselective		
Phenoxybenzamine (irreversible)	Pheochromocytoma (used preoperatively) to prevent catecholamine (hypertensive) crisis	Orthostatic hypotension, reflex tachycardia
Phentolamine (reversible)	Give to patients on MAO inhibitors who eat tyramine-containing foods	
α₁ selective (-osin ending)		
Prazosin, terazosin, doxazosin, tamsulosin	Urinary symptoms of BPH; PTSD (prazosin); hypertension (except tamsulosin)	1st-dose orthostatic hypotension, dizziness, headache
α₂ selective		
Mirtazapine	Depression	Sedation, ↑ serum cholesterol, ↑ appetite

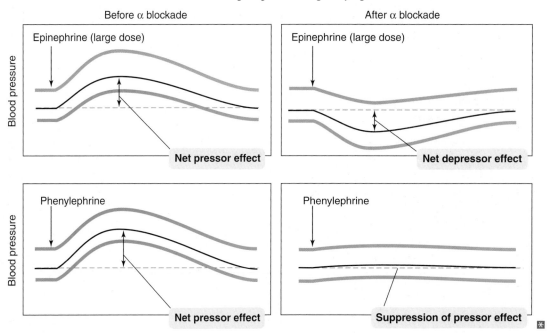

α-blockade of epinephrine vs. phenylephrine

Shown above are the effects of an α-blocker (e.g., phentolamine) on blood pressure responses to epinephrine and phenylephrine. The epinephrine response exhibits reversal of the mean blood pressure change, from a net increase (the α response) to a net decrease (the β_2 response). The response to phenylephrine is suppressed but not reversed because phenylephrine is a "pure" α-agonist without β action.

β-blockers	Metoprolol, acebutolol, betaxolol, carvedilol, esmolol, atenolol, nadolol, timolol, pindolol, labetalol.	
APPLICATION	EFFECTS	NOTES
Angina pectoris	↓ heart rate and contractility, resulting in ↓ O_2 consumption	
MI	β-blockers (metoprolol, carvedilol, and bisoprolol) ↓ mortality	
SVT (metoprolol, esmolol)	↓ AV conduction velocity (class II antiarrhythmic)	
Hypertension	↓ cardiac output, ↓ renin secretion (due to $β_1$-receptor blockade on JGA cells)	
CHF	Slows progression of chronic failure	
Glaucoma (timolol)	↓ secretion of aqueous humor	
TOXICITY	Impotence, cardiovascular adverse effects (bradycardia, AV block, CHF), CNS adverse effects (seizures, sedation, sleep alterations), dyslipidemia (metoprolol), and asthmatics/COPDers (may cause exacerbation)	Avoid in cocaine users due to risk of unopposed α-adrenergic receptor agonist activity Despite theoretical concern of masking hypoglycemia in diabetics, benefits likely outweigh risks; not contraindicated
SELECTIVITY	$β_1$-selective antagonists ($β_1 > β_2$)—acebutolol (partial agonist), atenolol, betaxolol, esmolol, metoprolol	Selective antagonists mostly go from **A** to **M** ($β_1$ with 1st half of alphabet)
	Nonselective antagonists ($β_1 = β_2$)—nadolol, pindolol (partial agonist), propranolol, timolol	Nonselective antagonists mostly go from **N** to **Z** ($β_2$ with 2nd half of alphabet)
	Nonselective α- and β-antagonists—carvedilol, labetalol	Nonselectives α- and β-antagonists have modified suffixes (instead of "-olol")
	Nebivolol combines cardiac-selective $β_1$-adrenergic blockade with stimulation of $β_3$-receptors, which activate nitric oxide synthase in the vasculature	

▶ PHARMACOLOGY–TOXICITIES AND SIDE EFFECTS

Specific antidotes

TOXIN	ANTIDOTE/TREATMENT
Acetaminophen	N-acetylcysteine (replenishes glutathione)
AChE inhibitors, organophosphates	Atropine followed by pralidoxime
Amphetamines (basic)	NH_4Cl (acidify urine)
Antimuscarinic, anticholinergic agents	Physostigmine salicylate, control hyperthermia
Benzodiazepines	Flumazenil
β-blockers	Glucagon
Carbon monoxide	100% O_2, hyperbaric O_2
Copper, arsenic, gold	Penicillamine
Cyanide	Nitrite + thiosulfate, hydroxocobalamin
Digitalis	Anti-dig Fab fragments
Heparin	Protamine sulfate
Iron	Deferoxamine, deferasirox
Lead	EDTA, dimercaprol, succimer, penicillamine
Mercury, arsenic, gold	Dimercaprol (BAL), succimer
Methanol, ethylene glycol (antifreeze)	Fomepizole > ethanol, dialysis
Methemoglobin	Methylene blue, vitamin C
Opioids	Naloxone
Salicylates	$NaHCO_3$ (alkalinize urine), dialysis
TCAs	$NaHCO_3$ (plasma alkalinization)
tPA, streptokinase, urokinase	Aminocaproic acid
Warfarin	Vitamin K, plasma (if active bleeding)

Drug reactions–cardiovascular

DRUG REACTION	CAUSAL AGENTS	NOTES
Coronary vasospasm	Cocaine, sumatriptan, ergot alkaloids	
Cutaneous flushing	Vancomycin, Adenosine, Niacin, Ca^{2+} channel blockers	VANC
Dilated cardiomyopathy	Doxorubicin, daunorubicin	
Torsades de pointes	Class III (e.g., sotalol) and class IA (e.g., quinidine) antiarrhythmics, macrolide antibiotics, antipsychotics, TCAs	

Drug reactions—endocrine/reproductive

DRUG REACTION	CAUSAL AGENTS	NOTES
Adrenocortical insufficiency	HPA suppression 2° to glucocorticoid withdrawal	
Hot flashes	Tamoxifen, clomiphene	
Hyperglycemia	Tacrolimus, Protease inhibitors, Niacin, HCTZ, β-blockers, Corticosteroids	Taking Pills Necessitates Having Blood Checked
Hypothyroidism	Lithium, amiodarone, sulfonamides	

Drug reactions—GI

DRUG REACTION	CAUSAL AGENTS	NOTES
Acute cholestatic hepatitis, jaundice	Erythromycin	
Diarrhea	Metformin, Erythromycin, Colchicine, Orlistat, Acarbose	Might Excite Colon On Accident
Focal to massive hepatic necrosis	Halothane, *Amanita phalloides* (death cap mushroom), Valproic acid, Acetaminophen	Liver "HAVAc"
Hepatitis	INH	
Pancreatitis	Didanosine, Corticosteroids, Alcohol, Valproic acid, Azathioprine, Diuretics (furosemide, HCTZ)	Drugs Causing A Violent Abdominal Distress
Pseudomembranous colitis	Clindamycin, ampicillin, cephalosporins	Antibiotics predispose to superinfection by resistant C. *difficile*

Drug reactions—hematologic

DRUG REACTION	CAUSAL AGENTS	NOTES
Agranulocytosis	Dapsone, Clozapine, Carbamazepine, Colchicine, Methimazole, Propylthiouracil	Drugs CCCrush Myeloblasts and Promyelocytes
Aplastic anemia	Carbamazepine, Methimazole, NSAIDs, Benzene, Chloramphenicol, Propylthiouracil	Can't Make New Blood Cells Properly
Direct Coombs-positive hemolytic anemia	Methyldopa, penicillin	
Gray baby syndrome	Chloramphenicol	
Hemolysis in G6PD deficiency	INH, Sulfonamides, Dapsone, Primaquine, Aspirin, Ibuprofen, Nitrofurantoin	Hemolysis IS D PAIN
Megaloblastic anemia	Phenytoin, Methotrexate, Sulfa drugs	Having a blast with PMS
Thrombocytopenia	Heparin, cimetidine	
Thrombotic complications	OCPs (e.g., estrogens)	

Drug reactions–musculoskeletal/skin/connective tissue

DRUG REACTION	CAUSAL AGENTS	NOTES
Fat redistribution	Protease inhibitors, Glucocorticoids	Fat PiG
Gingival hyperplasia	Phenytoin, verapamil, cyclosporine, nifedipine	
Hyperuricemia (gout)	Pyrazinamide, Thiazides, Furosemide, Niacin, Cyclosporine	Painful Tophi and Feet Need Care
Myopathy	Fibrates, niacin, colchicine, hydroxychloroquine, interferon-α, penicillamine, statins, glucocorticoids	
Osteoporosis	Corticosteroids, heparin	
Photosensitivity	Sulfonamides, Amiodarone, Tetracyclines, 5-FU	SAT For Photo
Rash (Stevens-Johnson syndrome)	Anti-epileptic drugs (ethosuximide, carbamazepine, lamotrigine, phenytoin, phenobarbital), Allopurinol, Sulfa drugs, Penicillin	Steven Johnson has epileptic Allergy to Sulfa drugs and Penicillin
SLE-like syndrome	Sulfa drugs, Hydralazine, INH, Procainamide, Phenytoin, Etanercept	Having lupus is "SHIPP-E"
Teeth discoloration	Tetracyclines	
Tendonitis, tendon rupture, and cartilage damage	Fluoroquinolones	

Drug reactions–neurologic

DRUG REACTION	CAUSAL AGENTS	NOTES
Cinchonism	Quinidine, quinine	
Parkinson-like syndrome	Antipsychotics, Reserpine, Metoclopramide	Cogwheel rigidity of ARM
Seizures	INH (vitamin B_6 deficiency), Bupropion, Imipenem/cilastatin, Tramadol, Enflurane, Metoclopramide	With seizures, I BITE My tongue
Tardive dyskinesia	Antipsychotics, metoclopramide	

Drug reactions–renal/genitourinary

DRUG REACTION	CAUSAL AGENTS	NOTES
Diabetes insipidus	Lithium, demeclocycline	
Fanconi syndrome	Expired tetracycline	
Hemorrhagic cystitis	Cyclophosphamide, ifosfamide	Prevent by coadministering with mesna
Interstitial nephritis	Methicillin, NSAIDs, furosemide	
SIADH	Carbamazepine, Cyclophosphamide, SSRIs	Can't Concentrate Serum Sodium

Drug reactions–respiratory

DRUG REACTION	CAUSAL AGENTS	NOTES
Dry cough	ACE inhibitors	
Pulmonary fibrosis	Bleomycin, Amiodarone, Busulfan, Methotrexate	Breathing Air Badly from Medications

Drug reactions–multiorgan

DRUG REACTION	CAUSAL AGENTS
Antimuscarinic	Atropine, TCAs, H_1-blockers, antipsychotics
Disulfiram-like reaction	Metronidazole, certain cephalosporins, griseofulvin, procarbazine, 1st-generation sulfonylureas
Nephrotoxicity/ ototoxicity	Aminoglycosides, vancomycin, loop diuretics, cisplatin

Cytochrome P-450 interactions (selected)	**Inducers (+)**	**Substrates**	**Inhibitors (–)**
	Chronic alcohol use	Anti-epileptics	Acute alcohol abuse
	Modafinil	Antidepressants	Gemfibrozil
	St. John's wort	Antipsychotics	Ciprofloxacin
	Phenytoin	Anesthetics	Isoniazid
	Phenobarbital	Theophylline	Grapefruit juice
	Nevirapine	Warfarin	Quinidine
	Rifampin	Statins	Amiodarone
	Griseofulvin	OCPs	Ketoconazole
	Carbamazepine		Macrolides
			Sulfonamides
			Cimetidine
			Ritonavir
	Chronic alcoholic Mona Steals Phen-Phen and Never Refuses Greasy Carbs	Always, Always, Always, Always Think When Starting Others	A cute Gentleman "Cipped" Iced Grapefruit juice Quickly And Kept Munching on Soft Cinammon Rolls

| **Sulfa drugs** | Probenecid, Furosemide, Acetazolamide, Celecoxib, Thiazides, Sulfonamide antibiotics, Sulfasalazine, Sulfonylureas. Patients with sulfa allergies may develop fever, urinary tract infection, Stevens-Johnson syndrome, hemolytic anemia, thrombocytopenia, agranulocytosis, and urticaria (hives). Symptoms range from mild to life threatening. | Popular FACTSSS |

▶ PHARMACOLOGY–MISCELLANEOUS

Drug names

ENDING	CATEGORY	EXAMPLE
Antimicrobial		
-azole	Ergosterol synthesis inhibitor	Ketoconazole
-bendazole	Antiparasitic/antihelmintic	Mebendazole
-cillin	Peptidoglycan synthesis inhibitor	Ampicillin
-cycline	Protein synthesis inhibitor	Tetracycline
-ivir	Neuraminidase inhibitor	Oseltamivir
-navir	Protease inhibitor	Ritonavir
-ovir	DNA polymerase inhibitor	Acyclovir
-thromycin	Macrolide antibiotic	Azithromycin
CNS		
-ane	Inhalational general anesthetic	Halothane
-azine	Typical antipsychotic	Thioridazine
-barbital	Barbiturate	Phenobarbital
-caine	Local anesthetic	Lidocaine
-etine	SSRI	Fluoxetine
-ipramine	TCA	Imipramine
-triptan	$5\text{-HT}_{1B/1D}$ agonists	Sumatriptan
-triptyline	TCA	Amitriptyline
-zepam	Benzodiazepine	Diazepam
-zolam	Benzodiazepine	Alprazolam
Autonomic		
-chol	Cholinergic agonist	Bethanechol/carbachol
-curium or -curonium	Non-depolarizing paralytic	Atracurium or vecuronium
-olol	β-blocker	Propranolol
-stigmine	AChE inhibitor	Neostigmine
-terol	β_2-agonist	Albuterol
-zosin	α_1-antagonist	Prazosin
Cardiovascular		
-afil	PDE-5 inhibitor	Sildenafil
-dipine	Dihydropyridine CCB	Amlodipine
-pril	ACE inhibitor	Captopril
-sartan	Angiotensin-II receptor blocker	Losartan
-statin	HMG-CoA reductase inhibitor	Atorvastatin
Other		
-dronate	Bisphosphonate	Alendronate
-glitazone	PPAR-γ activator	Rosiglitazone
-prazole	Proton pump inhibitor	Omeprazole
-prost	Prostaglandin analog	Latanoprost
-tidine	H_2-antagonist	Cimetidine
-tropin	Pituitary hormone	Somatotropin
-ximab	Chimeric monoclonal Ab	Basiliximab
-zumab	Humanized monoclonal Ab	Daclizumab

High-Yield Organ Systems

"*Symptoms, then, are in reality nothing but the cry from suffering organs.*"

—Jean-Martin Charcot

"*Man is an intelligence in servitude to his organs.*"

—Aldous Huxley

▶ APPROACHING THE ORGAN SYSTEMS

In this section, we have divided the High-Yield Facts into the major **Organ Systems**. Within each Organ System are several subsections, including **Embryology, Anatomy, Physiology, Pathology,** and **Pharmacology.** As you progress through each Organ System, refer back to information in the previous subsections to organize these basic science subsections into a "vertically integrated" framework for learning. Below is some general advice for studying the organ systems by these subsections.

Embryology

Relevant embryology is included in each organ system subsection. Embryology tends to correspond well with the relevant anatomy, especially with regard to congenital malformations.

Anatomy

Several topics fall under this heading, including gross anatomy, histology, and neuroanatomy. Do not memorize all the small details; however, do not ignore anatomy altogether. Review what you have already learned and what you wish you had learned. Many questions require two or more steps. The first step is to identify a structure on anatomic cross section, electron micrograph, or photomicrograph. The second step may require an understanding of the clinical significance of the structure.

When studying, stress clinically important material. For example, be familiar with gross anatomy and radiologic anatomy related to specific diseases (e.g., Pancoast tumor, Horner syndrome), traumatic injuries (e.g., fractures, sensory and motor nerve deficits), procedures (e.g., lumbar puncture), and common surgeries (e.g., cholecystectomy). There are also many questions on the exam involving x-rays, CT scans, and neuro MRI scans. Many students suggest browsing through a general radiology atlas, pathology atlas, and histology atlas. Focus on learning basic anatomy at key levels in the body (e.g., sagittal brain MRI; axial CT of the midthorax, abdomen, and pelvis). Basic neuroanatomy (especially pathways, blood supply, and functional anatomy), associated neuropathology, and neurophysiology have good yield. Please note that many of the photographic images in this book are for illustrative purposes and are not necessarily reflective of Step 1 emphasis.

Physiology

The portion of the examination dealing with physiology is broad and concept oriented and thus does not lend itself as well to fact-based review. Diagrams are often the best study aids, especially given the increasing number of questions requiring the interpretation of diagrams. Learn to apply basic physiologic relationships in a variety of ways (e.g., the Fick equation, clearance equations). You are seldom asked to perform complex calculations. Hormones are the focus of many questions, so learn their sites of production and action as well as their regulatory mechanisms.

A large portion of the physiology tested on the USMLE Step 1 is clinically relevant and involves understanding physiologic changes associated with pathologic processes (e.g., changes in pulmonary function with COPD). Thus, it is worthwhile to review the physiologic changes that are found with common pathologies of the major organ systems (e.g., heart, lungs, kidneys, GI tract) and endocrine glands.

Pathology

Questions dealing with this discipline are difficult to prepare for because of the sheer volume of material involved. Review the basic principles and hallmark characteristics of the key diseases. Given the clinical orientation of Step 1, it is no longer sufficient to know only the "buzz word" associations of certain diseases (e.g., café-au-lait macules and neurofibromatosis); you must also know the clinical descriptions of these findings.

Given the clinical slant of the USMLE Step 1, it is also important to review the classic presenting signs and symptoms of diseases as well as their associated laboratory findings. Delve into the signs, symptoms, and pathophysiology of major diseases that have a high prevalence in the United States (e.g., alcoholism, diabetes, hypertension, heart failure, ischemic heart disease, infectious disease). Be prepared to think one step beyond the simple diagnosis to treatment or complications.

The examination includes a number of color photomicrographs and photographs of gross specimens that are presented in the setting of a brief clinical history. However, read the question and the choices carefully before looking at the illustration, because the history will help you identify the pathologic process. Flip through an illustrated pathology textbook, color atlases, and appropriate Web sites in order to look at the pictures in the days before the exam. Pay attention to potential clues such as age, sex, ethnicity, occupation, recent activities and exposures, and specialized lab tests.

Pharmacology

Preparation for questions on pharmacology is straightforward. Memorizing all the key drugs and their characteristics (e.g., mechanisms, clinical use, and important side effects) is high yield. Focus on understanding the prototype drugs in each class. Avoid memorizing obscure derivatives. Learn the "classic" and distinguishing toxicities of the major drugs. Do not bother with drug dosages or trade names. Reviewing associated biochemistry, physiology, and microbiology can be useful while studying pharmacology. There is a strong emphasis on ANS, CNS, antimicrobial, and cardiovascular agents as well as NSAIDs. Much of the material is clinically relevant. Newer drugs on the market are also fair game.

▶ NOTES

Cardiovascular

"As for me, except for an occasional heart attack, I feel as young as I ever did."

—Robert Benchley

"Hearts will never be practical until they are made unbreakable."
—The Wizard of Oz

"As the arteries grow hard, the heart grows soft."

—H. L. Mencken

"Nobody has ever measured, not even poets, how much the heart can hold."

—Zelda Fitzgerald

"Only from the heart can you touch the sky."

—Rumi

"It is not the size of the man but the size of his heart that matters."
—Evander Holyfield

▶ CARDIOVASCULAR–EMBRYOLOGY

Heart embryology	EMBRYONIC STRUCTURE	GIVES RISE TO
	Truncus arteriosus (TA)	Ascending aorta and pulmonary trunk
	Bulbus cordis	Smooth parts (outflow tract) of left and right ventricles
	Primitive atria	Trabeculated part of left and right atria
	Primitive ventricle	Trabeculated part of left and right ventricles
	Primitive pulmonary vein	Smooth part of left atrium
	Left horn of sinus venosus (SV)	Coronary sinus
	Right horn of SV	Smooth part of right atrium
	Right common cardinal vein and right anterior cardinal vein	SVC

Heart morphogenesis	First functional organ in vertebrate embryos; beats spontaneously by week 4 of development.	
Cardiac looping	Primary heart tube loops to establish left-right polarity; begins in week 4 of gestation.	Defect in left-right dynein (involved in L/R asymmetry) can lead to dextrocardia, as seen in Kartagener syndrome (primary ciliary dyskinesia).

Septation of the chambers

Atria

❶ Septum primum grows toward endocardial cushions, narrowing foramen primum.

❷ Foramen secundum forms in septum primum (foramen primum disappears).

❸ Septum secundum develops as foramen secundum maintains right-to-left shunt.

❹ Septum secundum expands and covers most of the foramen secundum. The residual foramen is the foramen ovale.

❺ Remaining portion of septum primum forms valve of foramen ovale.

6. (Not shown) Septum secundum and septum primum fuse to form the atrial septum.

7. (Not shown) Foramen ovale usually closes soon after birth because of ↑ LA pressure.

Patent foramen ovale—caused by failure of septum primum and septum secundum to fuse after birth; most are left untreated. Can lead to paradoxical emboli (venous thromboemboli that enter systemic arterial circulation), similar to those resulting from an ASD.

Heart morphogenesis *(continued)*

Ventricles	❶ Muscular ventricular septum forms. Opening is called interventricular foramen. ❷ Aorticopulmonary septum rotates and fuses with muscular ventricular septum to form membranous interventricular septum, closing interventricular foramen. ❸ Growth of endocardial cushions separates atria from ventricles and contributes to both atrial septation and membranous portion of the interventricular septum.	Ventricular septal defect (VSD)—most commonly occurs in the membranous septum; acyanotic at birth due to left-to-right shunt.

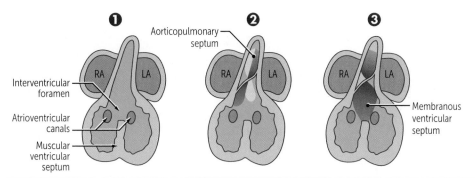

Outflow tract formation	Truncus arteriosus rotates; neural crest and endocardial cell migrations → truncal and bulbar ridges that spiral and fuse to form aorticopulmonary septum → ascending aorta and pulmonary trunk.	Conotruncal abnormalities: ▪ Transposition of great vessels. ▪ Tetralogy of Fallot. ▪ Persistent truncus arteriosus.
Valve development	Aortic/pulmonary: derived from endocardial cushions of outflow tract. Mitral/tricuspid: derived from fused endocardial cushions of the AV canal.	Valvular anomalies may be stenotic, regurgitant, atretic (e.g., tricuspid atresia), or displaced (e.g., Ebstein anomaly).

Fetal erythropoiesis	Fetal erythropoiesis occurs in: ▪ Yolk sac (3–8 weeks) ▪ Liver (6 weeks–birth) ▪ Spleen (10–28 weeks) ▪ Bone marrow (18 weeks to adult)	**Y**oung **L**iver **S**ynthesizes **B**lood.
Hemoglobin development	Fetal hemoglobin (HbF) = $\alpha_2\gamma_2$. Adult hemoglobin (HbA) = $\alpha_2\beta_2$. HbF has higher affinity for oxygen due to less avid binding of 2,3-BPG. This allows HbF to extract oxygen from (HbA) maternal hemoglobin across the placenta.	From fetal to adult hemoglobin: **A**lpha **A**lways; **G**amma **G**oes, **B**ecomes **B**eta.

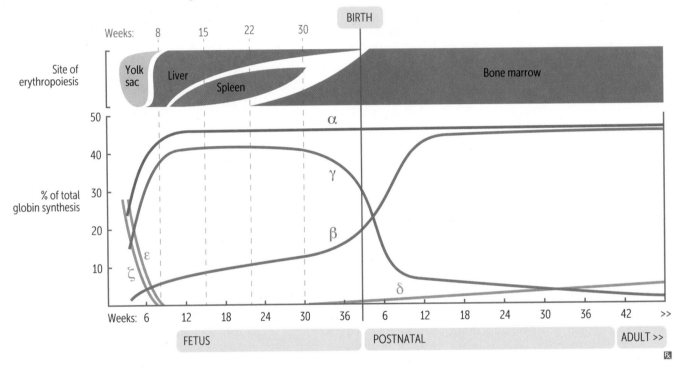

Fetal circulation

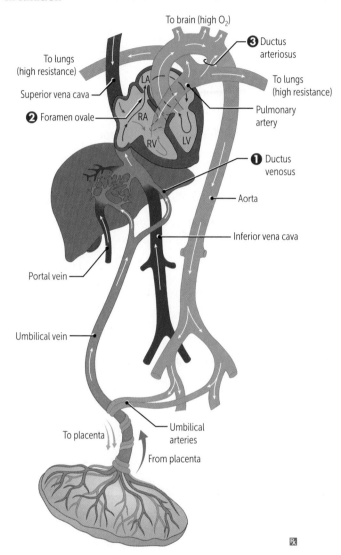

To brain (high O₂)

To lungs (high resistance)

Superior vena cava

❷ Foramen ovale

To lungs (high resistance)

Pulmonary artery

❸ Ductus arteriosus

LA

RA

RV

LV

❶ Ductus venosus

Aorta

Inferior vena cava

Portal vein

Umbilical vein

Umbilical arteries

To placenta

From placenta

Blood in umbilical vein has a P_{O_2} of ≈ 30 mmHg and is ≈ 80% saturated with O_2. Umbilical arteries have low O_2 saturation.

3 important shunts:

❶ Blood entering the fetus through the umbilical vein is conducted via the **ductus venosus** into the IVC to bypass the hepatic circulation.

❷ Most highly oxygenated blood reaching the heart via the IVC is diverted through the **foramen ovale** and pumped out the aorta to the head and body.

❸ Deoxygenated blood entering the RA from the SVC goes: RA → RV → main PA → patent ductus arteriosus → descending aorta; due to high fetal pulmonary artery resistance (due partly to low O_2 tension).

At birth, infant takes a breath; ↓ resistance in pulmonary vasculature causes ↑ left atrial pressure vs. right atrial pressure; foramen ovale closes (now called fossa ovalis); ↑ in O_2 (from respiration) and ↓ in prostaglandins (from placental separation) → closure of ductus arteriosus.

Indomethacin helps close PDA (patent) → DA remnant (i.e., ligamentum arteriosum). Prostaglandins E_1 and E_2 keep PDA open.

Fetal-postnatal derivatives

Umbilical vein	Ligamentum teres hepatis	Contained in falciform ligament.
UmbiLical arteries	MediaL umbilical ligaments	
Ductus arteriosus	Ligamentum arteriosum	
Ductus venosus	Ligamentum venosum	
Foramen ovale	Fossa ovalis	
AllaNtois	Urachus-mediaN umbilical ligament	The urachus is the part of the allantoic duct between the bladder and the umbilicus. Urachal cyst or sinus is a remnant.
Notochord	Nucleus pulposus of intervertebral disc	

▸ **CARDIOVASCULAR–ANATOMY**

Coronary artery anatomy

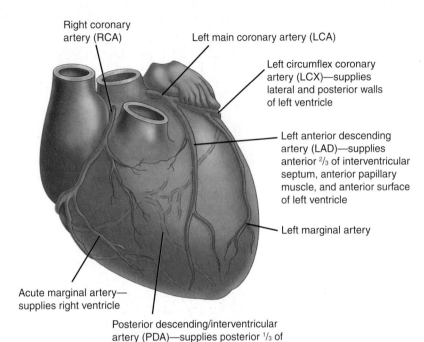

Right coronary artery (RCA)

Left main coronary artery (LCA)

Left circumflex coronary artery (LCX)—supplies lateral and posterior walls of left ventricle

Left anterior descending artery (LAD)—supplies anterior 2/3 of interventricular septum, anterior papillary muscle, and anterior surface of left ventricle

Left marginal artery

Acute marginal artery— supplies right ventricle

Posterior descending/interventricular artery (PDA)—supplies posterior 1/3 of interventricular septum and posterior walls of ventricles

SA and AV nodes are usually supplied by RCA. Infarct may cause nodal dysfunction (bradycardia or heart block).

Right-dominant circulation = 85% = PDA arises from RCA.

Left-dominant circulation = 8% = PDA arises from LCX.

Codominant circulation = 7% = PDA arises from both LCX and RCA.

Coronary artery occlusion most commonly occurs in the LAD.

Coronary blood flow peaks in early diastole.

The most posterior part of the heart is the left atrium; enlargement can cause dysphagia (due to compression of the esophagus) or hoarseness (due to compression of the left recurrent laryngeal nerve, a branch of the vagus).

▸ **CARDIOVASCULAR–PHYSIOLOGY**

Cardiac output

CO = stroke volume (SV) × heart rate (HR).

Fick principle:

$$CO = \frac{\text{rate of } O_2 \text{ consumption}}{\text{arterial } O_2 \text{ content} - \text{venous } O_2 \text{ content}}$$

Mean arterial pressure (MAP) = CO × TPR.

MAP = ⅔ diastolic pressure + ⅓ systolic pressure.

Pulse pressure = systolic pressure – diastolic pressure. Pulse pressure is proportional to SV, inversely proportional to arterial compliance.

SV = EDV – ESV.

During the early stages of exercise, CO is maintained by ↑ HR and ↑ SV. During the late stages of exercise, CO is maintained by ↑ HR only (SV plateaus).

Diastole is preferentially shortened with ↑ HR; less filling time → ↓ CO (e.g., ventricular tachycardia).

↑ pulse pressure in hyperthyroidism, aortic regurgitation, arteriosclerosis, obstructive sleep apnea (↑ sympathetic tone), exercise (transient).

↓ pulse pressure in aortic stenosis, cardiogenic shock, cardiac tamponade, and advanced heart failure.

Cardiac output variables

Stroke volume	Stroke Volume affected by Contractility, Afterload, and Preload. ↑ SV when ↑ contractility, ↑ preload, or ↓ afterload.	SV CAP.
Contractility	Contractility (and SV) ↑ with: • Catecholamines (↑ activity of Ca^{2+} pump in sarcoplasmic reticulum). • ↑ intracellular Ca^{2+}. • ↓ extracellular Na^+ (↓ activity of Na^+/Ca^{2+} exchanger). • Digitalis (blocks Na^+/K^+ pump → ↑ intracellular Na^+ → ↓ Na^+/Ca^{2+} exchanger activity → ↑ intracellular Ca^{2+}). Contractility (and SV) ↓ with: • β_1-blockade (↓ cAMP). • Heart failure with systolic dysfunction. • Acidosis. • Hypoxia/hypercapnea (↓ P_{O_2}/↑ P_{CO_2}). • Non-dihydropyridine Ca^{2+} channel blockers.	SV ↑ in anxiety, exercise, and pregnancy. A failing heart has ↓ SV (both systolic and diastolic dysfunction). Myocardial O_2 demand is ↑ by: • ↑ afterload (∝ arterial pressure). • ↑ contractility. • ↑ HR. • ↑ ventricular diameter (↑ wall tension).
Preload	Preload approximated by ventricular EDV; depends on venous tone and circulating blood volume.	VEnodilators (e.g., nitroglycerin) ↓ prEload.
Afterload	Afterload approximated by MAP. Relation of LV size and afterload → Laplace's law: $$\text{Wall tension} = \frac{\text{pressure} \times \text{radius}}{2 \times \text{wall thickness}}$$ LV compensates for ↑ afterload by thickening (hypertrophy) to ↓ wall tension.	VAsodilators (e.g., hydrAlazine) ↓ Afterload (Arterial). ACE inhibitors and ARBs ↓ both preload and afterload. Chronic hypertension (↑ MAP) → LV hypertrophy.
Ejection fraction	$$EF = \frac{SV}{EDV} = \frac{EDV - ESV}{EDV}$$ Left ventricular EF is an index of ventricular contractility; normal EF is ≥ 55%.	EF ↓ in systolic heart failure; EF is normal in diastolic heart failure.

Starling curve

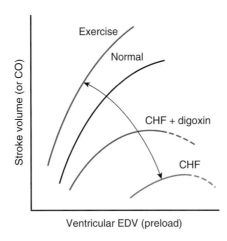

Force of contraction is proportional to end-diastolic length of cardiac muscle fiber (preload).

↑ contractility with catecholamines, digoxin.

↓ contractility with loss of myocardium (e.g., MI), β-blockers, calcium channel blockers, dilated cardiomyopathy.

Resistance, pressure, flow

$\Delta P = Q \times R$

Similar to Ohm's law: $\Delta V = IR$

Resistance

$$= \frac{\text{driving pressure } (\Delta P)}{\text{flow } (Q)} = \frac{8\eta \ (\text{viscosity}) \times \text{length}}{\pi r^4}$$

Total resistance of vessels in series:

$TR = R_1 + R_2 + R_3 \ldots$

Total resistance of vessels in parallel:

$$\frac{1}{TR} = \frac{1}{R_1} + \frac{1}{R_2} + \frac{1}{R_3} \ldots$$

Viscosity depends mostly on hematocrit

Viscosity ↑ in:

- Polycythemia
- Hyperproteinemic states (e.g., multiple myeloma)
- aHereditary spherocytosis

Viscosity ↓ in anemia

Pressure gradient drives flow from high pressure to low pressure.

Resistance is directly proportional to viscosity and vessel length and inversely proportional to the radius to the 4th power.

Arterioles account for most of TPR → regulate capillary flow.

Cardiac and vascular function curves

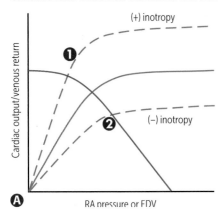

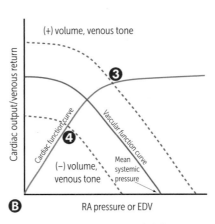

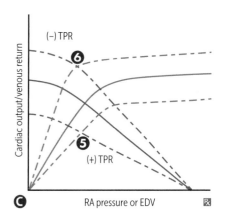

Intersection of curves = operating point of heart (i.e., venous return and CO are equal).

CURVE	EFFECT	EXAMPLES
Ⓐ Inotropy	Changes in contractility → altered CO for a given RA pressure (preload).	❶ Catecholamines, digoxin ⊕ ❷ Uncompensated heart failure, narcotic overdose ⊖
Ⓑ Venous return	Changes in circulating volume or venous tone → altered RA pressure for a given CO. Mean systemic pressure (x-intercept) changes with volume/venous tone.	❸ Fluid infusion, sympathetic activity ⊕ ❹ Acute hemorrhage, spinal anesthesia ⊖
Ⓒ Total peripheral resistance	Changes in TPR → altered CO at a given RA pressure; however, mean systemic pressure (x-intercept) is unchanged.	❺ Vasopressors ⊕ ❻ Exercise, AV shunt ⊖

Changes often occur in tandem, and may be reinforcing (exercise ↑ inotropy and ↓ TPR to maximize CO) or compensatory (heart failure ↓ inotropy → fluid retention to ↑ preload to maintain CO).

Pressure-volume loops and cardiac cycle

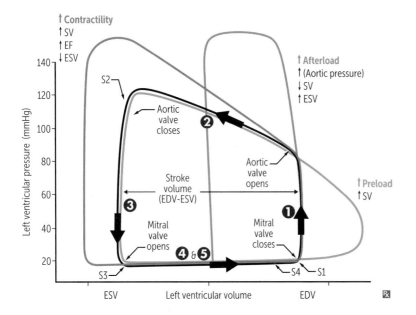

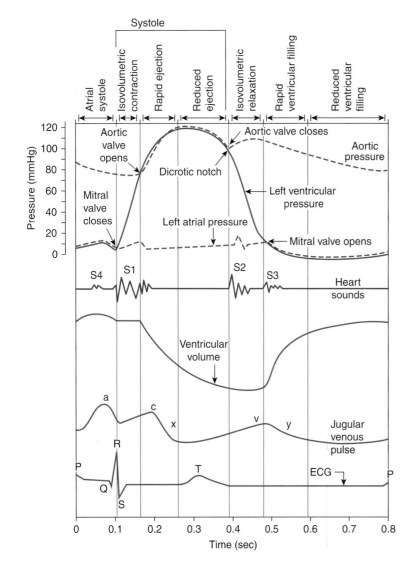

The black loop represents normal cardiac physiology.

Phases—left ventricle:
❶ Isovolumetric contraction—period between mitral valve closing and aortic valve opening; period of highest O_2 consumption
❷ Systolic ejection—period between aortic valve opening and closing
❸ Isovolumetric relaxation—period between aortic valve closing and mitral valve opening
❹ Rapid filling—period just after mitral valve opening
❺ Reduced filling—period just before mitral valve closing

Sounds:
S1—mitral and tricuspid valve closure. Loudest at mitral area.
S2—aortic and pulmonary valve closure. Loudest at left sternal border.
S3—in early diastole during rapid ventricular filling phase. Associated with ↑ filling pressures (e.g., mitral regurgitation, CHF) and more common in dilated ventricles (but normal in children and pregnant women).
S4 ("atrial kick")—in late diastole. High atrial pressure. Associated with ventricular hypertrophy. Left atrium must push against stiff LV wall.

Jugular venous pulse (JVP):
a wave—atrial contraction.
c wave—RV contraction (closed tricuspid valve bulging into atrium).
x descent—atrial relaxation and downward displacement of closed tricuspid valve during ventricular contraction. Absent in tricuspid regurgitation.
v wave—↑ right atrial pressure due to filling against closed tricuspid valve.
y descent—blood flow from RA to RV.

Splitting

Normal splitting	Inspiration → drop in intrathoracic pressure → ↑ venous return to the RV → ↑ RV stroke volume → ↑ RV ejection time → delayed closure of pulmonic valve. ↓ pulmonary impedance (↑ capacity of the pulmonary circulation) also occurs during inspiration, which contributes to delayed closure of pulmonic valve.	Expiration Inspiration	$\|$ $\|\|$ S1 A2 P2 $\|$ $\|$ $\|$
Wide splitting	Seen in conditions that delay RV emptying (pulmonic stenosis, right bundle branch block). Delay in RV emptying causes delayed pulmonic sound (regardless of breath). An exaggeration of normal splitting.	Expiration Inspiration	$\|$ $\|$ $\|$ S1 A2 P2 $\|$ $\|$ $\|$
Fixed splitting	Seen in ASD. ASD → left-to-right shunt → ↑ RA and RV volumes → ↑ flow through pulmonic valve such that, regardless of breath, pulmonic closure is greatly delayed.	Expiration Inspiration	$\|$ $\|$ $\|$ S1 A2 P2 $\|$ $\|$ $\|$
Paradoxical splitting	Seen in conditions that delay LV emptying (aortic stenosis, left bundle branch block). Normal order of valve closure is reversed so that P2 sound occurs before delayed A2 sound. Therefore on inspiration, P2 closes later and moves closer to A2, thereby "paradoxically" eliminating the split.	Expiration Inspiration	$\|$ $\|$ $\|$ S1 P2 A2 $\|$ $\|\|$

Auscultation of the heart

Where to listen: APT M

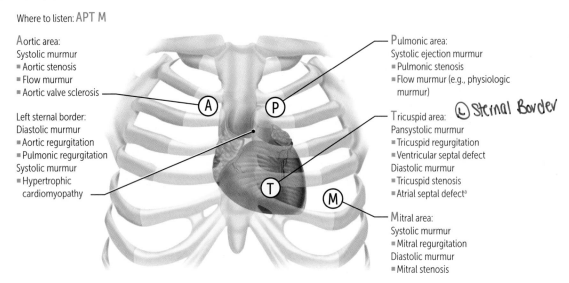

Aortic area:
Systolic murmur
- Aortic stenosis
- Flow murmur
- Aortic valve sclerosis

Left sternal border:
Diastolic murmur
- Aortic regurgitation
- Pulmonic regurgitation
Systolic murmur
- Hypertrophic cardiomyopathy

Pulmonic area:
Systolic ejection murmur
- Pulmonic stenosis
- Flow murmur (e.g., physiologic murmur)

Tricuspid area: (L) Sternal Border
Pansystolic murmur
- Tricuspid regurgitation
- Ventricular septal defect
Diastolic murmur
- Tricuspid stenosis
- Atrial septal defect[a]

Mitral area:
Systolic murmur
- Mitral regurgitation
Diastolic murmur
- Mitral stenosis

[a] ASD commonly presents with a pulmonary flow murmur (↑ flow through pulmonary valve) and a diastolic rumble (↑ flow across tricuspid); blood flow across the actual ASD does not cause a murmur because there is no pressure gradient. The murmur later progresses to a louder diastolic murmur of pulmonic regurgitation from dilatation of the pulmonary artery.

BEDSIDE MANEUVER	EFFECT
Inspiration	↑ intensity of right heart sounds
Hand grip (↑ systemic vascular resistance)	↑ intensity of MR, AR, VSD murmurs ↓ intensity of AS, hypertrophic cardiomyopathy murmurs MVP: ↑ murmur intensity, later onset of click/murmur
Valsalva (phase II), standing (↓ venous return)	↓ intensity of most murmurs (including AS) ↑ intensity of hypertrophic cardiomyopathy murmur MVP: ↓ murmur intensity, earlier onset of click/murmur
Rapid squatting (↑ venous return, ↑ preload, ↑ afterload with prolonged squatting)	↓ intensity of hypertrophic cardiomyopathy murmur ↑ intensity of AS murmur MVP: ↑ murmur intensity, later onset of click/murmur

Systolic heart sounds include aortic/pulmonic stenosis, mitral/tricuspid regurgitation, ventricular septal defect.
Diastolic heart sounds include aortic/pulmonic regurgitation, mitral/tricuspid stenosis.

MVP = mitral valve prolapse

Heart murmurs

Systolic

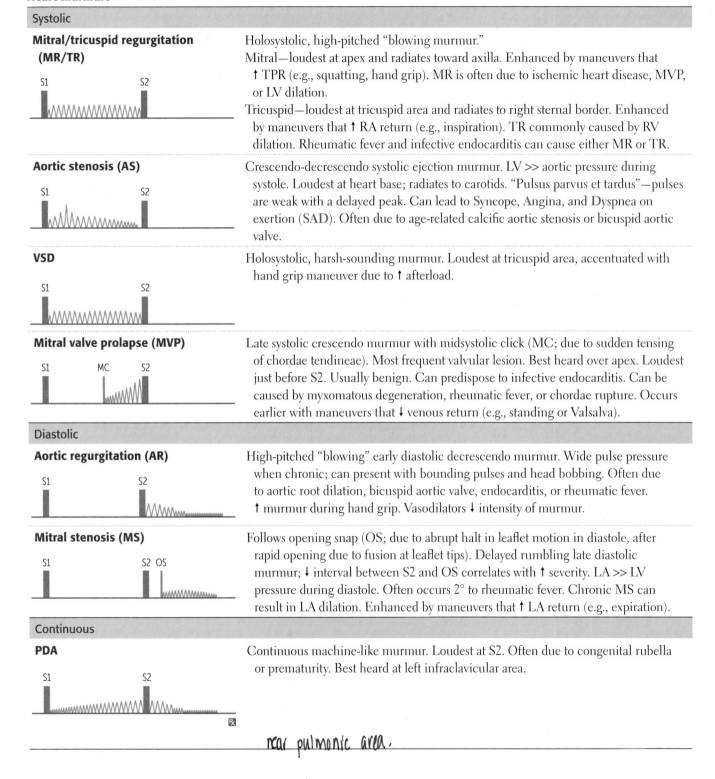

Mitral/tricuspid regurgitation (MR/TR)

Holosystolic, high-pitched "blowing murmur."

Mitral—loudest at apex and radiates toward axilla. Enhanced by maneuvers that ↑ TPR (e.g., squatting, hand grip). MR is often due to ischemic heart disease, MVP, or LV dilation.

Tricuspid—loudest at tricuspid area and radiates to right sternal border. Enhanced by maneuvers that ↑ RA return (e.g., inspiration). TR commonly caused by RV dilation. Rheumatic fever and infective endocarditis can cause either MR or TR.

Aortic stenosis (AS)

Crescendo-decrescendo systolic ejection murmur. LV >> aortic pressure during systole. Loudest at heart base; radiates to carotids. "Pulsus parvus et tardus"—pulses are weak with a delayed peak. Can lead to Syncope, Angina, and Dyspnea on exertion (SAD). Often due to age-related calcific aortic stenosis or bicuspid aortic valve.

VSD

Holosystolic, harsh-sounding murmur. Loudest at tricuspid area, accentuated with hand grip maneuver due to ↑ afterload.

Mitral valve prolapse (MVP)

Late systolic crescendo murmur with midsystolic click (MC; due to sudden tensing of chordae tendineae). Most frequent valvular lesion. Best heard over apex. Loudest just before S2. Usually benign. Can predispose to infective endocarditis. Can be caused by myxomatous degeneration, rheumatic fever, or chordae rupture. Occurs earlier with maneuvers that ↓ venous return (e.g., standing or Valsalva).

Diastolic

Aortic regurgitation (AR)

High-pitched "blowing" early diastolic decrescendo murmur. Wide pulse pressure when chronic; can present with bounding pulses and head bobbing. Often due to aortic root dilation, bicuspid aortic valve, endocarditis, or rheumatic fever. ↑ murmur during hand grip. Vasodilators ↓ intensity of murmur.

Mitral stenosis (MS)

Follows opening snap (OS; due to abrupt halt in leaflet motion in diastole, after rapid opening due to fusion at leaflet tips). Delayed rumbling late diastolic murmur; ↓ interval between S2 and OS correlates with ↑ severity. LA >> LV pressure during diastole. Often occurs 2° to rheumatic fever. Chronic MS can result in LA dilation. Enhanced by maneuvers that ↑ LA return (e.g., expiration).

Continuous

PDA

Continuous machine-like murmur. Loudest at S2. Often due to congenital rubella or prematurity. Best heard at left infraclavicular area.

near pulmonic area.

Ventricular action potential

Also occurs in bundle of His and Purkinje fibers.

Phase 0 = rapid upstroke and depolarization—voltage-gated Na⁺ channels open.

Phase 1 = initial repolarization—inactivation of voltage-gated Na⁺ channels. Voltage-gated K⁺ channels begin to open.

Phase 2 = plateau—Ca^{2+} influx through voltage-gated Ca^{2+} channels balances K⁺ efflux. Ca^{2+} influx triggers Ca^{2+} release from sarcoplasmic reticulum and myocyte contraction.

Phase 3 = rapid repolarization—massive K⁺ efflux due to opening of voltage-gated slow K⁺ channels and closure of voltage-gated Ca^{2+} channels.

Phase 4 = resting potential—high K⁺ permeability through K⁺ channels.

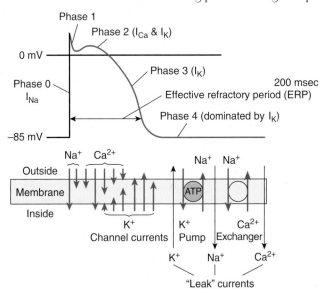

In contrast to skeletal muscle:
- Cardiac muscle action potential has a plateau, which is due to Ca^{2+} influx and K⁺ efflux; myocyte contraction occurs due to Ca^{2+}-induced Ca^{2+} release from the sarcoplasmic reticulum.
- Cardiac nodal cells spontaneously depolarize during diastole, resulting in automaticity due to I_f channels ("funny current" channels responsible for a slow, mixed Na⁺/K⁺ inward current).
- Cardiac myocytes are electrically coupled to each other by gap junctions.

Pacemaker action potential

Occurs in the SA and AV nodes. Key differences from the ventricular action potential include:

Phase 0 = upstroke—opening of voltage-gated Ca^{2+} channels. Fast voltage-gated Na^+ channels are permanently inactivated because of the less negative resting voltage of these cells. Results in a slow conduction velocity that is used by the AV node to prolong transmission from the atria to ventricles.

Phase 2 is absent.

Phase 3 = inactivation of the Ca^{2+} channels and ↑ activation of K^+ channels → ↑ K^+ efflux.

Phase 4 = slow diastolic depolarization—membrane potential spontaneously depolarizes as Na^+ conductance ↑ (I_f different from I_{Na} in phase 0 of ventricular action potential). Accounts for automaticity of SA and AV nodes. The slope of phase 4 in the SA node determines HR. ACh/adenosine ↓ the rate of diastolic depolarization and ↓ HR, while catecholamines ↑ depolarization and ↑ HR. Sympathetic stimulation ↑ the chance that I_f channels are open and thus ↑ HR.

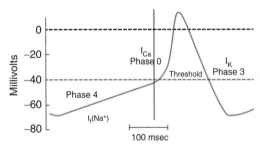

Electrocardiogram

P wave—atrial depolarization. Atrial repolarization is masked by QRS complex.

PR interval—conduction delay through AV node (normally < 200 msec).

QRS complex—ventricular depolarization (normally < 120 msec).

QT interval—mechanical contraction of the ventricles.

T wave—ventricular repolarization. T-wave inversion may indicate recent MI.

ST segment—isoelectric, ventricles depolarized.

U wave—caused by hypokalemia, bradycardia.

Speed of conduction—Purkinje > atria > ventricles > AV node.

Pacemakers—SA > AV > bundle of His/ Purkinje/ventricles.

Conduction pathway—SA node → atria → AV node → common bundle → bundle branches → Purkinje fibers → ventricles.

SA node "pacemaker" inherent dominance with slow phase of upstroke.

AV node—100-msec delay—atrioventricular delay; allows time for ventricular filling.

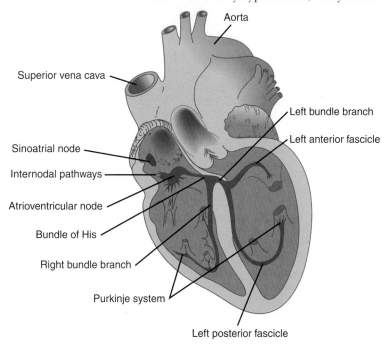

Aorta
Superior vena cava
Sinoatrial node
Internodal pathways
Atrioventricular node
Bundle of His
Right bundle branch
Purkinje system
Left posterior fascicle
Left bundle branch
Left anterior fascicle

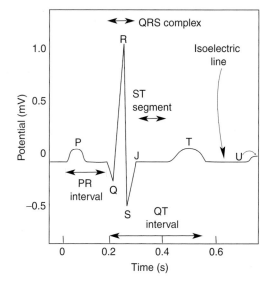

QRS complex
Isoelectric line
ST segment
PR interval
QT interval
Potential (mV)
Time (s)

Torsades de pointes 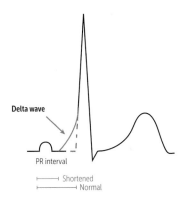	Polymorphic ventricular tachycardia, characterized by shifting sinusoidal waveforms on ECG; can progress to ventricular fibrillation. Long QT interval predisposes to torsades de pointes. Caused by drugs, ↓ K⁺, ↓ Mg²⁺, other abnormalities. Treatment includes magnesium sulfate.	Some Risky Meds Can Prolong QT: Sotalol Risperidone (antipsychotics) Macrolides Chloroquine Protease inhibitors (-navir) Quinidine (class Ia; also class III) Thiazides

Torsades de pointes

Polymorphic ventricular tachycardia, characterized by shifting sinusoidal waveforms on ECG; can progress to ventricular fibrillation. Long QT interval predisposes to torsades de pointes. Caused by drugs, ↓ K⁺, ↓ Mg²⁺, other abnormalities. Treatment includes magnesium sulfate.

Some Risky Meds Can Prolong QT:
Sotalol
Risperidone (antipsychotics)
Macrolides
Chloroquine
Protease inhibitors (-navir)
Quinidine (class Ia; also class III)
Thiazides

Congenital long QT syndrome

Inherited disorder of myocardial repolarization, typically due to ion channel defects; ↑ risk of sudden cardiac death due to torsades de pointes. Includes:
- **Romano-Ward syndrome**—autosomal dominant, pure cardiac phenotype (no deafness).
- **Jervell and Lange-Nielsen syndrome**—autosomal recessive, sensorineural deafness.

Wolff-Parkinson-White syndrome

Most common type of ventricular pre-excitation syndrome. Abnormal fast accessory conduction pathway from atria to ventricle (bundle of Kent) bypasses the rate-slowing AV node. As a result, ventricles begin to partially depolarize earlier, giving rise to characteristic delta wave with shortened PR interval on ECG. May result in reentry circuit → supraventricular tachycardia.

Delta wave

PR interval

Shortened
Normal

ECG tracings

Atrial fibrillation	Chaotic and erratic baseline (irregularly irregular) with no discrete P waves in between irregularly spaced QRS complexes. Can result in atrial stasis and lead to thromboembolic stroke. Treatment includes rate control, anticoagulation, and possible pharmacological or electrical cardioversion.

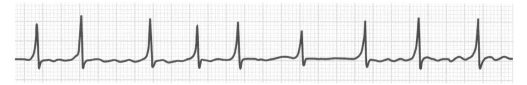

Atrial flutter	A rapid succession of identical, back-to-back atrial depolarization waves. The identical appearance accounts for the "sawtooth" appearance of the flutter waves. Pharmacologic conversion to sinus rhythm: class IA, IC, or III antiarrhythmics. Rate control: β-blocker or calcium channel blocker. Definitive treatment is catheter ablation.

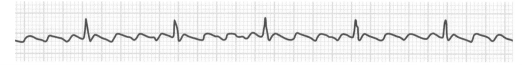

Ventricular fibrillation	A completely erratic rhythm with no identifiable waves. Fatal arrhythmia without immediate CPR and defibrillation.

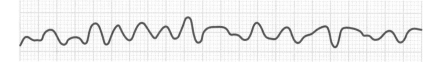

AV block

1st degree	The PR interval is prolonged (> 200 msec). Benign and asymptomatic. No treatment required.

Prolonged PR interval

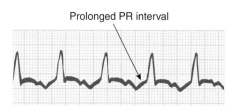

2nd degree

Mobitz type I (Wenckebach)	Progressive lengthening of the PR interval until a beat is "dropped" (a P wave not followed by a QRS complex). Usually asymptomatic.

Progressive increase in PR length before dropped beat

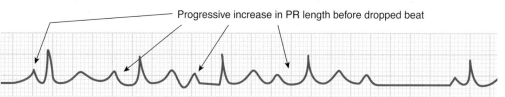

ECG tracings *(continued)*

Mobitz type II	Dropped beats that are not preceded by a change in the length of the PR interval (as in type I). It is often found as 2:1 block, where there are 2 or more P waves to 1 QRS response. May progress to 3rd-degree block. Often treated with pacemaker.

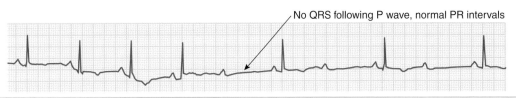

No QRS following P wave, normal PR intervals

3rd degree (complete)	The atria and ventricles beat independently of each other. Both P waves and QRS complexes are present, although the P waves bear no relation to the QRS complexes. The atrial rate is faster than the ventricular rate. Usually treated with pacemaker. Lyme disease can result in 3rd-degree heart block.

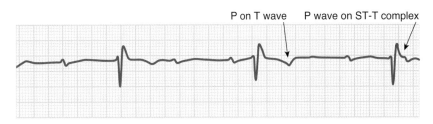

P on T wave   P wave on ST-T complex

Atrial natriuretic peptide	Released from **atrial myocytes** in response to ↑ blood volume and atrial pressure. Causes vasodilation and ↓ Na⁺ reabsorption at the renal collecting tubule. Constricts efferent renal arterioles and dilates afferent arterioles via cGMP, promoting diuresis and contributing to "aldosterone escape" mechanism.

B-type (brain) natriuretic peptide	Released from **ventricular myocytes** in response to ↑ tension. Similar physiologic action to ANP, with longer half-life. BNP blood test used for diagnosing heart failure (very good negative predictive value). Available in recombinant form (nesiritide) for treatment of heart failure.

Baroreceptors and chemoreceptors

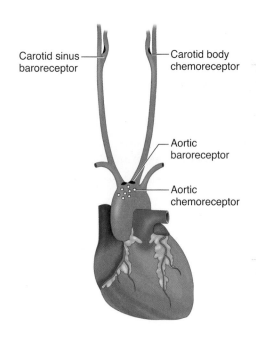

Carotid sinus baroreceptor

Carotid body chemoreceptor

Aortic baroreceptor

Aortic chemoreceptor

Receptors:

- Aortic arch transmits via vagus nerve to solitary nucleus of medulla (responds **only** to ↑ BP).
- Carotid sinus (dilated region at carotid bifurcation) transmits via glossopharyngeal nerve to solitary nucleus of medulla (responds to ↓ and ↑ in BP).

Baroreceptors:

- Hypotension—↓ arterial pressure → ↓ stretch → ↓ afferent baroreceptor firing → ↑ efferent sympathetic firing and ↓ efferent parasympathetic stimulation → vasoconstriction, ↑ HR, ↑ contractility, ↑ BP. Important in the response to severe hemorrhage.
- Carotid massage—↑ pressure on carotid sinus → ↑ stretch → ↑ afferent baroreceptor firing → ↑ AV node refractory period → ↓ HR.
- Contributes to Cushing reaction (triad of hypertension, bradycardia, and respiratory depression)—↑ intracranial pressure constricts arterioles → cerebral ischemia and reflex sympathetic ↑ in perfusion pressure (hypertension) → ↑ stretch → reflex baroreceptor induced–bradycardia.

Chemoreceptors:

- Peripheral—carotid and aortic bodies are stimulated by ↓ P_{O_2} (< 60 mmHg), ↑ P_{CO_2}, and ↓ pH of blood.
- Central—are stimulated by changes in pH and P_{CO_2} of brain interstitial fluid, which in turn are influenced by arterial CO_2. Do not directly respond to P_{O_2}.

Circulation through organs

Lung	Organ with largest blood flow (100% of cardiac output).
Liver	Largest share of systemic cardiac output.
Kidney	Highest blood flow per gram of tissue.
Heart	Largest arteriovenous O_2 difference because O_2 extraction is ~ 80%. Therefore ↑ O_2 demand is met by ↑ coronary blood flow, not by ↑ extraction of O_2.

Normal pressures

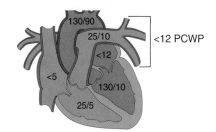

130/90
25/10
<12 PCWP
<12
<5
130/10
25/5

PCWP—pulmonary capillary wedge pressure (in mmHg) is a good approximation of left atrial pressure. In mitral stenosis, PCWP > LV diastolic pressure.

Measured with pulmonary artery catheter (Swan-Ganz catheter).

Autoregulation

How blood flow to an organ remains constant over a wide range of perfusion pressures.

ORGAN	FACTORS DETERMINING AUTOREGULATION
Heart	Local metabolites (vasodilatory)–CO_2, adenosine, NO
Brain	Local metabolites (vasodilatory)–CO_2 (pH)
Kidneys	Myogenic and tubuloglomerular feedback
Lungs	Hypoxia causes vasoconstriction
Skeletal muscle	Local metabolites—lactate, adenosine, K^+, H^+, CO_2
Skin	Sympathetic stimulation most important mechanism—temperature control

Note: the pulmonary vasculature is unique in that hypoxia causes vasoconstriction so that only well-ventilated areas are perfused. In other organs, hypoxia causes vasodilation.

Capillary fluid exchange

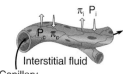

π_i P_i

P_c π_c

Interstitial fluid

Capillary

Starling forces determine fluid movement through capillary membranes:
- P_c = capillary pressure—pushes fluid out of capillary
- P_i = interstitial fluid pressure—pushes fluid into capillary
- π_c = plasma colloid osmotic pressure—pulls fluid into capillary
- π_i = interstitial fluid colloid osmotic pressure—pulls fluid out of capillary

Thus, net filtration pressure = $P_{net} = [(P_c - P_i) - (\pi_c - \pi_i)]$.

K_f = filtration constant (capillary permeability).

J_v = net fluid flow = $(K_f)(P_{net})$.

Edema—excess fluid outflow into interstitium commonly caused by:
- ↑ capillary pressure (↑ P_c; heart failure)
- ↓ plasma proteins (↓ π_c; nephrotic syndrome, liver failure)
- ↑ capillary permeability (↑ K_f; toxins, infections, burns)
- ↑ interstitial fluid colloid osmotic pressure (↑ π_i; lymphatic blockage)

▸ **CARDIOVASCULAR—PATHOLOGY**

Congenital heart diseases

RIGHT-TO-LEFT SHUNTS	Early cyanosis—"blue babies." Often diagnosed prenatally or become evident immediately after birth. Usually require urgent surgical correction and/or maintenance of a PDA.	The 5 Ts: 1. Truncus arteriosus (1 vessel) 2. Transposition (2 switched vessels) 3. Tricuspid atresia (3 = Tri) 4. Tetralogy of Fallot (4 = Tetra) 5. TAPVR (5 letters in the name)
Persistent truncus arteriosus	Failure of truncus arteriosus to divide into pulmonary trunk and aorta; most patients have accompanying VSD.	
D-transposition of great vessels	Aorta leaves RV (anterior) and pulmonary trunk leaves LV (posterior) → separation of systemic and pulmonary circulations. Not compatible with life unless a shunt is present to allow mixing of blood (e.g., VSD, PDA, or patent foramen ovale). Due to failure of the aorticopulmonary septum to spiral. Without surgical intervention, most infants die within the first few months of life.	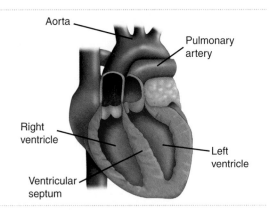 Aorta, Pulmonary artery, Right ventricle, Left ventricle, Ventricular septum
Tricuspid atresia	Absence of tricuspid valve and hypoplastic RV; requires both ASD and VSD for viability.	
Tetralogy of Fallot	Caused by anterosuperior displacement of the infundibular septum. Most common cause of early childhood cyanosis. ❶ Pulmonary infundibular stenosis (most important determinant for prognosis) ❷ RVH—boot-shaped heart on CXR ❸ Overriding aorta ❹ VSD Pulmonary stenosis forces right-to-left flow across VSD → early cyanotic "tet spells," RVH.	PROVe. Squatting: ↑ SVR, ↓ right-to-left shunt, improves cyanosis. Treatment: early surgical correction.
Total anomalous pulmonary venous return (TAPVR)	Pulmonary veins drain into right heart circulation (SVC, coronary sinus, etc.); associated with ASD and sometimes PDA to allow for right-to-left shunting to maintain CO.	

Congenital heart diseases (continued)

LEFT-TO-RIGHT SHUNTS	Late cyanosis—"blue kids."	Frequency: VSD > ASD > PDA.
Ventricular septal defect	Most common congenital cardiac defect. Asymptomatic at birth, may manifest weeks later or remain asymptomatic throughout life. Most self resolve; larger lesions may lead to LV overload and heart failure.	
Atrial septal defect	Defect in interatrial septum; loud S1; wide, fixed split S2. Usually occurs in septum secundum; septum primum defects usually occur with other anomalies. Symptoms range from none to heart failure. Distinct from patent foramen ovale in that septa are missing tissue rather than unfused.	
Patent ductus arteriosus Aorta — Ductus arteriosus (patent) — Pulmonary artery	In fetal period, shunt is right to left (normal). In neonatal period, ↓ lung resistance → shunt becomes left to right → progressive RVH and/or LVH and heart failure. Associated with a continuous, "machine-like" murmur. Patency is maintained by PGE synthesis and low O_2 tension. Uncorrected PDA can eventually result in late cyanosis in the lower extremities (differential cyanosis).	"**Endo**methacin" (indomethacin) **ends** patency of PDA; PGE k**EE**ps it open (may be necessary to sustain life in conditions such as transposition of the great vessels). PDA is normal in utero and normally closes only after birth.
Eisenmenger syndrome	Uncorrected left-to-right shunt (VSD, ASD, PDA) → ↑ pulmonary blood flow → pathologic remodeling of vasculature → pulmonary arteriolar hypertension. RVH occurs to compensate → shunt becomes right to left. Causes late cyanosis, clubbing, and polycythemia. Age of onset varies.	

OTHER ANOMALIES		
Coarctation of the aorta	Associated with bicuspid aortic valve, other heart defects.	
Infantile type	Aorta narrowing is proximal to insertion of ductus arteriosus (preductal). Associated with Turner syndrome. Can present with closure of the ductus arteriosus (reverse with PGE_2).	Infantile: in close to the heart.
Adult type	Aorta narrowing is distal to ligamentum arteriosum (postductal). Associated with notching of the ribs (collateral circulation), hypertension in upper extremities, and weak, delayed pulses in lower extremities (radiofemoral delay).	Adult: distal to ductus.

Congenital cardiac defect associations	DISORDER	DEFECT
	22q11 syndromes	Truncus arteriosus, tetralogy of Fallot
	Down syndrome	ASD, VSD, AV septal defect (endocardial cushion defect)
	Congenital rubella	Septal defects, PDA, pulmonary artery stenosis
	Turner syndrome	Bicuspid aortic valve, coarctation of aorta (preductal)
	Marfan syndrome	MVP, thoracic aortic aneurysm and dissection, aortic regurgitation
	Infant of diabetic mother	Transposition of great vessels

Hypertension	Defined as a systolic BP ≥ 140 mmHg and/or diastolic BP ≥ 90 mmHg
RISK FACTORS	↑ age, obesity, diabetes, smoking, genetics, black > white > Asian.
FEATURES	90% of hypertension is 1° (essential) and related to ↑ CO or ↑ TPR; remaining 10% mostly 2° to renal disease, including fibromuscular dysplasia in young patients **A**. Hypertensive emergency—severe hypertension (≥ 180/120 mmHg) with evidence of acute, ongoing target organ damage (e.g., papilledema, mental status changes).
PREDISPOSES TO	Atherosclerosis, LVH, stroke, CHF, renal failure **B**, retinopathy, and aortic dissection.

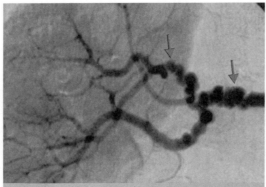

A **Fibromuscular dysplasia.** "String of beads" appearance (arrows) of the renal artery in fibromuscular dysplasia, a cause of hypertension in younger patients. ✶

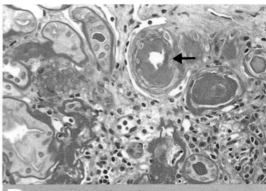

B **Hypertensive nephropathy.** Renal arterial hyalinosis (arrow) on PAS stain. ✶

Hyperlipidemia signs

Xanthomas	Plaques or nodules composed of lipid-laden histiocytes in the skin **A**, especially the eyelids (xanthelasma **B**).
Tendinous xanthoma	Lipid deposit in tendon **C**, especially Achilles.
Corneal arcus	Lipid deposit in cornea, appears early in life with hypercholesterolemia. Common in elderly (arcus senilis **D**).

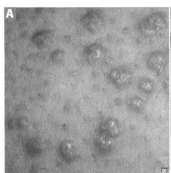 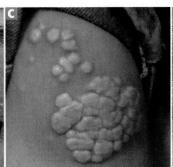 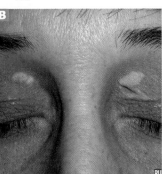 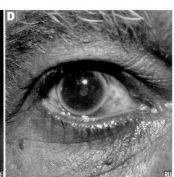

Arteriosclerosis

Mönckeberg (medial calcific sclerosis)	Uncommon. Calcification in the media of the arteries, especially radial or ulnar. Usually benign; "pipestem" arteries on x-ray **A**. Does not obstruct blood flow; intima not involved.
Arteriolosclerosis	Common. Two types: hyaline (thickening of small arteries in essential hypertension or diabetes mellitus **B**) and hyperplastic ("onion skinning" as seen in severe hypertension **C**).

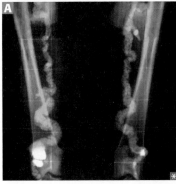 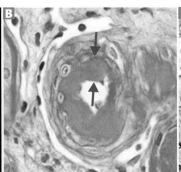 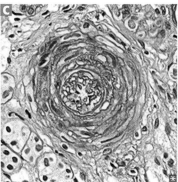

Atherosclerosis	Disease of elastic arteries and large- and medium-sized muscular arteries.
RISK FACTORS	Modifiable: smoking, hypertension, hyperlipidemia, diabetes. Non-modifiable: age, sex (↑ in men and postmenopausal women), and family history.
PROGRESSION 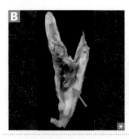	Inflammation important in pathogenesis. Endothelial cell dysfunction → macrophage and LDL accumulation → foam cell formation → fatty streaks → smooth muscle cell migration (involves PDGF and FGF), proliferation, and extracellular matrix deposition → fibrous plaque → complex atheromas **A**.
COMPLICATIONS	Aneurysms, ischemia, infarcts, peripheral vascular disease, thrombus, emboli.
LOCATION	Abdominal aorta > coronary artery > popliteal artery > carotid artery **B**.
SYMPTOMS	Angina, claudication, but can be asymptomatic.

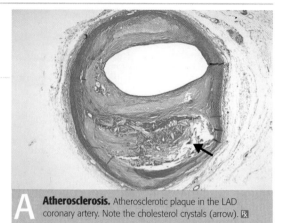

A **Atherosclerosis.** Atherosclerotic plaque in the LAD coronary artery. Note the cholesterol crystals (arrow). ℞

Aortic aneurysms	Localized pathologic dilation of the aorta. May cause pain, which is a sign of leaking, dissection, or imminent rupture.
Abdominal aortic aneurysm	Associated with atherosclerosis. Occurs more frequently in hypertensive male smokers > 50 years old **A**.
Thoracic aortic aneurysm	Associated with cystic medial degeneration due to hypertension (older patients) or Marfan syndrome (younger patients). Also historically associated with 3° syphilis (obliterative endarteritis of the vasa vasorum). **B**

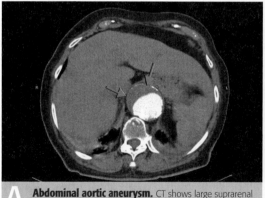

A **Abdominal aortic aneurysm.** CT shows large suprarenal aneurysm with eccentric mural thrombus (arrows). ℞

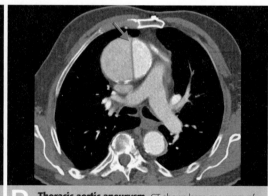

B **Thoracic aortic aneurysm.** CT shows large aneurysm of the ascending aorta, with dissection (arrow). ✦

Aortic dissection	Longitudinal intraluminal tear forming a false lumen 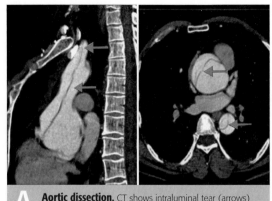. Associated with hypertension, bicuspid aortic valve, and inherited connective tissue disorders (e.g., Marfan syndrome). Can present with tearing chest pain, of sudden onset, radiating to the back +/– markedly unequal BP in arms. CXR shows mediastinal widening. The false lumen can be limited to the ascending aorta, propagate from the ascending aorta, or propagate from the descending aorta. Can result in pericardial tamponade, aortic rupture, and death.

Aortic dissection. CT shows intraluminal tear (arrows) forming a "flap" separating true and false lumen, involving the ascending and descending aorta (Stanford Type A).

Ischemic heart disease manifestations

Angina	Chest pain due to ischemic myocardium 2° to coronary artery narrowing or spasm; no myocyte necrosis. ▪ **Stable**—usually 2° to atherosclerosis; exertional chest pain in classic distribution (usually with ST depression on ECG), resolving with rest. ▪ **Variant angina (Prinzmetal)**—occurs at rest 2° to coronary artery spasm; transient ST elevation on ECG. Known triggers include tobacco, cocaine, and triptans, but trigger is often unknown. Treat with calcium channel blockers, nitrates, and smoking cessation (if applicable). ▪ **Unstable/crescendo**—thrombosis with incomplete coronary artery occlusion; ST depression on ECG (↑ in frequency or intensity of chest pain; any chest pain at rest).
Coronary steal syndrome	Distal to coronary stenosis, vessels are maximally dilated at baseline. Administration of vasodilators (e.g., dipyridamole, regadenoson) dilates normal vessels and shunts blood toward well-perfused areas → ↓ flow and ischemia in the poststenotic region. Principle behind pharmacologic stress tests.
Myocardial infarction	Most often acute thrombosis due to coronary artery atherosclerosis with complete occlusion of coronary artery and myocyte necrosis. If transmural, ECG will show ST elevations; if subendocardial, ECG may show ST depressions. Cardiac biomarkers are diagnostic.
Sudden cardiac death	Death from cardiac causes within 1 hour of onset of symptoms, most commonly due to a lethal arrhythmia (e.g., ventricular fibrillation). Associated with CAD (up to 70% of cases), cardiomyopathy (hypertrophic, dilated), and hereditary ion channelopathies (e.g., long QT syndrome).
Chronic ischemic heart disease	Progressive onset of CHF over many years due to chronic ischemic myocardial damage.

Evolution of MI

Commonly occluded coronary arteries: LAD > RCA > circumflex.

Symptoms: diaphoresis, nausea, vomiting, severe retrosternal pain, pain in left arm and/or jaw, shortness of breath, fatigue.

TIME	GROSS	LIGHT MICROSCOPE	COMPLICATIONS
0–4 hr	None	None	Arrhythmia, HF, cardiogenic shock, death.
4–12 hr	Occluded artery / Infarct / Dark mottling; pale with tetrazolium stain	Early coagulative necrosis, release of necrotic cell contents into blood; edema, hemorrhage, wavy fibers.	Arrhythmia, HF, cardiogenic shock, death.
12–24 hr		Neutrophil migration starts. Reperfusion injury may cause contraction bands (due to free radical damage).	Arrhythmia, HF, cardiogenic shock, death.
1–3 days	Hyperemia	Extensive coagulative necrosis. Tissue surrounding infarct shows acute inflammation with neutrophils.	Fibrinous pericarditis.
3–14 days	Hyperemic border; central yellow-brown softening—maximally yellow and soft by 10 days	Macrophages, then granulation tissue at margins.	Free wall rupture → tamponade; papillary muscle rupture → mitral regurgitation; interventricular septal rupture due to macrophage-mediated structural degradation. LV pseudoaneurysm (mural thrombus "plugs" hole in myocardium → "time bomb").
2 weeks to several months	Recanalized artery / Gray-white	Contracted scar complete.	Dressler syndrome, HF, arrhythmias, true ventricular aneurysm (outward bulge during contraction, "dyskinesia").

Diagnosis of MI

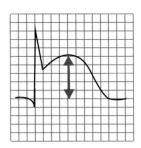

In the first 6 hours, ECG is the gold standard.

Cardiac troponin I rises after 4 hours and is ↑ for 7–10 days; more specific than other protein markers.

CK-MB is predominantly found in myocardium but can also be released from skeletal muscle. Useful in diagnosing reinfarction following acute MI because levels return to normal after 48 hours.

ECG changes can include ST elevation (STEMI, acute transmural infarct), ST depression (subendocardial infarct), and pathologic Q waves (evolving or old transmural infarct).

Types of infarcts

Transmural infarcts	Subendocardial infarcts
↑ necrosis	Due to ischemic necrosis of < 50% of ventricle wall
Affects entire wall	Subendocardium especially vulnerable to ischemia
ST elevation on ECG, Q waves	ST depression on ECG

ECG diagnosis of MI

INFARCT LOCATION	LEADS WITH Q WAVES
Anterior wall (LAD)	V1–V4
Anteroseptal (LAD)	V1–V2
Anterolateral (LAD or LCX)	V4–V6
Lateral wall (LCX)	I, aVL
InFerior wall (RCA)	II, III, aVF

MI complications

Cardiac arrhythmia—important cause of death before reaching hospital; common in first few days.

LV failure and pulmonary edema.

Cardiogenic shock (large infarct—high risk of mortality).

Ventricular free wall rupture → cardiac tamponade; papillary muscle rupture → severe mitral regurgitation; and interventricular septum rupture → VSD. Greatest risk 6–14 days postinfarct.

Ventricular pseudoaneurysm formation—↓ CO, risk of arrhythmia, embolus from mural thrombus; greatest risk approximately 1 week post-MI.

Postinfarction fibrinous pericarditis—friction rub (1–3 days post-MI).

Dressler syndrome—autoimmune phenomenon resulting in fibrinous pericarditis (several weeks post-MI).

Cardiomyopathies

Dilated cardiomyopathy	Most common cardiomyopathy (90% of cases). Often idiopathic or congenital. Other etiologies include chronic **A**lcohol abuse, wet **B**eriberi, **C**oxsackie B virus myocarditis, chronic **C**ocaine use, **C**hagas disease, **D**oxorubicin toxicity, hemochromatosis, and peripartum cardiomyopathy. Findings: heart failure, S3, dilated heart on echocardiogram, balloon appearance of heart on CXR. Treatment: Na⁺ restriction, ACE inhibitors, β-blockers, diuretics, digoxin, implantable cardioverter defibrillator (ICD), heart transplant.	Systolic dysfunction ensues. Eccentric hypertrophy (sarcomeres added in series). ABCCCD.
Hypertrophic cardiomyopathy	60–70% of cases are familial, autosomal dominant (commonly a β-myosin heavy-chain mutation). Rarely can be associated with Friedreich ataxia. Cause of sudden death in young athletes, due to ventricular arrhythmia. Findings: S4, systolic murmur. Treatment: Cessation of high-intensity athletics, use of β-blocker or non-dihydropyridine calcium channel blockers (e.g., verapamil). ICD if patient is high risk.	Diastolic dysfunction ensues. Marked ventricular hypertrophy 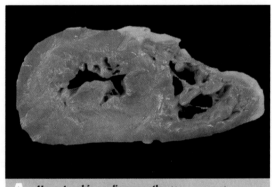, often septal predominance. Myofibrillar disarray and fibrosis. Obstructive HCM (subset): hypertrophied septum too close to anterior mitral leaflet → outflow obstruction → dyspnea, possible syncope. **A** **Hypertrophic cardiomyopathy.** Note concentric hypertrophy of the left ventricle.
Restrictive/infiltrative cardiomyopathy	Major causes include sarcoidosis, amyloidosis, postradiation fibrosis, endocardial fibroelastosis (thick fibroelastic tissue in endocardium of young children), **Löffler syndrome** (endomyocardial fibrosis with a prominent eosinophilic infiltrate), and hemochromatosis (dilated cardiomyopathy can also occur).	Diastolic dysfunction ensues. Can have low-voltage ECG despite thick myocardium (especially amyloid).

CHF

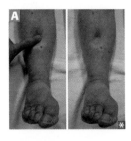

Clinical syndrome of cardiac pump dysfunction. Symptoms include dyspnea, orthopnea, and fatigue; signs include rales, JVD, and pitting edema **A**.

Systolic dysfunction—low EF, poor contractility, often 2° to ischemic heart disease or DCM.

Diastolic dysfunction—normal EF and contractility, impaired relaxation, ↓ compliance.

Right heart failure most often results from left heart failure. Isolated right heart failure is usually due to cor pulmonale.

ACE inhibitors, β-blockers (except in acute decompensated HF), angiotensin II receptor blockers, and spironolactone ↓ mortality. Thiazide or loop diuretics are used mainly for symptomatic relief. Hydralazine with nitrate therapy improves both symptoms and mortality in select patients.

ABNORMALITY	CAUSE
Cardiac dilation	Greater ventricular end-diastolic volume.
Dyspnea on exertion	Failure of CO to ↑ during exercise.
Left heart failure	
Pulmonary edema	↑ pulmonary venous pressure → pulmonary venous distention and transudation of fluid. Presence of hemosiderin-laden macrophages ("heart failure" cells) in the lungs.
Orthopnea	Shortness of breath when supine: ↑ venous return from redistribution of blood (immediate gravity effect) exacerbates pulmonary vascular congestion.
Paroxysmal nocturnal dyspnea	Breathless awakening from sleep: ↑ venous return from redistribution of blood, reabsorption of edema, etc.
Right heart failure	
Hepatomegaly (nutmeg liver)	↑ central venous pressure → ↑ resistance to portal flow. Rarely, leads to "cardiac cirrhosis."
Peripheral edema	↑ venous pressure → fluid transudation.
Jugular venous distention	↑ venous pressure.

Flow diagram:

↓ LV contractility → Pulmonary venous congestion → Pulmonary edema

↓ LV contractility → ↓ Cardiac output → ↑ Renin-angiotensin-aldosterone → ↑ Renal Na⁺ and H₂O reabsorption

Pulmonary venous congestion → ↓ RV output → ↑ Systemic venous pressure → Peripheral edema

↑ Systemic venous pressure → ↑ Preload, ↑ cardiac output (compensation) ← ↑ LV contractility ← ↑ Sympathetic activity

Bacterial endocarditis

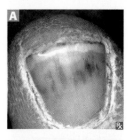

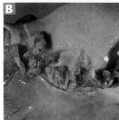

Fever (most common symptom), new murmur, Roth spots (round white spots on retina surrounded by hemorrhage), Osler nodes (tender raised lesions on finger or toe pads), Janeway lesions (small, painless, erythematous lesions on palm or sole), anemia, splinter hemorrhages A on nail bed. Multiple blood cultures necessary for diagnosis.

- **Acute**—*S. aureus* (high virulence). Large vegetations on previously normal valves B. Rapid onset.
- **Subacute**—viridans streptococci (low virulence). Smaller vegetations on congenitally abnormal or diseased valves. Sequela of dental procedures. Gradual onset.
- **Culture-negative**—most likely *Coxiella burnetii* and *Bartonella* spp.

Endocarditis may also be nonbacterial 2° to malignancy, hypercoagulable state, or lupus (marantic/thrombotic endocarditis). *S. bovis* is present in colon cancer, *S. epidermidis* on prosthetic valves.

Mitral valve is most frequently involved. Tricuspid valve endocarditis is associated with IV **drug** abuse (don't "**tri**" drugs). Associated with *S. aureus*, *Pseudomonas*, and *Candida*.

Complications: chordae rupture, glomerulonephritis, suppurative pericarditis, emboli.

♥ Bacteria **FROM JANE** ♥:
Fever
Roth spots
Osler nodes
Murmur
Janeway lesions
Anemia
Nail-bed hemorrhage
Emboli

Rheumatic fever

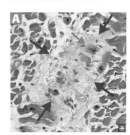

A consequence of pharyngeal infection with group A β-hemolytic streptococci. Early deaths due to myocarditis. Late sequelae include rheumatic heart disease, which affects heart valves—mitral > aortic >> tricuspid (high-pressure valves affected most). Early lesion is mitral valve regurgitation; late lesion is mitral stenosis. Associated with Aschoff bodies (granuloma with giant cells [blue arrows in A]), Anitschkow cells (enlarged macrophages with ovoid, wavy, rod-like nucleus [red arrow in A]), ↑ ASO titers.

Immune mediated (type II hypersensitivity); not a direct effect of bacteria. Antibodies to M protein cross-react with self antigens.

FEVERSS:
Fever
Erythema marginatum
Valvular damage (vegetation and fibrosis)
ESR ↑
Red-hot joints (migratory polyarthritis)
Subcutaneous nodules
St. Vitus' dance (Sydenham chorea)

Acute pericarditis

Commonly presents with sharp pain, aggravated by inspiration, and relieved by sitting up and leaning forward. Presents with friction rub. ECG changes include widespread ST-segment elevation and/or PR depression.

- **Fibrinous**—caused by Dressler syndrome, uremia, radiation. Presents with loud friction rub.
- **Serous**—viral pericarditis (often resolves spontaneously); noninfectious inflammatory diseases (e.g., rheumatoid arthritis, SLE).
- **Suppurative/purulent**—usually caused by bacterial infections (e.g., *Pneumococcus*, *Streptococcus*). Rare now with antibiotics.

Cardiac tamponade

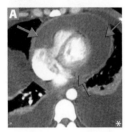

Compression of heart by fluid (e.g., blood, effusions) in pericardium **A**, leading to ↓ CO. Equilibration of diastolic pressures in all 4 chambers.

Findings: Beck triad (hypotension, distended neck veins, distant heart sounds), ↑ HR, pulsus paradoxus, Kussmaul sign. ECG shows low-voltage QRS and electrical alternans (due to "swinging" movement of heart in large effusion).

Pulsus paradoxus—↓ in amplitude of systolic blood pressure by ≥ 10 mmHg during inspiration. Seen in cardiac tamponade, asthma, obstructive sleep apnea, pericarditis, and croup.

Syphilitic heart disease

3° syphilis disrupts the vasa vasorum of the aorta with consequent atrophy of the vessel wall and dilation of the aorta and valve ring. May see calcification of the aortic root and ascending aortic arch. Leads to "tree bark" appearance of the aorta.

Can result in aneurysm of the ascending aorta or aortic arch and aortic insufficiency.

Cardiac tumors	Most common heart tumor is a metastasis (e.g., from melanoma, lymphoma).
Myxomas	Most common 1° cardiac tumor in adults 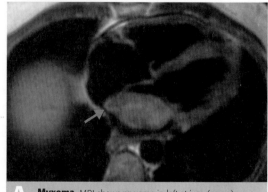. 90% occur in the atria (mostly left atrium). Myxomas are usually described as a "ball valve" obstruction in the left atrium (associated with multiple syncopal episodes).
Rhabdomyomas	Most frequent 1° cardiac tumor in children (associated with tuberous sclerosis).

A **Myxoma.** MRI shows myxoma in left atrium (arrow).

Kussmaul sign	↑ in JVP on inspiration instead of a normal ↓. Inspiration → negative intrathoracic pressure not transmitted to heart → impaired filling of right ventricle → blood backs up into venae cavae → JVD. May be seen with constrictive pericarditis, restrictive cardiomyopathies, right atrial or ventricular tumors.

Raynaud phenomenon	↓ blood flow to the skin due to arteriolar vasospasm in response to cold temperature or emotional stress. Most often in the fingers **A** and toes. Called **Raynaud disease** when 1° (idiopathic), **Raynaud syndrome** when 2° to a disease process such as mixed connective tissue disease, SLE, or CREST (limited form of systemic sclerosis) syndrome.	Affects small vessels.

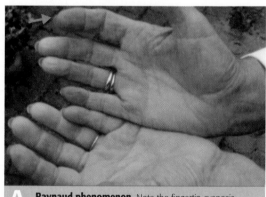

A **Raynaud phenomenon.** Note the fingertip cyanosis (arrow). ⊡

Vascular tumors

Strawberry hemangioma	Benign capillary hemangioma of infancy 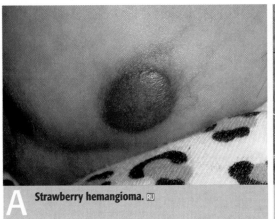. Appears in first few weeks of life (1/200 births); grows rapidly and regresses spontaneously at 5–8 years old.
Cherry hemangioma	Benign capillary hemangioma of the elderly 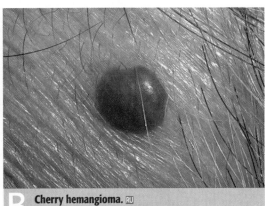. Does not regress. Frequency ↑ with age.
Pyogenic granuloma	Polypoid capillary hemangioma that can ulcerate and bleed. Associated with trauma and pregnancy.
Cystic hygroma	Cavernous lymphangioma of the neck. Associated with Turner syndrome.
Glomus tumor	Benign, painful, red-blue tumor under fingernails. Arises from modified smooth muscle cells of glomus body.
Bacillary angiomatosis	Benign capillary skin papules found in AIDS patients. Caused by *Bartonella henselae* infections. Frequently mistaken for Kaposi sarcoma.
Angiosarcoma	Rare blood vessel malignancy typically occurring in the head, neck, and breast areas. Usually in elderly, on sun-exposed areas. Associated with radiation therapy and arsenic exposure. Very aggressive and difficult to resect due to delay in diagnosis.
Lymphangiosarcoma	Lymphatic malignancy associated with persistent lymphedema (e.g., post–radical mastectomy).
Kaposi sarcoma	Endothelial malignancy most commonly of the skin, but also mouth, GI tract, and respiratory tract. Associated with HHV-8 and HIV. Frequently mistaken for bacillary angiomatosis.

A Strawberry hemangioma. RU

B Cherry hemangioma. RU

Vasculitis

	EPIDEMIOLOGY/PRESENTATION	PATHOLOGY/LABS
Large-vessel vasculitis		
Temporal (giant cell) arteritis	Generally elderly females. Unilateral headache (temporal artery), jaw claudication. May lead to irreversible blindness due to ophthalmic artery occlusion. Associated with polymyalgia rheumatica.	Most commonly affects branches of carotid artery. Focal granulomatous inflammation **A**. ↑ ESR. Treat with high-dose corticosteroids prior to temporal artery biopsy to prevent vision loss.
Takayasu arteritis	Asian females < 40 years old. "Pulseless disease" (weak upper extremity pulses), fever, night sweats, arthritis, myalgias, skin nodules, ocular disturbances.	Granulomatous thickening and narrowing of aortic arch (**B**) and proximal great vessels. ↑ ESR. Treat with corticosteroids.
Medium-vessel vasculitis		
Polyarteritis nodosa	Young adults. Hepatitis B seropositivity in 30% of patients. Fever, weight loss, malaise, headache. GI: abdominal pain, melena. Hypertension, neurologic dysfunction, cutaneous eruptions, renal damage.	Typically involves renal and visceral vessels, not pulmonary arteries. Immune complex mediated. Transmural inflammation of the arterial wall with fibrinoid necrosis. Innumerable microaneurysms **C** and spasm on arteriogram. Treat with corticosteroids, cyclophosphamide.
Kawasaki disease	Asian children < 4 years old. Fever, cervical lymphadenitis, conjunctival injection, changes in lips/oral mucosa ("strawberry tongue" **D**), hand-foot erythema, desquamating rash.	May develop coronary artery aneurysms **E**, thrombosis → MI, rupture. Treat with IV immunoglobulin and aspirin.
Buerger disease (thromboangiitis obliterans)	Heavy smokers, males < 40 years old. Intermittent claudication may lead to gangrene, autoamputation of digits, superficial nodular phlebitis. Raynaud phenomenon is often present.	Segmental thrombosing vasculitis. Treat with smoking cessation.
Small-vessel vasculitis		
Granulomatosis with polyangiitis (Wegener)	Upper respiratory tract: perforation of nasal septum, chronic sinusitis, otitis media, mastoiditis. Lower respiratory tract: hemoptysis, cough, dyspnea. Renal: hematuria, red cell casts.	Triad: ▪ Focal necrotizing vasculitis ▪ Necrotizing granulomas in the lung and upper airway ▪ Necrotizing glomerulonephritis. PR3-ANCA/c-ANCA **F** (anti-proteinase 3). CXR: large nodular densities. Treat with cyclophosphamide, corticosteroids.
Microscopic polyangiitis	Necrotizing vasculitis commonly involving lung, kidneys, and skin with pauci-immune glomerulonephritis and palpable purpura. Presentation similar to granulomatosis with polyangiitis but without nasopharyngeal involvement.	No granulomas. MPO-ANCA/p-ANCA **G** (anti-myeloperoxidase). Treat with cyclophosphamide and corticosteroids.

Vasculitis *(continued)*

	EPIDEMIOLOGY/PRESENTATION	PATHOLOGY/LABS
Small-vessel vasculitis *(continued)*		
Churg-Strauss syndrome	Asthma, sinusitis, palpable purpura, peripheral neuropathy (e.g., wrist/foot drop). Can also involve heart, GI, kidneys (pauci-immune glomerulonephritis).	Granulomatous, necrotizing vasculitis with eosinophilia H. MPO-ANCA/p-ANCA, ↑ IgE level.
Henoch-Schönlein purpura	Most common childhood systemic vasculitis. Often follows URI. Classic triad: ▪ Skin: palpable purpura on buttocks/legs I ▪ Arthralgias ▪ GI: abdominal pain, melena, multiple lesions of same age	Vasculitis 2° to IgA complex deposition. Associated with IgA nephropathy.

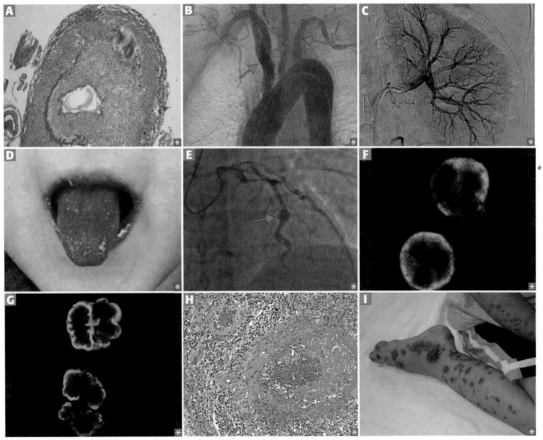

▶ **CARDIOVASCULAR–PHARMACOLOGY**

Antihypertensive therapy

Primary (essential) hypertension	Diuretics, ACE inhibitors, angiotensin II receptor blockers (ARBs), calcium channel blockers.	See the Renal chapter for more details about diuretics and ACE inhibitors/ARBs.
Hypertension with CHF	Diuretics, ACE inhibitors/ARBs, β-blockers (compensated CHF), aldosterone antagonists.	β-blockers must be used cautiously in decompensated CHF and are contraindicated in cardiogenic shock.
Hypertension with diabetes mellitus	ACE inhibitors/ARBs. Calcium channel blockers, diuretics, β-blockers, α-blockers.	ACE inhibitors/ARBs are protective against diabetic nephropathy.

Calcium channel blockers

Amlodipine, nimodipine, nifedipine (dihydropyridine); diltiazem, verapamil (non-dihydropyridine).

MECHANISM	Block voltage-dependent L-type calcium channels of cardiac and smooth muscle, thereby reduce muscle contractility. Vascular smooth muscle—amlodipine = nifedipine > diltiazem > verapamil. Heart—verapamil > diltiazem > amlodipine = nifedipine (verapamil = ventricle).
CLINICAL USE	Dihydropyridine (except nimodipine): hypertension, angina (including Prinzmetal), Raynaud phenomenon. Non-dihydropyridine: hypertension, angina, atrial fibrillation/flutter. Nimodipine: subarachnoid hemorrhage (prevents cerebral vasospasm).
TOXICITY	Cardiac depression, AV block, peripheral edema, flushing, dizziness, hyperprolactinemia, and constipation.

Hydralazine

MECHANISM	↑ cGMP → smooth muscle relaxation. Vasodilates arterioles > veins; afterload reduction.
CLINICAL USE	Severe hypertension, CHF. First-line therapy for hypertension in pregnancy, with methyldopa. Frequently coadministered with a β-blocker to prevent reflex tachycardia.
TOXICITY	Compensatory tachycardia (contraindicated in angina/CAD), fluid retention, nausea, headache, angina. Lupus-like syndrome.

Hypertensive emergency

	Commonly used drugs include nitroprusside, nicardipine, clevidipine, labetalol, and fenoldopam.
Nitroprusside	Short acting; ↑ cGMP via direct release of NO. Can cause cyanide toxicity (releases cyanide).
Fenoldopam	Dopamine D_1 receptor agonist—coronary, peripheral, renal, and splanchnic vasodilation. ↓ BP and ↑ natriuresis.

Nitroglycerin, isosorbide dinitrate

MECHANISM	Vasodilate by ↑ NO in vascular smooth muscle → ↑ in cGMP and smooth muscle relaxation. Dilate veins >> arteries. ↓ preload.
CLINICAL USE	Angina, acute coronary syndrome, pulmonary edema.
TOXICITY	Reflex tachycardia (treat with β-blockers), hypotension, flushing, headache, "Monday disease" in industrial exposure: development of tolerance for the vasodilating action during the work week and loss of tolerance over the weekend results in tachycardia, dizziness, and headache upon reexposure.

Antianginal therapy

Goal—reduction of myocardial O_2 consumption (MVO_2) by ↓ 1 or more of the determinants of MVO_2: end-diastolic volume, blood pressure, heart rate, contractility.

COMPONENT	NITRATES (AFFECT PRELOAD)	β-BLOCKERS (AFFECT AFTERLOAD)	NITRATES + β-BLOCKERS
End-diastolic volume	↓	↑	No effect or ↓
Blood pressure	↓	↓	↓
Contractility	↑ (reflex response)	↓	Little/no effect
Heart rate	↑ (reflex response)	↓	↓
Ejection time	↓	↑	Little/no effect
MVO_2	↓	↓	↓↓

Calcium channel blockers—nifedipine is similar to nitrates in effect; verapamil is similar to β-blockers in effect.
Pindolol and acebutolol—partial β-agonists contraindicated in angina.

Lipid-lowering agents

DRUG	EFFECT ON LDL "BAD CHOLESTEROL"	EFFECT ON HDL "GOOD CHOLESTEROL"	EFFECT ON TRIGLYCERIDES	MECHANISMS OF ACTION	SIDE EFFECTS/PROBLEMS
HMG-CoA reductase inhibitors (lovastatin, pravastatin, simvastatin, atorvastatin, rosuvastatin)	↓↓↓	↑	↓	Inhibit conversion of HMG-CoA to mevalonate, a cholesterol precursor	Hepatotoxicity (↑ LFTs), rhabdomyolysis (esp. when used with fibrates and niacin)
Niacin (vitamin B₃)	↓↓	↑↑	↓	Inhibits lipolysis in adipose tissue; reduces hepatic VLDL synthesis	Red, flushed face, which is ↓ by aspirin or long-term use Hyperglycemia (acanthosis nigricans) Hyperuricemia (exacerbates gout)
Bile acid resins (cholestyramine, colestipol, colesevelam)	↓↓	Slightly ↑	Slightly ↑	Prevent intestinal reabsorption of bile acids; liver must use cholesterol to make more	Patients hate it—tastes bad and causes GI discomfort, ↓ absorption of fat-soluble vitamins Cholesterol gallstones
Cholesterol absorption blockers (ezetimibe)	↓↓	—	—	Prevent cholesterol absorption at small intestine brush border	Rare ↑ LFTs, diarrhea
Fibrates (gemfibrozil, clofibrate, bezafibrate, fenofibrate)	↓	↑	↓↓↓	Upregulate LPL → ↑ TG clearance Activates PPAR-α to induce HDL synthesis	Myositis (↑ risk with concurrent statins), hepatotoxicity (↑ LFTs), cholesterol gallstones (esp. with concurrent bile acid resins)

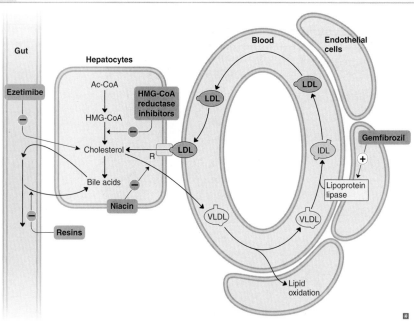

Cardiac glycosides	Digoxin—75% bioavailability, 20–40% protein bound, $t_{1/2}$ = 40 hours, urinary excretion.
MECHANISM	Direct inhibition of Na^+/K^+ ATPase leads to indirect inhibition of Na^+/Ca^{2+} exchanger/antiport. ↑ $[Ca^{2+}]_i$ → positive inotropy. Stimulates vagus nerve → ↓ HR.
CLINICAL USE	CHF (↑ contractility); atrial fibrillation (↓ conduction at AV node and depression of SA node).
TOXICITY	Cholinergic—nausea, vomiting, diarrhea, blurry yellow vision (think Van Gogh). ECG—↑ PR, ↓ QT, ST scooping, T-wave inversion, arrhythmia, AV block. Can lead to hyperkalemia, which indicates poor prognosis. Factors predisposing to toxicity—renal failure (↓ excretion), hypokalemia (permissive for digoxin binding at K^+-binding site on Na^+/K^+ ATPase), verapamil, amiodarone, quinidine (↓ digoxin clearance; displaces digoxin from tissue-binding sites).
ANTIDOTE	Slowly normalize K^+, cardiac pacer, anti-digoxin Fab fragments, Mg^{2+}.

Antiarrhythmics– **Na⁺ channel blockers** **(class I)**	Slow or block (↓) conduction (especially in depolarized cells). ↓ slope of phase 0 depolarization and ↑ threshold for firing in abnormal pacemaker cells. Are state dependent (selectively depress tissue that is frequently depolarized [e.g., tachycardia]). Hyperkalemia causes ↑ toxicity for all class I drugs.	
Class IA	Quinidine, Procainamide, Disopyramide. "The Queen Proclaims Diso's pyramid."	Class IA
MECHANISM	↑ AP duration, ↑ effective refractory period (ERP), ↑ QT interval.	
CLINICAL USE	Both atrial and ventricular arrhythmias, especially re-entrant and ectopic SVT and VT.	
TOXICITY	Cinchonism (headache, tinnitus with quinidine), reversible SLE-like syndrome (procainamide), heart failure (disopyramide), thrombocytopenia, torsades de pointes due to ↑ QT interval.	
Class IB	Lidocaine, Mexiletine.	Class IB
MECHANISM	↓ AP duration. Preferentially affect ischemic or depolarized Purkinje and ventricular tissue. Phenytoin can also fall into the IB category.	
CLINICAL USE	Acute ventricular arrhythmias (especially post-MI), digitalis-induced arrhythmias. IB is Best post-MI.	
TOXICITY	CNS stimulation/depression, cardiovascular depression.	
Class IC	Flecainide, Propafenone. "Can I have Fries, Please."	Class IC
MECHANISM	Significantly prolongs refractory period in AV node. Minimal effect on AP duration.	
CLINICAL USE	SVTs, including atrial fibrillation. Only as a last resort in refractory VT.	
TOXICITY	Proarrhythmic, especially post-MI (contraindicated). IC is Contraindicated in structural and ischemic heart disease.	

Antiarrhythmics–β-blockers (class II)	Metoprolol, propranolol, esmolol, atenolol, timolol, carvedilol.
MECHANISM	Decrease SA and AV nodal activity by ↓ cAMP, ↓ Ca^{2+} currents. Suppress abnormal pacemakers by ↓ slope of phase 4. AV node particularly sensitive—↑ PR interval. Esmolol very short acting.
CLINICAL USE	SVT, slowing ventricular rate during atrial fibrillation and atrial flutter.
TOXICITY	Impotence, exacerbation of COPD and asthma, cardiovascular effects (bradycardia, AV block, CHF), CNS effects (sedation, sleep alterations). May mask the signs of hypoglycemia. Metoprolol can cause dyslipidemia. Propranolol can exacerbate vasospasm in Prinzmetal angina. Contraindicated in cocaine users (risk of unopposed α-adrenergic receptor agonist activity). Treat overdose with glucagon.

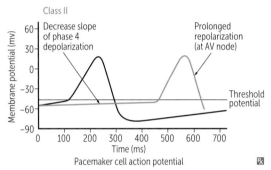

Class II

Decrease slope of phase 4 depolarization

Prolonged repolarization (at AV node)

Threshold potential

Pacemaker cell action potential

Antiarrhythmics–K⁺ channel blockers (class III)	Amiodarone, Ibutilide, Dofetilide, Sotalol.	"AIDS."
MECHANISM	↑ AP duration, ↑ ERP. Used when other antiarrhythmics fail. ↑ QT interval.	
CLINICAL USE	Atrial fibrillation, atrial flutter; ventricular tachycardia (amiodarone, sotalol).	
TOXICITY	Sotalol—torsades de pointes, excessive β blockade. Ibutilide—torsades de pointes. Amiodarone—pulmonary fibrosis, hepatotoxicity, hypothyroidism/hyperthyroidism (amiodarone is 40% iodine by weight), corneal deposits, skin deposits (blue/gray) resulting in photodermatitis, neurologic effects, constipation, cardiovascular effects (bradycardia, heart block, CHF).	Remember to check PFTs, LFTs, and TFTs when using amiodarone. Amiodarone has class I, II, III, and IV effects and alters the lipid membrane.

Class III

0 mV

Markedly prolonged repolarization (I_K)

85 mV

Cell action potential

Antiarrhythmics— Ca²⁺ channel blockers (class IV)	Verapamil, diltiazem.
MECHANISM	↓ conduction velocity, ↑ ERP, ↑ PR interval.
CLINICAL USE	Prevention of nodal arrhythmias (e.g., SVT), rate control in atrial fibrillation.
TOXICITY	Constipation, flushing, edema, CV effects (CHF, AV block, sinus node depression).

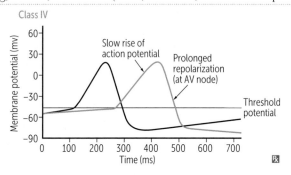

Other antiarrhythmics

Adenosine	↑ K⁺ out of cells → hyperpolarizing the cell and ↓ I_{Ca}. Drug of choice in diagnosing/abolishing supraventricular tachycardia. Very short acting (~ 15 sec). Adverse effects include flushing, hypotension, chest pain. Effects blocked by theophylline and caffeine.
Mg²⁺	Effective in torsades de pointes and digoxin toxicity.

Endocrine

"We have learned that there is an endocrinology of elation and despair, a chemistry of mystical insight, and, in relation to the autonomic nervous system, a meteorology and even . . . an astro-physics of changing moods."
—Aldous (Leonard) Huxley

"Chocolate causes certain endocrine glands to secrete hormones that affect your feelings and behavior by making you happy."
—Elaine Sherman, *Book of Divine Indulgences*

▶ **ENDOCRINE–EMBRYOLOGY**

Thyroid development

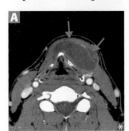

Thyroid diverticulum arises from floor of primitive pharynx, and descends into neck. Connected to tongue by thyroglossal duct, which normally disappears but may persist as pyramidal lobe of thyroid. Foramen cecum is normal remnant of thyroglossal duct. Most common ectopic thyroid tissue site is the tongue.

Thyroglossal duct cyst **A** presents as an anterior midline neck mass that moves with swallowing or protrusion of the tongue (vs. persistent cervical sinus leading to branchial cleft cyst in lateral neck).

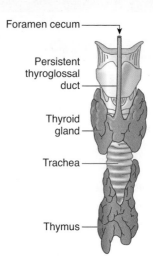

▶ **ENDOCRINE–ANATOMY**

Adrenal cortex and medulla

Adrenal cortex (derived from mesoderm) and medulla (derived from neural crest).

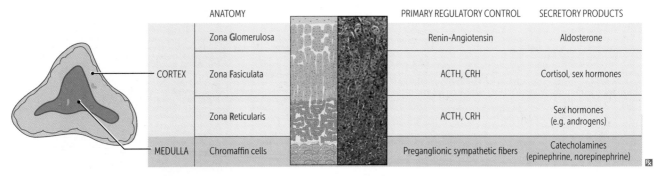

	ANATOMY		PRIMARY REGULATORY CONTROL	SECRETORY PRODUCTS
CORTEX	Zona **G**lomerulosa		Renin-Angiotensin	Aldosterone
	Zona **F**asiculata		ACTH, CRH	Cortisol, sex hormones
	Zona **R**eticularis		ACTH, CRH	Sex hormones (e.g. androgens)
MEDULLA	Chromaffin cells		Preganglionic sympathetic fibers	Catecholamines (epinephrine, norepinephrine)

GFR corresponds with **S**alt (Na⁺), **S**ugar (glucocorticoids), and **S**ex (androgens).
"The deeper you go, the sweeter it gets."
Pheochromocytoma—most common tumor of the adrenal medulla in adults. Episodic hypertension.
Neuroblastoma—most common tumor of the adrenal medulla in children. Rarely causes hypertension.

Adrenal gland drainage

Left adrenal gland → left adrenal vein → left renal vein → IVC.
Right adrenal gland → right adrenal vein → IVC.

Same as left and right gonadal vein.

Pituitary gland

Posterior pituitary (neurohypophysis)	Secretes vasopressin (antidiuretic hormone, or ADH) and oxytocin, made in the hypothalamus and shipped to posterior pituitary via neurophysins (carrier proteins). Derived from neuroectoderm.	
Anterior pituitary (adenohypophysis)	Secretes FSH, LH, ACTH, TSH, prolactin, GH, melanotropin (MSH). Derived from oral ectoderm (Rathke pouch). <ul><li>α subunit—hormone subunit common to TSH, LH, FSH, and hCG.</li><li>β subunit—determines hormone specificity.</li></ul>	Acidophils—GH, prolactin. **B-FLAT**: Basophils—FSH, LH, ACTH, TSH. **FLAT PiG**: FSH, LH, ACTH, TSH, Prolactin, GH.

Endocrine pancreas cell types	Islets of Langerhans are collections of α, β, and δ endocrine cells. Islets arise from pancreatic buds. α = glucagon (peripheral); β = insulin (central); δ = somatostatin (interspersed).	Insulin (β cells) inside. 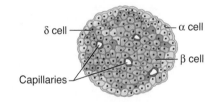

▶ ENDOCRINE–PHYSIOLOGY

Insulin

SYNTHESIS	Preproinsulin (synthesized in RER) → cleavage of "presignal" → proinsulin (stored in secretory granules) → cleavage of proinsulin → exocytosis of insulin and C-peptide equally. Insulin and C-peptide are ↑ in insulinoma, whereas exogenous insulin lacks C-peptide.

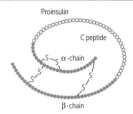

Proinsulin

C peptide

α-chain

β-chain

SOURCE	Released from pancreatic β cells.

FUNCTION	Binds insulin receptors (tyrosine kinase activity ❶), inducing glucose uptake (carrier-mediated transport) in insulin-dependent tissue ❷ and gene transcription. Anabolic effects of insulin: ▪ ↑ glucose transport in skeletal muscle and adipose tissue ▪ ↑ glycogen synthesis and storage ▪ ↑ triglyceride synthesis ▪ ↑ Na^+ retention (kidneys) ▪ ↑ protein synthesis (muscles, proteins) ▪ ↑ cellular uptake of K^+ and amino acids ▪ ↓ glucagon release **IN**sulin moves glucose **IN**to cells. Unlike glucose, insulin does not cross placenta.	Insulin-dependent glucose transporters: ▪ GLUT-4: adipose tissue, skeletal muscle Insulin-independent transporters: ▪ GLUT-1: RBCs, brain, cornea ▪ GLUT-5 (fructose): spermatocytes, GI tract ▪ GLUT-2 (bidirectional): β islet cells, liver, kidney, small intestine Brain utilizes glucose for metabolism normally and ketone bodies during starvation. RBCs always utilize glucose because they lack mitochondria for aerobic metabolism. **BRICK L** (insulin-independent glucose uptake): Brain, RBCs, Intestine, Cornea, Kidney, Liver.

REGULATION	Glucose is major regulator of insulin release. GH (causes insulin resistance → ↑ insulin release) and $β_2$-agonists → ↑ insulin. Glucose enters β cells ❸ → ↑ ATP generated from glucose metabolism ❹ closes K^+ channels ❺ and depolarizes β cell membrane ❻ → opens voltage-gated Ca^{2+} channels, resulting in Ca^{2+} influx ❼ and stimulating insulin exocytosis ❽.

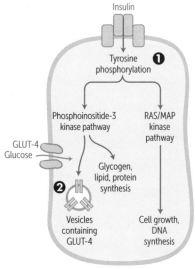

Glucose uptake–insulin-dependent

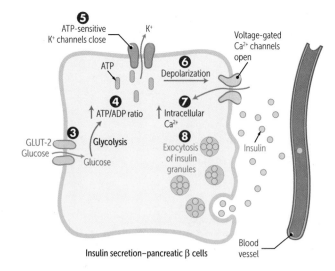

Insulin secretion–pancreatic β cells

Glucagon

SOURCE	Made by α cells of pancreas.
FUNCTION	Catabolic effects of glucagon: ■ Glycogenolysis, gluconeogenesis ■ Lipolysis and ketone production
REGULATION	Secreted in response to hypoglycemia. Inhibited by insulin, hyperglycemia, and somatostatin.

Hypothalamic-pituitary hormones

HORMONE	FUNCTION	CLINICAL NOTES
CRH	↑ ACTH, MSH, β-endorphin	↓ in chronic exogenous steroid use
Dopamine	↓ prolactin	Dopamine antagonists (e.g., antipsychotics) can cause galactorrhea
GnRH	↑ FSH, LH	Regulated by prolactin Tonic GnRH suppresses HPA axis Pulsatile GnRH leads to puberty, fertility
Prolactin	↓ GnRH	Pituitary prolactinoma → amenorrhea, osteoporosis
Somatostatin	↓ GH, TSH	Analogs used to treat acromegaly
TRH	↑ TSH, prolactin	

Prolactin

SOURCE	Secreted mainly by anterior pituitary.	
FUNCTION	Stimulates milk production in breast; inhibits ovulation in females and spermatogenesis in males by inhibiting GnRH synthesis and release.	Excessive amounts of prolactin associated with ↓ libido.
REGULATION	Prolactin secretion from anterior pituitary is tonically inhibited by dopamine from hypothalamus. Prolactin in turn inhibits its own secretion by ↑ dopamine synthesis and secretion from hypothalamus. TRH ↑ prolactin secretion.	Dopamine agonists (bromocriptine) inhibit prolactin secretion and can be used in treatment of prolactinoma. Dopamine antagonists (most antipsychotics) and estrogens (OCPs, pregnancy) stimulate prolactin secretion.

Growth hormone (somatotropin)

SOURCE	Secreted mainly by anterior pituitary.	
FUNCTION	Stimulates linear growth and muscle mass through IGF-1/somatomedin secretion. ↑ insulin resistance (diabetogenic).	
REGULATION	Released in pulses in response to growth hormone–releasing hormone (GHRH). Secretion ↑ during exercise and sleep. Secretion inhibited by glucose and somatostatin.	Excess secretion of GH (e.g., pituitary adenoma) may cause acromegaly (adults) or gigantism (children).

Antidiuretic hormone

SOURCE	Synthesized in hypothalamus (supraoptic nuclei), released by posterior pituitary.	
FUNCTION	Regulates serum osmolarity (V_2-receptors) and blood pressure (V_1-receptors). Primary function is serum osmolarity regulation (ADH ↓ serum osmolarity, ↑ urine osmolarity) via regulation of aquaporin channel transcription in principal cells of renal collecting duct.	ADH level is ↓ in central diabetes insipidus (DI), normal or ↑ in nephrogenic DI and 1° polydipsia. Nephrogenic DI can be caused by mutation in V_2-receptor. Desmopressin (ADH analog) = treatment for central DI.
REGULATION	Osmoreceptors in hypothalamus (1°); hypovolemia (2°).	

Adrenal steroids and congenital adrenal hyperplasias

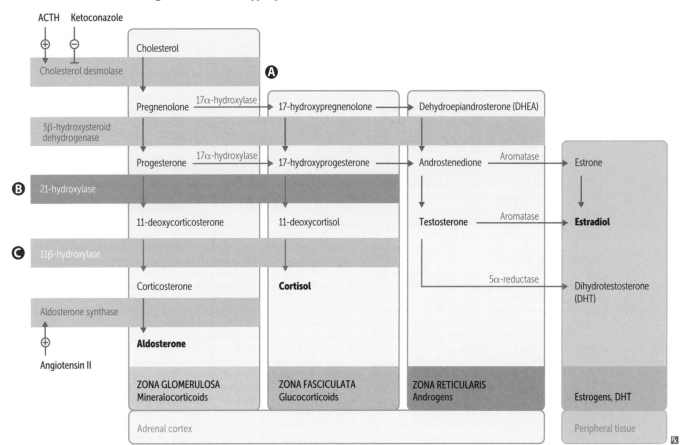

ENZYME DEFICIENCY	MINERALOCORTICOIDS	CORTISOL	SEX HORMONES	LABS	PRESENTATION
Ⓐ 17α-hydroxylase[a]	↑	↓	↓	**Hyper**tension, **Hypo**kalemia. ↓ DHT	XY: pseudo-hermaphroditism (ambiguous genitalia, undescended testes) XX: lack secondary sexual development
Ⓑ 21-hydroxylase[a]	↓	↓	↑	**Hypo**tension **Hyper**kalemia ↑ renin activity ↑ 17-hydroxy-progesterone	Most common Presents in infancy (salt wasting) or childhood (precocious puberty) XX: virilization
Ⓒ 11β-hydroxylase[a]	↓ aldosterone ↑ 11-deoxycorticosterone (results in ↑ BP)	↓	↑	**Hyper**tension (low-renin)	XX: virilization

[a]All congenital adrenal enzyme deficiencies are characterized by an enlargement of both adrenal glands due to ↑ ACTH stimulation (due to ↓ cortisol).

Cortisol

SOURCE	Adrenal zona fasciculata.	Bound to corticosteroid-binding globulin.

FUNCTION	↑ Blood pressure (upregulates α_1-receptors on arterioles → ↑ sensitivity to norepinephrine and epinephrine
	↑ Insulin resistance (diabetogenic)
	↑ Gluconeogenesis, lipolysis, and proteolysis
	↓ Fibroblast activity (causes striae)
	↓ Inflammatory and Immune responses:
	  ▪ Inhibits production of leukotrienes and prostaglandins
	  ▪ Inhibits leukocyte adhesion → neutrophilia
	  ▪ Blocks histamine release from mast cells
	  ▪ Reduces eosinophils
	  ▪ Blocks IL-2 production
	↓ Bone formation (↓ osteoblast activity)
		Cortisol is a **BIG FIB**.
		Exogenous corticosteroids can cause reactivation of TB and candidiasis (blocked IL-2 production).

REGULATION	CRH (hypothalamus) stimulates ACTH release (pituitary), causing cortisol production in adrenal zona fasciculata. Excess cortisol ↓ CRH, ACTH, and cortisol secretion.	Chronic stress induces prolonged secretion.

PTH

SOURCE	Chief cells of parathyroid.
FUNCTION	↑ bone resorption of Ca^{2+} and PO_4^{3-}. ↑ kidney reabsorption of Ca^{2+} in distal convoluted tubule. ↓ reabsorption of PO_4^{3-} in proximal convoluted tubule. ↑ 1,25-$(OH)_2$ D_3 (calcitriol) production by stimulating kidney 1α-hydroxylase.
	PTH ↑ serum Ca^{2+}, ↓ serum (PO_4^{3-}), ↑ urine (PO_4^{3-}). ↑ production of macrophage colony-stimulating factor and RANK-L (receptor activator of NF-κB ligand). RANK-L binds RANK on osteoblasts → osteoclast stimulation and ↑ Ca^{2+}. PTH = Phosphate Trashing Hormone. PTH-related peptide (PTHrP) functions like PTH and is commonly ↑ in malignancies (e.g., paraneoplastic syndrome).
REGULATION	↓ serum Ca^{2+} → ↑ PTH secretion. ↓ serum Mg^{2+} → ↑ PTH secretion. ↓↓ serum Mg^{2+} → ↓ PTH secretion. Common causes of ↓ Mg^{2+} include diarrhea, aminoglycosides, diuretics, and alcohol abuse.

Low ionized calcium
(+)
Four parathyroid glands

⊖ Feedback inhibition of PTH synthesis

⊖ Feedback inhibition of PTH secretion

PTH (1-84) released into circulation

Renal tubular cells → Bone

- Stimulates reabsorption of calcium
- Inhibits phosphate reabsorption
- Stimulates production of 1,25-$(OH)_2$ D_3

- Stimulates calcium release from bone mineral compartment
- Stimulates osteoblastic cells
- Stimulates bone resorption via indirect effect on osteoclasts
- Enhances bone matrix degradation

- Increases intestinal calcium absorption → Increases serum calcium

Calcium homeostasis

Low serum phosphorus → ↑ Conversion 25-(OH) D_3 → 1,25-$(OH)_2$ D_3

- Releases phosphate from matrix

- Increases intestinal phosphate reabsorption

Phosphate homeostasis

Calcium homeostasis	Plasma Ca^{2+} exists in three forms:	↑ in pH → ↑ affinity of albumin (negative charge) to bind Ca^{2+} → clinical manifestations of hypocalcemia (cramps, pain, paresthesias, carpopedal spasm).
	▪ Ionized (~45%)	
	▪ Bound to albumin (~40%)	
	▪ Bound to anions (~15%)	

Vitamin D (cholecalciferol)

SOURCE	D_3 from sun exposure in skin. D_2 ingested from plants. Both converted to 25-OH in liver and to 1,25-$(OH)_2$ (active form) in kidney.	Deficiency causes rickets in kids and osteomalacia in adults. Caused by malabsorption, ↓ sunlight, poor diet, chronic kidney failure.
FUNCTION	↑ absorption of dietary Ca^{2+} and PO_4^{3-} ↑ bone resorption → ↑ Ca^{2+} and PO_4^{3-}	24,25-$(OH)_2$ D_3 is an inactive form of vitamin D.
REGULATION	↑ PTH, ↓ $[Ca^{2+}]$, ↓ PO_4^{3-} cause ↑ 1,25-$(OH)_2$ production. 1,25-$(OH)_2$ feedback inhibits its own production.	PTH leads to ↑ Ca^{2+} reabsorption and ↓ PO_4^{3-} reabsorption in the kidney, whereas 1,25-$(OH)_2$ leads to ↑ absorption of both Ca^{2+} and PO_4^{3-} in the gut.

Calcitonin

SOURCE	Parafollicular cells (C cells) of thyroid.	Calcitonin opposes actions of PTH. Not important in normal Ca^{2+} homeostasis. Calcitonin tones down Ca^{2+} levels.
FUNCTION	↓ bone resorption of Ca^{2+}.	
REGULATION	↑ serum Ca^{2+} causes calcitonin secretion.	

Signaling pathways of endocrine hormones

cAMP	FSH, LH, ACTH, TSH, CRH, hCG, ADH (V_2-receptor), MSH, PTH, calcitonin, GHRH, glucagon	FLAT ChAMP
cGMP	ANP, NO (EDRF)	Think vasodilators
IP₃	GnRH, Oxytocin, ADH (V_1-receptor), TRH, Histamine (H_1-receptor), Angiotensin II, Gastrin	GOAT HAG
Steroid receptor	Vitamin D, Estrogen, Testosterone, T_3/T_4, Cortisol, Aldosterone, Progesterone	VETTT CAP
Intrinsic tyrosine kinase	Insulin, IGF-1, FGF, PDGF, EGF	MAP kinase pathway Think growth factors
Receptor-associated tyrosine kinase	Prolactin, Immunomodulators (e.g., cytokines IL-2, IL-6, IL-8, IFN), GH	JAK/STAT pathway Think acidophiles and cytokines PIG

Signaling pathway of steroid hormones

Steroid hormones are lipophilic and therefore must circulate bound to specific binding globulins, which ↑ their solubility.

In men, ↑ sex hormone–binding globulin (SHBG) lowers free testosterone → gynecomastia.

In women, ↓ SHBG raises free testosterone → hirsutism.

OCPs, pregnancy ↑ SHBG (free estrogen levels remain unchanged).

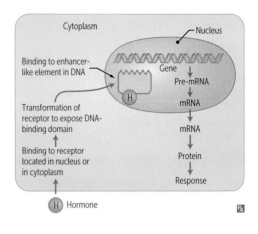

Thyroid hormones (T₃/T₄)

Iodine-containing hormones that control the body's metabolic rate.

SOURCE	Follicles of thyroid. Most T_3 formed in target tissues.	T_3 functions—4 B's: Brain maturation Bone growth β-adrenergic effects Basal metabolic rate ↑
FUNCTION	Bone growth (synergism with GH) CNS maturation ↑ β_1 receptors in heart = ↑ CO, HR, SV, contractility ↑ basal metabolic rate via ↑ Na^+/K^+-ATPase activity = ↑ O_2 consumption, RR, body temperature ↑ glycogenolysis, gluconeogenesis, lipolysis	Thyroxine-binding globulin (TBG) binds most T_3/T_4 in blood; only free hormone is active. ↓ TBG in hepatic failure; ↑ TBG in pregnancy or OCP use (estrogen ↑ TBG). T_4 is major thyroid product; converted to T_3 in peripheral tissue by 5'-deiodinase. T_3 binds receptors with greater affinity than T_4.
REGULATION	TRH (hypothalamus) stimulates TSH (pituitary), which stimulates follicular cells. Negative feedback by free T_3, T_4 to anterior pituitary ↓ sensitivity to TRH. Thyroid-stimulating immunoglobulins (TSIs), like TSH, stimulate follicular cells (e.g., Graves disease). Wolff-Chaikoff effect—excess iodine temporarily inhibits thyroid peroxidase → ↓ iodine organification → ↓ T_3/T_4 production.	Peroxidase is enzyme responsible for oxidation and organification of iodide as well as coupling of monoiodotyrosine (MIT) and di-iodotyrosine (DIT). Propylthiouracil inhibits both peroxidase and 5'-deiodinase. Methimazole inhibits peroxidase only.

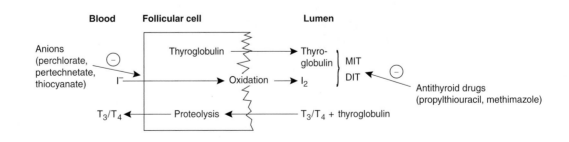

▶ **ENDOCRINE–PATHOLOGY**

Cushing syndrome

ETIOLOGY	↑ cortisol due to a variety of causes:
	  ▪ Exogenous corticosteroids—#1 cause, results in ↓ ACTH, bilateral adrenal atrophy.
	  ▪ Primary adrenal adenoma, hyperplasia, or carcinoma; results in ↓ ACTH, atrophy of uninvolved adrenal gland. Can also present as 1° aldosteronism (Conn syndrome).
	  ▪ ACTH-secreting pituitary adenoma (Cushing disease); paraneoplastic ACTH secretion (e.g., small cell lung cancer, bronchial carcinoids); results in ↑ ACTH, bilateral adrenal hyperplasia. Cushing disease is responsible for the majority of endogenous cases of Cushing syndrome.

FINDINGS	Hypertension, weight gain, moon facies, truncal obesity **B**, buffalo hump, hyperglycemia (insulin resistance), skin changes (thinning, striae), osteoporosis, amenorrhea, and immune suppression.
DIAGNOSIS	Screening tests include: ↑ free cortisol on 24-hr urinalysis, midnight salivary cortisol, and overnight low-dose dexamethasone suppression test: Measure serum ACTH. If ↓, suspect adrenal tumor. If ↑, distinguish between Cushing disease and ectopic ACTH secretion with a high-dose (8 mg) dexamethasone suppression test and CRH stimulation test. Ectopic secretion will not decrease with dexamethasone because the source is resistant to negative feedback; ectopic secretion will not increase with CRH because pituitary ACTH is suppressed.

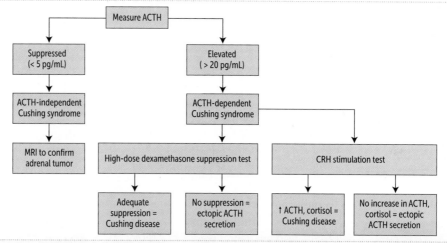

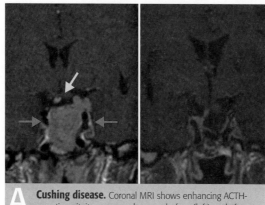

A   **Cushing disease.** Coronal MRI shows enhancing ACTH-secreting pituitary macroadenoma, before (left) and after (right) stereotactic radiosurgery. Note the elevated optic chiasm above the mass (yellow arrow) and the cavernous carotid arteries on both sides (red arrows). ✷

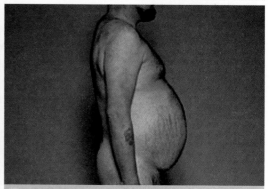

B   **Cushing disease.** Note the truncal obesity and abdominal striae.

Hyperaldosteronism

Primary	Caused by adrenal hyperplasia or an aldosterone-secreting adrenal adenoma (Conn syndrome), resulting in hypertension, hypokalemia, metabolic alkalosis, and **low** plasma renin. Normal Na^+ due to aldosterone escape = no edema due to aldosterone escape mechanism. May be bilateral or unilateral.	Treatment: surgery to remove the tumor and/or spironolactone, a K^+-sparing diuretic that acts as an aldosterone antagonist.
Secondary	Renal perception of low intravascular volume results in an overactive renin-angiotensin system. Due to renal artery stenosis, CHF, cirrhosis, or nephrotic syndrome. Associated with **high** plasma renin.	Treatment: spironolactone.

Addison disease

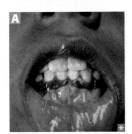

Chronic 1° adrenal insufficiency due to adrenal atrophy or destruction by disease (e.g., autoimmune, TB, metastasis). Deficiency of aldosterone and cortisol, causing hypotension (hyponatremic volume contraction), hyperkalemia, acidosis, and skin and mucosal hyperpigmentation **A** (due to MSH, a by-product of ↑ ACTH production from pro-opiomelanocortin (POMC). Characterized by **A**drenal **A**trophy and **A**bsence of hormone production; involves **A**ll **3** cortical divisions (spares medulla). Distinguish from 2° adrenal insufficiency (↓ pituitary ACTH production), which has no skin/mucosal hyperpigmentation and no hyperkalemia.

Waterhouse-Friderichsen syndrome

Acute 1° adrenal insufficiency due to adrenal hemorrhage associated with *Neisseria meningitidis* septicemia, DIC, and endotoxic shock.

Neuroblastoma

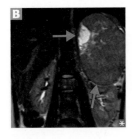

The most common tumor of the adrenal medulla in **children**, usually < 4 years old. Originates from neural crest cells **A**. Occurs anywhere along the sympathetic chain. Most common presentation is abdominal distension and a firm, irregular mass **B** that can cross the midline (vs. Wilms tumor, which is smooth and unilateral). Homovanillic acid (HVA), a breakdown product of dopamine, ↑ in urine. Bombesin ⊕. Less likely to develop hypertension. Associated with overexpression of N-*myc* oncogene.

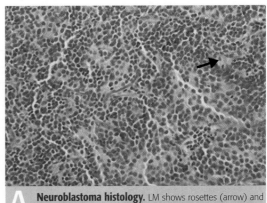

A **Neuroblastoma histology.** LM shows rosettes (arrow) and classic small, round, blue/purple nuclei. ℞

Pheochromocytoma

ETIOLOGY	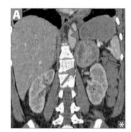 Most common tumor of the adrenal medulla in adults **A** **B**. Derived from chromaffin cells (arise from neural crest) **C**.	Rule of 10's: 10% malignant 10% bilateral 10% extra-adrenal 10% calcify 10% kids
SYMPTOMS	Most tumors secrete epinephrine, norepinephrine, and dopamine, which can cause episodic hypertension. Associated with von Hippel-Lindau disease, MEN 2A and 2B. Symptoms occur in "spells"—relapse and remit.	Episodic hyperadrenergic symptoms (**5 P's**): Pressure (↑ BP) Pain (headache) Perspiration Palpitations (tachycardia) Pallor
FINDINGS	Urinary VMA (a breakdown product of norepinephrine and epinephrine) and plasma catecholamines are ↑.	
TREATMENT	Irreversible α-antagonists (phenoxybenzamine) and β-blockers followed by tumor resection. α-blockade must be achieved before giving β-blockers to avoid a hypertensive crisis.	

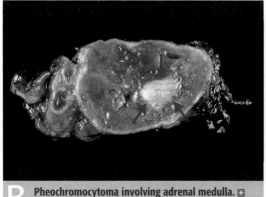

B **Pheochromocytoma involving adrenal medulla.** ✳

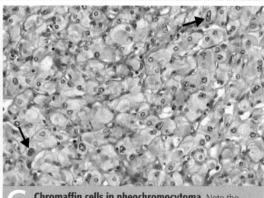

C **Chromaffin cells in pheochromocytoma.** Note the enlarged dysmorphic nuclei (arrows) typical of malignancy. ✳

Hypothyroidism vs. hyperthyroidism

	Hypothyroidism	**Hyperthyroidism**
SIGNS/SYMPTOMS	Cold intolerance (↓ heat production)	Heat intolerance (↑ heat production)
	Weight gain, ↓ appetite	Weight loss, ↑ appetite
	Hypoactivity, lethargy, fatigue, weakness	Hyperactivity
	Constipation	Diarrhea
	↓ reflexes	↑ reflexes
	Myxedema (facial/periorbital)	Pretibial myxedema (Graves disease), periorbital edema
	Dry, cool skin; coarse, brittle hair	Warm, moist skin; fine hair
	Bradycardia, dyspnea on exertion	Chest pain, palpitations, arrhythmias, ↑ number and sensitivity of β-adrenergic receptors
LAB FINDINGS	↑ TSH (sensitive test for 1° hypothyroidism)	↓ TSH (if 1°)
	↓ free T_3 and T_4	↑ free or total T_3 and T_4
	Hypercholesterolemia (due to ↓ LDL receptor expression)	Hypocholesterolemia (due to ↑ LDL receptor expression)

Hypothyroidism

Hashimoto thyroiditis	Most common cause of hypothyroidism in iodine-sufficient regions; an autoimmune disorder (anti-thyroid peroxidase, antithyroglobulin antibodies). Associated with HLA-DR5. ↑ risk of non-Hodgkin lymphoma. May be hyperthyroid early in course due to thyrotoxicosis during follicular rupture. Histologic findings: Hürthle cells, lymphoid aggregate with germinal centers **A**. Findings: moderately enlarged, **nontender** thyroid.	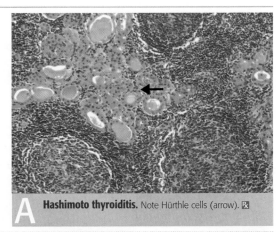 **Hashimoto thyroiditis.** Note Hürthle cells (arrow). ℞
Congenital hypothyroidism (cretinism) 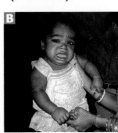	Severe fetal hypothyroidism due to maternal hypothyroidism, thyroid agenesis, thyroid dysgenesis (most common cause in U.S.), iodine deficiency, dyshormonogenic goiter. Findings: **P**ot-bellied, **P**ale, **P**uffy-faced child with **P**rotruding umbilicus, **P**rotuberant tongue, and **P**oor brain development: the 6 P's **B C**.	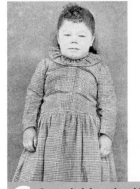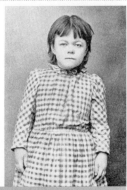 **Congenital hypothyroidism.** Patient with congenital hypothyroidism before (left) and after (right) treatment. ⊡

Hypothyroidism *(continued)*

Subacute thyroiditis (de Quervain)	Self-limited hypothyroidism often following a flu-like illness. May be hyperthyroid early in course. Histology: granulomatous inflammation. Findings: ↑ ESR, jaw pain, early inflammation, very **tender** thyroid. (de Quervain is associated with **pain**.)
Riedel thyroiditis	Thyroid replaced by fibrous tissue (hypothyroid). Fibrosis may extend to local structures (e.g., airway), mimicking anaplastic carcinoma. Considered a manifestation of IgG_4-related systemic disease. Findings: fixed, hard (rock-like), and **painless** goiter.
Other causes	Iodine deficiency 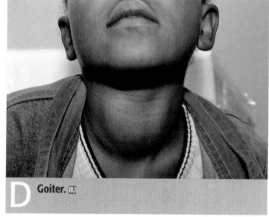, goitrogens, Wolff-Chaikoff effect, painless thyroiditis.

D Goiter. [RU]

Hyperthyroidism

Toxic multinodular goiter	Focal patches of hyperfunctioning follicular cells working independently of TSH due to mutation in TSH receptor 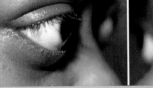. ↑ release of T_3 and T_4. Hot nodules are rarely malignant. **Jod-Basedow phenomenon**—thyrotoxicosis if a patient with iodine deficiency goiter is made iodine replete.
Graves disease	Most common cause of hyperthyroidism. Autoantibodies (IgG) stimulate TSH receptors on thyroid (hyperthyroidism, diffuse goiter), retro-orbital fibroblasts (exophthalmos: proptosis, extraocular muscle swelling 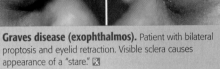), and dermal fibroblasts (pretibial myxedema). Often presents during stress (e.g., childbirth).
Thyroid storm	Stress-induced catecholamine surge seen as a serious complication of Graves disease and other hyperthyroid disorders. Presents with agitation, delirium, fever, diarrhea, coma, and tachyarrhythmia (cause of death). May see ↑ ALP due to ↑ bone turnover. Treat with the 3 P's: β-blockers (e.g., **P**ropranolol), **P**ropylthiouracil, corticosteroids (e.g., **P**rednisolone).

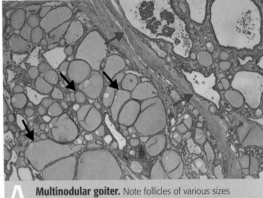

A **Multinodular goiter.** Note follicles of various sizes distended with colloid (black arrows) and lined by flattened epithelium with areas of fibrosis and hemorrhage (blue arrows).

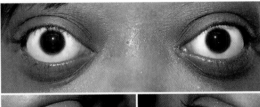

B **Graves disease (exophthalmos).** Patient with bilateral proptosis and eyelid retraction. Visible sclera causes appearance of a "stare." ℞

Thyroid cancer	Thyroidectomy is treatment option for thyroid cancers and hyperthyroidism. Complications of surgery include hoarseness (due to recurrent laryngeal nerve damage), hypocalcemia (due to removal of parathyroid glands), and transection of inferior thyroid artery.
Papillary carcinoma	Most common, excellent prognosis. Empty-appearing nuclei ("Orphan Annie" eyes) **A**, psammoma bodies, nuclear grooves. ↑ risk with *RET* and *BRAF* mutations, childhood irradiation.
Follicular carcinoma	Good prognosis, invades thyroid capsule (unlike follicular adenoma), uniform follicles.
Medullary carcinoma	From parafollicular "C cells"; produces calcitonin, sheets of cells in an amyloid stroma **B**. Associated with MEN 2A and 2B (*RET* mutations).
Undifferentiated/ anaplastic carcinoma	Older patients; invades local structures, very poor prognosis.
Lymphoma	Associated with Hashimoto thyroiditis.

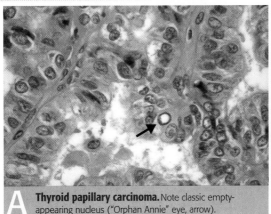

A **Thyroid papillary carcinoma.** Note classic empty-appearing nucleus ("Orphan Annie" eye, arrow).

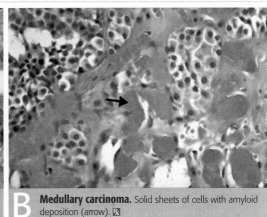

B **Medullary carcinoma.** Solid sheets of cells with amyloid deposition (arrow). ℞

Hyperparathyroidism

Primary	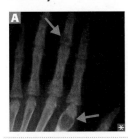 Usually an adenoma. **Hypercalcemia,** hypercalciuria (renal stones), hypophosphatemia, ↑ PTH, ↑ ALP, ↑ cAMP in urine. Most often asymptomatic. May present with weakness and constipation ("groans"), abdominal/flank pain (kidney stones, acute pancreatitis), depression ("psychiatric overtones").	**Osteitis fibrosa cystica**—cystic bone spaces filled with brown fibrous tissue **A** (bone pain). "Stones, bones, groans, and psychiatric overtones."
Secondary	2° hyperplasia due to ↓ gut Ca^{2+} absorption and ↑ PO_4^{3-}, most often in chronic renal disease (causes hypovitaminosis D → ↓ Ca^{2+} absorption). **Hypocalcemia,** hyperphosphatemia in chronic renal failure (vs. hypophosphatemia with most other causes), ↑ ALP, ↑ PTH.	**Renal osteodystrophy**—bone lesions due to 2° or 3° hyperparathyroidism due in turn to renal disease.
Tertiary	Refractory (autonomous) hyperparathyroidism resulting from chronic renal disease. ↑↑ PTH, ↑ Ca^{2+}.	

Hypoparathyroidism

Due to accidental surgical excision of parathyroid glands, autoimmune destruction, or DiGeorge syndrome. Findings: hypocalcemia, tetany.

Chvostek sign—tapping of facial nerve (tap the Cheek) → contraction of facial muscles.

Trousseau sign—occlusion of brachial artery with BP cuff (cuff the Triceps) → carpal spasm.

Pseudohypoparathyroidism (Albright hereditary osteodystrophy)—autosomal dominant unresponsiveness of kidney to PTH. Hypocalcemia, shortened 4th/5th digits, short stature.

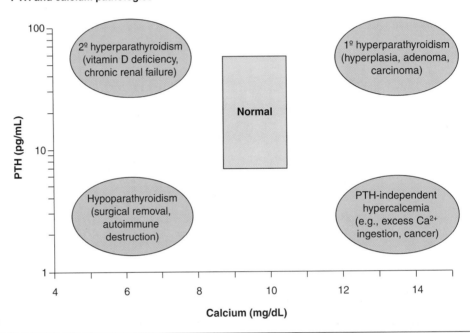

PTH and calcium pathologies

Pituitary adenoma

Most commonly prolactinoma (benign). Adenoma A may be functional (hormone producing) or nonfunctional (silent). Nonfunctional tumors present with mass effect (bitemporal hemianopia, hypopituitarism, headache). Functional tumor presentation is based on the hormone produced (e.g., prolactinoma: amenorrhea, galactorrhea, low libido, infertility; somatotropic adenoma: acromegaly). Treatment for prolactinoma: dopamine agonists (bromocriptine or cabergoline). .

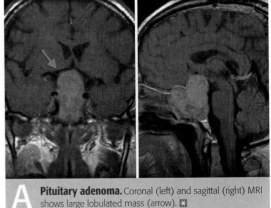

A **Pituitary adenoma.** Coronal (left) and sagittal (right) MRI shows large lobulated mass (arrow). ✱

Acromegaly	Excess GH in adults. Typically caused by pituitary adenoma.	
FINDINGS	Large tongue with deep furrows, deep voice, large hands and feet, coarse facial features A, impaired glucose tolerance (insulin resistance).	↑ GH in children → gigantism (↑ linear bone growth). Cardiac failure most common cause of death.
DIAGNOSIS	↑ serum IGF-1; failure to suppress serum GH following oral glucose tolerance test; pituitary mass seen on brain MRI.	
TREATMENT	Pituitary adenoma resection. If not cured, treat with octreotide (somatostatin analog) or pegvisomant (growth hormone receptor antagonist).	

A **Acromegaly.** Note marked coarsening of facial features over time. RU

Diabetes insipidus	Characterized by intense thirst and polyuria with inability to concentrate urine due to lack of ADH. Has a central or nephrogenic cause.	
	Central DI	**Nephrogenic DI**
ETIOLOGY	Pituitary tumor, autoimmune, trauma, surgery, ischemic encephalopathy, idiopathic	Hereditary (ADH receptor mutation), 2° to hypercalcemia, lithium, demeclocycline (ADH antagonist)
FINDINGS	↓ ADH Urine specific gravity < 1.006 Serum osmolarity > 290 mOsm/L Hyperosmotic volume contraction	Normal ADH levels Urine specific gravity < 1.006 Serum osmolarity > 290 mOsm/L Hyperosmotic volume contraction
DIAGNOSIS	Water restriction test[a]: > 50% ↑ in urine osmolarity	Water restriction test: no change in urine osmolarity
TREATMENT	Intranasal DDAVP Hydration	HCTZ, indomethacin, amiloride Hydration

[a]No water intake for 2–3 hr followed by hourly measurements of urine volume and osmolarity and plasma Na^+ concentration and osmolarity. DDAVP (ADH analog) is administered if normal values are not clearly reached.

SIADH

Syndrome of inappropriate antidiuretic hormone secretion:

- Excessive water retention
- Hyponatremia with continued urinary Na⁺ excretion
- Urine osmolarity > serum osmolarity

Body responds to water retention with ↓ aldosterone (hyponatremia) to maintain near-normal volume status. Very low serum sodium levels can lead to cerebral edema, seizures. Correct slowly to prevent central pontine myelinolysis.

Causes include:

- Ectopic ADH (small cell lung cancer)
- CNS disorders/head trauma
- Pulmonary disease
- Drugs (e.g., cyclophosphamide)

Treatment: fluid restriction, IV hypertonic saline, conivaptan, tolvaptan, demeclocycline.

Hypopituitarism

Undersecretion of pituitary hormones due to:

- Nonsecreting pituitary adenoma, craniopharyngioma
- **Sheehan syndrome** (ischemic infarct of pituitary following postpartum bleeding; usually presents with failure to lactate)
- **Empty sella syndrome** (atrophy or compression of pituitary, often idiopathic, common in obese women)
- Brain injury, hemorrhage (pituitary apoplexy)
- Radiation

Treatment: hormone replacement therapy (corticosteroids, thyroxine, sex steroids, human growth hormone).

Diabetes mellitus

ACUTE MANIFESTATIONS

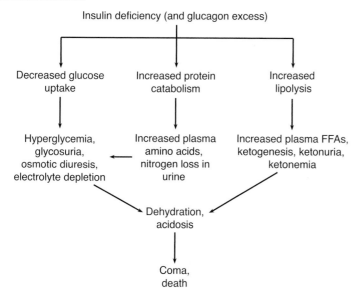

Insulin deficiency (and glucagon excess)

↓

Decreased glucose uptake | Increased protein catabolism | Increased lipolysis

↓

Hyperglycemia, glycosuria, osmotic diuresis, electrolyte depletion | Increased plasma amino acids, nitrogen loss in urine | Increased plasma FFAs, ketogenesis, ketonuria, ketonemia

↓

Dehydration, acidosis

↓

Coma, death

Polydipsia, polyuria, polyphagia, weight loss, DKA (type 1), hyperosmolar coma (type 2). Rarely, can be caused by unopposed secretion of GH and epinephrine.

CHRONIC MANIFESTATIONS

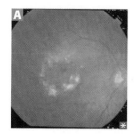

Nonenzymatic glycosylation:
- Small vessel disease (diffuse thickening of basement membrane) → retinopathy (hemorrhage, exudates, microaneurysms, vessel proliferation) , glaucoma, nephropathy (nodular sclerosis, progressive proteinuria, chronic renal failure, arteriolosclerosis leading to hypertension, Kimmelstiel-Wilson nodules)
- Large vessel atherosclerosis, CAD, peripheral vascular occlusive disease, and gangrene → limb loss, cerebrovascular disease. MI most common cause of death.

Osmotic damage (sorbitol accumulation in organs with aldose reductase and ↓ or absent sorbitol dehydrogenase):
- Neuropathy (motor, sensory, and autonomic degeneration)
- Cataracts

TESTS

Fasting serum glucose, oral glucose tolerance test, HbA_{1c} (reflects average blood glucose over prior 3 months).

Type 1 vs. type 2 diabetes mellitus

Variable	Type 1	Type 2
1° DEFECT	Autoimmune destruction of β cells	↑ resistance to insulin, progressive pancreatic β-cell failure
INSULIN NECESSARY IN TREATMENT	Always	Sometimes
AGE (EXCEPTIONS COMMONLY OCCUR)	< 30 yr	> 40 yr
ASSOCIATION WITH OBESITY	No	Yes
GENETIC PREDISPOSITION	Relatively weak (50% concordance in identical twins), polygenic	Relatively strong (90% concordance in identical twins), polygenic
ASSOCIATION WITH HLA SYSTEM	Yes (HLA-DR3 and 4)	No
GLUCOSE INTOLERANCE	Severe	Mild to moderate
INSULIN SENSITIVITY	High	Low
KETOACIDOSIS	Common	Rare
β-CELL NUMBERS IN THE ISLETS	↓	Variable (with amyloid deposits)
SERUM INSULIN LEVEL	↓	Variable
CLASSIC SYMPTOMS OF POLYURIA, POLYDIPSIA, POLYPHAGIA, WEIGHT LOSS	Common	Sometimes
HISTOLOGY	Islet leukocytic infiltrate	Islet amyloid polypeptide (IAPP) deposits

---

Diabetic ketoacidosis

One of the most important complications of diabetes (usually type 1). Usually due to ↑ insulin requirements from ↑ stress (e.g., infection). Excess fat breakdown and ↑ ketogenesis from ↑ free fatty acids, which are then made into ketone bodies (β-hydroxybutyrate > acetoacetate).

SIGNS/SYMPTOMS	Kussmaul respirations (rapid/deep breathing), nausea/vomiting, abdominal pain, psychosis/delirium, dehydration. Fruity breath odor (due to exhaled acetone).
LABS	Hyperglycemia, ↑ H^+, ↓ HCO_3^- (anion gap metabolic acidosis), ↑ blood ketone levels, leukocytosis. Hyperkalemia, but depleted intracellular K^+ due to transcellular shift from ↓ insulin.
COMPLICATIONS	Life-threatening mucormycosis (usually caused by *Rhizopus* infection), cerebral edema, cardiac arrhythmias, heart failure.
TREATMENT	IV fluids, IV insulin, and K^+ (to replete intracellular stores); glucose if necessary to prevent hypoglycemia.

Insulinoma

Tumor of β cells of pancreas → overproduction of insulin → hypoglycemia. Whipple triad of episodic CNS symptoms: lethargy, syncope, and diplopia. Symptomatic patients have ↓ blood glucose and ↑ C-peptide levels (vs. exogenous insulin use). Treatment: surgical resection.

Carcinoid syndrome	Rare syndrome caused by carcinoid tumors (neuroendocrine cells), especially metastatic small bowel tumors, which secrete high levels of serotonin (5-HT). Not seen if tumor is limited to GI tract (5-HT undergoes first-pass metabolism in liver). Results in recurrent diarrhea, cutaneous flushing, asthmatic wheezing, and right-sided valvular disease. ↑ 5-hydroxyindoleacetic acid (5-HIAA) in urine, niacin deficiency (pellagra). Treatment: resection, somatostatin analog (e.g., octreotide).	Rule of 1/3s: 1/3 metastasize 1/3 present with 2nd malignancy 1/3 are multiple Most common malignancy in the small intestine.

Zollinger-Ellison syndrome	Gastrin-secreting tumor of pancreas or duodenum. Acid hypersecretion causes recurrent ulcers in distal duodenum and jejunum. Presents with abdominal pain (peptic ulcer disease, distal ulcers), diarrhea (malabsorption). May be associated with MEN 1.

Multiple endocrine neoplasias

SUBTYPE	CHARACTERISTICS	COMMENTS
MEN 1 (Wermer syndrome)	Parathyroid tumors Pituitary tumors (prolactin or GH) Pancreatic endocrine tumors—Zollinger-Ellison syndrome, insulinomas, VIPomas, glucagonomas (rare) Commonly presents with kidney stones and stomach ulcers	MEN 1 = 3 P's (from cephalad to caudad: Pituitary, Parathyroid, and Pancreas; remember by drawing a diamond). MEN 2A = 2 P's (Parathyroids and Pheochromocytoma; remember by drawing a square). MEN 2B = 1 P (Pheochromocytoma; remember by drawing a triangle).
MEN 2A (Sipple syndrome)	Medullary thyroid carcinoma (secretes calcitonin) Pheochromocytoma Parathyroid hyperplasia	All **MEN** syndromes have autosomal **dominant** inheritance. "All **MEN** are **dominant**" (or so they think).
MEN 2B	Medullary thyroid carcinoma (secretes calcitonin) Pheochromocytoma Oral/intestinal ganglioneuromatosis (mucosal neuromas). Associated with marfanoid habitus.	Associated with *ret* gene mutation in MEN 2A and 2B.

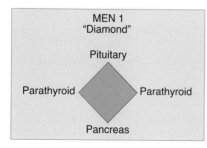

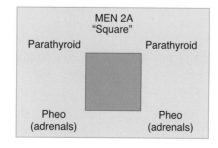

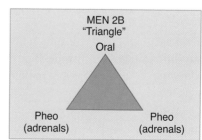

▶ **ENDOCRINE–PHARMACOLOGY**

Diabetes drugs

Treatment strategies:

DM1—low-sugar diet, insulin replacement

DM2—dietary modification and exercise for weight loss; oral agents, non-insulin injectables, insulin replacement

Gestational DM (GDM)—dietary modifications, exercise, insulin replacement if lifestyle modification fails

DRUG CLASSES	ACTION	CLINICAL USE	TOXICITIES
Insulin, rapid acting Lispro Aspart Glulisine	Bind insulin receptor (tyrosine kinase activity). Liver: ↑ glucose stored as glycogen. Muscle: ↑ glycogen, protein synthesis; ↑ K^+ uptake. Fat: ↑ TG storage.	DM1, DM2, GDM (postprandial glucose control).	Hypoglycemia, rare hypersensitivity reactions.
Insulin, short acting Regular		DM1, DM2, GDM, DKA (IV), hyperkalemia (+ glucose), stress hyperglycemia.	
Insulin, intermediate acting NPH		DM1, DM2, GDM.	
Insulin, long acting Glargine Detemir		DM1, DM2, GDM (basal glucose control).	
Biguanides Metformin	Exact mechanism is unknown. ↓ gluconeogenesis, ↑ glycolysis, ↑ peripheral glucose uptake (insulin sensitivity).	Oral. First-line therapy in type 2 DM. Can be used in patients without islet function.	GI upset; most serious adverse effect is lactic acidosis (thus contraindicated in renal failure).
Sulfonylureas First generation: Tolbutamide Chlorpropamide Second generation: Glyburide Glimepiride Glipizide	Close K^+ channel in β-cell membrane, so cell depolarizes → triggering of insulin release via ↑ Ca^{2+} influx.	Stimulate release of endogenous insulin in type 2 DM. Require some islet function, so useless in type 1 DM.	Risk of hypoglycemia ↑ in renal failure. First generation: disulfiram-like effects. Second generation: hypoglycemia.
Glitazones/ thiazolidinediones Pioglitazone Rosiglitazone	↑ insulin sensitivity in peripheral tissue. Binds to PPAR-γ nuclear transcription regulator.[a]	Used as monotherapy in type 2 DM or combined with above agents.	Weight gain, edema. Hepatotoxicity, heart failure.
α-glucosidase inhibitors Acarbose Miglitol	Inhibit intestinal brush-border α-glucosidases. Delayed sugar hydrolysis and glucose absorption → ↓ postprandial hyperglycemia.	Used as monotherapy in type 2 DM or in combination with above agents.	GI disturbances.

Diabetes drugs *(continued)*

DRUG CLASSES	ACTION	CLINICAL USE	TOXICITIES
Amylin analogs Pramlintide	↓ gastric emptying, ↓ glucagon.	Type 1 and type 2 DM.	Hypoglycemia, nausea, diarrhea.
GLP-1 analogs Exenatide Liraglutide	↑ insulin, ↓ glucagon release.	Type 2 DM.	Nausea, vomiting; pancreatitis.
DPP-4 inhibitors Linagliptin Saxagliptin Sitagliptin	↑ insulin, ↓ glucagon release.	Type 2 DM.	Mild urinary or respiratory infections.

[a]Genes activated by PPAR-γ regulate fatty acid storage and glucose metabolism. Activation of PPAR-γ ↑ insulin sensitivity and levels of adiponectin.

Propylthiouracil, methimazole

MECHANISM	Block thyroid peroxidase, inhibiting the oxidation of iodide and the organification (coupling) of iodine → inhibition of thyroid hormone synthesis. Propylthiouracil also blocks 5′-deiodinase, which ↓ peripheral conversion of T_4 to T_3.
CLINICAL USE	Hyperthyroidism. PTU blocks Peripheral conversion, used in Pregnancy.
TOXICITY	Skin rash, agranulocytosis (rare), aplastic anemia, hepatotoxicity (propylthiouracil). Methimazole is a possible teratogen (can cause aplasia cutis).

Levothyroxine, triiodothyronine

MECHANISM	Thyroxine replacement.
CLINICAL USE	Hypothyroidism, myxedema.
TOXICITY	Tachycardia, heat intolerance, tremors, arrhythmias.

Hypothalamic/pituitary drugs

DRUG	CLINICAL USE
GH	GH deficiency, Turner syndrome.
Somatostatin (octreotide)	Acromegaly, carcinoid, gastrinoma, glucagonoma, esophageal varices.
Oxytocin	Stimulates labor, uterine contractions, milk let-down; controls uterine hemorrhage.
ADH (DDAVP)	Pituitary (central, not nephrogenic) DI.

Demeclocycline

MECHANISM	ADH antagonist (member of the tetracycline family).
CLINICAL USE	SIADH.
TOXICITY	Nephrogenic DI, photosensitivity, abnormalities of bone and teeth.

Glucocorticoids	Hydrocortisone, prednisone, triamcinolone, dexamethasone, beclomethasone, fludrocortisone (mineralocorticoid and glucocorticoid activity).
MECHANISM	Metabolic, catabolic, anti-inflammatory, and immunosuppressive effects mediated by interactions with glucocorticoid response elements and inhibition of transcription factors such as NF-κB.
CLINICAL USE	Addison disease, inflammation, immune suppression, asthma.
TOXICITY	Iatrogenic Cushing syndrome—buffalo hump, moon facies, truncal obesity, muscle wasting, thin skin, easy bruisability, osteoporosis (treat with bisphosphonates), adrenocortical atrophy, peptic ulcers, diabetes (if chronic). Adrenal insufficiency when drug stopped abruptly after chronic use.

Gastrointestinal

"A good set of bowels is worth more to a man than any quantity of brains."
—Josh Billings

"Man should strive to have his intestines relaxed all the days of his life."
—Moses Maimonides

"The colon is the playing field for all human emotions."
—Cyrus Kapadia, MD

▸ **GASTROINTESTINAL–EMBRYOLOGY**

GI embryology

Foregut—pharynx to duodenum.
Midgut—duodenum to proximal $^2/_3$ of transverse colon.
Hindgut—distal $^1/_3$ of transverse colon to anal canal above pectinate line.
Developmental defects of anterior abdominal wall due to failure of:
- Rostral fold closure: sternal defects
- Lateral fold closure: omphalocele, gastroschisis
- Caudal fold closure: bladder exstrophy

Duodenal atresia—failure to recanalize (trisomy 21).
Jejunal, ileal, colonic atresia—due to vascular accident (apple peel atresia).
Midgut development:
- 6th week—midgut herniates through umbilical ring
- 10th week—returns to abdominal cavity + rotates around SMA

Pathology—malrotation of midgut, omphalocele, intestinal atresia or stenosis, volvulus.

Gastroschisis—extrusion of abdominal contents through abdominal folds; not covered by peritoneum.

Omphalocele—persistence of herniation of abdominal contents into umbilical cord, **sealed** by peritoneum 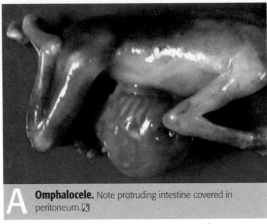.

A **Omphalocele.** Note protruding intestine covered in peritoneum.

SMA → superior mesenteric artery

Tracheoesophageal anomalies

Esophageal atresia (EA) with distal tracheoesophageal fistula (TEF) is the most common (85%). Results in drooling, choking, and vomiting with first feeding. TEF allows air to enter stomach (visible on CXR). Cyanosis is 2° to laryngospasm (to avoid reflux-related aspiration). Clinical test: failure to pass nasogastric tube into stomach.
In H-type it is a fistula alone. In pure atresia (isolated) EA the CXR shows gasless abdomen.

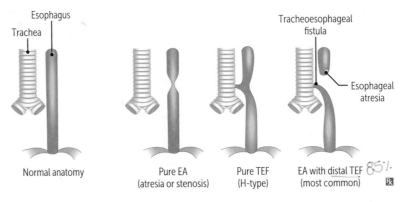

Esophagus
Trachea

Tracheoesophageal fistula

Esophageal atresia

Normal anatomy | Pure EA (atresia or stenosis) | Pure TEF (H-type) | EA with distal TEF (most common) 85%

Congenital pyloric stenosis

Hypertrophy of the pylorus causes obstruction. Palpable "olive" mass in epigastric region and nonbilious projectile vomiting at ≈ 2–6 weeks old. Treatment is surgical incision. Occurs in 1/600 live births, more often in firstborn males.

Pancreas and spleen embryology

⌐→ *also pharynx to duodenum.*

Pancreas—derived from foregut. Ventral pancreatic buds contribute to the pancreatic head and main pancreatic duct. The uncinate process is formed by the ventral bud alone. The dorsal pancreatic bud becomes everything else (body, tail, isthmus, and accessory pancreatic duct).

Annular pancreas—ventral pancreatic bud abnormally encircles 2nd part of duodenum; forms a ring of pancreatic tissue that may cause duodenal narrowing.

Pancreas divisum—ventral and dorsal parts fail to fuse at 8 weeks.

Spleen—arises in mesentery of stomach (hence is mesodermal) but is supplied by foregut (celiac artery).

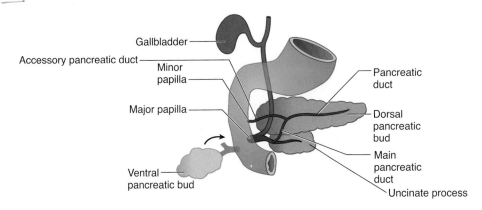

Gallbladder

Accessory pancreatic duct

Minor papilla

Major papilla

Ventral pancreatic bud

Pancreatic duct

Dorsal pancreatic bud

Main pancreatic duct

Uncinate process

▶ GASTROINTESTINAL–ANATOMY

Retroperitoneal structures

Retroperitoneal structures include GI structures that lack a mesentery and non-GI structures. Injuries to retroperitoneal structures can cause blood or gas accumulation in retroperitoneal space.

SAD PUCKER:
Suprarenal (adrenal) glands [not shown]
Aorta and IVC
Duodenum (2nd through 4th parts)
Pancreas (except tail)
Ureters [not shown]
Colon (descending and ascending)
Kidneys
Esophagus (lower $^2/_3$) [not shown]
Rectum (partially) [not shown]

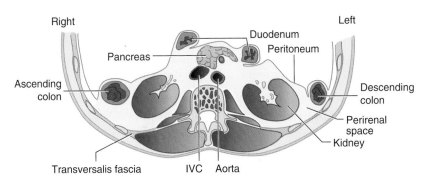

Right

Pancreas

Ascending colon

Transversalis fascia

IVC

Aorta

Duodenum

Peritoneum

Left

Descending colon

Perirenal space

Kidney

Important GI ligaments

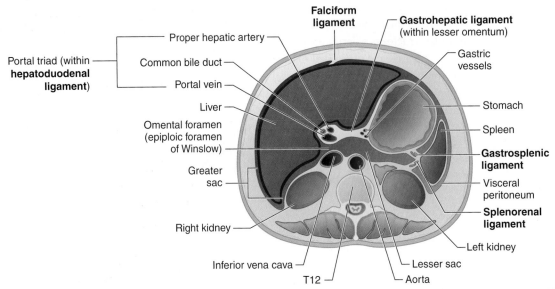

LIGAMENT	CONNECTS	STRUCTURES CONTAINED	NOTES
Falciform	Liver to anterior abdominal wall	Ligamentum teres hepatis (derivative of fetal umbilical vein)	Derivative of ventral mesentery
Hepatoduodenal	Liver to duodenum	Portal triad: proper hepatic artery, portal vein, common bile duct	Pringle maneuver—ligament may be compressed between thumb and index finger placed in omental foramen to control bleeding Borders the omental foramen, which connects the greater and lesser sacs
Gastrohepatic	Liver to lesser curvature of stomach	Gastric arteries	Separates greater and lesser sacs on the right May be cut during surgery to access lesser sac
Gastrocolic (not shown)	Greater curvature and transverse colon	Gastroepiploic arteries	Part of greater omentum
Gastrosplenic	Greater curvature and spleen	Short gastrics, left gastroepiploic vessels	Separates greater and lesser sacs on the left
Splenorenal	Spleen to posterior abdominal wall	Splenic artery and vein, tail of pancreas	

Digestive tract anatomy

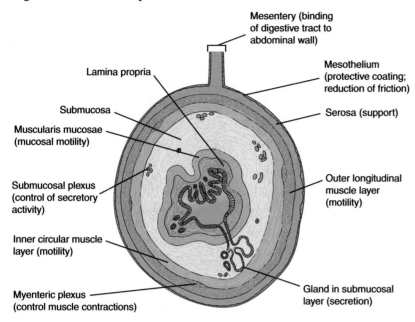

Lamina propria

Submucosa

Muscularis mucosae
(mucosal motility)

Submucosal plexus
(control of secretory
activity)

Inner circular muscle
layer (motility)

Myenteric plexus
(control muscle contractions)

Mesentery (binding
of digestive tract to
abdominal wall)

Mesothelium
(protective coating;
reduction of friction)

Serosa (support)

Outer longitudinal
muscle layer
(motility)

Gland in submucosal
layer (secretion)

Layers of gut wall (inside to outside—**MSMS**):
- Mucosa—epithelium (absorption), lamina propria (support), muscularis mucosa (motility)
- Submucosa—includes Submucosal nerve plexus (Meissner)
- Muscularis externa—includes Myenteric nerve plexus (Auerbach)
- Serosa (when intraperitoneal)/adventitia (when retroperitoneal)

Ulcers can extend into submucosa, inner or outer muscular layer. Erosions are in the mucosa only.

Frequencies of basal electric rhythm (slow waves):
- Stomach—3 waves/min
- Duodenum—12 waves/min
- Ileum—8–9 waves/min

Digestive tract histology

ORGAN	HISTOLOGY
Esophagus	Nonkeratinized stratified squamous epithelium.
Stomach	Gastric glands.
Duodenum	Villi and microvilli ↑ absorptive surface. Brunner glands (submucosa) and crypts of Lieberkühn.
Jejunum	Plicae circulares and crypts of Lieberkühn.
Ileum	Peyer patches (lamina propria, submucosa), plicae circulares (proximal ileum), and crypts of Lieberkühn. Largest number of goblet cells in the small intestine.
Colon	Colon has crypts of Lieberkühn but no villi; numerous goblet cells.

Abdominal aorta and branches

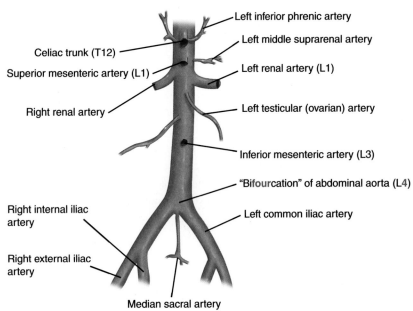

Left inferior phrenic artery

Left middle suprarenal artery

Celiac trunk (T12)

Left renal artery (L1)

Superior mesenteric artery (L1)

Right renal artery

Left testicular (ovarian) artery

Inferior mesenteric artery (L3)

"Bifourcation" of abdominal aorta (L4)

Right internal iliac artery

Left common iliac artery

Right external iliac artery

Median sacral artery

Arteries supplying GI structures branch **anteriorly.** Arteries supplying non-GI structures branch **laterally.**

Superior mesenteric artery (SMA) syndrome occurs when the transverse portion (third segment) of the duodenum is entrapped between SMA and aorta, causing intestinal obstruction.

GI blood supply and innervation

EMBRYONIC GUT REGION	ARTERY	PARASYMPATHETIC INNERVATION	VERTEBRAL LEVEL	STRUCTURES SUPPLIED
Foregut	Celiac	Vagus	T12/L1	Pharynx to proximal duodenum; liver, gallbladder, pancreas, spleen (mesoderm)
Midgut	SMA	Vagus	L1	Distal duodenum to proximal $^2/_3$ of transverse colon
Hindgut	IMA	Pelvic	L3	Distal $^1/_3$ of transverse colon to upper portion of rectum; splenic flexure is a watershed region

Celiac trunk

Branches of celiac trunk: common hepatic, splenic, left gastric. These constitute the main blood supply of the stomach.

Short gastrics have poor anastomoses if splenic artery is blocked.

Strong anastomoses exist between:
- Left and right gastroepiploics
- Left and right gastrics

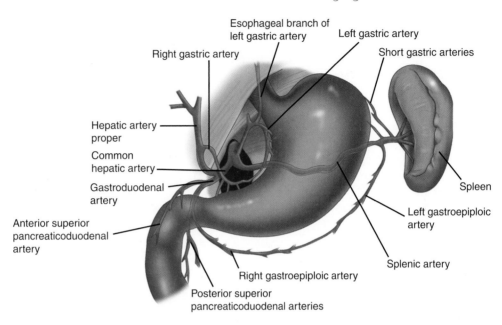

Collateral arterial circulation

If branches off of the abdominal aorta are blocked, these arterial anastomoses (origin) compensate:
- Superior epigastric (internal thoracic/mammary) ↔ inferior epigastric (external iliac)
- Superior pancreaticoduodenal (celiac trunk) ↔ inferior pancreaticoduodenal (SMA)
- Middle colic (SMA) ↔ left colic (IMA)
- Superior rectal (IMA) ↔ middle and inferior rectal (internal iliac)

Portosystemic anastomoses

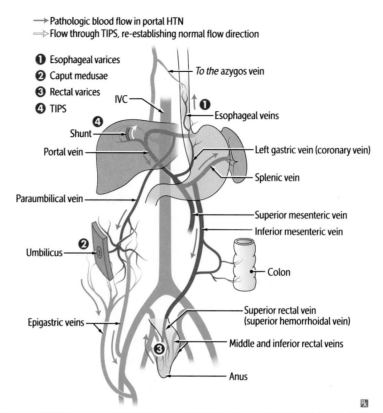

→ Pathologic blood flow in portal HTN
⇒ Flow through TIPS, re-establishing normal flow direction

❶ Esophageal varices
❷ Caput medusae
❸ Rectal varices
❹ TIPS

SITE OF ANASTOMOSIS	CLINICAL SIGN	PORTAL ↔ SYSTEMIC
❶ Esophagus	Esophageal varices	Left gastric ↔ esophageal
❷ Umbilicus	Caput medusae	Paraumbilical ↔ small epigastric veins of the anterior abdominal wall.
❸ Rectum	Anorectal varices (not internal hemorrhoids)	Superior rectal ↔ middle and inferior rectal

Varices of **gut**, **butt**, and **caput** (medusae) are commonly seen with portal hypertension.

Treatment with a transjugular intrahepatic portosystemic shunt (TIPS) ❹ between the portal vein and hepatic vein percutaneously relieves portal hypertension by shunting blood to the systemic circulation.

Pectinate (dentate) line   Formed where endoderm (hindgut) meets ectoderm.

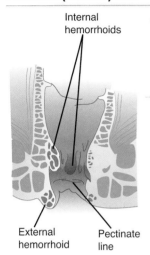

Internal hemorrhoids

External hemorrhoid

Pectinate line

Above pectinate line—internal hemorrhoids, adenocarcinoma. Arterial supply from superior rectal artery (branch of IMA). Venous drainage is to superior rectal vein → inferior mesenteric vein → portal system.

Below pectinate line—external hemorrhoids, anal fissures, squamous cell carcinoma. Arterial supply from inferior rectal artery (branch of internal pudendal artery). Venous drainage to inferior rectal vein → internal pudendal vein → internal iliac vein → IVC.

Internal hemorrhoids receive visceral innervation and are therefore **not painful**. Lymphatic drainage to deep nodes.

External hemorrhoids receive somatic innervation (inferior rectal branch of pudendal nerve) and are therefore **painful**. Lymphatic drainage to superficial inguinal nodes.

Anal fissure—tear in the anal mucosa below the Pectinate line. Pain while Pooping; blood on "toilet" paper Paper. Located Posteriorly since this area is Poorly Perfused.

Liver anatomy   Apical surface of hepatocytes faces bile canaliculi. Basolateral surface faces sinusoids.

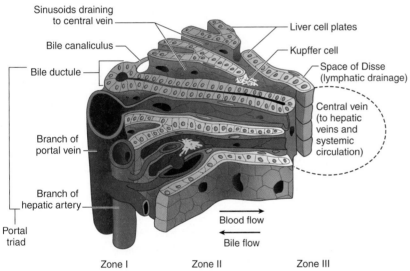

Sinusoids draining to central vein

Bile canaliculus

Bile ductule

Branch of portal vein

Branch of hepatic artery

Portal triad

Liver cell plates

Kupffer cell

Space of Disse (lymphatic drainage)

Central vein (to hepatic veins and systemic circulation)

Blood flow

Bile flow

Zone I   Zone II   Zone III

Zone I: periportal zone:
- Affected 1st by viral hepatitis
- Ingested toxins (e.g., cocaine)

Zone II: intermediate zone.

Zone III: pericentral vein (centrilobular) zone:
- Affected 1st by ischemia
- Contains cytochrome P-450 system
- Most sensitive to metabolic toxins
- Site of alcoholic hepatitis

Biliary structures

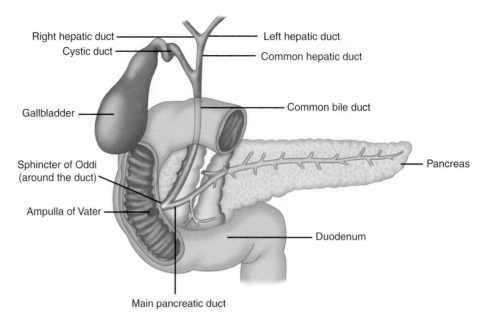

Right hepatic duct
Cystic duct
Gallbladder
Sphincter of Oddi (around the duct)
Ampulla of Vater
Main pancreatic duct
Left hepatic duct
Common hepatic duct
Common bile duct
Pancreas
Duodenum

Gallstones that reach the common channel at ampulla of Vater can block both the bile and pancreatic ducts.
Tumors that arise in the head of the pancreas (near the duodenum) can cause obstruction of the common bile duct.

Femoral region

ORGANIZATION	Lateral to medial: Nerve-Artery-Vein-Empty space-Lymphatics.	You go from **lateral to medial** to find your **NAVEL**.
Femoral triangle	Contains femoral vein, artery, nerve.	**Venous** near the **penis**.
Femoral sheath	Fascial tube 3–4 cm below inguinal ligament. Contains femoral vein, artery, and canal (deep inguinal lymph nodes) but not femoral nerve.	

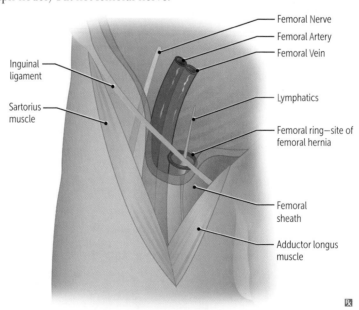

Inguinal ligament
Sartorius muscle
Femoral Nerve
Femoral Artery
Femoral Vein
Lymphatics
Femoral ring—site of femoral hernia
Femoral sheath
Adductor longus muscle

Inguinal canal

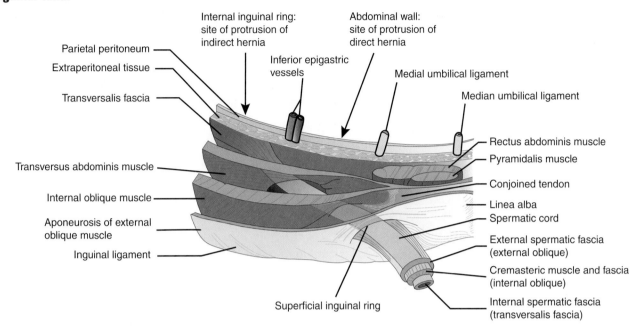

Parietal peritoneum

Extraperitoneal tissue

Transversalis fascia

Internal inguinal ring:
site of protrusion of
indirect hernia

Inferior epigastric
vessels

Abdominal wall:
site of protrusion of
direct hernia

Medial umbilical ligament

Median umbilical ligament

Rectus abdominis muscle

Pyramidalis muscle

Transversus abdominis muscle

Internal oblique muscle

Aponeurosis of external
oblique muscle

Inguinal ligament

Conjoined tendon

Linea alba

Spermatic cord

External spermatic fascia
(external oblique)

Cremasteric muscle and fascia
(internal oblique)

Internal spermatic fascia
(transversalis fascia)

Superficial inguinal ring

Hernias	A protrusion of peritoneum through an opening, usually a site of weakness.	
Diaphragmatic hernia	Abdominal structures enter the thorax; may occur in infants as a result of defective development of pleuroperitoneal membrane. Most commonly a **hiatal hernia**, in which stomach herniates upward through the esophageal hiatus of the diaphragm.	**Sliding hiatal hernia** is most common. Gastroesophageal junction is displaced ↑; "hourglass stomach." **Paraesophageal hernia**—gastroesophageal junction is normal. Fundus protrudes into the thorax.
Indirect inguinal hernia	Goes through the internal (deep) inguinal ring, external (superficial) inguinal ring, and into the scrotum. Enters internal inguinal ring lateral to inferior epigastric artery. Occurs in infants owing to failure of processus vaginalis to close (can form hydrocele). Much more common in males.	An indirect inguinal hernia follows the path of descent of the testes. Covered by all 3 layers of spermatic fascia.
Direct inguinal hernia	Protrudes through the inguinal (Hesselbach) triangle. Bulges directly through abdominal wall medial to inferior epigastric artery. Goes through the external (superficial) inguinal ring only. Covered by external spermatic fascia. Usually in older men.	MDs don't LIe: Medial to inferior epigastric artery = Direct hernia. Lateral to inferior epigastric artery = Indirect hernia.
Femoral hernia	Protrudes below inguinal ligament through femoral canal below and lateral to pubic tubercle. More common in females.	Leading cause of bowel incarceration.

Hesselbach triangle:
- Inferior epigastric vessels
- Lateral border of rectus abdominis
- Inguinal ligament

▸ GASTROINTESTINAL–PHYSIOLOGY

GI regulatory substances

REGULATORY SUBSTANCE	SOURCE	ACTION	REGULATION	NOTES
Cholecystokinin	I cells (duodenum, jejunum)	↑ pancreatic secretion ↑ gallbladder contraction ↓ gastric emptying ↑ sphincter of Oddi relaxation	↑ by fatty acids, amino acids	CCK acts on neural muscarinic pathways to cause pancreatic secretion.
Gastrin	G cells (antrum of stomach)	↑ gastric H^+ secretion ↑ growth of gastric mucosa ↑ gastric motility	↑ by stomach distention/alkalinization, amino acids, peptides, vagal stimulation ↓ by stomach pH < 1.5	↑↑ in Zollinger-Ellison syndrome. ↑ by chronic PPI use. Phenylalanine and tryptophan are potent stimulators.
Glucose-dependent insulinotropic peptide	K cells (duodenum, jejunum)	Exocrine: ↓ gastric H^+ secretion Endocrine: ↑ insulin release	↑ by fatty acids, amino acids, oral glucose	Also known as gastric inhibitory peptide (GIP). An oral glucose load is used more rapidly than the equivalent given by IV due to GIP secretion.
Motilin	Small intestine	Produces migrating motor complexes (MMCs)	↑ in fasting state	Motilin receptor agonists (e.g., erythromycin) are used to stimulate intestinal peristalsis.
Secretin	S cells (duodenum)	↑ pancreatic HCO_3^- secretion ↓ gastric acid secretion ↑ bile secretion	↑ by acid, fatty acids in lumen of duodenum	↑ HCO_3^- neutralizes gastric acid in duodenum, allowing pancreatic enzymes to function.
Somatostatin	D cells (pancreatic islets, GI mucosa)	↓ gastric acid and pepsinogen secretion ↓ pancreatic and small intestine fluid secretion ↓ gallbladder contraction ↓ insulin and glucagon release	↑ by acid ↓ by vagal stimulation	Inhibitory hormone. Antigrowth hormone effects (inhibits digestion and absorption of substances needed for growth).
Nitric oxide		↑ smooth muscle relaxation, including lower esophageal sphincter (LES)		Loss of NO secretion is implicated in ↑ LES tone of achalasia.
Vasoactive intestinal polypeptide (VIP)	Parasympathetic ganglia in sphincters, gallbladder, small intestine	↑ intestinal water and electrolyte secretion ↑ relaxation of intestinal smooth muscle and sphincters	↑ by distention and vagal stimulation ↓ by adrenergic input	VIPoma—non-α, non-β islet cell pancreatic tumor that secretes VIP. Copious Watery Diarrhea, Hypokalemia, and Achlorhydria (WDHA syndrome).

GI secretory products

PRODUCT	SOURCE	ACTION	REGULATION	NOTES
Intrinsic factor	Parietal cells (stomach)	Vitamin B_{12}–binding protein (required for B_{12} uptake in terminal ileum)		Autoimmune destruction of parietal cells → chronic gastritis and pernicious anemia.
Gastric acid	Parietal cells (stomach)	↓ stomach pH	↑ by histamine, ACh, gastrin ↓ by somatostatin, GIP, prostaglandin, secretin	**Gastrinoma:** gastrin-secreting tumor that causes high levels of acid secretion and ulcers refractory to medical therapy.
Pepsin	Chief cells (stomach)	Protein digestion	↑ by vagal stimulation, local acid	Inactive pepsinogen → pepsin by H^+.
HCO_3^-	Mucosal cells (stomach, duodenum, salivary glands, pancreas) and Brunner glands (duodenum)	Neutralizes acid	↑ by pancreatic and biliary secretion with secretin	HCO_3^- is trapped in mucus that covers the gastric epithelium.

Locations of GI secretory cells

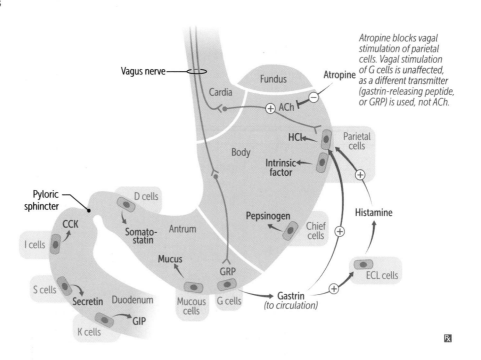

Atropine blocks vagal stimulation of parietal cells. Vagal stimulation of G cells is unaffected, as a different transmitter (gastrin-releasing peptide, or GRP) is used, not ACh.

Gastrin ↑ acid secretion primarily through its effects on enterochromaffin-like (ECL) cells (leading to histamine release) rather than through its direct effect on parietal cells.

Gastric parietal cell

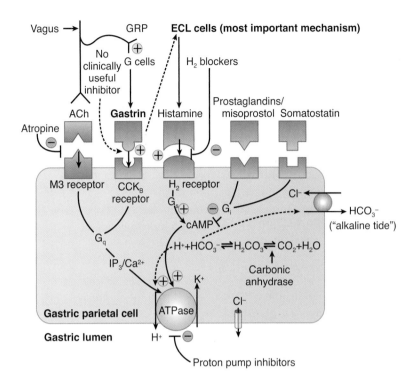

Brunner glands	Located in duodenal submucosa. Secrete alkaline mucus. Hypertrophy seen in peptic ulcer disease.

Pancreatic secretions	Isotonic fluid; low flow → high Cl^-, high flow → high HCO_3^-.

ENZYME	ROLE	NOTES
α-amylase	Starch digestion	Secreted in active form
Lipase, phospholipase A, colipase	Fat digestion	
Proteases	Protein digestion	Includes trypsin, chymotrypsin, elastase, carboxypeptidases Secreted as proenzymes also known as zymogens
Trypsinogen	Converted to active enzyme trypsin → activation of other proenzymes and cleaving of additional trypsinogen molecules into active trypsin (positive feedback loop)	Converted to trypsin by enterokinase/ enteropeptidase, a brush-border enzyme on the duodenal and jejunal mucosa

Carbohydrate absorption	Only monosaccharides (glucose, galactose, fructose) are absorbed by enterocytes. Glucose and galactose are taken up by SGLT1 (Na^+ dependent). Fructose is taken up by facilitated diffusion by GLUT-5. All are transported to blood by GLUT-2. D-xylose absorption test: distinguishes GI mucosal damage from other causes of malabsorption.

Vitamin/mineral absorption

Iron	Absorbed as Fe^{2+} in duodenum.	Iron Fist, Bro
Folate	Absorbed in jejunum and ileum.	
B$_{12}$	Absorbed in terminal ileum along with bile acids, requires intrinsic factor.	

Peyer patches	Unencapsulated lymphoid tissue 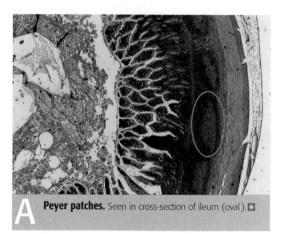 found in lamina propria and submucosa of ileum. Contain specialized M cells that sample and present antigens to immune cells. B cells stimulated in germinal centers of Peyer patches differentiate into IgA-secreting plasma cells, which ultimately reside in lamina propria. IgA receives protective secretory component and is then transported across the epithelium to the gut to deal with intraluminal antigen.	Think of **IgA**, the **I**ntra-gut **A**ntibody. And always say "secretory IgA."

A **Peyer patches.** Seen in cross-section of ileum (oval). ✳

Bile	Composed of bile salts (bile acids conjugated to glycine or taurine, making them water soluble), phospholipids, cholesterol, bilirubin, water, and ions. Cholesterol 7α-hydroxylase catalyzes rate-limiting step of bile synthesis. Functions: ▪ Digestion and absorption of lipids and fat-soluble vitamins ▪ Cholesterol excretion (body's only means of eliminating cholesterol) ▪ Antimicrobial activity (via membrane disruption)

Bilirubin

Product of heme metabolism. Bilirubin is removed from blood by liver, conjugated with glucuronate, and excreted in bile.

Direct bilirubin—conjugated with glucuronic acid; water soluble.

Indirect bilirubin—unconjugated; water insoluble.

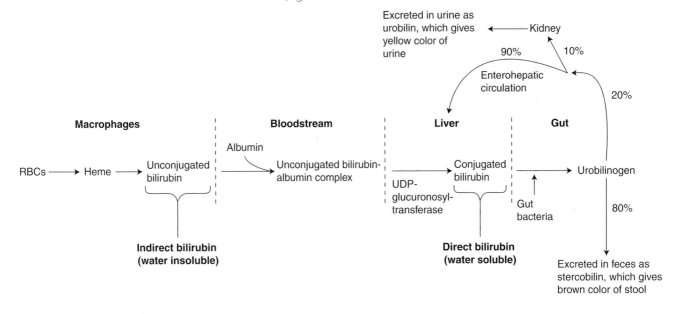

▸ GASTROINTESTINAL–PATHOLOGY

Salivary gland tumors

Generally benign and occur in parotid gland:
- **Pleomorphic adenoma** (benign mixed tumor) is the most common salivary gland tumor. Presents as a painless, mobile mass. It is composed of chondromyxoid stroma and epithelium and recurs if incompletely excised or ruptured intraoperatively.
- **Warthin tumor** (papillary cystadenoma lymphomatosum) is a benign cystic tumor with germinal centers.
- **Mucoepidermoid carcinoma** is the most common malignant tumor and has mucinous and squamous components. It typically presents as a painless, slow-growing mass.

Achalasia

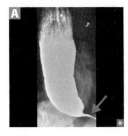

Failure of relaxation of LES due to loss of myenteric (Auerbach) plexus. High LES opening pressure and uncoordinated peristalsis → progressive dysphagia to solids and liquids (vs. obstruction—solids only). Barium swallow shows dilated esophagus with an area of distal stenosis. Associated with an ↑ risk of esophageal squamous cell carcinoma.

A-chalasia = absence of relaxation.

"Bird's beak" on barium swallow A.

2° achalasia may arise from Chagas disease.

Esophageal pathologies

Boerhaave syndrome	Transmural, usually distal esophageal rupture due to violent retching; surgical emergency.
Eosinophilic esophagitis	Infiltration of eosinophils in the esophagus in atopic patients. Food allergens → dysphagia, heartburn, strictures. Unresponsive to GERD therapy.
Esophageal strictures	Associated with lye ingestion and acid reflux.
Esophageal varices	Painless bleeding of dilated submucosal veins in lower $\frac{1}{3}$ of esophagus 2° to portal hypertension.
Esophagitis	Associated with reflux, infection in immunocompromised (*Candida*: white pseudomembrane; HSV-1: punched-out ulcers; CMV: linear ulcers), or chemical ingestion.
Gastroesophageal reflux disease	Commonly presents as heartburn and regurgitation upon lying down. May also present with nocturnal cough and dyspnea, adult-onset asthma. Decrease in LES tone.
Mallory-Weiss syndrome	Mucosal lacerations at the gastroesophageal junction due to severe vomiting. Leads to hematemesis. Usually found in alcoholics and bulimics.
Plummer-Vinson syndrome	Triad of **D**ysphagia (due to esophageal webs), **I**ron deficiency anemia, and **G**lossitis ("Plumbers" DIG).
Sclerodermal esophageal dysmotility	Esophageal smooth muscle atrophy → ↓ LES pressure and dysmotility → acid reflux and dysphagia → stricture, Barrett esophagus, and aspiration. Part of CREST syndrome.

Barrett esophagus	Glandular metaplasia—replacement of nonkeratinized (stratified) squamous epithelium with intestinal epithelium (nonciliated columnar with goblets cells) in the distal esophagus 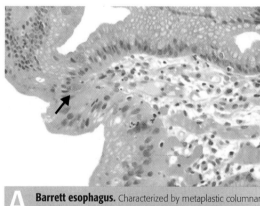. Due to chronic acid reflux (GERD). Associated with esophagitis, esophageal ulcers, and ↑ risk of esophageal adenocarcinoma.

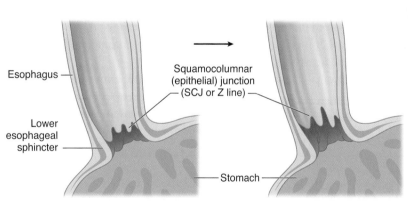

Esophagus

Lower esophageal sphincter

Squamocolumnar (epithelial) junction (SCJ or Z line)

Stomach

Barrett esophagus. Characterized by metaplastic columnar epithelium with goblet cells (arrow).

Esophageal cancer

Can be squamous cell carcinoma or adenocarcinoma. Typically presents with progressive dysphagia (first solids, then liquids) and weight loss; poor prognosis. Risk factors include:

- Achalasia
- Alcohol—squamous
- Barrett esophagus—adeno
- Cigarettes—both
- Diverticula (e.g., Zenker)—squamous
- Esophageal web—squamous
- Familial
- Fat (obesity)—adeno
- GERD—adeno
- Hot liquids—squamous

AABCDEFFGH.
Worldwide, squamous cell is more common.
In the United States, adenocarcinoma is more common.
Squamous cell—upper $2/3$.
Adenocarcinoma—lower $1/3$.

Gastritis

Acute gastritis (erosive)	Disruption of mucosal barrier → inflammation. Can be caused by stress, NSAIDs ($\downarrow$ PGE$_2$ → $\downarrow$ gastric mucosa protection), alcohol, uremia, burns (**Curling** ulcer—$\downarrow$ plasma volume → sloughing of gastric mucosa), and brain injury (**Cushing** ulcer—$\uparrow$ vagal stimulation → $\uparrow$ ACh → $\uparrow$ H$^+$ production).	Burned by the **Curling** iron. Always **Cushion** the brain. Especially common among alcoholics and patients taking daily NSAIDs (e.g., patients with rheumatoid arthritis).

Chronic gastritis (nonerosive)

Type A (fundus/body)	Autoimmune disorder characterized by Autoantibodies to parietal cells, pernicious Anemia, and Achlorhydria. Associated with other autoimmune disorders.	A comes before B: • Type **A**—**A**utoimmune; first part of the stomach (fundus/body). • Type **B**—*H. pylori* **B**acteria; second part of the stomach (antrum).
Type B (antrum)	Most common type. Caused by *H. pylori* infection. $\uparrow$ risk of MALT lymphoma and gastric adenocarcinoma.	

Ménétrier disease

Gastric hypertrophy with protein loss, parietal cell atrophy, and $\uparrow$ mucous cells. Precancerous. Rugae of stomach are so hypertrophied that they look like brain gyri.

Stomach cancer

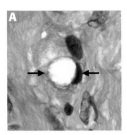

signet ring cell.

Almost always adenocarcinoma. Early aggressive local spread and node/liver metastases. Often presents with acanthosis nigricans.

- **Intestinal**—associated with *H. pylori* infection, dietary nitrosamines (smoked foods), tobacco smoking, achlorhydria, chronic gastritis. Commonly on lesser curvature; looks like ulcer with raised margins.
- **Diffuse**—not associated with *H. pylori*; signet ring cells **A**; stomach wall grossly thickened and leathery (linitis plastica).

Virchow node—involvement of left supraclavicular node by metastasis from stomach.
Krukenberg tumor—bilateral metastases to ovaries. Abundant mucus, signet ring cells.
Sister Mary Joseph nodule—subcutaneous periumbilical metastasis.

Peptic ulcer disease

	Gastric ulcer	**Duodenal ulcer**
Pain	Can be Greater with meals—weight loss	Decreases with meals—weight gain
H. pylori infection	In 70%	In almost 100%
Mechanism	↓ mucosal protection against gastric acid	↓ mucosal protection or ↑ gastric acid secretion
Other causes	NSAIDs	Zollinger-Ellison syndrome
Risk of carcinoma	↑	Generally benign
Other	Often occurs in older patients	Hypertrophy of Brunner glands

Ulcer complications

Hemorrhage	Gastric, duodenal (posterior > anterior). Ruptured gastric ulcer on the lesser curvature of the stomach → bleeding from left gastric artery. An ulcer on the posterior wall of the duodenum → bleeding from gastroduodenal artery.
Perforation	Duodenal (anterior > posterior). May see free air under the diaphragm A with referred pain to the shoulder. *due to imitation of the phrenic nerve.*

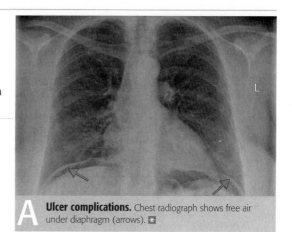

A **Ulcer complications.** Chest radiograph shows free air under diaphragm (arrows). ✷

Malabsorption syndromes	Can cause diarrhea, steatorrhea, weight loss, weakness, and vitamin and mineral deficiencies.	These Will Cause Devastating Absorption Problems.
		↳ acronym for the malabsorptive syndrome
Tropical sprue	Similar findings as celiac sprue (affects small bowel), but responds to antibiotics. Cause is unknown, but seen in residents of or recent visitors to tropics.	
Whipple disease	Infection with *Tropheryma whipplei* (gram positive); PAS ⊕ **foamy** macrophages in intestinal lamina propria, mesenteric nodes. **C**ardiac symptoms, **A**rthralgias, and **N**eurologic symptoms are common. Most often occurs in older men.	**Foamy** **W**hipped cream in a **CAN**.
Celiac sprue	Autoimmune-mediated intolerance of gliadin (wheat) leading to malabsorption and steatorrhea. Associated with HLA-DQ2, HLA-DQ8, and northern European descent. Findings include anti-endomysial, anti-tissue transglutaminase, and anti-gliadin antibodies; blunting of villi; and lymphocytes in the lamina propria **A**. ↓ mucosal absorption that primarily affects distal duodenum and/or proximal jejunum. Serum levels of tissue transglutaminase antibodies are used for diagnosis. Associated with dermatitis herpetiformis. Moderately ↑ risk of malignancy (e.g., T-cell lymphoma). Treatment: gluten-free diet.	**A** **Celiac sprue.** Blunting of villi (single arrow) and crypt hyperplasia (double arrows).
Disaccharidase deficiency	Most common is lactase deficiency → milk intolerance. Normal-appearing villi. Osmotic diarrhea. Since lactase is located at tips of intestinal villi, self-limited lactase deficiency can occur following injury (e.g., viral diarrhea).	Lactose tolerance test: ⊕ for lactase deficiency if: ▪ Administration of lactose produces symptoms, and ▪ Glucose rises < 20 mg/dL
Abetalipoproteinemia	↓ synthesis of apolipoprotein B → inability to generate chylomicrons → ↓ secretion of cholesterol, VLDL into bloodstream → fat accumulation in enterocytes.	Presents in early childhood with failure to thrive, steatorrhea, acanthocytosis, ataxia, night blindness.
Pancreatic insufficiency	Due to cystic fibrosis, obstructing cancer, and chronic pancreatitis. Causes malabsorption of fat and fat-soluble vitamins (vitamins A, D, E, K).	↑ neutral fat in stool. D-xylose absorption test: normal urinary excretion in pancreatic insufficiency; ↓ excretion with intestinal mucosa defects or bacterial overgrowth.

Inflammatory bowel diseases

	Crohn disease	Ulcerative colitis
POSSIBLE ETIOLOGY	Disordered response to intestinal bacteria.	Autoimmune.
LOCATION	Any portion of the GI tract, usually the terminal ileum and colon. **Skip** lesions, **rectal** sparing.	Colitis = colon inflammation. Continuous colonic lesions, always with rectal involvement.
GROSS MORPHOLOGY	Transmural inflammation → fistulas. **Cobblestone** mucosa, creeping **fat**, bowel wall thickening ("string sign" on barium swallow x-ray **A**), linear ulcers, fissures.	Mucosal and submucosal inflammation only. Friable mucosal pseudopolyps with freely hanging mesentery **B**. Loss of haustra → "lead pipe" appearance on imaging.
MICROSCOPIC MORPHOLOGY	Noncaseating **granulomas** and lymphoid aggregates (Th_1 mediated).	Crypt abscesses and ulcers, bleeding, no granulomas (Th_2 mediated).
COMPLICATIONS	Strictures (leading to obstruction), fistulas, perianal disease, malabsorption, nutritional depletion, colorectal cancer, gallstones.	Malnutrition, sclerosing cholangitis, toxic megacolon, colorectal carcinoma (worse with right-sided colitis or pancolitis).
INTESTINAL MANIFESTATION	Diarrhea that may or may not be bloody.	Bloody diarrhea.
EXTRAINTESTINAL MANIFESTATIONS	Migratory polyarthritis, erythema nodosum, ankylosing spondylitis, pyoderma gangrenosum, aphthous ulcers, uveitis, kidney stones.	Pyoderma gangrenosum, erythema nodosum, 1° sclerosing cholangitis, ankylosing spondylitis, apthous ulcers, uveitis.
TREATMENT	Corticosteroids, azathioprine, methotrexate, infliximab, adalimumab.	ASA preparations (sulfasalazine), 6-mercaptopurine, infliximab, colectomy.
	For **Crohn**, think of a **fat granny** and an old **crone skipping** down a **cobblestone** road away from the **wreck** (rectal sparing).	Ulcerative colitis causes **ULCCCERS**: Ulcers Large intestine Continuous, Colorectal carcinoma, Crypt abscesses Extends proximally Red diarrhea Sclerosing cholangitis

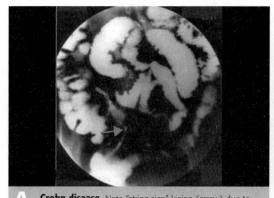

A **Crohn disease.** Note "string sign" lesion (arrow) due to wall thickening, which narrows the contrast-filled lumen. ✱

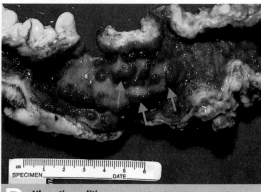

B **Ulcerative colitis.** Note pseudopolyps (arrows) with intervening ulcerated, inflamed mucosa. True polyps typically separated by healthy mucosa. ℞

String sign:
▸ Bowel wall thickening causing narrowing of the lumen.

Sclerosing cholangitis:
▸ leads to liver damage & need for an eventual liver transplant due to inflammation of the bile ducts → leading to their hardening & scarring from the chronic inflammation.

Irritable bowel syndrome	Recurrent abdominal pain associated with ≥ 2 of the following:
	▪ Pain improves with defecation
	▪ Change in stool frequency
	▪ Change in appearance of stool
	No structural abnormalities. Most common in middle-aged women. Chronic symptoms. May present with diarrhea, constipation, or alternating symptoms. Pathophysiology is multifaceted. Treat symptoms.

Appendicitis	Acute inflammation of the appendix due to obstruction by fecalith (in adults) or lymphoid hyperplasia (in children).
	Initial diffuse periumbilical pain migrates to McBurney point (¹⁄₃ the distance from anterior superior iliac spine to umbilicus). Nausea, fever; may perforate → peritonitis; may see psoas, obturator, and Rovsing signs.
	Differential: diverticulitis (elderly), ectopic pregnancy (use β-hCG to rule out).
	Treatment: appendectomy.

psoas = extend hip
obturator - int. rot. of hip.
Rovsing = press on ⓛ

Diverticula of the GI tract

Diverticulum	Blind pouch 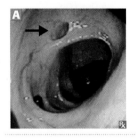 protruding from the alimentary tract that communicates with the lumen of the gut. Most diverticula (esophagus, stomach, duodenum, colon) are acquired and are termed "false" in that they lack or have an attenuated muscularis externa. Most often in sigmoid colon.	"True" diverticulum—all 3 gut wall layers outpouch (e.g., Meckel). "False" diverticulum or pseudodiverticulum— only mucosa and submucosa outpouch. Occur especially where vasa recta perforate muscularis externa.

＊Need muscularis externa to be a true diverticulum.

Diverticulosis	Many false diverticula of the colon, commonly sigmoid. Common (in ~50% of people > 60 years). Caused by ↑ intraluminal pressure and focal weakness in colonic wall. Associated with low-fiber diets.	Often asymptomatic or associated with vague discomfort. A common cause of hematochezia. Complications include diverticulitis, fistulas.

Diverticulitis	Inflammation of diverticula classically causing LLQ pain, fever, leukocytosis 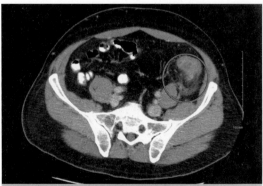. May perforate → peritonitis, abscess formation, or bowel stenosis. Give antibiotics. Stool occult blood is common +/– hematochezia. May also cause colovesical fistula (fistula with bladder) → pneumaturia. Sometimes called "left-sided appendicitis" due to overlapping clinical presentation.	

B **Diverticulitis.** CT shows inflammation surrounding segment of colon (circled) in left lower quadrant.

Zenker diverticulum

Pharyngoesophageal **false** diverticulum 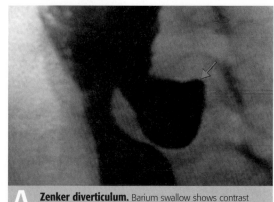. Herniation of mucosal tissue at Killian triangle between the thyropharyngeal and cricopharyngeal parts of the inferior pharyngeal constrictor. Presenting symptoms: dysphagia, obstruction, foul breath from trapped food particles (halitosis). Most common in elderly males.

A **Zenker diverticulum.** Barium swallow shows contrast filling false diverticulum (arrow) originating from posterior esophagus. ✳

Meckel diverticulum

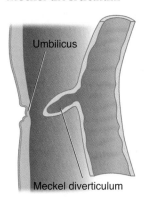

True diverticulum. Persistence of the vitelline duct. May contain ectopic acid–secreting gastric mucosa and/or pancreatic tissue. Most common congenital anomaly of the GI tract. Can cause melena, RLQ pain, intussusception, volvulus, or obstruction near the terminal ileum. Contrast with omphalomesenteric cyst = cystic dilation of vitelline duct.
Diagnosis: pertechnetate study for uptake by ectopic gastric mucosa.

The **five** 2's:
2 inches long.
2 feet from the ileocecal valve.
2% of population.
Commonly presents in first 2 years of life.
May have 2 types of epithelia (gastric/pancreatic).

Intussusception and volvulus

Intussusception

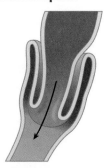

"Telescoping" of 1 bowel segment into distal segment, commonly at ileocecal junction. Compromised blood supply → intermittent abdominal pain often with "currant jelly" stools. Unusual in adults (associated with intraluminal mass or tumor that acts as lead point that is pulled into the lumen). Majority of cases occur in children (usually idiopathic; may be associated with recent enteric or respiratory viral infection). Abdominal emergency in early childhood.

Volvulus

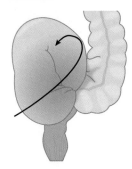

Twisting of portion of bowel around its mesentery; can lead to obstruction and infarction. Can occur throughout the GI tract. Midgut volvulus more common in infants and children. Sigmoid volvulus more common in elderly.

Hirschsprung disease

Congenital megacolon characterized by lack of ganglion cells/enteric nervous plexuses (Auerbach and Meissner plexuses) in segment on intestinal biopsy. Due to failure of neural crest cell migration. Associated with mutations in the *RET* gene.

Presents with bilious emesis, abdominal distention, and failure to pass meconium in the first 48 hours of life, ultimately manifesting as chronic constipation. Dilated portion of the colon proximal to the aganglionic segment, resulting in a "transition zone." Involves rectum.

Think of Hirsch**sprung** as a giant spring that has **sprung** in the colon. Risk ↑ with Down syndrome.

Diagnosed by rectal suction biopsy.

Treatment: resection.

Other intestinal disorders

Adhesion	Fibrous band of scar tissue; commonly forms after surgery; most common cause of small bowel obstruction. Can have well-demarcated necrotic zones.
Angiodysplasia	Tortuous dilation of vessels → hematochezia. Most often found in cecum, terminal ileum, and ascending colon. More common in older patients. Confirmed by angiography.
Duodenal atresia	Causes early bilious vomiting with proximal stomach distention ("double bubble" on X-ray) because of failure of small bowel recanalization. Associated with Down syndrome.
Ileus	Intestinal hypomotility without obstruction → constipation and ↓ flatus; distended/tympanic abdomen with ↓ bowel sounds. Associated with abdominal surgeries, opiates, hypokalemia, and sepsis.
Ischemic colitis	Reduction in intestinal blood flow causes ischemia. Pain after eating → weight loss. Commonly occurs at splenic flexure and distal colon. Typically affects elderly.
Meconium ileus	In cystic fibrosis, meconium plug obstructs intestine, preventing stool passage at birth.
Necrotizing enterocolitis	Necrosis of intestinal mucosa and possible perforation. Colon is usually involved, but can involve entire GI tract. In neonates, more common in preemies (↓ immunity).

Colonic polyps	Masses protruding into gut lumen → sawtooth appearance. 90% are non-neoplastic. Often rectosigmoid. Can be tubular **A** or villous **B**.
Adenomatous	Adenomatous polyps are precancerous. Malignant risk is associated with ↑ size, villous histology, ↑ epithelial dysplasia. Precursor to colorectal cancer (CRC). The more villous the polyp, the more likely it is to be malignant (**villous = villainous**). Polyp symptoms—often asymptomatic, lower GI bleed, partial obstruction, secretory diarrhea (villous adenomas).
Hyperplastic	Most common non-neoplastic polyp in colon (> 50% found in rectosigmoid colon).
Juvenile	Mostly sporadic lesions in children < 5 years old. 80% in rectum. If single, no malignant potential. Juvenile polyposis syndrome—multiple juvenile polyps in GI tract, ↑ risk of adenocarcinoma.
Hamartomatous	Peutz-Jeghers syndrome—autosomal dominant syndrome featuring multiple nonmalignant hamartomas throughout GI tract, along with hyperpigmented mouth, lips, hands, genitalia. Associated with ↑ risk of CRC and other visceral malignancies.

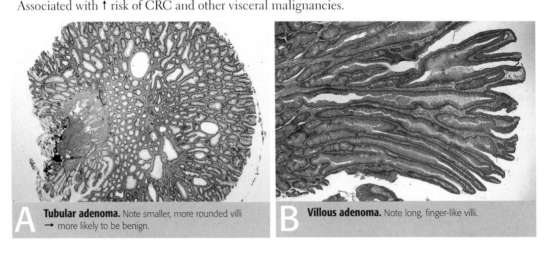

A **Tubular adenoma.** Note smaller, more rounded villi → more likely to be benign.

B **Villous adenoma.** Note long, finger-like villi.

Colorectal cancer

EPIDEMIOLOGY	Most patients are > 50 years old. ~ 25% have a family history.
GENETICS	**Familial adenomatous polyposis (FAP)**—autosomal dominant mutation of *APC* gene on chromosome 5q. 2-hit hypothesis. 100% progress to CRC unless colon is resected. Thousands of polyps arise starting at a young age; pancolonic; always involves rectum. **Gardner syndrome**—FAP + osseous and soft tissue tumors, congenital hypertrophy of retinal pigment epithelium. **Turcot syndrome**—FAP + malignant CNS tumor. Turcot = Turban. **Hereditary nonpolyposis colorectal cancer (HNPCC/Lynch syndrome)**—autosomal dominant mutation of DNA mismatch repair genes. ~ 80% progress to CRC. Proximal colon is always involved.
ADDITIONAL RISK FACTORS	IBD, tobacco use, large villous adenomas, juvenile polyposis syndrome, Peutz-Jeghers syndrome.
PRESENTATION	Rectosigmoid > ascending > descending. Ascending—exophytic mass, iron deficiency anemia, weight loss. Descending—infiltrating mass, partial obstruction, colicky pain, hematochezia. Rarely presents as *Streptococcus bovis* bacteremia.
DIAGNOSIS	Iron deficiency anemia in males (especially > 50 years old) and postmenopausal females raises suspicion. Screen patients > 50 years old with colonoscopy or stool occult blood test. "Apple core" lesion seen on barium enema x-ray **A**. CEA tumor marker: good for monitoring recurrence, not useful for screening.

Right side bleeds; left side obstructs.

A "Apple core" lesion. Seen here in the sigmoid colon (arrow). ℞

Molecular pathogenesis of CRC	There are 2 molecular pathways that lead to CRC: ▪ Microsatellite instability pathway (~15%): DNA mismatch repair gene mutations → sporadic and HNPCC syndrome. Mutations accumulate, but no defined morphologic correlates. ▪ APC/β-catenin (chromosomal instability) pathway (~85%) → sporadic cancer.	Order of gene events—AK-53.

Loss of *APC* gene   *K-RAS* mutation   Loss of tumor suppressor gene(s) (*p*53, DCC)

Normal colon → Colon at risk → Adenoma → Carcinoma

Decreased intercellular adhesion and increased proliferation   Unregulated intracellular signal transduction   Increased tumorigenesis

Cirrhosis and portal hypertension

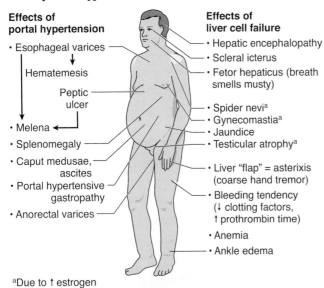

Effects of portal hypertension

- Esophageal varices
  ↓
  Hematemesis
  ↓
- Melena ←── Peptic ulcer
- Splenomegaly
- Caput medusae, ascites
- Portal hypertensive gastropathy
- Anorectal varices

ᵃDue to ↑ estrogen

Effects of liver cell failure

- Hepatic encephalopathy
- Scleral icterus
- Fetor hepaticus (breath smells musty)
- Spider neviᵃ
- Gynecomastiaᵃ
- Jaundice
- Testicular atrophyᵃ
- Liver "flap" = asterixis (coarse hand tremor)
- Bleeding tendency (↓ clotting factors, ↑ prothrombin time)
- Anemia
- Ankle edema

Cirrhosis—diffuse fibrosis and nodular regeneration destroys normal architecture of liver **A** **B**; ↑ risk for hepatocellular carcinoma (HCC).

Etiologies—alcohol (60–70%), viral hepatitis, biliary disease, hemochromatosis.

Portosystemic shunts partially alleviate portal hypertension:

- Esophageal varices
- Caput medusae

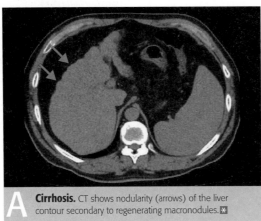

A Cirrhosis. CT shows nodularity (arrows) of the liver contour secondary to regenerating macronodules. ✳

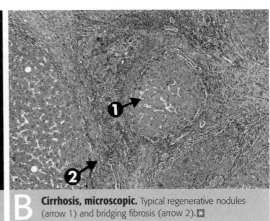

B Cirrhosis, microscopic. Typical regenerative nodules (arrow 1) and bridging fibrosis (arrow 2). ✳

Serum markers of liver and pancreas pathology

SERUM MARKER	MAJOR DIAGNOSTIC USE
Alkaline phosphatase (ALP)	Obstructive hepatobiliary disease, HCC, bone disease
Aminotransferases (AST and ALT) (often called "liver enzymes")	Viral hepatitis (ALT > AST) Alcoholic hepatitis (AST > ALT)
Amylase	Acute pancreatitis, mumps
Ceruloplasmin	↓ in Wilson disease
γ-glutamyl transpeptidase (GGT)	↑ in various liver and biliary diseases (just as ALP can), but **not** in bone disease; associated with alcohol use
Lipase	Acute pancreatitis (most specific)

Reye syndrome	Rare, often fatal childhood hepatoencephalopathy. Findings: mitochondrial abnormalities, fatty liver (microvesicular fatty change), hypoglycemia, vomiting, hepatomegaly, coma. Associated with viral infection (especially VZV and influenza B) that has been treated with aspirin. Mechanism: aspirin metabolites ↓ β-oxidation by reversible inhibition of mitochondrial enzyme. Avoid aspirin in children, except in those with Kawasaki disease.

Alcoholic liver disease

Hepatic steatosis	Reversible change with moderate alcohol intake. Macrovesicular fatty change 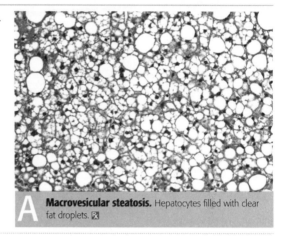 that may be reversible with alcohol cessation.	

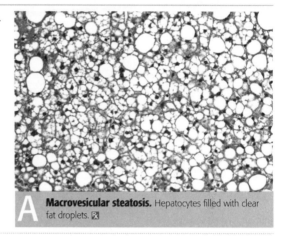

A **Macrovesicular steatosis.** Hepatocytes filled with clear fat droplets.

Alcoholic hepatitis	Requires sustained, long-term consumption. Swollen and necrotic hepatocytes with neutrophilic infiltration. Mallory bodies (intracytoplasmic eosinophilic inclusions) are present.	Make a toAST with alcohol: AST > ALT (ratio usually > 1.5).
Alcoholic cirrhosis	Final and irreversible form. Micronodular, irregularly shrunken liver with "hobnail" appearance. Sclerosis around central vein (zone III). Has manifestations of chronic liver disease (e.g., jaundice, hypoalbuminemia).	

Non-alcoholic fatty liver disease	Metabolic syndrome (insulin resistance) → fatty infiltration of hepatocytes → cellular "ballooning" and eventual necrosis. May cause cirrhosis and HCC. Independent of alcohol use.	ALT > AST (Lipids)

Hepatic encephalopathy	Cirrhosis → portosystemic shunts → ↓ NH_3 metabolism → neuropsychiatric dysfunction. Spectrum from disorientation/asterixis (mild) to difficult arousal or coma (severe). Triggers: ▪ ↑ NH_3 production (due to dietary protein, GI bleed, constipation, infection). ▪ ↓ NH_3 removal (due to renal failure, diuretics, post-TIPS). Treatment: lactulose (↑ NH_4^+ generation), low-protein diet, and rifaximin (kills intestinal bacteria).

Hepatocellular carcinoma/hepatoma

Most common 1° malignant tumor of the liver in adults 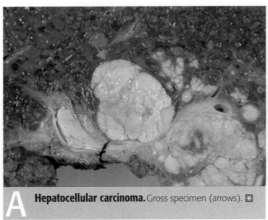. Associated with hepatitis B and C, Wilson disease, hemochromatosis, α_1-antitrypsin deficiency, alcoholic cirrhosis, and carcinogens (e.g., aflatoxin from *Aspergillus*). May lead to Budd-Chiari syndrome.

Findings: jaundice, tender hepatomegaly 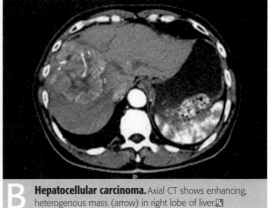, ascites, and anorexia. Spreads hematogenously.

Diagnosis: ↑ α-fetoprotein; ultrasound or contrast CT.

Hepatocellular carcinoma. Gross specimen (arrows). ✱

Hepatocellular carcinoma. Axial CT shows enhancing, heterogenous mass (arrow) in right lobe of liver.℞

Other liver tumors

Cavernous hemangioma	Common, benign liver tumor; typically occurs at age 30–50 years. Biopsy contraindicated because of risk of hemorrhage.
Hepatic adenoma	Rare, benign liver tumor, often related to oral contraceptive or anabolic steroid use; may regress spontaneously or rupture (abdominal pain and shock).
Angiosarcoma	Malignant tumor of endothelial origin; associated with exposure to arsenic, vinyl chloride.

Nutmeg liver

Due to backup of blood into liver. Commonly caused by right-sided heart failure and Budd-Chiari syndrome. The liver appears mottled like a nutmeg. If the condition persists, centrilobular congestion and necrosis can result in cardiac cirrhosis.

Budd-Chiari syndrome

Occlusion of IVC or hepatic veins with centrilobular congestion and necrosis, leading to congestive liver disease (hepatomegaly, ascites, abdominal pain, and eventual liver failure). May develop varices and have visible abdominal and back veins. Absence of JVD. Associated with hypercoagulable states, polycythemia vera, pregnancy, and HCC.

α₁-antitrypsin deficiency	Misfolded gene product protein aggregates in hepatocellular ER → cirrhosis with PAS ⊕ globules in liver. Codominant trait.	In lungs, ↓ α₁-antitrypsin → uninhibited elastase in alveoli → ↓ elastic tissue → panacinar emphysema.

Jaundice

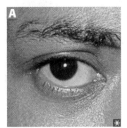

Abnormal yellowing of the skin and/or sclera **A** due to bilirubin deposition. Occurs at high bilirubin levels (> 2.5 mg/dL) in the blood 2° to ↑ production or defective metabolism.

	Unconjugated (indirect) hyperbilirubinemia	Conjugated (direct) hyperbilirubinemia	Mixed (direct and indirect) hyperbilirubinemia
URINE UROBILINOGEN	↑	↓	Normal/↑
DISEASES	Hemolytic, physiologic (newborns), Crigler-Najjar, Gilbert syndrome	Biliary tract obstruction: gallstones, pancreatic liver cancer, liver fluke Biliary tract disease: 1° sclerosing cholangitis, 1° biliary cirrhosis Excretion defect: Dubin-Johnson syndrome, Rotor syndrome	Hepatitis, cirrhosis

Physiologic neonatal jaundice	At birth, immature UDP-glucuronosyltransferase → unconjugated hyperbilirubinemia → jaundice/kernicterus. Treatment: phototherapy (converts unconjugated bilirubin to water-soluble form).

Hereditary hyperbilirubinemias

❶ **Gilbert syndrome**	Mildly ↓ UDP-glucuronosyltransferase conjugation activity → ↓ bilirubin uptake by hepatocytes. Asymptomatic or mild jaundice. Elevated unconjugated bilirubin without overt hemolysis. Bilirubin ↑ with fasting and stress.	Very common. No clinical consequences.
❷ **Crigler-Najjar syndrome, type I**	Absent UDP-glucuronosyltransferase. Presents early in life; patients die within a few years. Findings: jaundice, kernicterus (bilirubin deposition in brain), ↑ unconjugated bilirubin. Treatment: plasmapheresis and phototherapy.	Type II is less severe and responds to phenobarbital, which ↑ liver enzyme synthesis.
❸ **Dubin-Johnson syndrome**	Conjugated hyperbilirubinemia due to defective liver excretion. Grossly black liver. Benign.	❹ **Rotor syndrome** is similar but even milder and does not cause black liver.

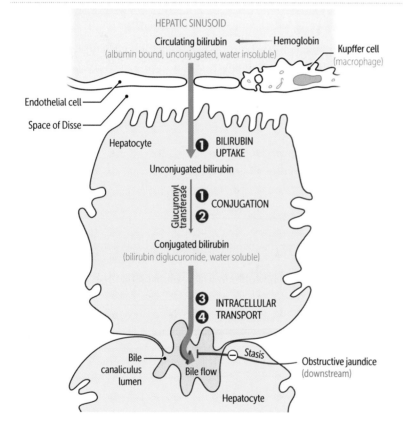

❶ **Gilbert** = problem with bilirubin uptake → unconjugated bilirubinemia

❷ **Crigler-Najjar** = problem with bilirubin conjugation → unconjugated bilirubinemia

❸ **Dubin-Johnson** = problem with excretion of conjugated bilirubin → conjugated bilirubinemia

❹ **Rotor** = mild conjugated hyperbilirubinemia

Wilson disease (hepatolenticular degeneration)

Inadequate hepatic copper excretion and failure of copper to enter circulation as ceruloplasmin. Leads to **copper** accumulation, especially in liver, brain, cornea, kidneys, and joints.

Characterized by:
  ↓ Ceruloplasmin, Cirrhosis, Corneal deposits (Kayser-Fleischer rings) 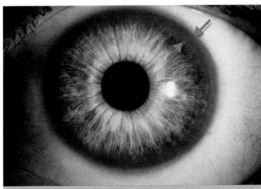, Copper accumulation, Carcinoma (hepatocellular)
  Hemolytic anemia
  Basal ganglia degeneration (parkinsonian symptoms)
  Asterixis
  Dementia, Dyskinesia, Dysarthria

Treat with penicillamine or trientine. Autosomal recessive inheritance (chromosome 13). Copper is normally excreted into bile by hepatocyte copper transporting ATPase (*ATP7B* gene).

"Copper is Hella BAD."

A **Kayser-Fleischer ring.** Note golden brown corneal ring (arrows).

Hemochromatosis

Hemosiderosis is the deposition of hemosiderin (iron); hemochromatosis is the disease caused by this iron deposition. Classic triad of micronodular Cirrhosis, Diabetes mellitus, and skin pigmentation → "bronze" diabetes. Results in CHF, testicular atrophy, and ↑ risk of HCC. Disease may be 1° (autosomal recessive) or 2° to chronic transfusion therapy (e.g., β-thalassemia major). ↑ ferritin, ↑ iron, ↓ TIBC → ↑ transferrin saturation.

Hemochromatosis Can Cause Deposits.
Total body iron may reach 50 g, enough to set off metal detectors at airports.
Primary hemochromatosis due to C282Y or H63D mutation on *HFE* gene. Associated with HLA-A3.
Iron loss through menstruation slows progression in women.
Treatment of hereditary hemochromatosis: repeated phlebotomy, deferasirox, deferoxamine.

Biliary tract disease

	Secondary biliary cirrhosis	Primary biliary cirrhosis	Primary sclerosing cholangitis
PATHOPHYSIOLOGY/ PATHOLOGY	Extrahepatic biliary obstruction (gallstone, biliary stricture, chronic pancreatitis, carcinoma of the pancreatic head) → ↑ pressure in intrahepatic ducts → injury/ fibrosis and bile stasis.	Autoimmune reaction → lymphocytic infiltrate + granulomas → destruction of intralobular bile ducts.	Unknown cause of concentric "onion skin" bile duct fibrosis → alternating strictures and dilation with "beading" of intra- and extrahepatic bile ducts on ERCP.
PRESENTATION	Pruritus, jaundice, dark urine, light stools, hepatosplenomegaly.	Same.	Same.
LABS	↑ conjugated bilirubin, ↑ cholesterol, ↑ ALP.	Same.	Same.
ADDITIONAL INFORMATION	Complicated by ascending cholangitis.	↑ serum mitochondrial antibodies, including IgM. Associated with other autoimmune conditions (e.g., CREST, Sjögren syndrome, rheumatoid arthritis, celiac disease).	Hypergammaglobulinemia (IgM). Associated with ulcerative colitis. Can lead to 2° biliary cirrhosis and cholangiocarcinoma.

Gallstones (cholelithiasis)

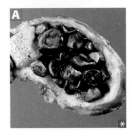

↑ cholesterol and/or bilirubin, ↓ bile salts, and gallbladder stasis all cause stones .

2 types of stones:

- Cholesterol stones (radiolucent with 10–20% opaque due to calcifications)—80% of stones. Associated with obesity, Crohn disease, cystic fibrosis, advanced age, clofibrate, estrogen therapy, multiparity, rapid weight loss, and Native American origin.
- Pigment stones (black = radiopaque, hemolysis; brown = radiolucent, infection)—seen in patients with chronic hemolysis, alcoholic cirrhosis, advanced age, and biliary infection.

Most often causes cholecystitis; also ascending cholangitis, acute pancreatitis, bile stasis.

Can also lead to **biliary colic**—neurohormonal activation (e.g., by CCK after a fatty meal) triggers contraction of the gallbladder, forcing a stone into the cystic duct. May present without pain (e.g., in diabetics).

Can cause fistula between gallbladder and small intestine, leading to air in the biliary tree. Gallstone may obstruct ileocecal valve → gallstone ileus.

Diagnose with ultrasound 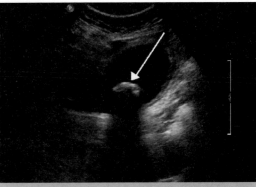. Treat with cholecystectomy if symptomatic.

Risk factors (4 F's):
1. Female
2. Fat
3. Fertile (pregnant)
4. Forty

Charcot triad of cholangitis:
- Jaundice
- Fever
- RUQ pain

B **Cholelithiasis.** Ultrasound of distended gallbladder containing large gallstone (arrow). ✱

Cholecystitis

Acute or chronic inflammation of gallbladder. Usually from cholelithiasis (gallstones 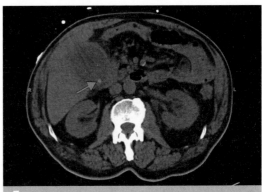); most commonly blocking the cystic duct → 2° infection; rarely ischemia or 1° infection (CMV). Murphy sign ⊕—inspiratory arrest on RUQ palpation due to pain. ↑ ALP if bile duct becomes involved (e.g., ascending cholangitis). Diagnose with ultrasound or HIDA.

A **Acute cholecystitis.** Axial CT shows thick-walled gallbladder with stone at neck (arrow). ✗

Porcelain gallbladder

Calcified gallbladder due to chronic cholecystitis; usually found incidentally on imaging A. Treatment: prophylactic cholecystectomy due to high rates of gallbladder carcinoma.

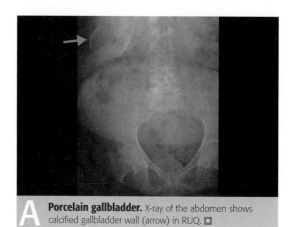

A **Porcelain gallbladder.** X-ray of the abdomen shows calcified gallbladder wall (arrow) in RUQ. ✳

Acute pancreatitis

Autodigestion of pancreas by pancreatic enzymes A.

Causes: idiopathic, Gallstones, Ethanol, Trauma, Steroids, Mumps, Autoimmune disease, Scorpion sting, Hypercalcemia/Hypertriglyceridemia (> 1000 mg/dL), ERCP, Drugs (e.g., sulfa drugs).

Clinical presentation: epigastric abdominal pain radiating to back, anorexia, nausea.

Labs: ↑ amylase, lipase (higher specificity).

Can lead to DIC, ARDS, diffuse fat necrosis, hypocalcemia (Ca^{2+} collects in pancreatic calcium soap deposits), pseudocyst formation, hemorrhage, infection, and multiorgan failure.

Complication: pancreatic pseudocyst (lined by granulation tissue, not epithelium; can rupture and hemorrhage).

GET SMASHED.

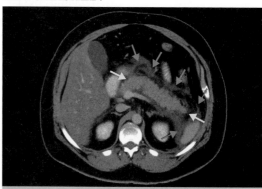

A **Acute pancreatitis.** Axial CT shows acute exudative pancreatitis with extensive fluid collections (red arrows) surrounding the pancreas (yellow arrows). ✳

Chronic pancreatitis

Chronic inflammation, atrophy, calcification of the pancreas A. Major causes are alcohol abuse and idiopathic.

Can lead to pancreatic insufficiency → steatorrhea, fat-soluble vitamin deficiency, diabetes mellitus, and ↑ risk of pancreatic adenocarcinoma.

Amylase and lipase may or may not be elevated (almost always elevated in acute pancreatitis).

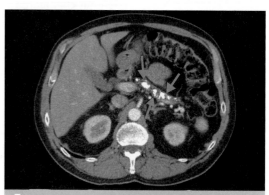

A **Chronic pancreatitis.** Near complete atrophy of the pancreas with residual coarse calcifications. ✳

Pancreatic adenocarcinoma

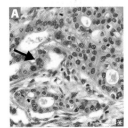

Prognosis averages 1 year; very aggressive tumor arising from pancreatic ducts (disorganized glandular structure with cellular infiltration 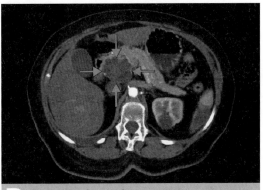...); already metastasized at presentation; tumors more common in pancreatic head (→ obstructive jaundice). Associated with CA-19-9 tumor marker (also CEA, less specific).

Risk factors:

- Tobacco use
- Chronic pancreatitis (especially > 20 years)
- Diabetes
- Age > 50 years
- Jewish and African-American males

Often presents with:

- Abdominal pain radiating to back
- Weight loss (due to malabsorption and anorexia)
- Migratory thrombophlebitis—redness and tenderness on palpation of extremities (**Trousseau syndrome**)
- Obstructive jaundice with palpable, nontender gallbladder (Courvoisier sign)

Treatment: Whipple procedure, chemotherapy, radiation therapy.

Pancreatic adenocarcinoma. Large lobulated low-density mass in the head of the pancreas (arrows).

GI therapy

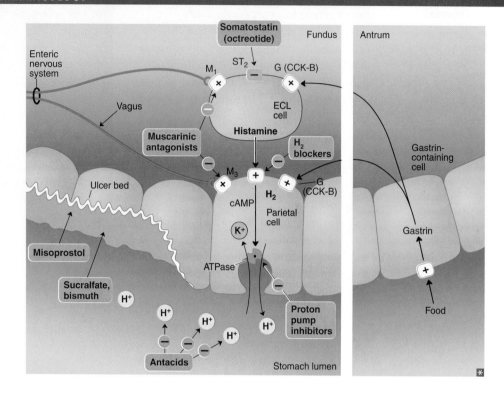

H₂ blockers	Cimetidine, ranitidine, famotidine, nizatidine.	Take H₂ blockers before you **dine**. Think "table for 2" to remember H_2.
MECHANISM	Reversible block of histamine H_2-receptors → ↓ H^+ secretion by parietal cells.	
CLINICAL USE	Peptic ulcer, gastritis, mild esophageal reflux.	
TOXICITY	Cimetidine is a potent inhibitor of cytochrome P-450 (multiple drug interactions); it also has antiandrogenic effects (prolactin release, gynecomastia, impotence, ↓ libido in males); can cross blood-brain barrier (confusion, dizziness, headaches) and placenta. Both cimetidine and ranitidine ↓ renal excretion of creatinine. Other H_2 blockers are relatively free of these effects.	

Proton pump inhibitors	Omeprazole, lansoprazole, esomeprazole, pantoprazole, dexlansoprazole.
MECHANISM	Irreversibly inhibit H^+/K^+ ATPase in stomach parietal cells.
CLINICAL USE	Peptic ulcer, gastritis, esophageal reflux, Zollinger-Ellison syndrome.
TOXICITY	Increased risk of *C. difficile* infection, pneumonia. Hip fractures, ↓ serum Mg^{2+} with long-term use.

Bismuth, sucralfate	
MECHANISM	Bind to ulcer base, providing physical protection and allowing HCO_3^- secretion to reestablish pH gradient in the mucous layer.
CLINICAL USE	↑ ulcer healing, travelers' diarrhea.

Misoprostol	
MECHANISM	A PGE_1 analog. ↑ production and secretion of gastric mucous barrier, ↓ acid production.
CLINICAL USE	Prevention of NSAID-induced peptic ulcers (NSAIDs block PGE_1 production); maintenance of a PDA. Also used to induce labor (ripens cervix).
TOXICITY	Diarrhea. Contraindicated in women of childbearing potential (abortifacient).

Octreotide	
MECHANISM	Long-acting somatostatin analog.
CLINICAL USE	Acute variceal bleeds, acromegaly, VIPoma, and carcinoid tumors.
TOXICITY	Nausea, cramps, steatorrhea.

Antacid use	Can affect absorption, bioavailability, or urinary excretion of other drugs by altering gastric and urinary pH or by delaying gastric emptying. All can cause hypokalemia. Overuse can also cause the following problems.	
Aluminum hydroxide	Constipation and hypophosphatemia; proximal muscle weakness, osteodystrophy, seizures	Alu**minimum** amount of feces.
Calcium carbonate	Hypercalcemia, rebound acid ↑	Can chelate and ↓ effectiveness of other drugs (e.g., tetracycline).
Magnesium hydroxide	Diarrhea, hyporeflexia, hypotension, cardiac arrest	**Mg** = **M**ust **g**o to the bathroom.

Osmotic laxatives

Magnesium hydroxide, magnesium citrate, polyethylene glycol, lactulose.

MECHANISM	Provide osmotic load to draw water out. Lactulose also treats hepatic encephalopathy since gut flora degrade it into metabolites (lactic acid and acetic acid) that promote nitrogen excretion as NH_4^+.
CLINICAL USE	Constipation.
TOXICITY	Diarrhea, dehydration; may be abused by bulimics.

Infliximab

MECHANISM	Monoclonal antibody to TNF-α.
CLINICAL USE	Crohn disease, ulcerative colitis, rheumatoid arthritis, ankylosing spondylitis, psoriasis.
TOXICITY	Infection (including reactivation of latent TB), fever, hypotension.

Sulfasalazine

MECHANISM	A combination of sulfapyridine (antibacterial) and 5-aminosalicylic acid (anti-inflammatory). Activated by colonic bacteria.
CLINICAL USE	Ulcerative colitis, Crohn disease.
TOXICITY	Malaise, nausea, sulfonamide toxicity, reversible oligospermia.

Ondansetron

MECHANISM	5-HT$_3$ antagonist; ↓ vagal stimulation. Powerful central-acting antiemetic.
CLINICAL USE	Control vomiting postoperatively and in patients undergoing cancer chemotherapy.
TOXICITY	Headache, constipation.

At a party but feeling queasy? Keep **on dancing** with **ondansetron**!

Metoclopramide

MECHANISM	D$_2$ receptor antagonist. ↑ resting tone, contractility, LES tone, motility. Does not influence colon transport time.
CLINICAL USE	Diabetic and post-surgery gastroparesis, antiemetic.
TOXICITY	↑ parkinsonian effects. Restlessness, drowsiness, fatigue, depression, nausea, diarrhea. Drug interaction with digoxin and diabetic agents. Contraindicated in patients with small bowel obstruction or Parkinson disease (D$_1$-receptor blockade).

Hematology and Oncology

"Of all that is written, I love only what a person has written with his own blood."

—Friedrich Nietzsche

"I used to get stressed out, but my cancer has put everything into perspective."

—Delta Goodrem

"The best blood will at some time get into a fool or a mosquito."

—Austin O'Malley

Study tip: When reviewing oncologic drugs, focus on mechanisms and side effects rather than details of clinical uses, which may be lower yield.

▶ HEMATOLOGY AND ONCOLOGY—ANATOMY

Erythrocyte

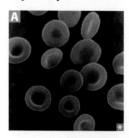

Carries O_2 to tissues and CO_2 to lungs. Anucleate and biconcave **A**, with large surface area-to-volume ratio for rapid gas exchange. Life span of 120 days. Source of energy is glucose (90% used in glycolysis, 10% used in HMP shunt). Membrane contains chloride-HCO_3^- antiporter, which allows RBCs to export HCO_3^- and transport CO_2 from the periphery to the lungs for elimination.

Eryth = red; *cyte* = cell.

Erythrocytosis = polycythemia = ↑ hematocrit.
Anisocytosis = varying sizes.
Poikilocytosis = varying shapes.

Reticulocyte = immature erythrocyte, marker of erythroid proliferation.

Platelet (thrombocyte)

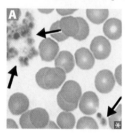

Involved in 1° hemostasis. Small cytoplasmic fragment **A** derived from megakaryocytes. Life span of 8–10 days. When activated by endothelial injury, aggregates with other platelets and interacts with fibrinogen to form platelet plug. Contains dense granules (ADP, calcium) and α granules (vWF, fibrinogen). Approximately ⅓ of platelet pool is stored in the spleen.

Thrombocytopenia or ↓ platelet function results in petechiae.
vWF receptor: GpIb.
Fibrinogen receptor: GpIIb/IIIa.

Leukocyte

Divided into granulocytes (neutrophil, eosinophil, basophil) and mononuclear cells (monocytes, lymphocytes). Responsible for defense against infections. Normally 4000–10,000 cells/mm³.
WBC differential from highest to lowest (normal ranges per USMLE):
    Neutrophils (54–62%)
    Lymphocytes (25–33%)
    Monocytes (3–7%)
    Eosinophils (1–3%)
    Basophils (0–0.75%)

Leuk = white; *cyte* = cell.

Neutrophils **L**ike **M**aking **E**verything **B**etter.

Neutrophil

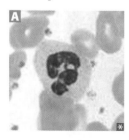

Acute inflammatory response cell. Increased in bacterial infections. Phagocytic. Multilobed nucleus **A**. Small, more numerous specific granules contain ALP, collagenase, lysozyme, and lactoferrin. Larger, less numerous azurophilic granules (lysosomes) contain proteinases, acid phosphatase, myeloperoxidase, and β-glucuronidase.

Hypersegmented polys (5 or more lobes) are seen in vitamin B_{12}/ folate deficiency.
↑ band cells (immature neutrophils) reflect states of ↑ myeloid proliferation (bacterial infections, CML).

Monocyte

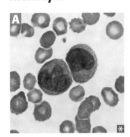

Differentiates into macrophages in tissues. Large, kidney-shaped nucleus A. Extensive "frosted glass" cytoplasm.

Mono = one (nucleus); *cyte* = cell.
Monocyte: in the blood.

Macrophage

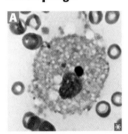

Phagocytoses bacteria, cellular debris, and senescent RBCs and scavenges damaged cells and tissues A. Long life in tissues. Macrophages differentiate from circulating blood monocytes. Activated by γ-interferon. Can function as antigen-presenting cell via MHC II. CD14 is a cell surface marker for macrophages.

Macro = large; *phage* = eater.
Important component of granuloma formation (e.g., TB, sarcoidosis).
Macrophage: in the tissue.

Eosinophil

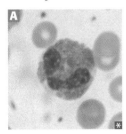

Defends against helminthic infections (major basic protein). Bilobate nucleus. Packed with large eosinophilic granules of uniform size A. Highly phagocytic for antigen-antibody complexes.
Produces histaminase and arylsulfatase (helps limit reaction following mast cell degranulation).

Eosin = a dye; *philic* = loving.
Causes of eosinophilia = **NAACP**:
   Neoplasia
   Asthma
   Allergic processes
   Connective tissue diseases
   Parasites (invasive)

Basophil

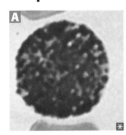

Mediates allergic reaction. Densely basophilic granules A containing heparin (anticoagulant), histamine (vasodilator), and leukotrienes.

Basophilic—staining readily with **basic** stains.
Isolated basophilia is uncommon, but can be a sign of myeloproliferative disease, particularly CML.

Mast cell

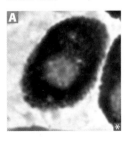

Mediates allergic reaction in local tissues. Mast cells resemble basophils structurally and functionally but are not the same cell type A. Can bind the Fc portion of IgE to membrane. IgE cross-links upon antigen binding, causing degranulation, which releases histamine, heparin, and eosinophil chemotactic factors.

Involved in type I hypersensitivity reactions. Cromolyn sodium prevents mast cell degranulation (used for asthma prophylaxis).

Dendritic cell

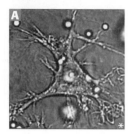

Highly phagocytic APCs . Functions as link between innate and adaptive immune systems. Expresses MHC class II and Fc receptor on surface. Called Langerhans cell in the skin.

Lymphocyte

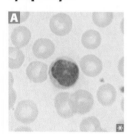

Divided into B cells, T cells, and NK cells. B cells and T cells mediate adaptive immunity. NK cells are part of the innate immune response. Round, densely staining nucleus with small amount of pale cytoplasm A.

B lymphocyte

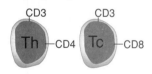

Part of humoral immune response. Arises from stem cells in bone marrow. Matures in marrow. Migrates to peripheral lymphoid tissue (follicles of lymph nodes, white pulp of spleen, unencapsulated lymphoid tissue). When antigen is encountered, B cells differentiate into plasma cells that produce antibodies, and memory cells. Can function as an APC via MHC II.

B = Bone marrow.

T lymphocyte

Mediates cellular immune response. Originates from stem cells in the bone marrow, but matures in the thymus. T cells differentiate into cytotoxic T cells (express CD8, recognize MHC I), helper T cells (express CD4, recognize MHC II), and regulatory T cells. CD28 (costimulatory signal) necessary for T-cell activation. The majority of circulating lymphocytes are T cells (80%).

T is for Thymus.
CD is for Cluster of Differentiation.
CD4+ helper T cells are the primary target of HIV.

$MHC \times CD = 8$ (e.g., $MHC\ 2 \times CD4 = 8$, and $MHC\ 1 \times CD8 = 8$).

Plasma cell

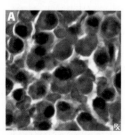

Produces large amounts of antibody specific to a particular antigen. Eccentric nucleus A, clock-face chromatin distribution, abundant RER, and well-developed Golgi apparatus.

Multiple myeloma is a plasma cell cancer.

▶ HEMATOLOGY AND ONCOLOGY–PHYSIOLOGY

Blood groups

A	A antigen on RBC surface and anti-B antibody in plasma.	Incompatible blood transfusions can cause immunologic response, hemolysis, renal failure, shock, and death.
B	B antigen on RBC surface and anti-A antibody in plasma.	Note: anti-A and anti-B antibodies—IgM (do not cross placenta); anti-Rh—IgG (cross placenta).
AB	A and B antigens on RBC surface; no antibodies in plasma; "universal recipient" of RBCs, "universal donor" of plasma.	
O	Neither A nor B antigen on RBC surface; both antibodies in plasma; "universal donor" of RBCs, "universal recipient" of plasma.	
Rh	Rh antigen on RBC surface. Rh− mothers exposed to fetal Rh+ blood (often during delivery) may make anti-Rh IgG. In subsequent pregnancies, anti-Rh IgG crosses the placenta, causing hemolytic disease of the newborn (erythroblastosis fetalis) in the next fetus that is Rh+.	Treatment: Rho(D) immune globulin for mother during every pregnancy to prevent initial sensitization of Rh− mother to Rh antigen.

Coagulation, complement, and kinin pathways

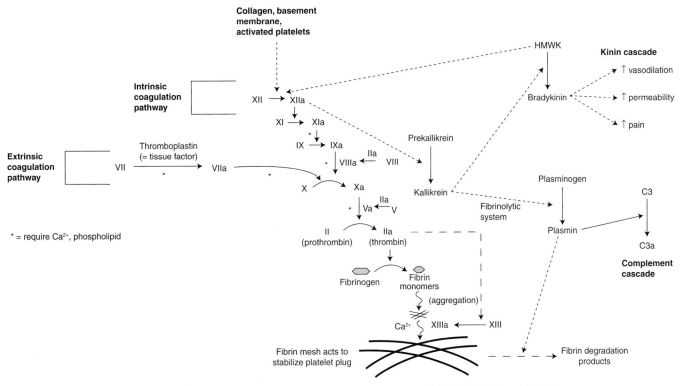

Note: Kallikrein activates bradykinin; ACE inactivates bradykinin.

Hemophilia A: deficiency of factor VIII.
Hemophilia B: deficiency of factor IX.

Coagulation cascade components

Procoagulation

Oxidized vitamin K —epoxide reductase→ reduced vitamin K —(acts as cofactor) +→ ⌠ precursors of II, VII, IX, X, C, S
  ⌡→ mature II, VII, IX, X, C, S

Warfarin inhibits the enzyme vitamin K epoxide reductase. Neonates lack enteric bacteria, which produce vitamin K.

Vitamin K deficiency: ↓ synthesis of factors II, VII, IX, X, protein C, protein S.

vWF carries/protects VIII.

Anticoagulation

thrombin-thrombomodulin complex (endothelial cells)   Protein S

Protein C ——————————→ activated protein C —→ cleaves and inactivates Va, VIIIa

Plasminogen —tPA→ plasmin —→ Fibrinolysis:
  1. cleavage of fibrin mesh
  2. destruction of coagulation factors

Antithrombin inhibits activated forms of factors II, VII, IX, X, XI, XII.

Heparin enhances the activity of antithrombin.

Principal targets of antithrombin: thrombin and factor Xa.

Factor V Leiden mutation produces a factor V resistant to inhibition by activated protein C.

tPA is used clinically as a thrombolytic.

Platelet plug formation (primary hemostasis)

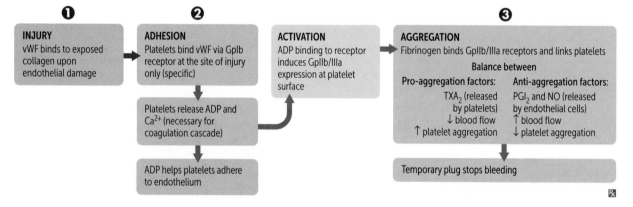

❶

INJURY
vWF binds to exposed collagen upon endothelial damage

❷

ADHESION
Platelets bind vWF via GpIb receptor at the site of injury only (specific)

Platelets release ADP and Ca²⁺ (necessary for coagulation cascade)

ADP helps platelets adhere to endothelium

ACTIVATION
ADP binding to receptor induces GpIIb/IIIa expression at platelet surface

❸

AGGREGATION
Fibrinogen binds GpIIb/IIIa receptors and links platelets

Balance between

Pro-aggregation factors:	Anti-aggregation factors:
TXA₂ (released by platelets)	PGI₂ and NO (released by endothelial cells)
↓ blood flow	↑ blood flow
↑ platelet aggregation	↓ platelet aggregation

Temporary plug stops bleeding

℞

Thrombogenesis

Formation of insoluble fibrin mesh.
Aspirin inhibits cyclooxygenase (TXA_2 synthesis).
Ticlopidine and clopidogrel inhibit ADP-induced expression of GpIIb/IIIa.
Abciximab inhibits GpIIb/IIIa directly.
Ristocetin activates vWF to bind to GpIb. Useful for diagnosis: normal platelet aggregation response is not seen in von Willebrand disease.

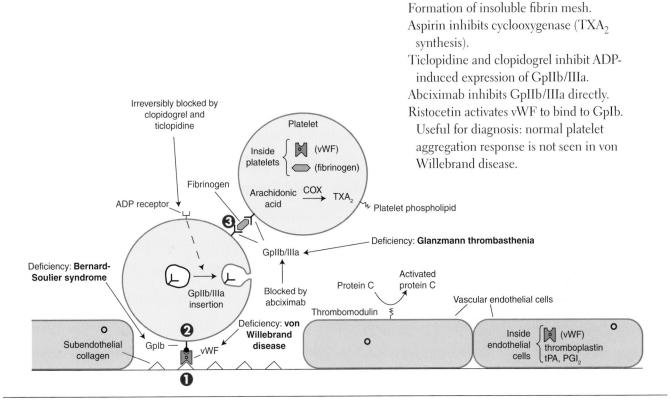

Erythrocyte sedimentation rate

Acute-phase reactants in plasma (e.g., fibrinogen) can cause RBC aggregation, thereby ↑ RBC sedimentation rate (RBC aggregates have a higher density than plasma).
↑ ESR → infections, autoimmune diseases (e.g., SLE, rheumatoid arthritis, temporal arteritis), malignant neoplasms, GI disease (ulcerative colitis), pregnancy.
↓ ESR → polycythemia, sickle cell anemia, CHF, microcytosis, hypofibrinogenemia.

▶ HEMATOLOGY AND ONCOLOGY–PATHOLOGY

Pathologic RBC forms

TYPE	EXAMPLE	ASSOCIATED PATHOLOGY	NOTES
Acanthocyte (spur cell)		Liver disease, abetalipoproteinemia (states of cholesterol dysregulation).	*Acantho* = spiny.
Basophilic stippling		Anemia of Chronic Disease, **alcohol** abuse, Lead poisoning, Thalassemias.	Basically, ACiD alcohol is LeThal.
Bite cell		G6PD deficiency.	
Elliptocyte		Hereditary elliptocytosis.	
Macro-ovalocyte		Megaloblastic anemia (also hypersegmented PMNs), marrow failure.	
Ringed sideroblast		Sideroblastic anemia. Excess iron in mitochondria = pathologic.	
Schistocyte, helmet cell		DIC, TTP/HUS, traumatic hemolysis (i.e., mechanical heart valve prosthesis).	

Pathologic RBC forms *(continued)*

TYPE	EXAMPLE	ASSOCIATED PATHOLOGY	NOTES
Sickle cell		Sickle cell anemia.	
Spherocyte		Hereditary spherocytosis, autoimmune hemolysis.	
Teardrop cell		Bone marrow infiltration (e.g., myelofibrosis).	RBC "sheds a tear" because it's been forced out of its home in the bone marrow.
Target cell		HbC disease, Asplenia, Liver disease, Thalassemia.	"HALT," said the hunter to his target.

Other RBC pathologies

TYPE	EXAMPLE	PROCESS	ASSOCIATED PATHOLOGY
Heinz bodies		Oxidation of hemoglobin sulfhydryl groups → denatured hemoglobin precipitation and phagocytic damage to RBC membrane → bite cells. Visualized with special stains such as crystal violet.	Seen in G6PD deficiency; Heinz body–like inclusions seen in α-thalassemia.
Howell-Jolly bodies		Basophilic nuclear remnants found in RBCs. Howell-Jolly bodies are normally removed from RBCs by splenic macrophages.	Seen in patients with functional hyposplenia or asplenia.

Anemias

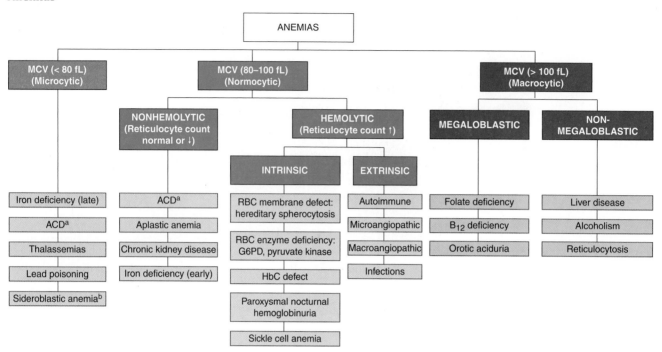

```
                                    ANEMIAS

        MCV (< 80 fL)              MCV (80–100 fL)                    MCV (> 100 fL)
        (Microcytic)               (Normocytic)                       (Macrocytic)

                        NONHEMOLYTIC          HEMOLYTIC          MEGALOBLASTIC      NON-
                        (Reticulocyte count   (Reticulocyte count ↑)               MEGALOBLASTIC
                        normal or ↓)

                                      INTRINSIC        EXTRINSIC

   Iron deficiency (late)   ACDᵃ        RBC membrane defect:   Autoimmune     Folate deficiency    Liver disease
                                        hereditary spherocytosis
   ACDᵃ                     Aplastic anemia                    Microangiopathic  B₁₂ deficiency     Alcoholism
                                        RBC enzyme deficiency:
   Thalassemias             Chronic kidney disease  G6PD, pyruvate kinase  Macroangiopathic  Orotic aciduria  Reticulocytosis
   Lead poisoning           Iron deficiency (early)  HbC defect            Infections
   Sideroblastic anemiaᵇ                  Paroxysmal nocturnal
                                          hemoglobinuria
                                          Sickle cell anemia
```

ᵃACD and iron deficiency anemia may first present as a normocytic anemia and then progress to a microcytic anemia.
ᵇCopper deficiency can cause a microcytic sideroblastic anemia.

Microcytic, hypochromic (MCV < 80 fL) anemia

	DESCRIPTION	FINDINGS
Iron deficiency	↓ iron due to chronic bleeding (GI loss, menorrhagia), malnutrition/absorption disorders or ↑ demand (e.g., pregnancy) → ↓ final step in heme synthesis.	↓ iron, ↑ TIBC, ↓ ferritin. Fatigue, conjunctival pallor **A**. Microcytosis and hypochromia **B**. May manifest as **Plummer-Vinson syndrome** (triad of iron deficiency anemia, esophageal webs, and atrophic glossitis).

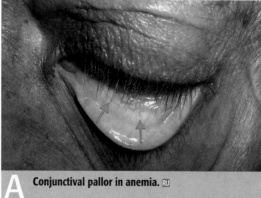

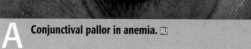

A **Conjunctival pallor in anemia.** RU

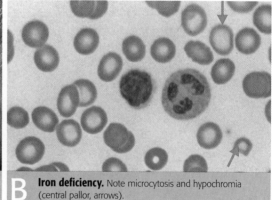

B **Iron deficiency.** Note microcytosis and hypochromia (central pallor, arrows).

α-thalassemia	Defect: α-globin gene deletions → ↓ α-globin synthesis. *cis* deletion prevalent in Asian populations; *trans* deletion prevalent in African populations.	4 allele deletion: No α-globin. Excess γ-globin forms γ₄ (Hb Barts). Incompatible with life (causes hydrops fetalis). 3 allele deletion: HbH disease. Very little α-globin. Excess β-globin forms β₄ (HbH). 1–2 allele deletion: no clinically significant anemia.

Microcytic, hypochromic (MCV < 80 fL) anemia *(continued)*

	DESCRIPTION	FINDINGS
β-thalassemia	Point mutations in splice sites and promoter sequences → ↓ β-globin synthesis. Prevalent in Mediterranean populations. 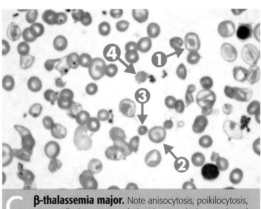 **β-thalassemia major.** Note anisocytosis, poikilocytosis, target cells (arrows 1 and 2), microcytosis (arrow 3), and schistocytes (arrow 4).	**β-thalassemia minor** (heterozygote): • β chain is underproduced. • Usually asymptomatic. • Diagnosis confirmed by ↑ HbA2 (> 3.5%) on electrophoresis. **β-thalassemia major** (homozygote): • β chain is absent → severe anemia **C** requiring blood transfusion (2° hemochromatosis). • Marrow expansion ("crew cut" on skull x-ray) → skeletal deformities. "Chipmunk" facies. • Extramedullary hematopoiesis (leads to hepatosplenomegaly). ↑ risk of parvovirus B19-induced aplastic crisis. Major → ↑ HbF ($\alpha_2\gamma_2$). HbF is protective in the infant and disease only becomes symptomatic after 6 months. **HbS/β-thalassemia heterozygote:** mild to moderate sickle cell disease depending on amount of β-globin production.
Lead poisoning 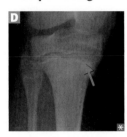	Lead inhibits ferrochelatase and ALA dehydratase → ↓ heme synthesis and ↑ RBC protoporphyrin. Also inhibits rRNA degradation, causing RBCs to retain aggregates of rRNA (basophilic stippling). High risk in old houses with chipped paint.	**LEAD:** **L**ead **L**ines on gingivae (Burton lines) and on metaphyses of long bones **D** on x-ray. **E**ncephalopathy and **E**rythrocyte basophilic stippling. **A**bdominal colic and sideroblastic **A**nemia. **D**rops—wrist and foot drop. Dimercaprol and EDTA are 1st line of treatment. Succimer used for chelation for kids (It "**succ**s" to be a kid who eats lead).
Sideroblastic anemia 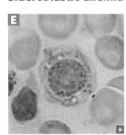	Defect in heme synthesis. Hereditary: X-linked defect in δ-ALA synthase gene. Causes: genetic, acquired (myelodysplastic syndromes), and reversible (alcohol is most common, lead, vitamin B_6 deficiency, copper deficiency, and isoniazid).	Ringed sideroblasts (**E** with iron-laden mitochondria) seen in bone marrow. ↑ iron, normal TIBC, ↑ ferritin. Treatment: pyridoxine (B_6, cofactor for δ-ALA synthase).

Macrocytic (MCV > 100 fL) anemia

	DESCRIPTION	FINDINGS
Megaloblastic anemia	Impaired DNA synthesis → maturation of nucleus of precursor cells in bone marrow delayed relative to maturation of cytoplasm. Abnormal cell division → pancytopenia.	
Folate deficiency	Causes: malnutrition (e.g., alcoholics), malabsorption, antifolates (e.g., methotrexate, trimethoprim, phenytoin), ↑ requirement (e.g., hemolytic anemia, pregnancy).	Hypersegmented neutrophils, glossitis, ↓ folate, ↑ homocysteine but normal methylmalonic acid. No neurologic symptoms (distinguishes from B_{12} deficiency).
B_{12} deficiency (cobalamin)	Causes: insufficient intake (e.g., strict vegans), malabsorption (e.g., Crohn disease), pernicious anemia, *Diphyllobothrium latum* (fish tapeworm), proton pump inhibitors.	Hypersegmented neutrophils **A**, glossitis, ↓ B_{12}, ↑ homocysteine, ↑ methylmalonic acid. **Neurologic symptoms:** subacute combined degeneration (due to involvement of B_{12} in fatty acid pathways and myelin synthesis): ▪ Peripheral neuropathy with sensorimotor dysfunction ▪ Dorsal columns (vibration/proprioception) ▪ Lateral corticospinal (spasticity) ▪ Dementia
Orotic aciduria	Inability to convert orotic acid to UMP (de novo pyrimidine synthesis pathway) because of defect in UMP synthase. Autosomal recessive. Presents in children as megaloblastic anemia that cannot be cured by folate or B_{12} with failure to thrive. No hyperammonemia (vs. ornithine transcarbamylase deficiency—↑ orotic acid with hyperammonemia).	Hypersegmented neutrophils, glossitis, orotic acid in urine. Treatment: uridine monophosphate to bypass mutated enzyme.
Nonmegaloblastic macrocytic anemias	Macrocytic anemia in which DNA synthesis is unimpaired. Causes: liver disease; alcoholism; reticulocytosis → ↑ MCV; drugs (5-FU, zidovudine, hydroxyurea).	Macrocytosis and bone marrow suppression can occur in the absence of folate/B_{12} deficiency.

Normocytic, normochromic anemia	Normocytic, normochromic anemias are classified as nonhemolytic or hemolytic. The hemolytic anemias are further classified according to the cause of the hemolysis (intrinsic vs. extrinsic to the RBC) and by the location of the hemolysis (intravascular vs. extravascular).
Intravascular hemolysis	Findings: ↓ haptoglobin, ↑ LDH, schistocytes and ↑ reticulocytes on peripheral blood smear; and urobilinogen in urine (e.g., paroxysmal nocturnal hemoglobinuria, mechanical destruction [aortic stenosis, prosthetic valve], microangiopathic hemolytic anemias).
Extravascular hemolysis	Findings: macrophage in spleen clears RBC. Spherocytes in peripheral smear, ↑ LDH plus ↑ unconjugated bilirubin, which causes jaundice (e.g., hereditary spherocytosis).

Nonhemolytic, normocytic anemia

	DESCRIPTION	FINDINGS
Anemia of chronic disease	Inflammation → ↑ hepcidin (released by liver, binds ferroportin on intestinal mucosal cells and macrophages, thus inhibiting iron transport) → ↓ release of iron from macrophages.	↓ iron, ↓ TIBC, ↑ ferritin. Can become microcytic, hypochromic
Aplastic anemia	Caused by failure or destruction of myeloid stem cells due to: ▪ Radiation and drugs (benzene, chloramphenicol, alkylating agents, antimetabolites) ▪ Viral agents (parvovirus B19, EBV, HIV, HCV) ▪ Fanconi anemia (DNA repair defect) ▪ Idiopathic (immune mediated, 1° stem cell defect); may follow acute hepatitis	Pancytopenia characterized by severe anemia, leukopenia, and thrombocytopenia. Normal cell morphology, but hypocellular bone marrow with fatty infiltration **A** (dry bone marrow tap). Symptoms: fatigue, malaise, pallor, purpura, mucosal bleeding, petechiae, infection. Treatment: withdrawal of offending agent, immunosuppressive regimens (antithymocyte globulin, cyclosporine), allogeneic bone marrow transplantation, RBC and platelet transfusion, G-CSF, or GM-CSF.
Chronic kidney disease	↓ EPO → ↓ hematopoiesis.	

Intrinsic hemolytic normocytic anemia

E = extravascular; I = intravascular.

	DESCRIPTION	FINDINGS
Hereditary spherocytosis (E)	Defect in proteins interacting with RBC membrane skeleton and plasma membrane (e.g., ankyrin, band 3, protein 4.2, spectrin). Less membrane causes small and round RBCs with no central pallor (↑ MCHC, ↑ red cell distribution width) → premature removal of RBCs by spleen.	Splenomegaly, aplastic crisis (parvovirus B19 infection). Labs: osmotic fragility test ⊕. Eosin-5-maleimide binding test useful for screening. Normal to ↓ MCV with abundance of cells; masks microcytia. Treatment: splenectomy.
G6PD deficiency (I/E)	Most common enzymatic disorder of RBCs. X-linked recessive. Defect in G6PD → ↓ glutathione → ↑ RBC susceptibility to oxidant stress. Hemolytic anemia following oxidant stress (classic causes: sulfa drugs, antimalarials, infections, **fava beans**).	Back pain, hemoglobinuria a few days after oxidant **stress.** Labs: blood smear shows RBCs with **Heinz** bodies and **bite** cells. "**Stress** makes me eat **bites** of **fava beans** with **Heinz** ketchup."
Pyruvate kinase deficiency (E)	Autosomal recessive. Defect in pyruvate kinase → ↓ ATP → rigid RBCs.	Hemolytic anemia in a newborn.
HbC defect (E)	Glutamic acid-to-lysine mutation at residue 6 in β-globin.	Patients with HbSC (1 of each mutant gene) have milder disease than have HbSS patients.
Paroxysmal nocturnal hemoglobinuria (I)	↑ complement-mediated RBC lysis (impaired synthesis of GPI anchor for decay-accelerating factor that protects RBC membrane from complement). Acquired mutation in a hematopoietic stem cell. Increased incidence of acute leukemias.	Triad: Coombs ⊖ hemolytic anemia, pancytopenia, and venous thrombosis. Labs: CD55/59 ⊖ RBCs on flow cytometry. Treatment: eculizumab.
Sickle cell anemia (E)	HbS point mutation causes a single amino acid replacement in β chain (substitution of glutamic acid with valine) at position 6. Pathogenesis: low O$_2$, dehydration, or acidosis precipitates sickling (deoxygenated HbS polymerizes), which results in anemia and vaso-occlusive disease. Newborns are initially asymptomatic because of ↑ HbF and ↓ HbS. Heterozygotes (sickle cell trait) have resistance to malaria. 8% of African Americans carry the HbS trait.	Sickled cells are crescent-shaped RBCs **A**. "Crew cut" on skull x-ray due to marrow expansion from ↑ erythropoiesis (also in thalassemias). Complications in sickle cell disease (SS): ▪ Aplastic crisis (due to parvovirus B19). ▪ Autosplenectomy (Howell-Jolly bodies) → ↑ risk of infection with encapsulated organisms; early splenic dysfunction occurs in childhood. ▪ Splenic sequestration crisis. ▪ *Salmonella* osteomyelitis. ▪ Painful crisis (vaso-occlusive): dactylitis. (painful hand swelling), acute chest syndrome (most common cause of death in adults), avascular necrosis, stroke. ▪ Renal papillary necrosis (due to low O$_2$ in papilla; also seen in heterozygotes) and microhematuria (medullary infarcts). Diagnosis: hemoglobin electrophoresis. Treatment: hydroxyurea (↑ HbF) and bone marrow transplantation.

Extrinsic hemolytic normocytic anemia

	DESCRIPTION	FINDINGS
Autoimmune hemolytic anemia	Warm agglutinin (IgG)—chronic anemia seen in SLE, CLL, or with certain drugs (e.g., α-methyldopa) ("**warm** weather is **GGG**reat"). Cold agglutinin (IgM)—acute anemia triggered by cold; seen in CLL, *Mycoplasma pneumonia* infections, or infectious mononucleosis ("**cold** ice cream—yu**MMM**"). Many warm and cold AIHA are idiopathic in etiology.	Autoimmune hemolytic anemias are usually Coombs ⊕. Direct Coombs test—anti-Ig antibody (Coombs reagent) added to patient's blood. RBCs agglutinate if RBCs are coated with Ig. Indirect Coombs test—normal RBCs added to patient's serum. If serum has anti-RBC surface Ig, RBCs agglutinate when anti-Ig antibodies (Coombs reagent) added.
Microangiopathic anemia	Pathogenesis: RBCs are damaged when passing through obstructed or narrowed vessel lumina. Seen in DIC, TTP-HUS, SLE, and malignant hypertension.	Schistocytes (helmet cells) are seen on blood smear due to mechanical destruction of RBCs.
Macroangiopathic anemia	Prosthetic heart valves and aortic stenosis may also cause hemolytic anemia 2° to mechanical destruction.	Schistocytes on peripheral blood smear.
Infections	↑ destruction of RBCs (e.g., malaria, *Babesia*).	

Lab values in anemia

	Iron deficiency	Chronic disease	Hemo-chromatosis	Pregnancy/OCP use
Serum iron	↓ (1°)	↓	↑ (1°)	—
Transferrin or TIBC (indirectly measures transferrin)	↑	↓[a]	↓	↑ (1°)[b]
Ferritin	↓	↑ (1°)	↑	—
% transferrin saturation (serum iron/TIBC)	↓↓	—	↑↑	↓

Transferrin—transports iron in blood.

Ferritin—1° iron storage protein of body.

[a] Evolutionary reasoning—pathogens use circulating iron to thrive. The body has adapted a system in which iron is stored within the cells of the body and prevents pathogens from acquiring circulating iron.

[b] Transferrin production is ↑ in pregnancy and by OCPs.

Leukopenias

CELL TYPE	CELL COUNT	CAUSES
Neutropenia	Absolute neutrophil count < 1500 cells/mm³	Sepsis/postinfection, drugs (including chemotherapy), aplastic anemia, SLE, radiation
Lymphopenia	Absolute lymphocyte count < 1500 cells/mm³ (< 3000 cells/mm³ in children)	HIV, DiGeorge syndrome, SCID, SLE, corticosteroids,[a] radiation, sepsis, postoperative
Eosinopenia		Cushing syndrome, corticosteroids[a]

[a] Corticosteroids cause neutrophilia, but eosinopenia and lymphopenia. Corticosteroids ↓ activation of neutrophil adhesion molecules, impairing migration out of the vasculature to sites of inflammation. In contrast, corticosteroids sequester eosinophils in lymph nodes and cause apoptosis of lymphocytes.

Heme synthesis, porphyrias, and lead poisoning

The porphyrias are hereditary or acquired conditions of defective heme synthesis that lead to the accumulation of heme precursors. Lead inhibits specific enzymes needed in heme synthesis, leading to a similar condition.

CONDITION	AFFECTED ENZYME	ACCUMULATED SUBSTRATE	PRESENTING SYMPTOMS
Lead poisoning	Ferrochelatase and ALA dehydratase	Protoporphyrin, δ-ALA (blood)	Microcytic anemia, GI and kidney disease. Children—exposure to lead paint → mental deterioration. Adults—environmental exposure (battery/ammunition/radiator factory) → headache, memory loss, demyelination.
Acute intermittent porphyria	Porphobilinogen deaminase	Porphobilinogen, δ-ALA, coporphobilinogen (urine)	Symptoms (5 P's): <ul><li>Painful abdomen</li><li>Port wine–colored urine</li><li>Polyneuropathy</li><li>Psychological disturbances</li><li>Precipitated by drugs, alcohol, and starvation</li></ul> Treatment: glucose and heme, which inhibit ALA synthase.
Porphyria cutanea tarda 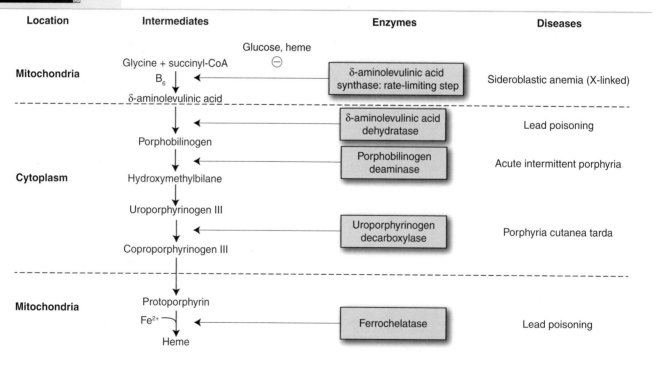	Uroporphyrinogen decarboxylase	Uroporphyrin (tea-colored urine)	Blistering cutaneous photosensitivity A. Most common porphyria.

Location	Intermediates	Enzymes	Diseases
Mitochondria	Glycine + succinyl-CoA ↓ B₆ δ-aminolevulinic acid	Glucose, heme ⊖ δ-aminolevulinic acid synthase: rate-limiting step	Sideroblastic anemia (X-linked)
Cytoplasm	Porphobilinogen ↓ Hydroxymethylbilane ↓ Uroporphyrinogen III ↓ Coproporphyrinogen III	δ-aminolevulinic acid dehydratase Porphobilinogen deaminase Uroporphyrinogen decarboxylase	Lead poisoning Acute intermittent porphyria Porphyria cutanea tarda
Mitochondria	Protoporphyrin ↓ Fe²⁺ Heme	Ferrochelatase	Lead poisoning

↓ heme → ↑ ALA synthase activity
↑ heme → ↓ ALA synthase activity

Coagulation disorders

PT—tests function of common and extrinsic pathway (factors I, II, V, VII, and X). Defect → ↑ PT.
PTT—tests function of common and intrinsic pathway (all factors except VII and XIII). Defect → ↑ PTT.

DISORDER	PT	PTT	MECHANISM AND COMMENTS
Hemophilia A or B	—	↑	Intrinsic pathway coagulation defect. ▪ A: deficiency of factor VIII → ↑ PTT. ▪ B: deficiency of factor IX → ↑ PTT. Macrohemorrhage in hemophilia—hemarthroses (bleeding into joints), easy bruising, ↑ PTT. Treatment: recombinant factor VIII (in hemophilia A).
Vitamin K deficiency	↑	↑	General coagulation defect. Bleeding time normal. ↓ synthesis of factors II, VII, IX, X, protein C, protein S.

Platelet disorders

Defects in platelet plug formation → ↑ bleeding time (BT).
Platelet abnormalities → microhemorrhage: mucous membrane bleeding, epistaxis, petechiae, purpura, ↑ bleeding time, possible ↓ platelet count (PC).

DISORDER	PC	BT	MECHANISM AND COMMENTS
Bernard-Soulier syndrome	↓	↑	Defect in platelet plug formation. ↓ GpIb → defect in platelet-to-vWF adhesion.
Glanzmann thrombasthenia	—	↑	Defect in platelet plug formation. ↓ GpIIb/IIIa → defect in platelet-to-platelet aggregation. Labs: blood smear shows no platelet clumping.
Immune thrombocytopenia	↓	↑	Defect: anti-GpIIb/IIIa antibodies → splenic macrophage consumption of platelet/antibody complex. May be triggered by viral illness. ↓ platelet survival. Labs: ↑ megakaryocytes on bone marrow biopsy.
Thrombotic thrombocytopenic purpura	↓	↑	Inhibition or deficiency of ADAMTS 13 (vWF metalloprotease) → ↓ degradation of vWF multimers. Pathogenesis: ↑ large vWF multimers → ↑ platelet adhesion → ↑ platelet aggregation and thrombosis. ↓ platelet survival. Labs: schistocytes, ↑ LDH. Symptoms: pentad of neurologic and renal symptoms, fever, thrombocytopenia, and microangiopathic hemolytic anemia. Treatment: exchange transfusion and steroids.

Mixed platelet and coagulation disorders

DISORDER	PC	BT	PT	PTT	MECHANISM AND COMMENTS
von Willebrand disease	—	↑	—	— or ↑	Intrinsic pathway coagulation defect: ↓ vWF → normal or ↑ PTT (depends on severity; vWF acts to carry/protect factor VIII). Defect in platelet plug formation: ↓ vWF → defect in platelet-to-vWF adhesion. Mild but most common inherited bleeding disorder. Autosomal dominant. Diagnosed in most cases by ristocetin cofactor assay (↓ agglutination is diagnostic). Treatment: DDAVP, which releases vWF stored in endothelium.
DIC	↓	↑	↑	↑	Widespread activation of clotting leads to a deficiency in clotting factors, which creates a bleeding state. Causes: Sepsis (gram-negative), Trauma, Obstetric complications, acute Pancreatitis, Malignancy, Nephrotic syndrome, Transfusion (**STOP** Making New Thrombi). Labs: schistocytes, ↑ fibrin split products (D-dimers), ↓ fibrinogen, ↓ factors V and VIII.

Hereditary thrombosis syndromes leading to hypercoagulability

DISEASE	DESCRIPTION
Factor V Leiden	Production of mutant factor V that is resistant to degradation by activated protein C. Most common cause of inherited hypercoagulability in whites.
Prothrombin gene mutation	Mutation in 3′ untranslated region → ↑ production of prothrombin → ↑ plasma levels and venous clots.
Antithrombin deficiency	Inherited deficiency of antithrombin: has no direct effect on the PT, PTT, or thrombin time but diminishes the increase in PTT following heparin administration. Can also be acquired: renal failure/nephrotic syndrome → antithrombin loss in urine → ↑ factors II and X.
Protein C or S deficiency	↓ ability to inactivate factors V and VIII. ↑ risk of thrombotic skin necrosis with hemorrhage following administration of warfarin. Skin and subcutaneous tissue necrosis after warfarin administration → think protein C deficiency. "Protein C Cancels Coagulation."

Blood transfusion therapy

COMPONENT	DOSAGE EFFECT	CLINICAL USE
Packed RBCs	↑ Hb and O_2 carrying capacity	Acute blood loss, severe anemia
Platelets	↑ platelet count (↑ ~5000/mm³/unit)	Stop significant bleeding (thrombocytopenia, qualitative platelet defects)
Fresh frozen plasma	↑ coagulation factor levels	DIC, cirrhosis, warfarin overdose, exchange transfusion in TTP/HUS
Cryoprecipitate	Contains fibrinogen, factor VIII, factor XIII, vWF, and fibronectin	Treat coagulation factor deficiencies involving fibrinogen and factor VIII

Blood transfusion risks include infection transmission (low), transfusion reactions, iron overload, hypocalcemia (citrate is a calcium chelator), and hyperkalemia (RBCs may lyse in old blood units).

Leukemia vs. lymphoma

Leukemia	Lymphoid or myeloid neoplasms with widespread involvement of bone marrow. Tumor cells are usually found in peripheral blood.
Lymphoma	Discrete tumor masses arising from lymph nodes. Presentations often blur definitions.

Leukemoid reaction

Acute inflammatory response to infection. ↑ WBC count with ↑ neutrophils and neutrophil precursors such as band cells (left shift); ↑ leukocyte ALP. Contrast with CML (also ↑ WBC count with left shift, but ↓ leukocyte ALP).

Hodgkin vs. non-Hodgkin lymphoma

Hodgkin	Non-Hodgkin
Localized, single group of nodes; extranodal rare; contiguous spread (stage is strongest predictor of prognosis). Prognosis is much better than with non-Hodgkin lymphoma.	Multiple, peripheral nodes; extranodal involvement common; noncontiguous spread
Characterized by Reed-Sternberg cells	Majority involve B cells (except those of lymphoblastic T-cell origin)
Bimodal distribution–young adulthood and > 55 years; more common in men except for nodular sclerosing type	Peak incidence for certain subtypes at 20–40 years old
50% of cases associated with EBV	May be associated with HIV and immunosuppression
Constitutional ("B") signs/symptoms—low-grade fever, night sweats, weight loss	Fewer constitutional signs/symptoms

Reed-Sternberg cells   Distinctive tumor giant cell seen in Hodgkin disease; binucleate or bilobed with the 2 halves as mirror images ("owl eyes" A). RS cells are CD15+ and CD30+ B-cell origin. Necessary but not sufficient for a diagnosis of Hodgkin disease. Better prognosis with strong stromal or lymphocytic reaction against RS cells. Nodular sclerosing form most common (affects women and men equally). Lymphocyte-rich form has best prognosis. Lymphocyte mixed or depleted forms have poor prognosis.

2 owl eyes × 15 = 30.

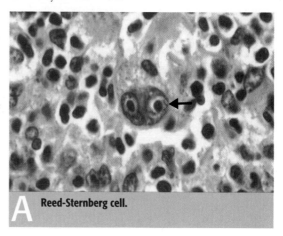

A   Reed-Sternberg cell.

Non-Hodgkin lymphoma

TYPE	OCCURS IN	GENETICS	COMMENTS
Neoplasms of mature B cells			
Burkitt lymphoma	Adolescents or young adults	t(8;14)—translocation of c-*myc* (8) and heavy-chain Ig (14)	"Starry sky" appearance A, sheets of lymphocytes with interspersed macrophages (arrows). Associated with EBV. Jaw lesion B in endemic form in Africa; pelvis or abdomen in sporadic form.
Diffuse large B-cell lymphoma	Usually older adults, but 20% in children	t(14;18)	Most common type of non-Hodgkin lymphoma in adults.
Mantle cell lymphoma	Older males	t(11;14)—translocation of cyclin D1 (11) and heavy-chain Ig (14)	CD5+.
Follicular lymphoma	Adults	t(14;18)—translocation of heavy-chain Ig (14) and *bcl*-2 (18)	Indolent course; *bcl*-2 inhibits apoptosis. Presents with painless "waxing and waning" lymphadenopathy.
Neoplasms of mature T cells			
Adult T-cell lymphoma	Adults	Caused by HTLV-1 (associated with IV drug abuse)	Adults present with cutaneous lesions; especially affects populations in Japan, West Africa, and the Caribbean. Lytic bone lesions, hypercalcemia.
Mycosis fungoides/ Sézary syndrome	Adults		Adults present with cutaneous patches C/ plaques/tumors with potential to spread to lymph nodes and viscera. Circulating malignant cells seen in Sézary syndrome. Indolent, CD4+.

Multiple myeloma

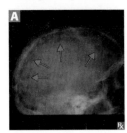

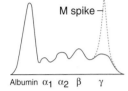

Monoclonal plasma cell ("fried egg" appearance) cancer that arises in the marrow and produces large amounts of IgG (55%) or IgA (25%). Most common 1° tumor arising within bone in the elderly (> 40–50 years old). Associated with:

- ↑ susceptibility to infection
- Primary amyloidosis (AL)
- Punched-out lytic bone lesions on x-ray **A**
- M spike on serum protein electrophoresis
- Ig light chains in urine (Bence Jones protein)
- Rouleaux formation (RBCs stacked like poker chips in blood smear)

Numerous plasma cells with "clock face" chromatin and intracytoplasmic inclusions containing immunoglobulin **B**.

Distinguish from **Waldenström macroglobulinemia** → M spike = IgM (→ hyperviscosity symptoms); no lytic bone lesions.

Monoclonal gammopathy of undetermined significance (MGUS)—monoclonal expansion of plasma cells with serum monoclonal protein < 3g/dL ("M spike") and bone marrow with < 10% monoclonal plasma cells. Asymptomatic precursor to multiple myeloma. Patients with MGUS develop multiple myeloma at a rate of 1–2% per year.

Think **CRAB**:
  Hyper**C**alcemia
  Renal insufficiency
  Anemia
  Bone lytic lesions/Back pain
Multiple Myeloma: Monoclonal M protein spike

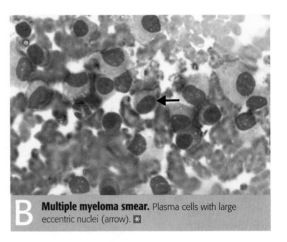

B **Multiple myeloma smear.** Plasma cells with large eccentric nuclei (arrow). ✳

Myelodysplastic syndromes

Stem cell disorders involving ineffective hematopoiesis → defects in cell maturation of all non-lymphoid lineages. Caused by de novo mutations or environmental exposure (e.g., radiation, benzene, chemotherapy). Risk of transformation to AML.

Pseudo–Pelger-Huet anomaly—neutrophils with bilobed nuclei (two nuclear masses connected with a thin filament of chromatin) typically seen after chemotherapy.

Leukemias   Unregulated growth of leukocytes in bone marrow → ↑ or ↓ number of circulating leukocytes in blood and marrow failure → anemia (↓ RBCs), infections (↓ mature WBCs), and hemorrhage (↓ platelets); leukemic cell infiltrates in liver, spleen, and lymph nodes are possible.

TYPE	PERIPHERAL BLOOD SMEAR	COMMENTS
Lymphoid neoplasms		
Acute lymphoblastic leukemia/lymphoma (ALL)		Age: < 15 years. T-cell ALL can present as mediastinal mass (leukemic infiltration of the thymus). Associated with Down syndrome. Peripheral blood and bone marrow have ↑↑↑ lymphoblasts A. TdT+ (marker of pre-T and pre-B cells), CD10+ (pre-B cells only). Most responsive to therapy. May spread to CNS and testes. t(12;21) → better prognosis.
Small lymphocytic lymphoma (SLL)/ chronic lymphocytic leukemia (CLL)		Age: > 60 years. CD20+, CD5+ B-cell neoplasm. Often asymptomatic, progresses slowly; smudge cells B in peripheral blood smear; autoimmune hemolytic anemia. SLL same as CLL except CLL has ↑ peripheral blood lymphocytosis or bone marrow involvement.
Hairy cell leukemia		Age: Adults. Mature B-cell tumor in the elderly. Cells have filamentous, hair-like projections C. Stains TRAP (tartrate-resistant acid phosphatase ⊕). TRAP stain largely replaced with flow cytometry. Causes marrow fibrosis → dry tap on aspiration. Treatment: cladribine (2-CDA), an adenosine analog (inhibits adenosine deaminase).

Leukemias *(continued)*

TYPE	PERIPHERAL BLOOD SMEAR	COMMENTS
Myeloid neoplasms		
Acute myelogenous leukemia (AML)	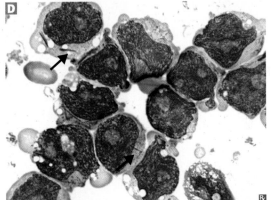	Age: median onset 65 years. Auer rods **D**; peroxidase ⊕ cytoplasmic inclusions seen mostly in M3 AML; ↑↑↑ circulating myeloblasts on peripheral smear; adults. Risk factors: prior exposure to alkylating chemotherapy, radiation, myeloproliferative disorders, Down syndrome. t(15;17) → M3 AML subtype responds to all-*trans* retinoic acid (vitamin A), inducing differentiation of myeloblasts; DIC is a common presentation in M3 AML and can be induced by chemotherapy due to release of Auer rods.
Chronic myelogenous leukemia (CML)	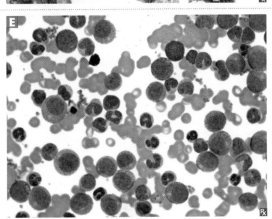	Age: peak incidence 45–85 years, median age at diagnosis 64 years. Defined by the Philadelphia chromosome (t[9;22], *bcr-abl*); myeloid stem cell proliferation; presents with ↑ neutrophils, metamyelocytes, basophils **E**; splenomegaly; may accelerate and transform to AML or ALL ("blast crisis"). Very low leukocyte alkaline phosphatase (LAP) as a result of low activity in mature granulocytes (vs. leukemoid reaction, in which LAP is ↑). Responds to imatinib (a small-molecule inhibitor of the *bcr-abl* tyrosine kinase).

Chromosomal translocations

TRANSLOCATION	ASSOCIATED DISORDER	
t(9;22) (**Philadelphia** chromosome)	CML (*bcr-abl* hybrid)	Philadelphia CreaML cheese.
t(8;14)	Burkitt lymphoma (c-*myc* activation)	
t(11;14)	Mantle cell lymphoma (cyclin D1 activation)	
t(14;18)	Follicular lymphomas (*bcl-2* activation)	
t(15;17)	M3 type of AML (responsive to all-*trans* retinoic acid)	

Langerhans cell histiocytosis

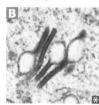

Proliferative disorders of dendritic (Langerhans) cells from monocyte lineage. Presents in a child as lytic bone lesions A and skin rash or as recurrent otitis media with a mass involving the mastoid bone. Cells are functionally immature and do not efficiently stimulate primary T lymphocytes via antigen presentation. Cells express S-100 (mesodermal origin) and CD1a. Birbeck granules ("tennis rackets" on EM) are characteristic B.

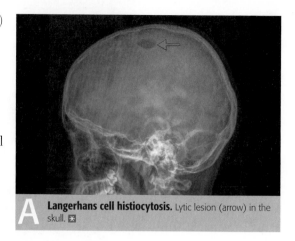

A **Langerhans cell histiocytosis.** Lytic lesion (arrow) in the skull. ✳

Chronic myeloproliferative disorders	The myeloproliferative disorders represent an often-overlapping spectrum, but the classic findings are described below. *JAK2* is involved in hematopoietic growth factor signaling. Mutations are implicated in myeloproliferative disorders other than CML.

Polycythemia vera 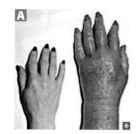	Hematocrit > 55%, somatic (non-hereditary) mutation in *JAK2* gene. Often presents as intense itching after hot shower. Rare but classic symptom is erythromelalgia (severe, burning pain and reddish or bluish coloration) due to episodic blood clots in vessels of the extremities **A**. 2° polycythemia is via natural or artificial ↑ in EPO levels.
Essential thrombocytosis 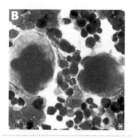	Similar to polycythemia vera, but specific for overproduction of abnormal platelets → bleeding, thrombosis. Bone marrow contains enlarged megakaryocytes **B**.
Myelofibrosis 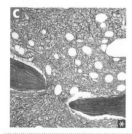	Fibrotic obliteration of bone marrow **C**. **Teardrop** RBCs and immature forms of the myeloid line. "Bone marrow is **crying** because it's fibrosed."
CML	*bcr-abl* transformation leads to ↑ cell division and inhibition of apoptosis. Treatment: imatinib (Gleevec).

	RBCs	WBCs	PLATELETS	PHILADELPHIA CHROMOSOME	*JAK2* MUTATIONS
Polycythemia vera	↑	↑	↑	⊖	⊕
Essential thrombocytosis	–	–	↑	⊖	⊕ (30–50%)
Myelofibrosis	↓	Variable	Variable	⊖	⊕ (30–50%)
CML	↓	↑	↑	⊕	⊖

Polycythemia

	PLASMA VOLUME	RBC MASS	O₂ SATURATION	EPO LEVELS	ASSOCIATIONS
Relative	↓	–	–	–	↓ plasma volume (dehydration, burns).
Appropriate absolute	–	↑	↓	↑	Lung disease, congenital heart disease, high altitude.
Inappropriate absolute	–	↑	–	↑	Renal cell carcinoma, Wilms tumor, cyst, hepatocellular carcinoma, hydronephrosis. Due to ectopic EPO.
Polycythemia vera	↑	↑↑	–	↓	Due to negative feedback.

▶ HEMATOLOGY AND ONCOLOGY–PHARMACOLOGY

Heparin

MECHANISM	Cofactor for the activation of antithrombin, ↓ thrombin, and ↓ factor Xa. Short half-life.
CLINICAL USE	Immediate anticoagulation for PE, acute coronary syndrome, MI, DVT. Used during pregnancy (does not cross placenta). Follow PTT.
TOXICITY	Bleeding, thrombocytopenia (HIT), osteoporosis, drug-drug interactions. For rapid reversal (antidote), use protamine sulfate (positively charged molecule that binds negatively charged heparin).
NOTES	Low-molecular-weight heparins (e.g., enoxaparin, dalteparin) act more on factor Xa, have better bioavailability and 2–4 times longer half-life. Can be administered subcutaneously and without laboratory monitoring. Not easily reversible. **Heparin-induced thrombocytopenia** (HIT)—development of IgG antibodies against heparin bound to platelet factor 4 (PF4). Antibody-heparin-PF4 complex activates platelets → thrombosis and thrombocytopenia.

Argatroban, bivalirudin	Derivatives of hirudin, the anticoagulant used by leeches; inhibit thrombin directly. Used instead of heparin for anticoagulating patients with HIT.

Warfarin (Coumadin)

MECHANISM	Interferes with normal synthesis and γ-carboxylation of vitamin K–dependent clotting factors II, VII, IX, and X and proteins C and S. Metabolized by the cytochrome P-450 pathway. In laboratory assay, has effect on **EX**trinsic pathway and ↑ **PT**. Long half-life.	The **EX-PresidenT** went to **war**(farin).
CLINICAL USE	Chronic anticoagulation (after STEMI, venous thromboembolism prophylaxis, and prevention of stroke in atrial fibrillation). Not used in pregnant women (because warfarin, unlike heparin, can cross the placenta). Follow PT/INR values.	
TOXICITY	Bleeding, teratogenic, skin/tissue necrosis **A**, drug-drug interactions.	For reversal of warfarin overdose, give vitamin K. For rapid reversal of severe warfarin overdose, give fresh frozen plasma.

Direct factor Xa inhibitors	Apixaban, rivaroxaban.
MECHANISM	Bind and directly inhibit the activity of factor Xa.
CLINICAL USE	Treatment and prophylaxis of DVT and PE (rivaroxaban), stroke prophylaxis in patients with atrial fibrillation. Oral agents do not usually require coagulation monitoring.
TOXICITY	Bleeding (no specific reversal agent available).

Heparin vs. warfarin

	Heparin	Warfarin
STRUCTURE	Large anionic, acidic polymer	Small lipid-soluble molecule
ROUTE OF ADMINISTRATION	Parenteral (IV, SC)	Oral
SITE OF ACTION	Blood	Liver
ONSET OF ACTION	Rapid (seconds)	Slow, limited by half-lives of normal clotting factors
MECHANISM OF ACTION	Activates antithrombin, which ↓ the action of IIa (thrombin) and factor Xa	Impairs the synthesis of vitamin K–dependent clotting factors II, VII, IX, and X (vitamin K antagonist)
DURATION OF ACTION	Acute (hours)	Chronic (days)
INHIBITS COAGULATION IN VITRO	Yes	No
TREATMENT OF ACUTE OVERDOSE	Protamine sulfate	IV vitamin K and fresh frozen plasma
MONITORING	PTT (intrinsic pathway)	PT/INR (extrinsic pathway)
CROSSES PLACENTA	No	Yes (teratogenic)

Thrombolytics

Alteplase (tPA), reteplase (rPA), tenecteplase (TNK-tPA).

MECHANISM	Directly or indirectly aid conversion of plasminogen to plasmin, which cleaves thrombin and fibrin clots. ↑ PT, ↑ PTT, no change in platelet count.
CLINICAL USE	Early MI, early ischemic stroke, direct thrombolysis of severe PE.
TOXICITY	Bleeding. Contraindicated in patients with active bleeding, history of intracranial bleeding, recent surgery, known bleeding diatheses, or severe hypertension. Treat toxicity with aminocaproic acid, an inhibitor of fibrinolysis. Fresh frozen plasma and cryoprecipitate can also be used to correct factor deficiencies.

Aspirin (ASA)

MECHANISM	Irreversibly inhibits cyclooxygenase (both COX-1 and COX-2) enzyme by covalent acetylation. Platelets cannot synthesize new enzyme, so effect lasts until new platelets are produced: ↑ bleeding time, ↓ TXA_2 and prostaglandins. No effect on PT or PTT.
CLINICAL USE	Antipyretic, analgesic, anti-inflammatory, antiplatelet (↓ aggregation).
TOXICITY	Gastric ulceration, tinnitus (CN VIII). Chronic use can lead to acute renal failure, interstitial nephritis, and upper GI bleeding. Reye syndrome in children with viral infection. Overdose causes respiratory alkalosis initially, which is then superimposed by metabolic acidosis.

ADP receptor inhibitors

Clopidogrel, ticlopidine, prasugrel, ticagrelor.

MECHANISM	Inhibit platelet aggregation by irreversibly blocking ADP receptors. Inhibit fibrinogen binding by preventing glycoprotein IIb/IIIa from binding to fibrinogen.
CLINICAL USE	Acute coronary syndrome; coronary stenting. ↓ incidence or recurrence of thrombotic stroke.
TOXICITY	Neutropenia (ticlopidine). TTP/HUS may be seen.

Cilostazol, dipyridamole

MECHANISM	Phosphodiesterase III inhibitor; ↑ cAMP in platelets, thus inhibiting platelet aggregation; vasodilators.
CLINICAL USE	Intermittent claudication, coronary vasodilation, prevention of stroke or TIAs (combined with aspirin), angina prophylaxis.
TOXICITY	Nausea, headache, facial flushing, hypotension, abdominal pain.

GP IIb/IIIa inhibitors

GP IIb/IIIa inhibitors	Abciximab, eptifibatide, tirofiban.
MECHANISM	Bind to the glycoprotein receptor IIb/IIIa on activated platelets, preventing aggregation. Abciximab is made from monoclonal antibody Fab fragments.
CLINICAL USE	Unstable angina, percutaneous transluminal coronary angioplasty.
TOXICITY	Bleeding, thrombocytopenia.

Cancer drugs–cell cycle

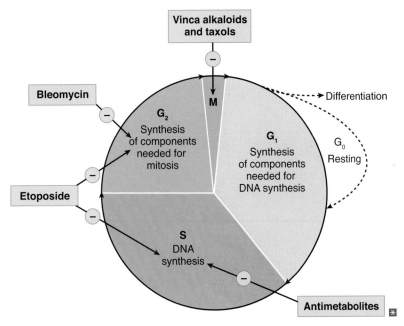

Antineoplastics

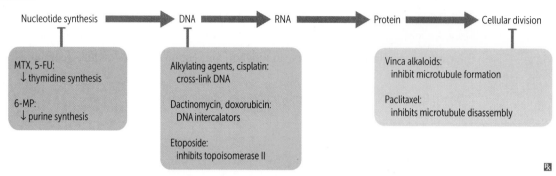

Antimetabolites

DRUG	MECHANISM[a]	CLINICAL USE	TOXICITY
Methotrexate (MTX)	Folic acid analog that inhibits dihydrofolate reductase → ↓ dTMP → ↓ DNA and ↓ protein synthesis.	Cancers: leukemias, lymphomas, choriocarcinoma, sarcomas. Non-neoplastic: abortion, ectopic pregnancy, rheumatoid arthritis, psoriasis, IBD.	Myelosuppression, which is reversible with leucovorin (folinic acid) "rescue." Macrovesicular fatty change in liver. Mucositis. Teratogenic.
5-fluorouracil (5-FU)	Pyrimidine analog bioactivated to 5F-dUMP, which covalently complexes folic acid. This complex inhibits thymidylate synthase → ↓ dTMP → ↓ DNA and ↓ protein synthesis.	Colon cancer, pancreatic cancer, basal cell carcinoma (topical).	Myelosuppression, which is not reversible with leucovorin. Overdose: "rescue" with uridine. Photosensitivity.
Cytarabine (arabinofuranosyl cytidine)	Pyrimidine analog → inhibition of DNA polymerase.	Leukemias, lymphomas.	Leukopenia, thrombocytopenia, megaloblastic anemia. CYTarabine causes panCYTopenia.
Azathioprine 6-mercaptopurine (6-MP) 6-thioguanine (6-TG)	Purine (thiol) analogs → ↓ de novo purine synthesis. Activated by HGPRT.	Preventing organ rejection, RA, SLE (azathioprine). Leukemia, IBD (6-MP, 6-TG).	Bone marrow, GI, liver. Azathioprine and 6-MP are metabolized by xanthine oxidase; thus both have ↑ toxicity with allopurinol, which inhibits their metabolism.

[a]All are S-phase specific.

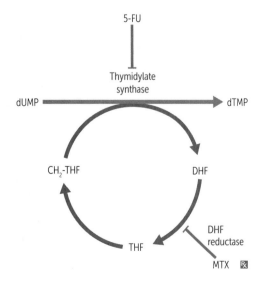

Antitumor antibiotics

DRUG	MECHANISM	CLINICAL USE	TOXICITY
Dactinomycin (actinomycin D)	Intercalates in DNA.	Wilms tumor, Ewing sarcoma, rhabdomyosarcoma. Used for childhood tumors ("children act out").	Myelosuppression.
Doxorubicin (Adriamycin), daunorubicin	Generate free radicals. Intercalate in DNA → breaks in DNA → ↓ replication.	Solid tumors, leukemias, lymphomas.	Cardiotoxicity (dilated cardiomyopathy), myelosuppression, alopecia. Toxic to tissues following extravasation. Dexrazoxane (iron chelating agent), used to prevent cardiotoxicity.
Bleomycin	Induces free radical formation, which causes breaks in DNA strands.	Testicular cancer, Hodgkin lymphoma.	Pulmonary fibrosis, skin changes, mucositis. Minimal myelosuppression.

Alkylating agents

DRUG	MECHANISM	CLINICAL USE	TOXICITY
Cyclophosphamide, ifosfamide	Covalently X-link (interstrand) DNA at guanine N-7. Require bioactivation by liver.	Solid tumors, leukemia, lymphomas, and some brain cancers.	Myelosuppression; hemorrhagic cystitis, partially prevented with mesna (thiol group of mesna binds toxic metabolites).
Nitrosoureas (carmustine, lomustine, semustine, streptozocin)	Require bioactivation. Cross blood-brain barrier → CNS. Cross-links DNA.	Brain tumors (including glioblastoma multiforme).	CNS toxicity (convulsions, dizziness, ataxia).
Busulfan	Cross-links DNA.	CML. Also used to ablate patient's bone marrow before bone marrow transplantation.	Severe myelosuppression (in almost all cases), pulmonary fibrosis, hyperpigmentation.

Microtubule inhibitors

DRUG	MECHANISM	CLINICAL USE	TOXICITY
Vincristine, vinblastine	Vinca alkaloids that bind β-tubulin, inhibit its polymerization into microtubules, thereby preventing mitotic spindle formation (M-phase arrest).	Solid tumors, leukemias, and lymphomas.	Vincristine—neurotoxicity (areflexia, peripheral neuritis), paralytic ileus. Vinblastine blasts bone marrow (suppression).
Paclitaxel, other taxols	Hyperstabilize polymerized microtubules in M phase so that mitotic spindle cannot break down (anaphase cannot occur). "It is taxing to stay polymerized."	Ovarian and breast carcinomas.	Myelosuppression, alopecia, hypersensitivity.

Cisplatin, carboplatin

MECHANISM	Cross-link DNA.
CLINICAL USE	Testicular, bladder, ovary, and lung carcinomas.
TOXICITY	Nephrotoxicity and acoustic nerve damage. Prevent nephrotoxicity with amifostine (free radical scavenger) and chloride diuresis.

Etoposide, teniposide

MECHANISM	Etoposide inhibits topoisomerase II → ↑ DNA degradation.
CLINICAL USE	Solid tumors (particularly testicular and small cell lung cancer), leukemias, lymphomas.
TOXICITY	Myelosuppression, GI irritation, alopecia.

Irinotecan, topotecan

MECHANISM	Inhibit topoisomerase I and prevent DNA unwinding and replication.
CLINICAL USE	Colon cancer (irinotecan); ovarian and small cell lung cancers (topotecan).
TOXICITY	Severe myelosuppression, diarrhea.

Hydroxyurea

MECHANISM	Inhibits ribonucleotide reductase → ↓ DNA Synthesis (S-phase specific).
CLINICAL USE	Melanoma, CML, sickle cell disease (↑ HbF).
TOXICITY	Bone marrow suppression, GI upset.

Prednisone, prednisolone

MECHANISM	May trigger apoptosis. May even work on nondividing cells.
CLINICAL USE	Most commonly used glucocorticoids in cancer chemotherapy. Used in CLL, non-Hodgkin lymphomas (part of combination chemotherapy regimen). Also used as immunosuppressants (e.g., autoimmune diseases).
TOXICITY	Cushing-like symptoms; weight gain, central obesity, muscle breakdown, cataracts, acne, osteoporosis, hypertension, peptic ulcers, hyperglycemia, psychosis.

Tamoxifen, raloxifene

MECHANISM	Selective estrogen receptor modulators (SERMs)—receptor antagonists in breast and agonists in bone. Block the binding of estrogen to ER ⊕ cells.
CLINICAL USE	Breast cancer treatment (tamoxifen only) and prevention. Raloxifene also useful to prevent osteoporosis.
TOXICITY	Tamoxifen—partial agonist in endometrium, which ↑ the risk of endometrial cancer; "hot flashes." Raloxifene—no ↑ in endometrial carcinoma because it is an endometrial antagonist.

Trastuzumab (Herceptin)

MECHANISM	Monoclonal antibody against HER-2 (*c-erbB2*), a tyrosine kinase receptor. Helps kill breast cancer cells that overexpress HER-2, through inhibition of HER2-initiated cellular signaling and antibody-dependent cytotoxicity.
CLINICAL USE	HER-2 ⊕ breast cancer and gastric cancer (tras2umab).
TOXICITY	Cardiotoxicity. "**HEART**ceptin" damages the **HEART**.

Imatinib (Gleevec)

MECHANISM	Tyrosine kinase inhibitor of *bcr-abl* (Philadelphia chromosome fusion gene in CML) and c-*Kit* (common in GI stromal tumors).
CLINICAL USE	CML, GI stromal tumors.
TOXICITY	Fluid retention.

Rituximab

MECHANISM	Monoclonal antibody against CD20, which is found on most B-cell neoplasms.
CLINICAL USE	Non-Hodgkin lymphoma, rheumatoid arthritis (with MTX), ITP.
TOXICITY	↑ risk of progressive multifocal leukoencephalopathy.

Vemurafenib

MECHANISM	Small molecule inhibitor of forms of the B-Raf kinase with the V600E mutation.
CLINICAL USE	Metastatic melanoma.

Bevacizumab

MECHANISM	Monoclonal antibody against VEGF. Inhibits angiogenesis.
CLINICAL USE	Solid tumors (colorectal cancer, renal cell carcinoma).
TOXICITY	Hemorrhage and impaired wound healing.

Common chemotoxicities

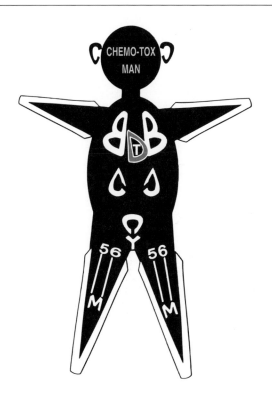

Cisplatin/Carboplatin → acoustic nerve damage (and nephrotoxicity)

Vincristine → peripheral neuropathy
Bleomycin, Busulfan → pulmonary fibrosis
Doxorubicin → cardiotoxicity
Trastuzumab → cardiotoxicity
Cisplatin/Carboplatin → nephrotoxic (and acoustic nerve damage)

CYclophosphamide → hemorrhagic cystitis

5-FU → myelosuppression
6-MP → myelosuppression

Methotrexate → myelosuppression

▶ NOTES

Musculoskeletal, Skin, and Connective Tissue

"Rigid, the skeleton of habit alone upholds the human frame."
—Virginia Woolf

"Beauty may be skin deep, but ugly goes clear to the bone."
—Redd Foxx

"The function of muscle is to pull and not to push, except in the case of the genitals and the tongue."
—Leonardo da Vinci

▶ MUSCULOSKELETAL, SKIN, AND CONNECTIVE TISSUE—ANATOMY AND PHYSIOLOGY

Epidermis layers

From surface to base:
- Stratum Corneum (keratin)
- Stratum Lucidum
- Stratum Granulosum
- Stratum Spinosum (spines = desmosomes)
- Stratum Basale (stem cell site)

Californians Like Girls in String Bikinis.

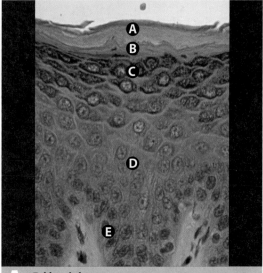

A **Epidermis layers.** A, Stratum corneum; B, stratum lucidum; C, stratum granulosum; D, stratum spinosum; E, stratum basale. ℞

Epithelial cell junctions

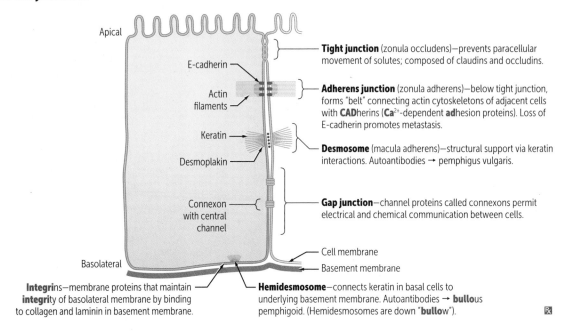

Apical

E-cadherin

Actin filaments

Keratin

Desmoplakin

Connexon with central channel

Basolateral

Cell membrane

Basement membrane

Tight junction (zonula occludens)—prevents paracellular movement of solutes; composed of claudins and occludins.

Adherens junction (zonula adherens)—below tight junction, forms "belt" connecting actin cytoskeletons of adjacent cells with **CAD**herins (**Ca**$^{2+}$-dependent **ad**hesion proteins). Loss of E-cadherin promotes metastasis.

Desmosome (macula adherens)—structural support via keratin interactions. Autoantibodies → pemphigus vulgaris.

Gap junction—channel proteins called connexons permit electrical and chemical communication between cells.

Integrins—membrane proteins that maintain **integri**ty of basolateral membrane by binding to collagen and laminin in basement membrane.

Hemidesmosome—connects keratin in basal cells to underlying basement membrane. Autoantibodies → **bullo**us pemphigoid. (Hemidesmosomes are down "**bull**ow"). ℞

Knee injury	Presents with acute knee pain and signs of joint injury/instability: ▪ Anterior drawer sign → ACL injury ▪ Posterior drawer sign → PCL injury ▪ Abnormal passive abduction (valgus stress) → MCL injury ▪ Abnormal passive adduction (varus stress) → LCL injury ▪ McMurray test: pain on external rotation → medial meniscus; pain on internal rotation → lateral meniscus. **Unhappy triad**—common injury in contact sports due to lateral force applied to a planted leg. Classically, consists of damage to the ACL, MCL, and medial meniscus (attached to MCL); however, lateral meniscus injury is more common.	"Anterior" and "posterior" in ACL and PCL refer to sites of tibial attachment. 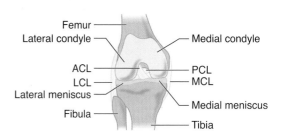
Clinically important landmarks	Pudendal nerve block (to relieve pain of delivery)—ischial spine. Appendix—$2/3$ of the distance between the umbilicus and the anterior superior iliac spine (ASIS), just proximal to the ASIS (McBurney point). Lumbar puncture—iliac crest.	
Rotator cuff muscles	Shoulder muscles that form the rotator cuff: ▪ Supraspinatus (suprascapular nerve)—abducts arm initially (before the action of the deltoid); most common rotator cuff injury. ▪ Infraspinatus (suprascapular nerve)—laterally rotates arm; pitching injury. ▪ Teres minor (axillary nerve)—adducts and laterally rotates arm. ▪ Subscapularis (subscapular nerve)—medially rotates and adducts arm. Innervated primarily by C5-C6.	S**I**t**S** (small t is for teres **minor**). 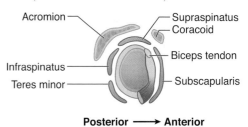

Wrist bones

Scaphoid, Lunate, Triquetrum, Pisiform, Hamate, Capitate, Trapezoid, Trapezium 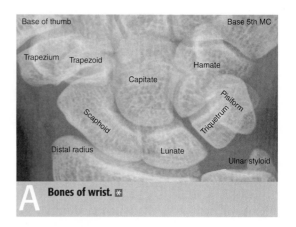. (So Long To Pinky, Here Comes The Thumb).

Scaphoid (palpated in anatomical snuff box) is the most commonly fractured carpal bone and is prone to avascular necrosis owing to retrograde blood supply.

Dislocation of lunate may cause acute carpal tunnel syndrome.

A fall on an outstretched hand that damages the hook of the hamate can cause ulnar nerve injury.

Carpal tunnel syndrome: entrapment of median nerve in carpal tunnel; nerve compression → paresthesia, pain, and numbness in distribution of median nerve.

Guyon canal syndrome: Compression of the ulnar nerve at the wrist or hand, classically seen in cyclists due to pressure from handlebars.

Base of thumb — Base 5th MC
Trapezium Trapezoid Hamate Capitate Scaphoid Pisiform Triquetrum Distal radius Lunate Ulnar styloid

A **Bones of wrist.** ✴

Brachial plexus lesions

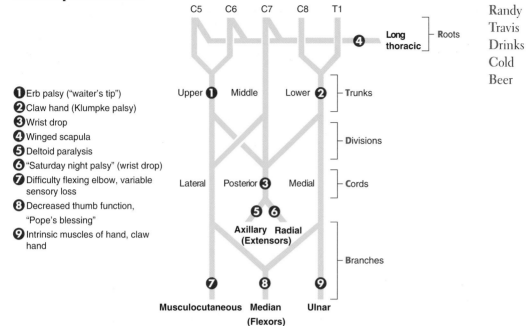

❶ Erb palsy ("waiter's tip")
❷ Claw hand (Klumpke palsy)
❸ Wrist drop
❹ Winged scapula
❺ Deltoid paralysis
❻ "Saturday night palsy" (wrist drop)
❼ Difficulty flexing elbow, variable sensory loss
❽ Decreased thumb function, "Pope's blessing"
❾ Intrinsic muscles of hand, claw hand

Randy
Travis
Drinks
Cold
Beer

CONDITION	INJURY	CAUSES	MUSCLE DEFICIT	FUNCTIONAL DEFICIT	PRESENTATION
Erb palsy ("waiter's tip")	Traction or tear of **upper** ("**Erb**-er") trunk: C5-C6 roots	Infants—lateral traction on neck during delivery Adults—trauma	Deltoid, supraspinatus	Abduction (arm hangs by side)	
			Infraspinatus	Lateral rotation (arm medially rotated)	
			Biceps brachii	Flexion, supination (arm extended and pronated)	
Klumpke palsy	Traction or tear of **lower** trunk: C8-T1 root	Infants—upward force on arm during delivery Adults—trauma (e.g., grabbing a tree branch to break a fall)	Intrinsic hand muscles: lumbricals, interossei, thenar, hypothenar	Total claw hand: lumbricals normally flex MCP joints and extend DIP and PIP joints	
Thoracic outlet syndrome	Compression of **lower** trunk and subclavian vessels	Cervical rib injury; Pancoast tumor	Same as Klumpke palsy	Atrophy of intrinsic hand muscles; ischemia, pain, and edema due to vascular compression	
Winged scapula	Lesion of long thoracic nerve	Axillary node dissection after mastectomy, stab wounds	Serratus anterior	Inability to anchor scapula to thoracic cage → cannot abduct arm above horizontal position	

Upper extremity nerves

NERVE	CAUSES OF INJURY	PRESENTATION
Axillary (C5-C6)	Fractured surgical neck of humerus; anterior dislocation of humerus	Flattened deltoid Loss of arm abduction at shoulder (> 15 degrees) Loss of sensation over deltoid muscle and lateral arm
Musculocutaneous (C5-C7)	Upper trunk compression	Loss of forearm flexion and supination Loss of sensation over lateral forearm
Radial (C5-T1)	Midshaft fracture of humerus; compression of axilla (e.g., due to crutches or sleeping with arm over chair ("Saturday night palsy"))	Wrist drop: loss of elbow, wrist, and finger extension ↓ grip strength (wrist extension necessary for maximal action of flexors) Loss of sensation over posterior arm/forearm and dorsal hand
Median (C5-T1)	Supracondylar fracture of humerus (proximal lesion); carpal tunnel syndrome and wrist laceration (distal lesion)	"Ape hand" and "Pope's blessing" Loss of wrist and lateral finger flexion, thumb opposition, lumbricals of 2nd and 3rd digits Loss of sensation over thenar eminence and dorsal and palmar aspects of lateral 3½ fingers with proximal lesion Tinel sign (tingling on percussion) in carpal tunnel syndrome
Ulnar (C8-T1)	Fracture of medial epicondyle of humerus "funny bone" (proximal lesion); fractured hook of hamate (distal lesion)	"Ulnar claw" on digit extension Radial deviation of wrist upon flexion (proximal lesion) Loss of flexion of wrist and medial fingers, abduction and adduction of fingers (interossei), actions of medial 2 lumbrical muscles Loss of sensation over medial 1½ fingers including hypothenar eminence
Recurrent branch of median nerve (C5-T1)	Superficial laceration of palm	"Ape hand" Loss of thenar muscle group: opposition, abduction, and flexion of thumb No loss of sensation

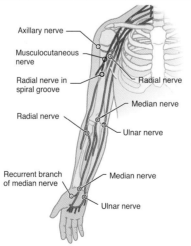

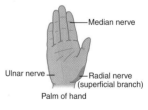

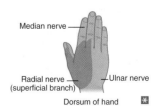

Distortions of the hand

At rest, a balance exists between the extrinsic flexors and extensors of the hand, as well as the intrinsic muscles of the hand—particularly the lumbrical muscles (flexion of MCP, extension of DIP and PIP joints).

"Clawing"—seen best with **distal** lesions of median or ulnar nerves. Remaining extrinsic flexors of the digits exaggerate the loss of the lumbricals → fingers extend at MCP, flex at DIP and PIP joints.

Deficits less pronounced in **proximal** lesions; deficits present during voluntary flexion of the digits.

PRESENTATION				
CONTEXT	Extending fingers/at rest	Making a fist	Extending fingers / at rest	Making a fist
LOCATION OF LESION	Distal ulnar nerve	Proximal median nerve	Distal median nerve	Proximal ulnar nerve
SIGN	"Ulnar claw"	"Pope's blessing"	"Median claw"	"OK gesture" (with digits 1–3 flexed)

Note: Atrophy of the thenar eminence (unopposable thumb → "ape hand") can be seen in median nerve lesions, while atrophy of the hypothenar eminence can be seen in ulnar nerve lesions.

Hand muscles

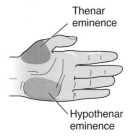

Thenar eminence

Hypothenar eminence

Thenar (median)—**O**pponens pollicis, **A**bductor pollicis brevis, **F**lexor pollicis brevis.

Hypothenar (ulnar)—**O**pponens digiti minimi, **A**bductor digiti minimi, **F**lexor digiti minimi brevis.

Dorsal interosseous muscles—abduct the fingers.

Palmar interosseous muscles—adduct the fingers.

Lumbrical muscles—flex at the MCP joint, extend PIP and DIP joints.

Both groups perform the same functions: **O**ppose, **A**bduct, and **F**lex (**OAF**).

DAB = **D**orsals **AB**duct.

PAD = **P**almars **AD**duct.

Lower extremity nerves

NERVE	CAUSE OF INJURY	PRESENTATION
Obturator (L2–L4)	Pelvic surgery	↓ thigh sensation (medial) and ↓ adduction.
Femoral (L2–L4)	Pelvic fracture	↓ thigh flexion and leg extension.
Common peroneal (L4–S2)	Trauma or compression of lateral aspect of leg, fibular neck fracture	Foot drop—inverted and plantarflexed at rest, loss of eversion and dorsiflexion. "Steppage gait." Loss of sensation on dorsum of foot.
Tibial (L4–S3)	Knee trauma, Baker cyst (proximal lesion); tarsal tunnel syndrome (distal lesion)	Inability to curl toes and loss of sensation on sole of foot. In proximal lesions, foot everted at rest with loss of inversion and plantarflexion.
Superior gluteal (L4–S1)	Posterior hip dislocation, polio	Trendelenburg sign/gait—pelvis tilts because weight-bearing leg cannot maintain alignment of pelvis through hip abduction (superior nerve → medius and minimus). Lesion is contralateral to the side of the hip that drops, ipsilateral to extremity on which the patient stands.
Inferior gluteal (L5–S2)	Posterior hip dislocation	Difficulty climbing stairs, rising from seated position. Loss of hip extension (inferior nerve → maximus).

PED = Peroneal Everts and Dorsiflexes; if injured, foot drop**PED**.
TIP = Tibial Inverts and Plantarflexes; if injured, can't stand on **TIP**toes.
Sciatic nerve (L4–S3)—posterior thigh, splits into common peroneal and tibial nerves.

Neurovascular pairing   Nerves and arteries are frequently named together by the bones/regions with which they are associated. The following are exceptions to this naming convention.

LOCATION	NERVE	ARTERY
Axilla/lateral thorax	Long thoracic	Lateral thoracic
Surgical neck of humerus	Axillary	Posterior circumflex
Midshaft of humerus	Radial	Deep brachial
Distal humerus/ cubital fossa	Median	Brachial
Popliteal fossa	Tibial	Popliteal
Posterior to medial malleolus	Tibial	Posterior tibial

Muscle conduction to contraction

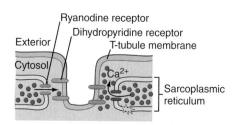

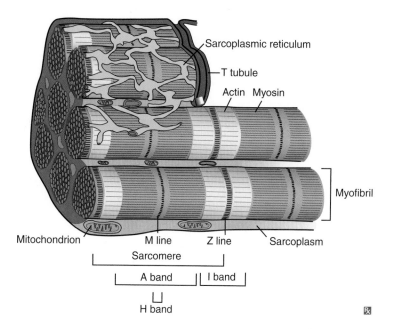

Muscle contraction

1. Action potential depolarization opens presynaptic voltage-gated Ca^{2+} channels, inducing neurotransmitter release.
2. Postsynaptic ligand binding leads to muscle cell depolarization in the motor end plate.
3. Depolarization travels along muscle cell and down the T tubule.
4. Depolarization of the voltage-sensitive dihydropyridine receptor, mechanically coupled to the ryanodine receptor on the sarcoplasmic reticulum, induces a conformational change, causing Ca^{2+} release from sarcoplasmic reticulum.
5. Released Ca^{2+} binds to troponin C, causing a conformational change that moves tropomyosin out of the myosin-binding groove on actin filaments.
6. Myosin releases bound ADP and subsequently, inorganic PO_4^{3-} → displacement of myosin on the actin filament (power stroke). Contraction results in shortening of **H** and **I** bands and between **Z** lines (**HIZ** shrinkage), but the A band remains the same length (**A** band is **A**lways the same length).

Types of muscle fibers

Type 1 muscle	Slow twitch; red fibers resulting from ↑ mitochondria and myoglobin concentration (↑ oxidative phosphorylation) → sustained contraction.	Think "1 slow red ox."
Type 2 muscle	Fast twitch; white fibers resulting from ↓ mitochondria and myoglobin concentration (↑ anaerobic glycolysis); weight training results in hypertrophy of fast-twitch muscle fibers.	

Smooth muscle contraction

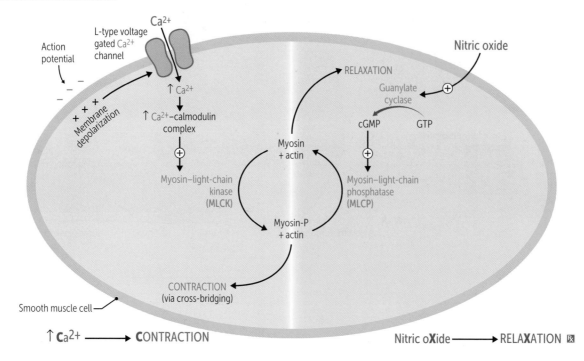

Bone formation

Endochondral ossification	Bones of axial and appendicular skeleton, and base of the skull. Cartilaginous model of bone is first made by chondrocytes. Osteoclasts and osteoblasts later replace with woven bone and then remodel to lamellar bone. In adults, woven bone occurs after fractures and in Paget disease.
Membranous ossification	Bones of calvarium and facial bones. Woven bone formed directly without cartilage. Later remodeled to lamellar bone.

Cell biology of bone

Osteoblasts	Build bone by secreting collagen and catalyzing mineralization. Differentiate from mesenchymal stem cells in periosteum.
Osteoclasts	Multinucleated cells that dissolve bone by secreting acid and collagenases. Differentiate from monocytes/macrophages.
Parathyroid hormone	At low, intermittent levels, exerts anabolic effects (building bone) on osteoblasts and osteoclasts (indirect). Chronic high PTH levels (1° hyperparathyroidism) cause catabolic effects (osteitis fibrosa cystica).
Estrogen	Estrogen inhibits apoptosis in bone-forming osteoblasts and induces apoptosis in bone-resorbing osteoclasts. Under estrogen deficiency (surgical or postmenopausal), excess remodeling cycles and bone resorption lead to osteoporosis.

▸ MUSCULOSKELETAL, SKIN, AND CONNECTIVE TISSUE—PATHOLOGY

Achondroplasia	Failure of longitudinal bone growth (endochondral ossification) → short limbs. Membranous ossification is not affected → large head relative to limbs. Constitutive activation of fibroblast growth factor receptor (FGFR3) actually inhibits chondrocyte proliferation. > 85% of mutations occur sporadically and are associated with advanced paternal age, but the condition also demonstrates autosomal dominant inheritance. Common cause of dwarfism. Normal life span and fertility.

Osteoporosis	Trabecular (spongy) bone loses mass and interconnections despite normal bone mineralization and lab values (serum Ca^{2+} and PO_4^{3-}). Diagnosis by a bone mineral density test (DEXA) with a T-score of ≤ -2.5. Can be caused by long-term exogenous steroid use. Can lead to **vertebral crush fractures**—acute back pain, loss of height, kyphosis.	
Type I	Postmenopausal: ↑ bone resorption due to ↓ estrogen levels.	Femoral neck fracture, distal radius (Colles) fracture.
Type II	Senile osteoporosis: affects men and women > 70 years old.	Prophylaxis: regular weight-bearing exercise and adequate calcium and vitamin D intake throughout adulthood. Treatment: bisphosphonates, PTH, SERMs, rarely calcitonin; denosumab (monoclonal antibody against RANKL).

Mild compression fracture　　　Normal vertebrae

Osteopetrosis (marble bone disease)

Failure of normal bone resorption due to defective osteoclasts → thickened, dense bones that are prone to fracture. Bone fills marrow space → pancytopenia, extramedullary hematopoiesis. Mutations (e.g., carbonic anhydrase II) impair ability of osteoclast to generate acidic environment necessary for bone resorption. X-rays show bone-in-bone appearance 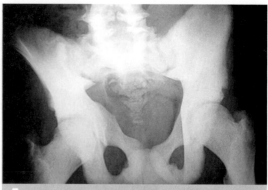. Can result in cranial nerve impingement and palsies as a result of narrowed foramina. Bone marrow transplant is potentially curative as osteoclasts are derived from monocytes.

Osteopetrosis. Radiograph of the pelvis shows diffusely dense bones. ✱

Osteomalacia/rickets

Vitamin D deficiency. Osteomalacia in adults; rickets in children. Due to defective mineralization/calcification of osteoid → soft bones that bow out. ↓ vitamin D → ↓ serum calcium → ↑ PTH secretion → ↓ serum PO_4^{3-}. Hyperactivity of osteoblasts → ↑ ALP (osteoblasts require alkaline environment).

Paget disease of bone (osteitis deformans)

Common, localized disorder of bone remodeling caused by ↑ in both osteoblastic and osteoclastic activity. Serum Ca^{2+}, phosphorus, and PTH levels are normal. ↑ ALP. Mosaic pattern of woven and lamellar bone 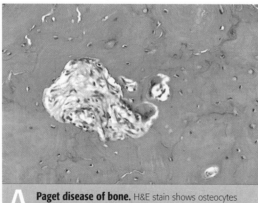; long bone chalk-stick fractures. ↑ blood flow from ↑ arteriovenous shunts may cause high-output heart failure. ↑ risk of osteogenic sarcoma.

Hat size can be increased 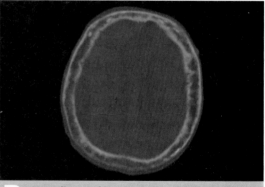; hearing loss is common due to auditory foramen narrowing. Stages of Paget disease:
- Lytic—osteoclasts
- Mixed—osteoclasts + osteoblasts
- Sclerotic—osteoblasts
- Quiescent—minimal osteoclast/osteoblast activity

Paget disease of bone. H&E stain shows osteocytes within lacunae (scattered small white dots) and chaotic, mosaic pattern (lacy purple lines) of bone remodeling. ✱

Paget disease of bone. Note marked thickening of calvarium. ✱

Osteonecrosis (avascular necrosis)

Infarction of bone and marrow, usually very painful. Caused by trauma, high-dose corticosteroids, alcoholism, sickle cell. Most common site is femoral head (due to insufficiency of medial circumflex femoral artery).

Lab values in bone disorders

DISORDER	SERUM Ca^{2+}	PO_4^{3-}	ALP	PTH	COMMENTS
Osteoporosis	—	—	—	—	↓ bone mass
Osteopetrosis	—/↓	—	—	—	Dense, brittle bones. Ca^{2+} ↓ in severe, malignant disease
Paget disease	—	—	↑	—	Abnormal "mosaic" bone architecture
Osteomalacia/rickets	↓	↓	↑	↑	Soft bones
Hypervitaminosis D	↑	↑	—	↓	Caused by over-supplementation or granulomatous disease (e.g., sarcoidosis)
Osteitis fibrosa cystica					"Brown tumors" due to fibrous replacement of bone, subperiosteal thinning
1° hyperparathyroidism	↑	↓	↑	↑	Idiopathic or parathyroid hyperplasia, adenoma, carcinoma
2° hyperparathyroidism	↓	↑	↑	↑	Often as compensation for ESRD (↓ PO_4^{3-} excretion and production of activated vitamin D)

Primary bone tumors

TUMOR TYPE	EPIDEMIOLOGY/LOCATION	CHARACTERISTICS
Benign tumors		
Giant cell tumor	20–40 years old. Epiphyseal end of long bones.	Locally aggressive benign tumor often around knee. "Soap bubble" appearance on x-ray A. Multinucleated giant cells.
Osteochondroma (exostosis)	Most common benign tumor. Males < 25 years old.	Mature bone with cartilaginous cap. Rarely transforms to chondrosarcoma.
Malignant tumors		
Osteosarcoma (osteogenic sarcoma)	2nd most common 1° malignant bone tumor (after multiple myeloma). Bimodal distribution: 10–20 years old (1°), > 65 (2°). Predisposing factors: Paget disease of bone, bone infarcts, radiation, familial retinoblastoma, Li-Fraumeni syndrome (germline *P53* mutation). Metaphysis of long bones, often around knee B C.	Codman triangle (from elevation of periosteum) or sunburst pattern on x-ray. Aggressive. Treat with surgical en bloc resection (with limb salvage) and chemotherapy. **Osteosarcoma.** Lucent lesion on x-ray B now better seen on MRI as heterogeneous mass with periosteal elevation. ✱
Ewing sarcoma	Boys < 15 years old. Commonly appears in diaphysis of long bones, pelvis, scapula, and ribs.	Anaplastic small blue cell malignant tumor D. Extremely aggressive with early metastases, but responsive to chemotherapy. "Onion skin" appearance in bone. Associated with t(11;22) translocation. 11 + 22 = 33 (Patrick **Ewing**'s jersey number).

Primary bone tumors *(continued)*

TUMOR TYPE	EPIDEMIOLOGY/LOCATION	CHARACTERISTICS
Malignant tumors *(continued)*		
Chondrosarcoma	Rare, malignant, cartilaginous tumor. Men 30–60 years old. Usually located in pelvis, spine, scapula, humerus, tibia, or femur.	Malignant cartilaginous tumor. May be of 1° origin or from osteochondroma. Expansile glistening mass within the medullary cavity.

Osteochondroma (exostosis)

Giant cell tumor (soap bubble)

Benign

Malignant

Ewing sarcoma

Chondrosarcoma

Osteosarcoma (Codman triangle)

Epiphysis   Metaphysis   Diaphysis   Metaphysis   Epiphysis

Osteoarthritis and rheumatoid arthritis

	Osteoarthritis	Rheumatoid arthritis
ETIOLOGY	Mechanical—joint wear and tear destroys articular cartilage.	Autoimmune—inflammatory destruction of synovial joints. Mediated by cytokines and type III and type IV hypersensitivity reactions.
JOINT FINDINGS	Subchondral cysts, sclerosis , osteophytes (bone spurs), eburnation (polished, ivory-like appearance of bone), Heberden nodes (DIP), and Bouchard nodes (PIP). No MCP involvement.	Pannus formation in joints (MCP, PIP), subcutaneous rheumatoid nodules (fibrinoid necrosis), ulnar deviation of fingers, subluxation **B**, Baker cyst (in popliteal fossa). No DIP involvement.
PREDISPOSING FACTORS	Age, obesity, joint deformity, trauma.	Females > males. 80% have ⊕ rheumatoid factor (anti-IgG antibody); anti–cyclic citrullinated peptide antibody is more specific. Strong association with HLA-DR4.
CLASSIC PRESENTATION	Pain in weight-bearing joints after use (e.g., at the end of the day), improving with rest. Knee cartilage loss begins medially ("bowlegged"). Noninflammatory. No systemic symptoms.	Morning stiffness lasting > 30 minutes and improving with use, symmetric joint involvement, systemic symptoms (fever, fatigue, pleuritis, pericarditis).
TREATMENT	NSAIDs, intra-articular glucocorticoids.	NSAIDs, glucocorticoids, disease-modifying agents (methotrexate, sulfasalazine, TNF-α inhibitors).

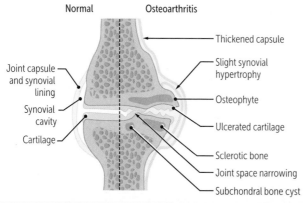

Normal   Osteoarthritis

Joint capsule and synovial lining
Synovial cavity
Cartilage

Thickened capsule
Slight synovial hypertrophy
Osteophyte
Ulcerated cartilage
Sclerotic bone
Joint space narrowing
Subchondral bone cyst

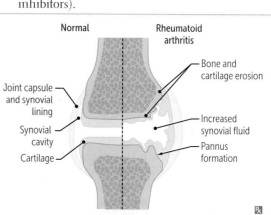

Normal   Rheumatoid arthritis

Joint capsule and synovial lining
Synovial cavity
Cartilage

Bone and cartilage erosion
Increased synovial fluid
Pannus formation

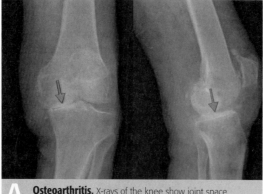

A **Osteoarthritis.** X-rays of the knee show joint space narrowing and sclerosis (arrows).

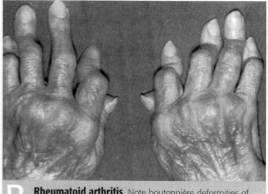

B **Rheumatoid arthritis.** Note boutonnière deformities of PIP joints with ulnar deviation.

Sjögren syndrome	Autoimmune disorder characterized by destruction of exocrine glands (especially lacrimal and salivary). Predominantly affects females 40–60 years old. Findings:	Can be a 1° disorder or a 2° syndrome associated with other autoimmune disorders (e.g., rheumatoid arthritis). Complications—dental caries; mucosa-associated lymphoid tissue (MALT) lymphoma (may present as unilateral parotid enlargement).

Findings:
- Xerophthalmia (↓ tear production and subsequent corneal damage)
- Xerostomia (↓ saliva production)
- Presence of antinuclear antibodies: SS-A (anti-Ro) and/or SS-B (anti-La)
- Bilateral parotid enlargement

Gout

FINDINGS	Acute inflammatory monoarthritis caused by precipitation of monosodium urate crystals in joints 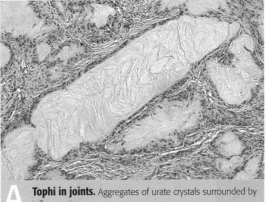. Associated with hyperuricemia, which can be caused by:

- Underexcretion of uric acid (90% of patients)—largely idiopathic; can be exacerbated by certain medications (e.g., thiazide diuretics).
- Overproduction of uric acid (10% of patients)—Lesch-Nyhan syndrome, PRPP excess, ↑ cell turnover (e.g., tumor lysis syndrome), von Gierke disease.

Crystals are needle shaped and ⊖ birefringent (yellow under parallel light, blue under perpendicular light). More common in males.

SYMPTOMS	Asymmetric joint distribution. Joint is swollen, red, and painful 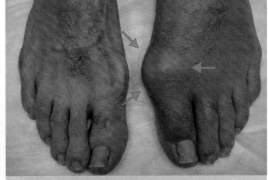. Classic manifestation is painful MTP joint of the big toe (podagra). Tophus formation (often on external ear, olecranon bursa, or Achilles tendon). Acute attack tends to occur after a large meal or alcohol consumption (alcohol metabolites compete for same excretion sites in kidney as uric acid, causing ↓ uric acid secretion and subsequent buildup in blood).

TREATMENT	Acute: NSAIDs (e.g., indomethacin), glucocorticoids, colchicine. Chronic (preventive): xanthine oxidase inhibitors (e.g., allopurinol, febuxostat).

A **Tophi in joints.** Aggregates of urate crystals surrounded by inflammation.

B **Gout.** Left big toe (podagra) is swollen and red. ✺

Pseudogout

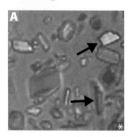

Presents with pain and effusion in a joint, caused by deposition of calcium pyrophosphate crystals within the joint space (chondrocalcinosis on x-ray). Forms basophilic, rhomboid crystals that are weakly positively birefringent **A**. Usually affects large joints (classically the knee). > 50 years old; both sexes affected equally. Diseases that may be associated with pseudogout include hemochromatosis, hyperparathyroidism, and hypoparathyroidism. Treatment includes NSAIDs for sudden, severe attacks; steroids; and colchicine.

Gout—crystals are yellow when parallel (||) to the light.
Pseudogout—crystals are blue when parallel (||) to the light.

Infectious arthritis

S. aureus, *Streptococcus*, and *Neisseria gonorrhoeae* are common causes. Gonococcal arthritis is an STD that presents as a migratory arthritis with an asymmetric pattern. Affected joint is swollen, red, and painful. STD = Synovitis (e.g., knee), Tenosynovitis (e.g., hand), and Dermatitis (e.g., pustules).

Seronegative spondyloarthropathies

Arthritis without rheumatoid factor (no anti-IgG antibody). Strong association with HLA-B27 (gene that codes for HLA MHC class I). Occurs more often in males. **PAIR**

Psoriatic arthritis	Joint pain and stiffness associated with psoriasis. Asymmetric and patchy involvement. Dactylitis ("sausage fingers" **A**), "pencil-in-cup" **B** deformity on x-ray. Seen in fewer than ⅓ of patients with psoriasis.	
Ankylosing spondylitis	Chronic inflammatory disease of spine and sacroiliac joints → ankylosis (stiff spine due to fusion of joints), uveitis, and aortic regurgitation.	Bamboo spine (vertebral fusion) **C**.
Inflammatory bowel disease	Crohn disease and ulcerative colitis are often accompanied by ankylosing spondylitis or peripheral arthritis.	
Reactive arthritis (Reiter syndrome)	Classic triad: ▪ Conjunctivitis and anterior uveitis ▪ Urethritis ▪ Arthritis	"Can't see, can't pee, can't bend my knee." Post-GI (*Shigella*, *Salmonella*, *Yersinia*, *Campylobacter*) or *Chlamydia* infections.

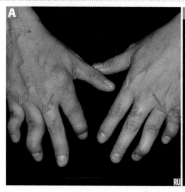
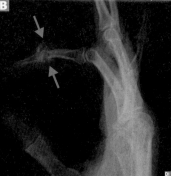
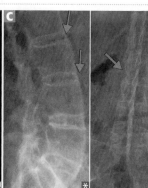

Systemic lupus erythematosus

SYMPTOMS	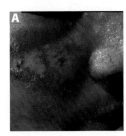 Classic presentation: rash, joint pain, and fever, most commonly in a female of reproductive age and African descent. **Libman-Sacks endocarditis**—wart-like vegetations on both sides of valve. Lupus nephritis (type III hypersensitivity reaction): <ul><li>Nephritic—diffuse proliferative glomerulonephritis.</li><li>Nephrotic—membranous glomerulonephritis.</li></ul>	**RASH OR PAIN:** Rash (malar 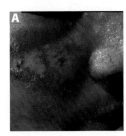 or discoid) Arthritis Soft tissues/serositis Hematologic disorders (e.g., cytopenias) Oral/nasopharyngeal ulcers Renal disease, Raynaud phenomenon Photosensitivity, Positive VDRL/RPR Antinuclear antibodies Immunosuppressants Neurologic disorders (e.g. seizures, psychosis) Common causes of death in SLE: <ul><li>Cardiovascular disease</li><li>Infections</li><li>Renal disease</li></ul>

FINDINGS	Antinuclear antibodies (ANA)—sensitive, not specific. Anti-dsDNA antibodies—specific, poor prognosis (renal disease). Anti-Smith antibodies—specific, not prognostic (directed against snRNPs). Antihistone antibodies—sensitive for drug-induced lupus. Anticardiolipin antibodies—false positive on tests for syphilis, prolonged PTT (paradoxically, ↑ risk of arteriovenous thromboembolism). ↓ C3, C4, and CH_{50} due to immune complex formation.
TREATMENT	NSAIDs, steroids, immunosuppressants, hydroxychloroquine.

Sarcoidosis

Characterized by immune-mediated, widespread noncaseating granulomas 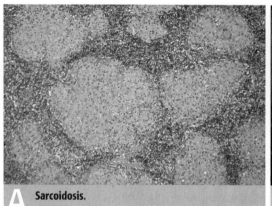 and elevated serum ACE levels. Common in black females. Often asymptomatic except for enlarged lymph nodes. Incidental findings on CXR of **bilateral hilar adenopathy** and/or reticular opacities 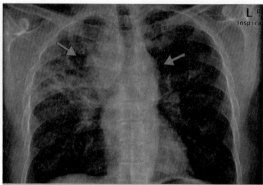.
Associated with restrictive lung disease (interstitial fibrosis), erythema nodosum, lupus pernio, Bell palsy, epithelioid granulomas containing microscopic Schaumann and asteroid bodies, uveitis, and hypercalcemia (due to ↑ 1α-hydroxylase–mediated vitamin D activation in macrophages). Treatment: steroids.

A **Sarcoidosis.**

B **Sarcoidosis.** Bilateral suprahilar adenopathy (arrows) and right upper lung reticular opacity on CXR. ✚

Polymyalgia rheumatica

SYMPTOMS	Pain and stiffness in shoulders and hips, often with fever, malaise, and weight loss. Does not cause muscular weakness. More common in women > 50 years old; associated with temporal (giant cell) arteritis.
FINDINGS	↑ ESR, ↑ C-reactive protein, normal CK.
TREATMENT	Rapid response to low-dose corticosteroids.

Fibromyalgia

Most commonly seen in females 20–50 years old. Chronic, widespread musculoskeletal pain associated with stiffness, paresthesias, poor sleep, and fatigue. Treat with regular exercise, antidepressants (TCAs, SNRIs), and anticonvulsants.

Polymyositis/dermatomyositis

SYMPTOMS

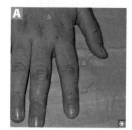

Polymyositis—progressive symmetric proximal muscle weakness, characterized by endomysial inflammation with CD8+ T cells. Most often involves shoulders.

Dermatomyositis—similar to polymyositis, but also involves malar rash (similar to SLE), Gottron papules **A**, heliotrope (erythematous periorbital) rash, "shawl and face" rash **B**, "mechanic's hands." ↑ risk of occult malignancy. Perimysial inflammation and atrophy with CD4+ T cells.

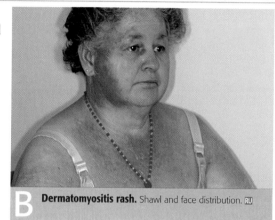

B **Dermatomyositis rash.** Shawl and face distribution. RU

FINDINGS | ↑ CK, ⊕ ANA, ⊕ anti-Jo-1, ⊕ anti-SRP, ⊕ anti-Mi-2 antibodies.

TREATMENT | Steroids.

Neuromuscular junction diseases

	Myasthenia gravis	Lambert-Eaton myasthenic syndrome
FREQUENCY	Most common NMJ disorder	Uncommon
PATHOPHYSIOLOGY	Autoantibodies to postsynaptic ACh receptor	Autoantibodies to presynaptic Ca^{2+} channel → ↓ ACh release
CLINICAL	Ptosis, diplopia, weakness Worsens with muscle use	Proximal muscle weakness, autonomic symptoms (dry mouth, impotence) Improves with muscle use
ASSOCIATED WITH	Thymoma, thymic hyperplasia	Small cell lung cancer
AChE INHIBITOR ADMINISTRATION	Reversal of symptoms	Minimal effect

Myositis ossificans

Metaplasia of skeletal muscle to bone following muscular trauma **A**. Most often seen in upper or lower extremity. May present as suspicious "mass" at site of known trauma or as incidental finding on radiography.

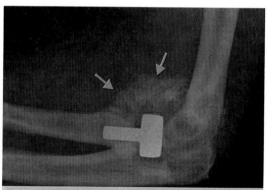

A **Myositis ossificans.** Heterotopic ossification of elbow (arrows) after injury and prosthetic radial head replacement.

Scleroderma (systemic sclerosis)

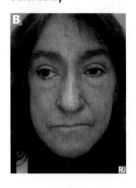

Excessive fibrosis and collagen deposition throughout the body. Commonly sclerosis of skin, manifesting as puffy and taut skin A B with absence of wrinkles. Also sclerosis of renal, pulmonary (most common cause of death), cardiovascular, and GI systems. 75% female. 2 major types:

- **Diffuse scleroderma**—widespread skin involvement, rapid progression, early visceral involvement. Associated with anti-Scl-70 antibody (anti-DNA topoisomerase I antibody).

- **Limited scleroderma**—limited skin involvement confined to fingers and face. Also with **CREST** involvement: **C**alcinosis, **R**aynaud phenomenon, **E**sophageal dysmotility, **S**clerodactyly, and **T**elangiectasia. More benign clinical course. Associated with anti**C**entromere antibody (**C** for **CREST**).

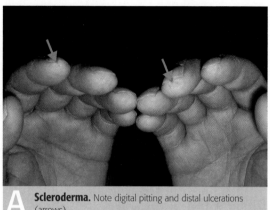

A **Scleroderma.** Note digital pitting and distal ulcerations (arrows).

Dermatologic macroscopic terms (morphology)

LESION	CHARACTERISTICS	EXAMPLES
Macule	Flat lesion with well-circumscribed change in skin color < 1 cm	Freckle, labial macule **A**
Patch	Macule > 1 cm	Large birthmark (congenital nevus) **B**
Papule	Elevated solid skin lesion < 1 cm	Mole (nevus) **C**, acne
Plaque	Papule > 1 cm	Psoriasis **D**
Vesicle	Small fluid-containing blister < 1 cm	Chickenpox (varicella), shingles (zoster) **E**
Bulla	Large fluid-containing blister > 1 cm	Bullous pemphigoid **F**
Pustule	Vesicle containing pus	Pustular psoriasis **G**
Wheal	Transient smooth papule or plaque	Hives (urticaria) **H**
Scale	Flaking off of stratum corneum	Eczema, psoriasis, SCC **I**
Crust	Dry exudate	Impetigo **J**

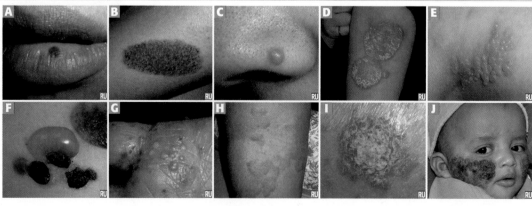

Dermatologic microscopic terms

LESION	CHARACTERISTICS	EXAMPLES
Hyperkeratosis	↑ thickness of stratum corneum	Psoriasis, calluses
Parakeratosis	Hyperkeratosis with retention of nuclei in stratum corneum	Psoriasis
Spongiosis	Epidermal accumulation of edematous fluid in intercellular spaces	Eczematous dermatitis
Acantholysis	Separation of epidermal cells	Pemphigus vulgaris
Acanthosis	Epidermal hyperplasia (↑ spinosum)	Acanthosis nigricans

Pigmented skin disorders

Albinism	Normal melanocyte number with ↓ melanin production 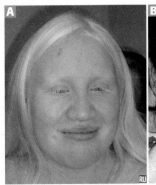 due to ↓ tyrosinase activity or defective tyrosine transport. Can also be caused by failure of neural crest cell migration during development. ↑ risk of skin cancer.
Melasma (chloasma)	Hyperpigmentation associated with pregnancy ("mask of pregnancy" 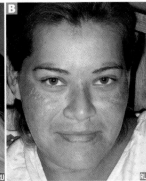) or OCP use.
Vitiligo	Irregular areas of complete depigmentation 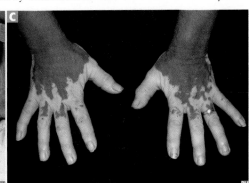. Caused by autoimmune destruction of melanocytes.

Common skin disorders

Verrucae	Warts; caused by HPV. Soft, tan-colored, cauliflower-like papules **A**. Epidermal hyperplasia, hyperkeratosis, koilocytosis. Condyloma acuminatum on genitals **B**.
Melanocytic nevus	Common mole. Benign, but melanoma can arise in congenital or atypical moles. Intradermal nevi are papular **C**. Junctional nevi are flat macules **D**.
Urticaria	Hives. Pruritic wheals that form after mast cell degranulation **E**. Characterized by superficial dermal edema and lymphatic channel dilation.
Ephelis	Freckle. Normal number of melanocytes, ↑ melanin pigment **F**.
Atopic dermatitis (eczema)	Pruritic eruption, commonly on skin flexures. Often associated with other atopic diseases (asthma, allergic rhinitis). Usually starts on the face in infancy **G** and often appears in the antecubital fossae **H** thereafter.
Allergic contact dermatitis	Type IV hypersensitivity reaction that follows exposure to allergen. Lesions occur at site of contact (e.g., nickel **I**, poison ivy, neomycin **J**).
Psoriasis	Papules and plaques with silvery scaling **K**, especially on knees and elbows. Acanthosis with parakeratotic scaling (nuclei still in stratum corneum). ↑ stratum spinosum, ↓ stratum granulosum. Auspitz sign (arrow in **L**)—pinpoint bleeding spots from exposure of dermal papillae when scales are scraped off. Can be associated with nail pitting and psoriatic arthritis.
Seborrheic keratosis	Flat, greasy, pigmented squamous epithelial proliferation with keratin-filled cysts (horn cysts) **M**. Looks "stuck on" **N O**. Lesions occur on head, trunk, and extremities. Common benign neoplasm of older persons. Leser-Trélat sign—sudden appearance of multiple seborrheic keratoses, indicating an underlying malignancy (e.g., GI, lymphoid).

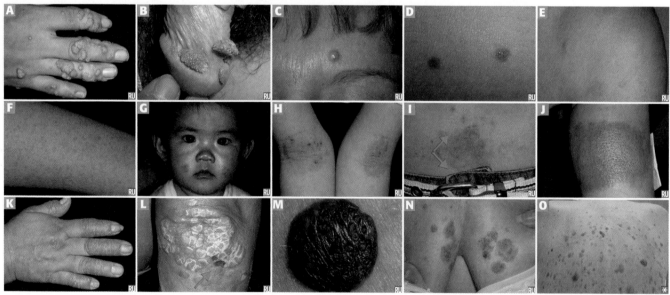

Infectious skin disorders

Impetigo	Very superficial skin infection. Usually from S. *aureus* or S. *pyogenes*. Highly contagious. Honey-colored crusting **A**. Bullous impetigo **B** has bullae and is usually caused by S. *aureus*.
Cellulitis	Acute, painful, spreading infection of dermis and subcutaneous tissues. Usually from S. *pyogenes* or S. *aureus*. Often starts with a break in skin from trauma or another infection **C**.
Necrotizing fasciitis	Deeper tissue injury, usually from anaerobic bacteria or S. *pyogenes*. Results in crepitus from methane and CO_2 production. "Flesh-eating bacteria." Causes bullae and a purple color to the skin **D**.
Staphylococcal scalded skin syndrome	Exotoxin destroys keratinocyte attachments in the stratum granulosum only (vs. toxic epidermal necrolysis, which destroys the epidermal-dermal junction). Characterized by fever and generalized erythematous rash with sloughing of the upper layers of the epidermis that heals completely. Seen in newborns and children **E**.
Hairy leukoplakia	White, painless plaques on the tongue that cannot be scraped off **F**. EBV mediated. Occurs in HIV-positive patients.

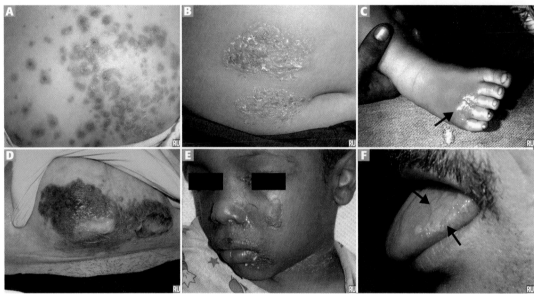

Blistering skin disorders

Pemphigus vulgaris

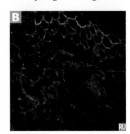

Potentially fatal autoimmune skin disorder with IgG antibody against desmoglein (component of desmosomes).

Flaccid intraepidermal bullae 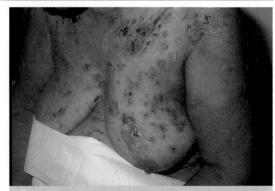 caused by acantholysis (keratinocytes in stratum spinosum are connected by desmosomes); oral mucosa also involved.

Immunofluorescence reveals antibodies around epidermal cells in a reticular (net-like) pattern B.

Nikolsky sign ⊕ (separation of epidermis upon manual stroking of skin).

A **Pemphigus vulgaris.** Note multiple crusty and weepy erythematous erosions where blisters have broken. ✲

Bullous pemphigoid

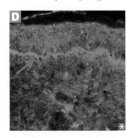

Less severe than pemphigus vulgaris. Involves IgG antibody against hemidesmosomes (epidermal basement membrane; antibodies are "**bullow**" the epidermis).

Tense blisters **C** containing eosinophils affect skin but spare oral mucosa.

Immunofluorescence reveals linear pattern at epidermal-dermal junction **D**.

Nikolsky sign ⊖.

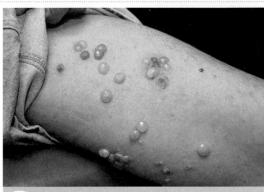

C **Bullous pemphigoid.** Note multiple intact, tense bullae. RU

Dermatitis herpetiformis

Pruritic papules, vesicles, and bullae (often found on elbows) **E**. Deposits of IgA at the tips of dermal papillae. Associated with celiac disease.

E **Dermatitis herpetiformis.** Papules and vesicles on an erythematous base. ✲

Blistering skin disorders *(continued)*

Erythema multiforme	Associated with infections (e.g., *Mycoplasma pneumoniae*, HSV), drugs (e.g., sulfa drugs, β-lactams, phenytoin), cancers, and autoimmune disease. Presents with multiple types of lesions—macules, papules, vesicles, and target lesions (look like targets with multiple rings and a dusky center showing epithelial disruption) **F**.	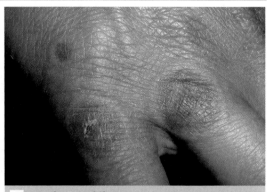 **F** **Erythema multiforme.** Note target lesions in patient with erythema multiforme secondary to HSV. RU
Stevens-Johnson syndrome	Characterized by fever, bulla formation and necrosis, sloughing of skin, and a high mortality rate. Typically 2 mucous membranes are involved **G**, and skin lesions may appear like targets as seen in erythema multiforme. Usually associated with adverse drug reaction. A more severe form of Stevens-Johnson syndrome with > 30% of the body surface area involved is **toxic epidermal necrolysis** **H** **I**.	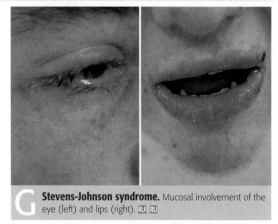 **G** **Stevens-Johnson syndrome.** Mucosal involvement of the eye (left) and lips (right). RU, RU

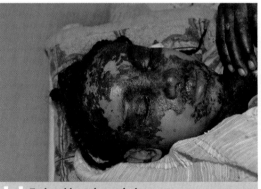

H **Toxic epidermal necrolysis.** Note epidermal sloughing of skin leading to depigmentation. RU

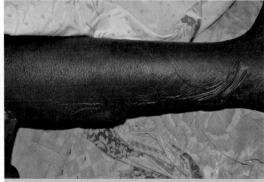

I **Toxic epidermal necrolysis.** Large bullae with skin sloughing in sheets. RU

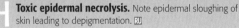

Miscellaneous skin disorders

Acanthosis nigricans	Epidermal hyperplasia causing symmetrical, hyperpigmented, velvety thickening of skin, especially on neck or in axilla 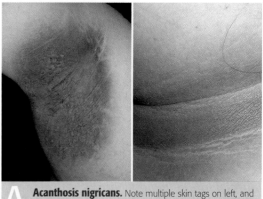. Associated with hyperinsulinemia (e.g., diabetes, obesity, Cushing syndrome) and visceral malignancy (e.g., gastric adenocarcinoma).	

A Acanthosis nigricans. Note multiple skin tags on left, and velvety appearance on right. RU, RU

Actinic keratosis	Premalignant lesions caused by sun exposure. Small, rough, erythematous or brownish papules or plaques 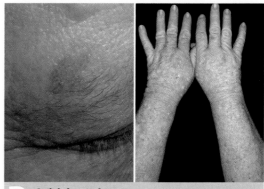. Risk of squamous cell carcinoma is proportional to degree of epithelial dysplasia.

B Actinic keratosis. Large actinic keratosis (AK) over the eyebrow (left). RU Multiple AKs on hands and forearms (right). RU

Erythema nodosum	Painful inflammatory lesions of subcutaneous fat, usually on anterior shins. Often idiopathic, but can be associated with sarcoidosis, coccidioidomycosis, histoplasmosis, TB, streptococcal infections, leprosy, and Crohn disease 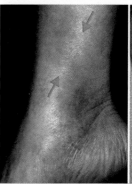.

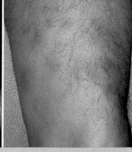

C Erythema nodosum Lesions on leg in patient with streptococcal infection (left) and patient with leprosy and erythema nodosum leprosum (right). RU, RU

Miscellaneous skin disorders (continued)

Lichen Planus	Pruritic, Purple, Polygonal Planar Papules and Plaques are the 6 P's of lichen Planus 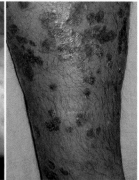. Mucosal involvement manifests as Wickham striae (reticular white lines). Sawtooth infiltrate of lymphocytes at dermal-epidermal junction. Associated with hepatitis C.

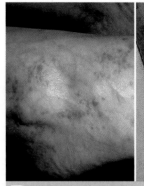

D **Lichen planus.** Appearance on light skin (left) and dark skin (right). RU, RU

Pityriasis rosea	"Herald patch" followed days later by "Christmas tree" distribution **E**. Multiple plaques with collarette scale. Self-resolving in 6–8 weeks.

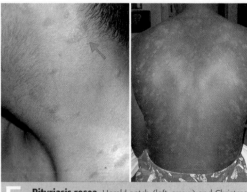

E **Pityriasis rosea.** Herald patch (left, arrow) and Christmas tree distribution (right). RU, RU

Sunburn	Acute cutaneous inflammatory reaction due to excessive UV irradiation. Causes DNA mutations, inducing apoptosis of keratinocytes. UVA is dominant in tanning and photoaging, UVB in sunburn. Can lead to impetigo **F** and skin cancers (basal cell carcinoma, squamous cell carcinoma, and melanoma).

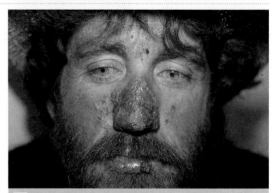

F **Sunburn with impetigo.** Disruption of normal skin integrity led to secondary bacterial infection (impetigo). RU

Skin cancer

Basal cell carcinoma

Most common skin cancer. Found in sun-exposed areas of body. Locally invasive, but almost never metastasizes. Pink, pearly nodules, commonly with telangiectasias, rolled borders, and central crusting or ulceration A. BCCs also appear as nonhealing ulcers with infiltrating growth B or as a scaling plaque (superficial BCC) C. Basal cell tumors have "palisading" nuclei D.

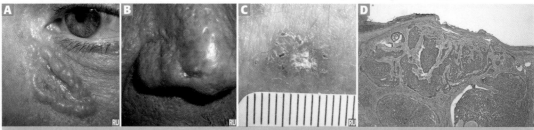

Basal cell carcinoma. Appearance includes A rolled borders, B nonhealing ulcer, or C scaling plaque. Histology D reveals nests of basaloid cells in dermis.

Squamous cell carcinoma

Second most common skin cancer. Associated with excessive exposure to sunlight, immunosuppression, and occasionally arsenic exposure. Commonly appears on face E, lower lip F, ears, and hands. Locally invasive, but may spread to lymph nodes and will rarely metastasize. Ulcerative red lesions with frequent scale. Associated with chronic draining sinuses. Histopathology: keratin "pearls" G.

Actinic keratosis, a scaly plaque, is a precursor to squamous cell carcinoma.

Keratoacanthoma is a variant that grows rapidly (4–6 weeks) and may regress spontaneously over months H.

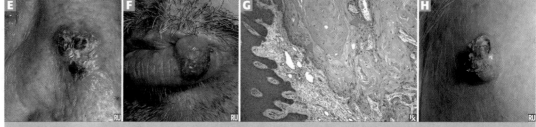

Squamous cell carcinoma. Commonly seen on faces E and lips F. Histology reveals keratin "pearls" G. Keratoacanthoma H is a variant.

Melanoma

Common tumor with significant risk of metastasis. S-100 tumor marker. Associated with sunlight exposure; fair-skinned persons are at ↑ risk. Depth of tumor correlates with risk of metastasis. Look for the **ABCDEs**: **A**symmetry, **B**order irregularity, **C**olor variation, **D**iameter > 6 mm, and **E**volution over time. At least 4 different types of melanoma I J K L. Often driven by activating mutation in BRAF kinase. Primary treatment is excision with appropriately wide margins. Metastatic or unresectable melanoma in patients with *BRAF* V600E mutation may benefit from vemurafenib, a BRAF kinase inhibitor.

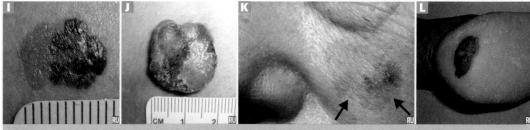

Melanoma. Multiple variants, including superficial spreading melanoma I, nodular melanoma J, lentigo maligna melanoma K, and acrolentiginous melanoma L.

▶ MUSCULOSKELETAL, SKIN, AND CONNECTIVE TISSUE–PHARMACOLOGY

Arachidonic acid products

Lipoxygenase pathway yields Leukotrienes. LTB_4 is a **neutrophil** chemotactic agent. LTC_4, D_4, and E_4 function in bronchoconstriction, vasoconstriction, contraction of smooth muscle, and ↑ vascular permeability.

PGI_2 inhibits platelet aggregation and promotes vasodilation.

L for Lipoxygenase and Leukotriene. **Neutrophils arrive "B4" others.**

Platelet-Gathering Inhibitor.

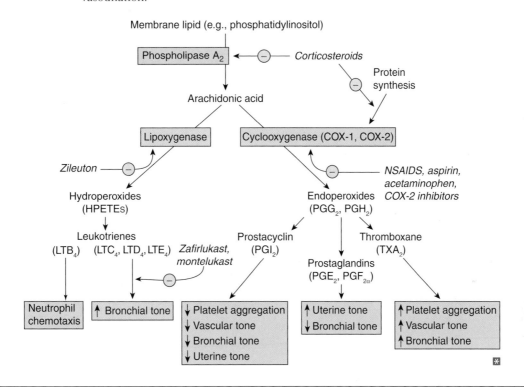

Aspirin

MECHANISM	Irreversibly inhibits cyclooxygenase (both COX-1 and COX-2) by covalent acetylation, which ↓ synthesis of both thromboxane A_2 (TXA_2) and prostaglandins. ↑ bleeding time until new platelets are produced (~ 7 days). No effect on PT, PTT. A type of NSAID.
CLINICAL USE	Low dose (< 300 mg/day): ↓ platelet aggregation. Intermediate dose (300–2400 mg/day): antipyretic and analgesic. High dose (2400–4000 mg/day): anti-inflammatory.
TOXICITY	Gastric ulceration, tinnitus (CN VIII). Chronic use can lead to acute renal failure, interstitial nephritis, and upper GI bleeding. Risk of Reye syndrome in children treated with aspirin for viral infection. Also stimulates respiratory centers, causing hyperventilation and respiratory alkalosis.

NSAIDs	Ibuprofen, naproxen, indomethacin, ketorolac, diclofenac.
MECHANISM	Reversibly inhibit cyclooxygenase (both COX-1 and COX-2). Block PG synthesis.
CLINICAL USE	Antipyretic, analgesic, anti-inflammatory. Indomethacin is used to close a PDA.
TOXICITY	Interstitial nephritis, gastric ulcer (PGs protect gastric mucosa), renal ischemia (PGs vasodilate afferent arteriole).

COX-2 inhibitors (celecoxib)	
MECHANISM	Reversibly inhibit specifically the cyclooxygenase (COX) isoform 2, which is found in inflammatory cells and vascular endothelium and mediates inflammation and pain; spares COX-1, which helps maintain the gastric mucosa. Thus, should not have the corrosive effects of other NSAIDs on the GI lining. Spares platelet function as TXA_2 production is dependent on COX-1.
CLINICAL USE	Rheumatoid arthritis and osteoarthritis; patients with gastritis or ulcers.
TOXICITY	↑ risk of thrombosis. Sulfa allergy.

Acetaminophen	
MECHANISM	Reversibly inhibits cyclooxygenase, mostly in CNS. Inactivated peripherally.
CLINICAL USE	Antipyretic, analgesic, but not anti-inflammatory. Used instead of aspirin to avoid Reye syndrome in children with viral infection.
TOXICITY	Overdose produces hepatic necrosis; acetaminophen metabolite (NAPQI) depletes glutathione and forms toxic tissue adducts in liver. N-acetylcysteine is antidote—regenerates glutathione.

Bisphosphonates	Alendronate, other -dronates.
MECHANISM	Pyrophosphate analogs; bind hydroxyapatite in bone, inhibiting osteoclast activity.
CLINICAL USE	Osteoporosis, hypercalcemia, Paget disease of bone.
TOXICITY	Corrosive esophagitis (patients are advised to take with water and remain upright for 30 minutes), osteonecrosis of the jaw.

Gout drugs

Chronic gout drugs (preventive)

Allopurinol	Inhibits xanthine oxidase, ↓ conversion of xanthine to uric acid. Also used in lymphoma and leukemia to prevent tumor lysis–associated urate nephropathy. ↑ concentrations of azathioprine and 6-MP (both normally metabolized by xanthine oxidase). Do not give salicylates; all but the highest doses depress uric acid clearance. Even high doses (5–6 g/day) have only minor uricosuric activity.
Febuxostat	Inhibits xanthine oxidase.
Probenecid	Inhibits reabsorption of uric acid in PCT (also inhibits secretion of penicillin).

Acute gout drugs

NSAIDs	Naproxen, indomethacin.
Glucocorticoids	Oral or intraarticular.
Colchicine	Binds and stabilizes tubulin to inhibit microtubule polymerization, impairing leukocyte chemotaxis and degranulation. Acute and prophylactic value. GI side effects.

Diet → Purines ← Nucleic acids

Hypoxanthine

Xanthine oxidase

Xanthine — **Allopurinol, Febuxostat**

Xanthine oxidase

Plasma uric acid → Urate crystals deposited in joints → Gout

Tubular reabsorption

Probenecid and high-dose salicylates

Tubular secretion

Diuretics and low-dose salicylates

Urine

TNF-α inhibitors	All TNF-α inhibitors predispose to infection, including reactivation of latent TB, since TNF blockade prevents activation of macrophages and destruction of phagocytosed microbes.

DRUG	MECHANISM	CLINICAL USE
Etanercept	Fusion protein (receptor for TNF-α + IgG$_1$ Fc), produced by recombinant DNA. Etanercept is a TNF decoy receptor.	Rheumatoid arthritis, psoriasis, ankylosing spondylitis
Infliximab, adalimumab	Anti-TNF-α monoclonal antibody	IBD, rheumatoid arthritis, ankylosing spondylitis, psoriasis

▶ NOTES

Neurology

"Estimated amount of glucose used by an adult human brain each day, expressed in M&Ms: 250."

—Harper's Index

"He has two neurons held together by a spirochete."

—Anonymous

"I never came upon any of my discoveries through the process of rational thinking."

—Albert Einstein

"I like nonsense; it wakes up the brain cells."

—Dr. Seuss

▶ NEUROLOGY–EMBRYOLOGY

Neural development

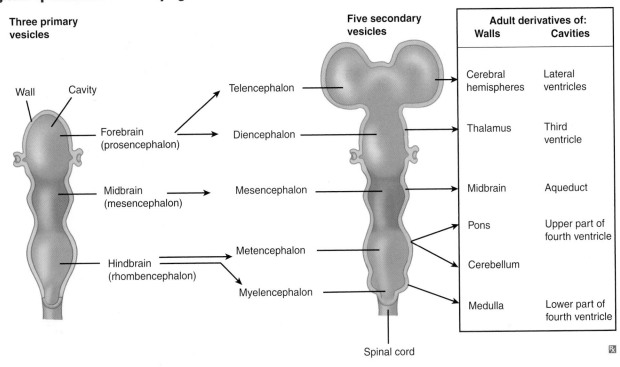

Day 18

Day 21

Notochord induces overlying ectoderm to differentiate into neuroectoderm and form the neural plate.

Neural plate gives rise to the neural tube and neural crest cells.

Notochord becomes nucleus pulposus of the intervertebral disc in adults.

Alar plate (dorsal): sensory
Basal plate (ventral): motor ⎤ Same orientation as spinal cord.

Regional specification of developing brain

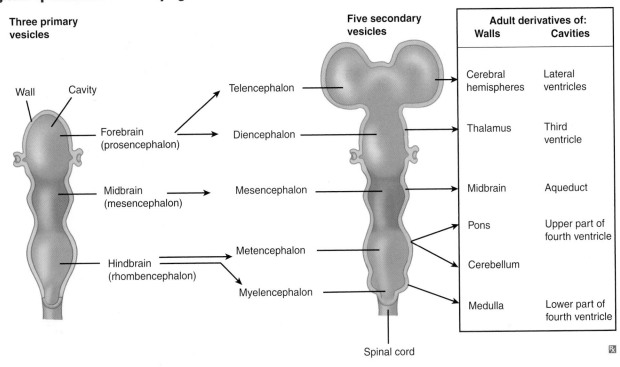

Three primary vesicles	Five secondary vesicles	Adult derivatives of:	
		Walls	**Cavities**
Forebrain (prosencephalon)	Telencephalon	Cerebral hemispheres	Lateral ventricles
	Diencephalon	Thalamus	Third ventricle
Midbrain (mesencephalon)	Mesencephalon	Midbrain	Aqueduct
Hindbrain (rhombencephalon)	Metencephalon	Pons	Upper part of fourth ventricle
		Cerebellum	
	Myelencephalon	Medulla	Lower part of fourth ventricle

Spinal cord

CNS/PNS origins

Neuroectoderm—CNS neurons; ependymal cells (inner lining of ventricles, make CSF); oligodendroglia; astrocytes.

Neural crest—PNS neurons, Schwann cells.

Mesoderm—**M**icroglia (like **M**acrophages, originate from **M**esoderm).

Neural tube defects	Neuropores fail to fuse (4th week) → persistent connection between amniotic cavity and spinal canal. Associated with low folic acid intake before conception and during pregnancy. Elevated α-fetoprotein (AFP) in amniotic fluid and maternal serum. ↑ acetylcholinesterase (AChE) in amniotic fluid is a helpful confirmatory test (fetal AChE in CSF transudates across defect into the amniotic fluid).
Spina bifida occulta	Failure of bony spinal canal to close, but no structural herniation. Usually seen at lower vertebral levels. Dura is intact. Associated with tuft of hair or skin dimple at level of bony defect.
Meningocele	Meninges (but not the spinal cord) herniate through spinal canal defect. Normal AFP.
Meningomyelocele	Meninges and spinal cord herniate through spinal canal defect.

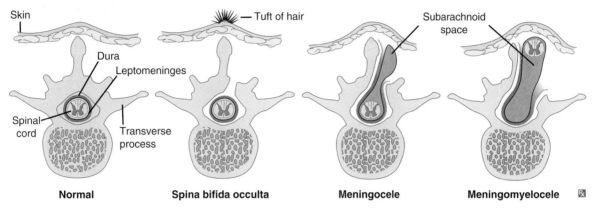

Normal   Spina bifida occulta   Meningocele   Meningomyelocele

Forebrain anomalies

Anencephaly	Malformation of anterior neural tube resulting in no forebrain, open calvarium ("frog-like appearance"). Clinical findings: ↑ AFP; polyhydramnios (no swallowing center in brain). Associated with maternal diabetes (type I). Maternal folate supplementation ↓ risk.
Holoprosencephaly	Failure of left and right hemispheres to separate; usually occurs during weeks 5–6. Complex multifactorial etiology that may be related to mutations in sonic hedgehog signaling pathway. Moderate form has cleft lip/palate, most severe form results in cyclopia.

Posterior fossa malformations

Chiari II (Arnold-Chiari malformation)	Significant herniation of cerebellar tonsils and vermis through foramen magnum with aqueductal stenosis and hydrocephalus. Often presents with lumbosacral myelomeningocele and paralysis below the defect.
Dandy-Walker	Agenesis of cerebellar vermis with cystic enlargement of 4th ventricle (fills the enlarged posterior fossa). Associated with hydrocephalus and spina bifida.

Syringomyelia   Cystic cavity (syrinx) within the spinal cord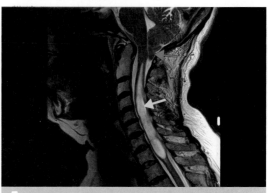
(if central canal → hydromyelia). Crossing
anterior spinal commissural fibers are typically
damaged first. Results in a "cape-like,"
bilateral loss of pain and temperature sensation
in upper extremities (fine touch sensation is
preserved).

Syrinx = tube, as in syringe.
Most common at C8–T1.
Associated with Chiari I malformation
(> 3–5 mm cerebellar tonsillar ectopia;
congenital, usually asymptomatic in
childhood, manifests with headaches and
cerebellar symptoms).

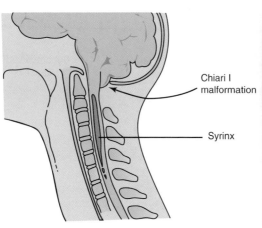

Chiari I
malformation

Syrinx

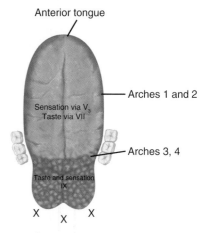

A   **Syringomyelia.** MRI of cervical spine shows low-lying
cerebellar tonsils (Chiari I, red arrow) and fluid-filled cavity in
spinal cord (syrinx, yellow arrow). ✴

Tongue development   1st and 2nd branchial arches form anterior $^2/_3$
(thus sensation via CN V_3, taste via CN VII).
3rd and 4th branchial arches form posterior $^1/_3$
(thus sensation and taste mainly via CN IX,
extreme posterior via CN X).
Motor innervation is via CN XII.
Muscles of the tongue are derived from occipital
myotomes.

Taste—CN VII, IX, X (solitary nucleus).
Pain—CN V_3, IX, X.
Motor—CN XII.

Anterior tongue

Arches 1 and 2

Sensation via V_3
Taste via VII

Arches 3, 4

Taste and sensation
IX

X   X   X

Posterior tongue

▶ NEUROLOGY–ANATOMY AND PHYSIOLOGY

Neurons

Signal-transmitting cells of the nervous system. Permanent cells—do not divide in adulthood (and, as a general rule, have no progenitor stem cell population).

Signal-relaying cells with dendrites (receive input), cell bodies, and axons (send output). Cell bodies and dendrites can be stained via the Nissl substance (stains RER). RER is not present in the axon.

If an axon is injured, it undergoes Wallerian degeneration—degeneration distal to the injury and axonal retraction proximally; allows for potential regeneration of axon (if in PNS).

Astrocytes

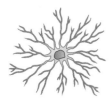

Physical support, repair, K^+ metabolism, removal of excess neurotransmitter, component of blood-brain barrier, glycogen fuel reserve buffer. Reactive gliosis in response to neural injury. Astrocyte marker—GFAP. Derived from neuroectoderm.

Microglia

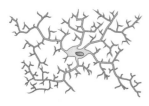

CNS phagocytes. Mesodermal origin. Not readily discernible in Nissl stains. Have small irregular nuclei and relatively little cytoplasm. Scavenger cells of the CNS. Respond to tissue damage by differentiating into large phagocytic cells. Part of the mononuclear phagocyte system.

HIV-infected microglia fuse to form multinucleated giant cells in the CNS.

Myelin

↑ conduction velocity of signals transmitted down axons. Results in saltatory conduction of action potential between nodes of Ranvier, where there are high concentrations of Na^+ channels. CNS—oligodendrocytes; PNS—Schwann cells.

Wraps and insulates axons: ↑ space constant and ↑ conduction velocity.

Oligodendroglia

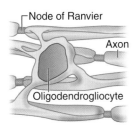

— Node of Ranvier

Axon

Oligodendrogliocyte

Myelinates the axons of neurons in the CNS. Each oligodendrocyte can myelinate many axons (~30). Predominant type of glial cell in white matter.

Derived from neuroectoderm.

"Fried egg" appearance on H&E stain.

Injured in multiple sclerosis, progressive multifocal leukoencephalopathy (PML), and leukodystrophies.

Schwann cells

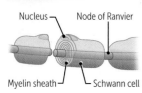

Each Schwann cell myelinates only 1 PNS axon. Also promote axonal regeneration. Derived from neural crest.

↑ conduction velocity via saltatory conduction between nodes of Ranvier, where there are high concentrations of Na⁺ channels.

Destroyed in Guillain-Barré syndrome.

Acoustic neuroma—type of schwannoma. Typically located in internal acoustic meatus (CN VIII). If bilateral, strongly associated with neurofibromatosis type 2.

Sensory corpuscles

RECEPTOR TYPE	DESCRIPTION	LOCATION	SENSES
Free nerve endings	C—slow, unmyelinated fibers Aδ—fast, myelinated fibers	All skin, epidermis, some viscera	Pain and temperature
Meissner corpuscles	Large, myelinated fibers; adapt quickly	Glabrous (hairless) skin	Dynamic, fine/light touch; position sense
Pacinian corpuscles	Large, myelinated fibers; adapt quickly	Deep skin layers, ligaments, and joints	Vibration, pressure
Merkel discs	Large, myelinated fibers; adapt slowly	Basal epidermal layer, hair follicles	Pressure, deep static touch (e.g., shapes, edges), position sense

Peripheral nerve

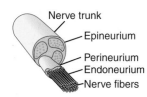

Endoneurium—invests single nerve fiber layers (inflammatory infiltrate in Guillain-Barré syndrome).

Perineurium (Permeability barrier)—surrounds a fascicle of nerve fibers. Must be rejoined in microsurgery for limb reattachment.

Epineurium—dense connective tissue that surrounds entire nerve (fascicles and blood vessels).

Endo = inner.
Peri = around.
Epi = outer.

Neurotransmitters

TYPE	CHANGE IN DISEASE	LOCATIONS OF SYNTHESIS[a]
Norepinephrine	↑ in anxiety ↓ in depression	Locus ceruleus (pons)
Dopamine	↑ in Huntington disease ↓ in Parkinson disease ↓ in depression	Ventral tegmentum and SNc (midbrain)
5-HT	↑ in Parkinson disease ↓ in anxiety ↓ in depression	Raphe nucleus (pons, medulla, midbrain)
ACh	↑ in Parkinson disease ↓ in Alzheimer disease ↓ in Huntington disease	Basal nucleus of Meynert
GABA	↓ in anxiety ↓ in Huntington disease	Nucleus accumbens

[a]Locus ceruleus—stress and panic. Nucleus accumbens and septal nucleus—reward center, pleasure, addiction, fear.

Blood-brain barrier

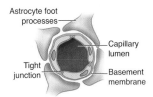

Astrocyte foot processes
Capillary lumen
Tight junction
Basement membrane

Prevents circulating blood substances from reaching the CSF/CNS. Formed by 3 structures:
- Tight junctions between nonfenestrated capillary endothelial cells
- Basement membrane
- Astrocyte foot processes

Glucose and amino acids cross slowly by carrier-mediated transport mechanism.

Nonpolar/lipid-soluble substances cross rapidly via diffusion.

A few specialized brain regions with fenestrated capillaries and no blood-brain barrier allow molecules in the blood to affect brain function (e.g., area postrema—vomiting after chemo, OVLT—osmotic sensing) or neurosecretory products to enter circulation (e.g., neurohypophysis—ADH release).

Other notable barriers include:
- Blood-testis barrier
- Maternal-fetal blood barrier of placenta

Infarction and/or neoplasm destroys endothelial cell tight junctions → vasogenic edema.

Hypothalamic inputs and outputs permeate the blood-brain barrier.

Helps prevent bacterial infection from spreading into the CNS. Also restricts drug delivery to brain.

Hypothalamus	The hypothalamus wears **TAN HATS**—Thirst and water balance, Adenohypophysis control (regulates anterior pituitary), Neurohypophysis releases hormones produced in the hypothalamus, Hunger, Autonomic regulation, Temperature regulation, Sexual urges. Inputs (areas not protected by blood-brain barrier): OVLT (organum vasculosum of the lamina terminalis; senses change in osmolarity), area postrema (responds to emetics). Supraoptic nucleus makes ADH. Paraventricular nucleus makes oxytocin. ADH and oxytocin: made by hypothalamus but stored and released by posterior pituitary.	
Lateral area	Hunger. Destruction → anorexia, failure to thrive (infants). Inhibited by leptin.	If you zap your **lateral** nucleus, you shrink **lateral**ly.
Ventromedial area	Satiety. Destruction (e.g., craniopharyngioma) → hyperphagia. Stimulated by leptin.	If you zap your **ventromedial** nucleus, you grow **ventral**ly and **medial**ly.
Anterior hypothalamus	Cooling, parasympathetic.	Anterior nucleus = cool off (cooling, p**A**rasympathetic). A/C = anterior cooling.
Posterior hypothalamus	Heating, sympathetic.	Posterior nucleus = get fired up (heating, sympathetic). If you zap your posterior hypothalamus, you become a poikilotherm (cold-blooded, like a snake).
Suprachiasmatic nucleus	Circadian rhythm.	You need **sleep** to be **charismatic** (chiasmatic).

Sleep physiology

Sleep cycle is regulated by the circadian rhythm, which is driven by SCN of hypothalamus. Circadian rhythm controls nocturnal release of ACTH, prolactin, melatonin, and norepinephrine: Suprachiasmatic nucleus (SCN) → norepinephrine release → pineal gland → melatonin. SCN is regulated by environment (e.g., light).

Two stages: rapid-eye movement (REM) and non-REM. Extraocular movements during REM sleep due to activity of PPRF (paramedian pontine reticular formation/conjugate gaze center). REM sleep occurs every 90 minutes, and duration ↑ through the night.

Alcohol, benzodiazepines, and barbiturates are associated with ↓ REM sleep and delta wave sleep; norepinephrine also ↓ REM sleep.

Treat bedwetting (sleep enuresis) with oral desmopressin acetate (DDAVP), which mimics ADH; preferred over imipramine because of the latter's adverse effects.

Benzodiazepines are useful for night terrors and sleepwalking.

SLEEP STAGE (% OF TOTAL SLEEP TIME IN YOUNG ADULTS)	DESCRIPTION	EEG WAVEFORM
Awake (eyes open)	Alert, active mental concentration	Beta (highest frequency, lowest amplitude)
Awake (eyes closed)		Alpha
Non-REM sleep		
Stage N1 (5%)	Light sleep	Theta
Stage N2 (45%)	Deeper sleep; when bruxism occurs	Sleep spindles and K complexes
Stage N3 (25%)	Deepest non-REM sleep (slow-wave sleep); when sleepwalking, night terrors, and bedwetting occur	Delta (lowest frequency, highest amplitude)
REM sleep (25%)	Loss of motor tone, ↑ brain O_2 use, ↑ and variable pulse and blood pressure; when dreaming and penile/clitoral tumescence occur; may serve a memory processing function	Beta At night, BATS Drink Blood

Awake · Stage N1 · Stage N2 · Stage N3 · REM

EEG · K-complex · Sleep spindle · 50 µV · 1 s

Posterior pituitary (neurohypophysis)

Receives hypothalamic axonal projections from supraoptic (ADH) and paraventricular (oxytocin) nuclei.

Oxytocin: *oxys* = quick; *tocos* = birth.
Adenohypophysis = Anterior pituitary.

Thalamus   Major relay for all ascending sensory information except olfaction.

NUCLEUS	INPUT	INFO	DESTINATION	MNEMONIC
VPL	Spinothalamic and dorsal columns/medial lemniscus	Pain and temperature; pressure, touch, vibration, and proprioception	1° somatosensory cortex	
VPM	Trigeminal and gustatory pathway	Face sensation and taste	1° somatosensory cortex	Makeup goes on the face (VPM)
LGN	CN II	Vision	Calcarine sulcus	Lateral = Light
MGN	Superior olive and inferior colliculus of tectum	Hearing	Auditory cortex of temporal lobe	Medial = Music
VL	Basal ganglia, cerebellum	Motor	Motor cortex	

Limbic system   Collection of neural structures involved in   The famous 5 F's.
emotion, long-term memory, olfaction,
behavior modulation, and autonomic nervous
system function.
Structures include hippocampus, amygdala,
fornix, mammillary bodies, and cingulate
gyrus. Responsible for Feeding, Fleeing,
Fighting, Feeling, and Sex.

Cerebellum   Modulates movement; aids in coordination and balance.
Input:
- Contralateral cortex via middle cerebellar peduncle.
- Ipsilateral proprioceptive information via inferior cerebellar peduncle from the spinal cord (input nerves = climbing and mossy fibers).

Output:
- Sends information to contralateral cortex to modulate movement. Output nerves = Purkinje cells → deep nuclei of cerebellum → contralateral cortex via the superior cerebellar peduncle.
- Deep nuclei (lateral → medial)—Dentate, Emboliform, Globose, Fastigial ("Don't Eat Greasy Foods").

Lateral lesions—voluntary movement of extremities; when injured, propensity to fall toward injured (ipsilateral) side.

Medial lesions—Lesions involving midline structures (vermal cortex, fastigial nuclei) and/or the flocculonodular lobe result in truncal ataxia, nystagmus, and head tilting. These patients also may have a wide-based (cerebellar) gait and deficits in truncal coordination. Generally, midline lesions result in bilateral motor deficits affecting axial and proximal limb musculature.

Basal ganglia

Important in voluntary movements and making postural adjustments.

Receives cortical input, provides negative feedback to cortex to modulate movement.

Striatum = putamen (motor) + caudate (cognitive).

Lentiform = putamen + globus pallidus.

D_1-Receptor = D1Rect pathway.

Indirect = Inhibitory.

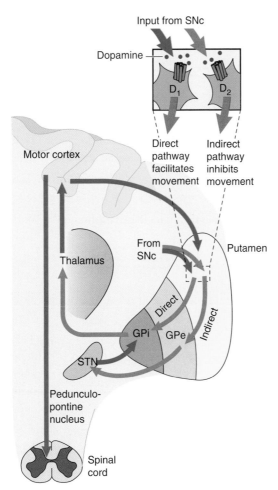

■ Stimulatory
■ Inhibitory

SNc	Substantia nigra pars compacta
GPe	Globus pallidus externus
GPi	Globus pallidus internus
STN	Subthalamic nucleus
D_1	Dopamine D_1 receptor
D_2	Dopamine D_2 receptor

Excitatory pathway—cortical inputs stimulate the striatum, stimulating the release of GABA, which disinhibits the thalamus via the GPi/SNr (↑ motion).

Inhibitory pathway—cortical inputs stimulate the striatum, which disinhibits STN via GPe, and STN stimulates GPi/SNr to inhibit the thalamus (↓ motion).

Dopamine binds to D_1, stimulating the excitatory pathway, and to D_2, inhibiting the inhibitory pathway → ↑ motion.

Parkinson disease

Degenerative disorder of CNS associated with Lewy bodies (composed of α-synuclein—intracellular eosinophilic inclusion) and loss of dopaminergic neurons (i.e., depigmentation) of the substantia nigra pars compacta.

Parkinson **TRAPS** your body—Tremor (at rest—e.g., pill-rolling tremor), cogwheel Rigidity, Akinesia (or bradykinesia), Postural instability and Shuffling gait.

Huntington disease

Autosomal dominant trinucleotide repeat disorder on chromosome 4. Symptoms manifest between ages 20 and 50; characterized by choreiform movements, aggression, depression, and dementia (sometimes initially mistaken for substance abuse). ↓ levels of GABA and ACh in the brain. Neuronal death via NMDA-R binding and glutamate toxicity. Atrophy of caudate nuclei can be seen on imaging.

Expansion of **CAG** repeats (anticipation). Caudate loses ACh and GABA.

Movement disorders

DISORDER	PRESENTATION	CHARACTERISTIC LESION	NOTES
Hemiballismus	Sudden, wild flailing of 1 arm +/– ipsilateral leg	Contralateral subthalamic nucleus (e.g., lacunar stroke)	"Half-of-body ballistic." Contralateral lesion.
Chorea	Sudden, jerky, purposeless movements	Basal ganglia (e.g., Huntington)	*Chorea* = dancing.
Athetosis	Slow, writhing movements; especially seen in fingers	Basal ganglia (e.g., Huntington)	Writhing, snake-like movement.
Myoclonus	Sudden, brief, uncontrolled muscle contraction		Jerks; hiccups; common in metabolic abnormalities such as renal and liver failure.
Dystonia	Sustained, involuntary muscle contractions		Writer's cramp; blepharospasm (sustained eyelid twitch).
Essential tremor (postural tremor)	Action tremor; exacerbated by holding posture/limb position		Genetic predisposition. Patients often self-medicated with EtOH, which ↓ tremor amplitude. Treatment: β-blockers, primidone.
Resting tremor	Uncontrolled movement of distal appendages (most noticeable in hands); tremor alleviated by intentional movement	Parkinson disease	Occurs at rest; "pill-rolling tremor" of Parkinson disease.
Intention tremor	Slow, zigzag motion when pointing/extending toward a target	Cerebellar dysfunction	

Cerebral cortex functions

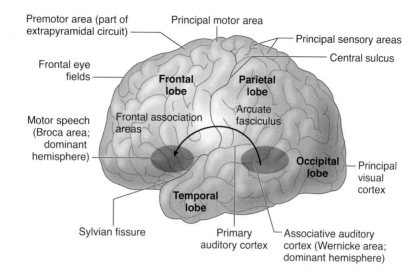

Homunculus

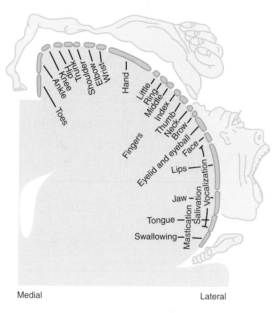

Topographical representation of motor (shown) and sensory areas in the cerebral cortex. Distorted appearance is due to certain body regions that are more richly innervated and thus have ↑ cortical representation.

Common brain lesions

AREA OF LESION	CONSEQUENCE	NOTES
Amygdala (bilateral)	**Klüver-Bucy syndrome** (hyperorality, hypersexuality, disinhibited behavior)	Associated with HSV-1.
Frontal lobe	Disinhibition and deficits in concentration, orientation, and judgment; may have reemergence of primitive reflexes	
Right parietal-temporal cortex	Spatial neglect syndrome (agnosia of the contralateral side of the world)	
Left parietal-temporal cortex	Agraphia, acalculia, finger agnosia, and left-right disorientation	Gerstmann syndrome.
Reticular activating system (midbrain)	Reduced levels of arousal and wakefulness (e.g., coma)	
Mammillary bodies (bilateral)	**Wernicke-Korsakoff syndrome**: confusion, ophthalmoplegia, ataxia; memory loss (anterograde and retrograde amnesia), confabulation, personality changes	Associated with thiamine (B_1) deficiency and excessive EtOH use; can be precipitated by giving glucose without B_1 to a B_1-deficient patient. Wernicke problems come in a **CAN** of beer: **C**onfusion, **A**taxia, **N**ystagmus.
Basal ganglia	May result in tremor at rest, chorea, or athetosis	Parkinson disease.
Cerebellar hemisphere	Intention tremor, limb ataxia, and loss of balance; damage to the cerebellum results in ipsilateral deficits; fall toward side of lesion	Cerebellar hemispheres are **laterally** located—affect **lateral** limbs.
Cerebellar vermis	Truncal ataxia, dysarthria	Vermis is **centrally** located—affects **central** body.
Subthalamic nucleus	Contralateral hemiballismus	
Hippocampus (bilateral)	Anterograde amnesia—inability to make new memories	
Paramedian pontine reticular formation	Eyes look away from side of lesion	
Frontal eye fields	Eyes look toward lesion	

Central pontine myelinolysis	A variant of the osmotic demyelination syndrome. Acute paralysis, dysarthria, dysphagia, diplopia, and loss of consciousness. Can cause "locked-in syndrome." Massive axonal demyelination in pontine white matter tracts 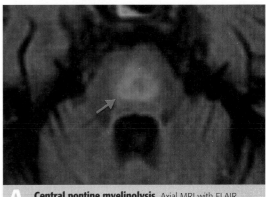 2° to osmotic forces and edema. Commonly iatrogenic, caused by overly rapid correction of hyponatremia.	Correcting serum Na⁺ too fast: ▪ "From low to high, your pons will die" (CPM) ▪ "From high to low, your brain will blow" (cerebral edema/herniation)

A **Central pontine myelinolysis.** Axial MRI with FLAIR shows abnormal increased signal in central pons (arrow). ✕

Aphasia	Aphasia = higher-order inability to speak (language deficit). Dysarthria = motor inability to speak (movement deficit).	
Broca	Nonfluent aphasia with intact comprehension. Broca area—inferior frontal gyrus of frontal lobe.	Broca Broken Boca (boca = mouth in Spanish).
Wernicke	Fluent aphasia with impaired comprehension and repetition. Wernicke area—superior temporal gyrus of temporal lobe.	Wernicke is Wordy but makes no sense. Wernicke = "What?"
Global	Nonfluent aphasia with impaired comprehension. Both Broca and Wernicke areas affected.	
Conduction	Poor repetition but fluent speech, intact comprehension. Can be caused by damage to left superior temporal lobe and/or left supramarginal gyrus.	Can't repeat phrases such as, "No ifs, ands, or buts."
Transcortical motor	Nonfluent aphasia with good comprehension and repetition.	
Transcortical sensory	Poor comprehension with fluent speech and repetition.	
Mixed transcortical	Nonfluent speech, poor comprehension, good repetition.	

Circle of Willis   System of anastomoses between anterior and posterior blood supplies to brain.

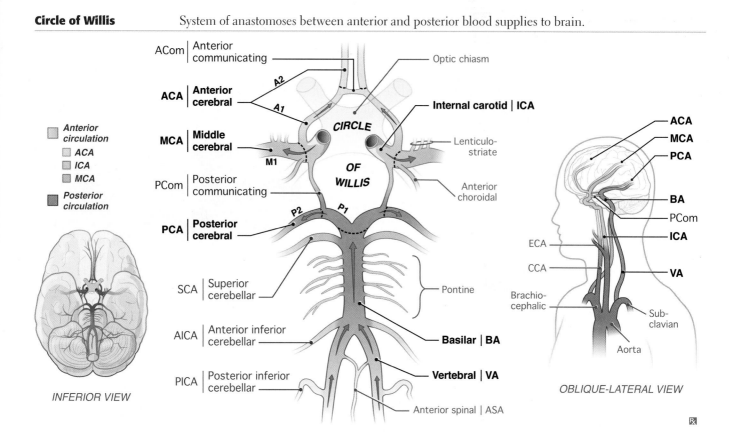

ACom | Anterior communicating — Optic chiasm

A2

ACA | **Anterior cerebral**   **Internal carotid | ICA**

A1

CIRCLE

MCA | **Middle cerebral**   Lenticulo-striate

M1   *OF*

PCom | Posterior communicating   *WILLIS*

Anterior choroidal

P2   P1

PCA | **Posterior cerebral**

Anterior circulation
☐ ACA
☐ ICA
☐ MCA
■ Posterior circulation

SCA | Superior cerebellar   Pontine

AICA | Anterior inferior cerebellar   **Basilar | BA**

PICA | Posterior inferior cerebellar   **Vertebral | VA**

Anterior spinal | ASA

INFERIOR VIEW

ACA
MCA
PCA
BA
PCom
ECA   **ICA**
CCA   **VA**
Brachio-cephalic
Sub-clavian
Aorta

OBLIQUE-LATERAL VIEW

Cerebral arteries–cortical distribution

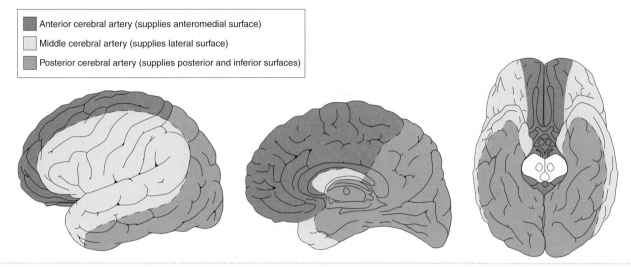

■ Anterior cerebral artery (supplies anteromedial surface)
☐ Middle cerebral artery (supplies lateral surface)
■ Posterior cerebral artery (supplies posterior and inferior surfaces)

Watershed zones	Between anterior cerebral/middle cerebral, posterior cerebral/middle cerebral arteries. Damage in severe hypotension → upper leg/upper arm weakness, defects in higher-order visual processing.

Regulation of cerebral perfusion	Brain perfusion relies on tight autoregulation. Cerebral perfusion is primarily driven by P_{CO_2} (P_{O_2} also modulates perfusion in severe hypoxia).	Therapeutic hyperventilation (↓ P_{CO_2}) helps ↓ intracranial pressure in cases of acute cerebral edema (stroke, trauma) via ↓ cerebral perfusion by vasoconstriction.

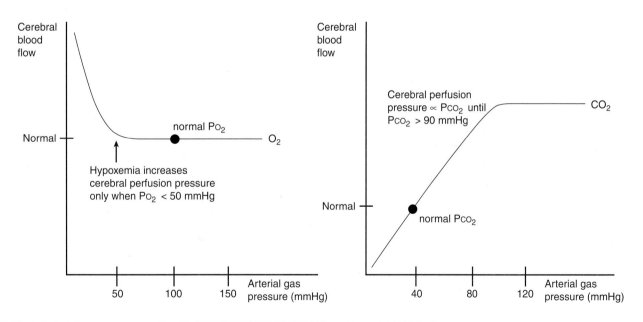

Effects of strokes

ARTERY	AREA OF LESION	SYMPTOMS	NOTES
Anterior circulation			
MCA	Motor cortex—upper limb and face.	Contralateral paralysis—upper limb and face.	
	Sensory cortex—upper limb and face.	Contralateral loss of sensation—upper and lower limbs, and face.	
	Temporal lobe (Wernicke area); frontal lobe (Broca area).	Aphasia if in dominant (usually left) hemisphere. Hemineglect if lesion affects nondominant (usually right) side.	
ACA	Motor cortex—lower limb.	Contralateral paralysis—lower limb.	
	Sensory cortex—lower limb.	Contralateral loss of sensation—lower limb.	
Lenticulo-striate artery	Striatum, internal capsule.	Contralateral hemiparesis/hemiplegia.	Common location of lacunar infarcts, 2° to unmanaged hypertension.
Posterior circulation			
ASA	Lateral corticospinal tract.	Contralateral hemiparesis—upper and lower limbs.	Stroke commonly bilateral. **Medial medullary syndrome**—caused by infarct of paramedian branches of ASA and vertebral arteries.
	Medial lemniscus. Caudal medulla—hypoglossal nerve.	↓ contralateral proprioception. Ipsilateral hypoglossal dysfunction (tongue deviates ipsilaterally).	
PICA	Lateral medulla—vestibular nuclei, lateral spinothalamic tract, spinal trigeminal nucleus, nucleus ambiguus, sympathetic fibers, inferior cerebellar peduncle.	Vomiting, vertigo, nystagmus; ↓ pain and temperature sensation from ipsilateral face and contralateral body; **dysphagia**, **hoarseness**, ↓ gag reflex; ipsilateral Horner syndrome; ataxia, dysmetria.	**Lateral medullary (Wallenberg) syndrome**. Nucleus ambiguus effects are specific to PICA lesions. "Don't **pick a (PICA) horse (hoarseness)** that **can't eat (dysphagia)**."
AICA	Lateral pons—cranial nerve nuclei; vestibular nuclei, facial nucleus, spinal trigeminal nucleus, cochlear nuclei, sympathetic fibers.	Vomiting, vertigo, nystagmus. **Paralysis** of face, ↓ lacrimation, salivation, ↓ taste from anterior ⅔ of tongue, ↓ corneal reflex. Face—↓ pain and temperature sensation. Ipsilateral ↓ hearing. Ipsilateral Horner syndrome.	**Lateral pontine syndrome**. Facial nucleus effects are specific to AICA lesions. "**Facial droop** means AICA's **pooped**."
	Middle and inferior cerebellar peduncles.	Ataxia, dysmetria.	
PCA	Occipital cortex, visual cortex.	Contralateral hemianopia with macular sparing.	
Basilar artery	Pons, medulla, lower midbrain, corticospinal and corticobulbar tracts, ocular cranial nerve nuclei, paramedian pontine reticular formation.	Preserved consciousness and blinking, quadriplegia, loss of voluntary facial, mouth, and tongue movements.	"Locked-in syndrome."

Effects of strokes *(continued)*

ARTERY	AREA OF LESION	SYMPTOMS	NOTES
Communicating arteries			
ACom	Most common lesion is aneurysm. Can lead to stroke. Saccular (berry) aneurysm can impinge cranial nerves.	Visual field defects.	Lesions are typically aneurysms, not strokes.
PCom	Common site of saccular aneurysm.	CN III palsy—eye is "down and out" with ptosis and pupil dilation.	Lesions are typically aneurysms, not strokes.

Aneurysms	In general, an abnormal dilation of artery due to weakening of vessel wall.

Berry aneurysm	Occurs at the bifurcations in the circle of Willis 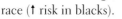. Most common site is junction of the anterior communicating artery and anterior cerebral artery. Rupture (most common complication) leads to subarachnoid hemorrhage ("worst headache of life") or hemorrhagic stroke. Can also cause bitemporal hemianopia via compression of optic chiasm. Associated with ADPKD, Ehlers-Danlos syndrome, and Marfan syndrome. Other risk factors: advanced age, hypertension, smoking, race (↑ risk in blacks).	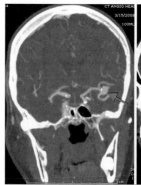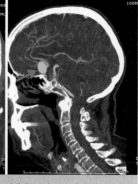 **A** **Berry aneurysm.** Coronal (left) and sagittal (right) contrast CT shows berry aneurysm (arrows). ✖
Charcot-Bouchard microaneurysm	Associated with chronic hypertension; affects small vessels (e.g., in basal ganglia, thalamus).	

Central post-stroke pain syndrome	Neuropathic pain due to thalamic lesions. Initial sensation of numbness and tingling followed in weeks to months by allodynia (ordinarily painless stimuli cause pain) and dysaesthesia. Occurs in 10% of stroke patients.

Intracranial hemorrhage

Epidural hematoma	Rupture of middle meningeal artery (branch of maxillary artery), often 2° to fracture of temporal bone. Lucid interval. Rapid expansion under systemic arterial pressure → transtentorial herniation, CN III palsy. CT shows biconvex (lentiform), hyperdense blood collection **A** **not crossing suture lines. Can cross falx, tentorium.**

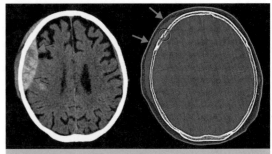

A **Epidural hematoma.** Axial CT of the brain shows lens-shaped collection of epidural blood (left, arrows), with bone windows showing associated skull fracture (right, circle) and scalp hematoma (arrows). ✳, ✳

Subdural hematoma	Rupture of bridging veins. Slow venous bleeding (less pressure = hematoma develops over time). Seen in elderly individuals, alcoholics, blunt trauma, shaken baby (predisposing factors: brain atrophy, shaking, whiplash). Crescent-shaped hemorrhage that **crosses suture lines** **B**. Midline shift. **Cannot cross falx, tentorium.**

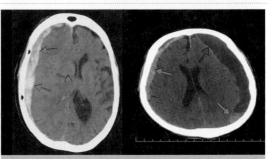

B **Subdural hematoma.** Axial CTs show crescent-shaped subdural blood collections. Left image shows acute bleed with midline shift (subfalcine herniation, arrows). ✳ Right image shows "acute on chronic" hemorrhage (red arrows, acute; blue arrow, chronic). ✗

Subarachnoid hemorrhage	Rupture of an aneurysm (such as a berry [saccular] aneurysm, as seen in Marfan, Ehlers-Danlos, ADPKD) or an AVM. Rapid time course. Patients complain of "worst headache of my life (WHOML)." Bloody or yellow (xanthochromic) spinal tap. 2–3 days afterward, risk of vasospasm due to blood breakdown (not visible on CT, treat with nimodipine) and rebleed (visible on CT) **C**.

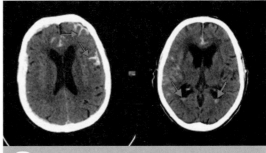

C **Subarachnoid hemorrhage.** Axial CT of the brain shows subarachnoid blood in the sulci (left, arrows) and intraventricular blood (right, arrows) layering in the posterior horn of the lateral ventricles. ✗, ✗

Intraparenchymal (hypertensive) hemorrhage	Most commonly caused by systemic hypertension **D**. Also seen with amyloid angiopathy, vasculitis, and neoplasm. Typically occurs in basal ganglia and internal capsule (Charcot-Bouchard aneurysm of lenticulostriate vessels), but can be lobar.

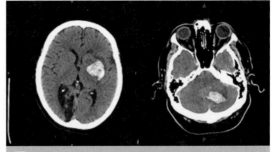

D **Hypertensive hemorrhage.** Axial CT of the brain shows intraparenchymal hemorrhage in the basal ganglia (left) and cerebellum (right). ✗, ✗

Ischemic brain disease/stroke

Irreversible damage begins after 5 minutes of hypoxia. Most vulnerable—hippocampus, neocortex, cerebellum, watershed areas. Irreversible neuronal injury.

Stroke imaging: bright on diffusion-weighted MRI in 3–30 minutes (highest sensitivity for early ischemia), dark abnormality on noncontrast CT in ~ 12–24 hours. Absence of bright areas on noncontrast CT highly accurate to exclude hemorrhage (contraindication for tPA).

Ischemic **hypoxia**—"**hypo**campus" is most vulnerable.

TIME SINCE ISCHEMIC EVENT	12–48 HOURS	24–72 HOURS	3–5 DAYS	1–2 WEEKS	> 2 WEEKS
Histologic features	Red neurons	Necrosis + neutrophils	Macrophages	Reactive gliosis + vascular proliferation	Glial scar

Hemorrhagic stroke

Intracerebral bleeding, often due to hypertension, anticoagulation, and cancer (abnormal vessels can bleed). May be 2° to ischemic stroke followed by reperfusion (↑ vessel fragility). Basal ganglia are most common site of intracerebral hemorrhage.

Ischemic stroke

Acute blockage of vessels → disruption of blood flow and subsequent ischemia. Results in liquefactive necrosis.

3 types:

- Thrombotic—due to a clot forming directly at the site of infarction (commonly the MCA **A**), usually over an atherosclerotic plaque.
- Embolic—an embolus from another part of the body obstructs a vessel. Can affect multiple vascular territories. Often cardioembolic.
- Hypoxic—due to hypoperfusion or hypoxemia. Common during cardiovascular surgeries, tends to affect watershed areas.

Treatment—tPA (if within 3–4.5 hr of onset and no hemorrhage/risk of hemorrhage). Reduce risk with medical therapy (e.g., aspirin, clopidogrel); optimum control of blood pressure, blood sugars, and lipids; and treat conditions that ↑ risk (e.g., atrial fibrillation).

Transient ischemic attack

Brief, reversible episode of focal neurologic dysfunction lasting < 24 hours without acute infarction (⊖ MRI), with the majority resolving in < 15 minutes; deficits due to focal ischemia.

Dural venous sinuses

Large venous channels that run through the dura. Drain blood from cerebral veins and receive CSF from arachnoid granulations. Empty into internal jugular vein.

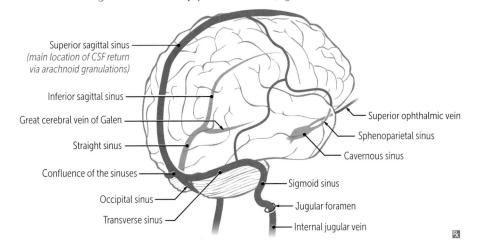

Superior sagittal sinus *(main location of CSF return via arachnoid granulations)*

Inferior sagittal sinus

Great cerebral vein of Galen

Straight sinus

Confluence of the sinuses

Occipital sinus

Transverse sinus

Superior ophthalmic vein

Sphenoparietal sinus

Cavernous sinus

Sigmoid sinus

Jugular foramen

Internal jugular vein

Ventricular system

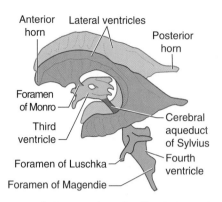

Anterior horn · Lateral ventricles · Posterior horn · Foramen of Monro · Third ventricle · Cerebral aqueduct of Sylvius · Foramen of Luschka · Fourth ventricle · Foramen of Magendie

Lateral ventricle → 3rd ventricle via right and left interventricular foramina of Monro.

3rd ventricle → 4th ventricle via cerebral aqueduct (of Sylvius).

4th ventricle → subarachnoid space via:
- Foramina of Luschka = Lateral.
- Foramen of Magendie = Medial.

CSF is made by ependymal cells of choroid plexus; it is reabsorbed by arachnoid granulations and then drains into dural venous sinuses.

Hydrocephalus

Communicating (nonobstructive)	
Communicating hydrocephalus	↓ CSF absorption by arachnoid granulations, which can lead to ↑ intracranial pressure, papilledema, and herniation (e.g., arachnoid scarring post-meningitis).
Normal pressure hydrocephalus 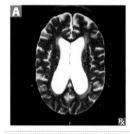	Does not result in increased subarachnoid space volume. Expansion of ventricles **A** distorts the fibers of the corona radiata and leads to clinical triad of **urinary incontinence, ataxia, and cognitive dysfunction** (sometimes reversible). "Wet, wobbly, and wacky."
Hydrocephalus ex vacuo	Appearance of ↑ CSF in atrophy (e.g., Alzheimer disease, advanced HIV, Pick disease). Intracranial pressure is normal; triad is not seen. Apparent increase in CSF observed on imaging is actually result of ↓ neural tissue due to neuronal atrophy.

Noncommunicating (obstructive)	
Noncommunicating hydrocephalus	Caused by a structural blockage of CSF circulation within the ventricular system (e.g., stenosis of the aqueduct of Sylvius).

Spinal nerves

There are 31 spinal nerves in total: 8 cervical, 12 thoracic, 5 lumbar, 5 sacral, 1 coccygeal.
Nerves C1–C7 exit above the corresponding vertebra. All other nerves exit below (e.g., C3 exits above the 3rd cervical vertebra; L2 exits below the 2nd lumbar vertebra).

31, just like 31 flavors of Baskin-Robbins ice cream!

Vertebral disc herniation—nucleus pulposus (soft central disc) herniates through annulus fibrosus (outer ring); usually occurs posterolaterally at L4–L5 or L5–S1.

Spinal cord–lower extent

In adults, spinal cord extends to lower border of L1–L2 vertebrae. Subarachnoid space (which contains the CSF) extends to lower border of S2 vertebra. Lumbar puncture is usually performed between L3–L4 or L4–L5 (level of cauda equina).

Goal of lumbar puncture is to obtain sample of CSF without damaging spinal cord. To **keep** the cord **alive**, keep the spinal needle between **L3** and **L5**.

Spinal cord and associated tracts

Legs (**L**umbosacral) are **L**ateral in **L**ateral corticospinal, spinothalamic tracts.
Dorsal column is organized as you are, with hands at sides. Arms outside, legs inside.

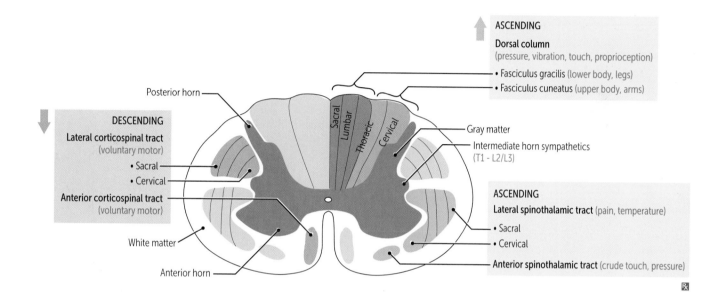

ASCENDING
Dorsal column (pressure, vibration, touch, proprioception)
• Fasciculus gracilis (lower body, legs)
• Fasciculus cuneatus (upper body, arms)

Posterior horn

Sacral
Lumbar
Thoracic
Cervical

Gray matter

DESCENDING
Lateral corticospinal tract (voluntary motor)
• Sacral
• Cervical
Anterior corticospinal tract (voluntary motor)

White matter

Anterior horn

Intermediate horn sympathetics (T1 - L2/L3)

ASCENDING
Lateral spinothalamic tract (pain, temperature)
• Sacral
• Cervical
Anterior spinothalamic tract (crude touch, pressure)

Spinal tract anatomy and functions   Remember, ascending tracts synapse and then cross.

TRACT AND FUNCTION	1ST-ORDER NEURON	SYNAPSE 1	2ND-ORDER NEURON	SYNAPSE 2	3RD-ORDER NEURON
Dorsal column Ascending: pressure, vibration, fine touch, and proprioception	Sensory nerve ending → cell body in dorsal root ganglion → enters spinal cord, ascends ipsilaterally in dorsal column	Ipsilateral nucleus cuneatus or gracilis (medulla)	Decussates in medulla → ascends contralaterally in medial lemniscus	VPL (thalamus)	Sensory cortex
Spinothalamic tract Ascending Lateral: pain, temperature Anterior: crude touch, pressure	Sensory nerve ending (Aδ and C fibers) (cell body in dorsal root ganglion) → enters spinal cord	Ipsilateral gray matter (spinal cord)	Decussates at anterior white commissure → ascends contralaterally	VPL (thalamus)	Sensory cortex
Lateral corticospinal tract Descending: voluntary movement of contralateral limbs	UMN: cell body in 1° motor cortex → descends ipsilaterally (through internal capsule), most fibers decussate at caudal medulla (pyramidal decussation) → descends contralaterally	Cell body of anterior horn (spinal cord)	LMN: leaves spinal cord	NMJ	

Motor neuron signs

SIGN	UMN LESION	LMN LESION	COMMENTS
Weakness	+	+	Lower MN = everything **lowered** (less muscle mass, ↓ muscle tone, ↓ reflexes, downgoing toes).
Atrophy	–	+	
Fasciculations	–	+	Upper MN = everything **up** (tone, DTRs, toes).
Reflexes	↑	↓	
Tone	↑	↓	Fasciculations = muscle twitching.
Babinski	+	–	Positive Babinski is normal in infants.
Spastic paralysis	+	–	
Flaccid paralysis	–	+	
Clasp knife spasticity	+	–	

Spinal cord lesions

AREA AFFECTED	DISEASE	CHARACTERISTICS
	Poliomyelitis and spinal muscular atrophy (Werdnig-Hoffmann disease)	LMN lesions only, due to destruction of anterior horns; flaccid paralysis.
	Multiple sclerosis	Due to demyelination; mostly white matter of cervical region; random and asymmetric lesions, due to demyelination; scanning speech, intention tremor, nystagmus.
	Amyotrophic lateral sclerosis	Combined UMN and LMN deficits with no sensory, cognitive, or oculomotor deficits; both UMN and LMN signs. Can be caused by defect in superoxide dismutase 1. Commonly presents as fasciculations with eventual atrophy and weakness of hands; fatal. Riluzole treatment modestly ↑ survival by ↓ presynaptic glutamate release. Commonly known as Lou Gehrig disease. Stephen Hawking is a well-known patient who highlights the lack of cognitive deficit. For **Lou** Gehrig disease, give ri**lou**zole.
Posterior spinal arteries / Anterior spinal artery	Complete occlusion of anterior spinal artery	Spares dorsal columns and Lissauer tract; upper thoracic ASA territory is a watershed area, as artery of Adamkiewicz supplies ASA below ~T8.
	Tabes dorsalis	Caused by 3° syphilis. Results from degeneration (demyelination) of dorsal columns and roots → impaired sensation and proprioception and progressive sensory ataxia (inability to sense or feel the legs → poor coordination). Associated with Charcot joints, shooting pain, Argyll Robertson pupils (small bilateral pupils that further constrict to accommodation and convergence, not to light). Exam will demonstrate absence of DTRs and ⊕ Romberg.
	Syringomyelia	Syrinx expands and damages anterior white commissure of spinothalamic tract (2nd-order neurons) → bilateral loss of pain and temperature sensation (usually C8–T1); seen with Chiari I malformation; can expand and affect other tracts.
	Vitamin B_{12} or vitamin E deficiency	Subacute combined degeneration—demyelination of dorsal columns, lateral corticospinal tracts, and spinocerebellar tracts; ataxic gait, paresthesia, impaired position and vibration sense.

Poliomyelitis	Caused by poliovirus (fecal-oral transmission). Replicates in the oropharynx and small intestine before spreading via the bloodstream to the CNS. Infection causes destruction of cells in anterior horn of spinal cord (LMN death).
SYMPTOMS	LMN lesion signs—weakness, hypotonia, flaccid paralysis, fasciculations, hyporeflexia, and muscle atrophy. Signs of infection—malaise, headache, fever, nausea, etc.
FINDINGS	CSF with ↑ WBCs and slight ↑ of protein (with no change in CSF glucose). Virus recovered from stool or throat.

Spinal muscular atrophy (Werdnig-Hoffmann disease)	Congenital degeneration of anterior horns of spinal cord → LMN lesion. "Floppy baby" with marked hypotonia and tongue fasciculations. Infantile type has median age of death of 7 months. Autosomal recessive inheritance.

Friedreich ataxia	Autosomal recessive trinucleotide repeat disorder (GAA) on chromosome 9 in gene that encodes frataxin (iron binding protein). Leads to impairment in mitochondrial functioning. Degeneration of multiple spinal cord tracts → muscle weakness and loss of DTRs, vibratory sense, and proprioception. **Staggering** gait, frequent **falling**, nystagmus, dysarthria, pes cavus, hammer toes, **hypertrophic cardiomyopathy** (cause of death). Presents in childhood with kyphoscoliosis.

Friedreich is Fratastic (**frataxin**): he's your favorite **frat** brother, always stumbling, **staggering**, and **falling**, but has a **big heart**.

Brown-Séquard syndrome 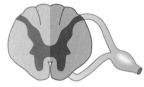 Lesion	Hemisection of spinal cord. Findings: <ul><li>Ipsilateral UMN signs below the level of the lesion (due to corticospinal tract damage)</li><li>Ipsilateral loss of tactile, vibration, proprioception sense 1–2 levels below the level of the lesion (due to dorsal column damage)</li><li>Contralateral pain and temperature loss below the level of the lesion (due to spinothalamic tract damage)</li><li>Ipsilateral loss of all sensation at the level of the lesion</li><li>Ipsilateral LMN signs (e.g., flaccid paralysis) at the level of the lesion</li></ul> If lesion occurs above T1, patient may present with Horner syndrome due to damage of oculosympathetic pathway.

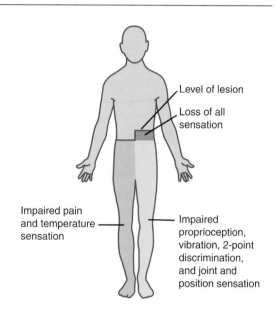

Level of lesion
Loss of all sensation
Impaired pain and temperature sensation
Impaired proprioception, vibration, 2-point discrimination, and joint and position sensation

Horner syndrome

Sympathectomy of face:

- Ptosis (slight drooping of eyelid: superior tarsal muscle)
- Anhidrosis (absence of sweating) and flushing (rubor) of affected side of face
- Miosis (pupil constriction)

Associated with lesion of spinal cord above T1 (e.g., Pancoast tumor, Brown-Séquard syndrome [cord hemisection], late-stage syringomyelia).

PAM is horny (Horner).
Ptosis, **a**nhidrosis, and **m**iosis (rhyming).

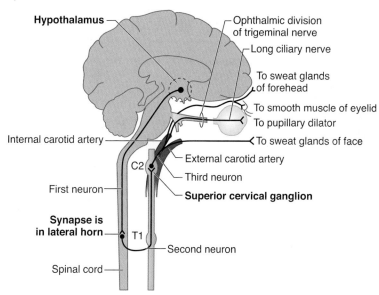

The 3-neuron oculosympathetic pathway projects from the hypothalamus to the intermediolateral column of the spinal cord, then to the superior cervical (sympathetic) ganglion, and finally to the pupil, the smooth muscle of the eyelids, and the sweat glands of the forehead and face. Interruption of any of these pathways results in Horner syndrome.

Landmark dermatomes

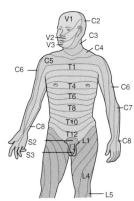

C2—posterior half of a skull "cap."
C3—high turtleneck shirt.
C4—low-collar shirt.
T4—at the nipple.
T7—at the xiphoid process.
T10—at the umbilicus (important for early appendicitis pain referral).
L1—at the inguinal ligament.
L4—includes the kneecaps.
S2, S3, S4—erection and sensation of penile and anal zones.

Diaphragm and gallbladder pain referred to the right shoulder via the phrenic nerve.

T4 at the **teat pore**.

T10 at the belly **butt**en.

L1 is **IL** (**I**nguinal **L**igament).
Down on **ALL 4**'s (**L4**).
"**S2, 3, 4** keep the penis off the **floor**."

Clinical reflexes

Biceps = C5 nerve root.
Triceps = C7 nerve root.
Patella = L4 nerve root.
Achilles = S1 nerve root.

Reflexes count up in order:
  S1, 2—"buckle my shoe" (Achilles reflex)
  L3, 4—"kick the door" (patellar reflex)
  C5, 6—"pick up sticks" (biceps reflex)
  C7, 8—"lay them straight" (triceps reflex)
Additional reflexes:
  L1, L2—"testicles move" (cremaster reflex)
  S3, S4—"winks galore" (anal wink reflex)

C5, 6
C7, 8
L3, 4
S1, 2

Primitive reflexes

CNS reflexes that are present in a healthy infant, but are absent in a neurologically intact adult. Normally disappear within 1st year of life. These "primitive" reflexes are inhibited by a mature/ developing frontal lobe. They may reemerge in adults following frontal lobe lesions → loss of inhibition of these reflexes.

Moro reflex	"Hang on for life" reflex—abduct/extend limbs when startled, and then draw together
Rooting reflex	Movement of head toward one side if cheek or mouth is stroked (nipple seeking)
Sucking reflex	Sucking response when roof of mouth is touched
Palmar reflex	Curling of fingers if palm is stroked
Plantar reflex	Dorsiflexion of large toe and fanning of other toes with plantar stimulation Babinski sign—presence of this reflex in an adult, which may signify a UMN lesion
Galant reflex	Stroking along one side of the spine while newborn is in ventral suspension (face down) causes lateral flexion of lower body toward stimulated side

---

Brain stem—ventral view

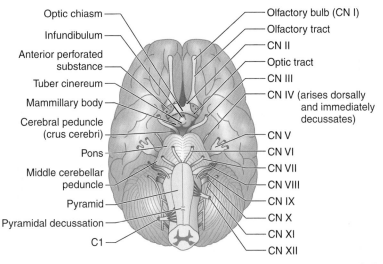

Optic chiasm — Olfactory bulb (CN I)
Infundibulum — Olfactory tract
Anterior perforated substance — CN II
Tuber cinereum — Optic tract
Mammillary body — CN III
Cerebral peduncle (crus cerebri) — CN IV (arises dorsally and immediately decussates)
Pons — CN V
Middle cerebellar peduncle — CN VI
Pyramid — CN VII
Pyramidal decussation — CN VIII
C1 — CN IX
— CN X
— CN XI
— CN XII

CNs that lie medially at brain stem: **III, VI, XII.** 3(×2) = 6(×2) = 12 (Motor = Medial).

Brain stem—dorsal view (cerebellum removed)

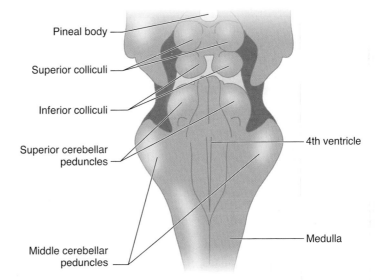

Pineal body

Superior colliculi

Inferior colliculi

Superior cerebellar peduncles

Middle cerebellar peduncles

4th ventricle

Medulla

Pineal gland—melatonin secretion, circadian rhythms.

Superior colliculi—conjugate vertical gaze center.

Inferior colliculi—auditory.

Parinaud syndrome—paralysis of conjugate vertical gaze due to lesion in superior colliculi (e.g., pinealoma).

Your eyes are **above** your ears, and the superior colliculus (visual) is **above** the inferior colliculus (auditory).

Cranial nerves

NERVE	CN	FUNCTION	TYPE	MNEMONIC
Olfactory	I	Smell (only CN without thalamic relay to cortex)	Sensory	Some
Optic	II	Sight	Sensory	Say
Oculomotor	III	Eye movement (SR, IR, MR, IO), pupillary constriction (sphincter pupillae: Edinger-Westphal nucleus, muscarinic receptors), accommodation, eyelid opening (levator palpebrae)	Motor	Marry
Trochlear	IV	Eye movement (SO)	Motor	Money
Trigeminal	V	Mastication, facial sensation (ophthalmic, maxillary, mandibular divisions), somatosensation from anterior $^2/_3$ of tongue	Both	But
Abducens	VI	Eye movement (LR)	Motor	My
Facial	VII	Facial movement, taste from anterior $^2/_3$ of tongue, lacrimation, salivation (submandibular and sublingual glands), eyelid closing (orbicularis oculi), stapedius muscle in ear (note: nerve courses through the parotid gland, but does not innervate it)	Both	Brother
Vestibulocochlear	VIII	Hearing, balance	Sensory	Says
Glossopharyngeal	IX	Taste and somatosensation from posterior $^1/_3$ of tongue, swallowing, salivation (parotid gland), monitoring carotid body and sinus chemo- and baroreceptors, and stylopharyngeus (elevates pharynx, larynx)	Both	Big
Vagus	X	Taste from epiglottic region, swallowing, soft palate elevation, midline uvula, talking, coughing, thoracoabdominal viscera, monitoring aortic arch chemo- and baroreceptors	Both	Brains
Accessory	XI	Head turning, shoulder shrugging (SCM, trapezius)	Motor	Matter
Hypoglossal	XII	Tongue movement	Motor	Most

Cranial nerve nuclei

Located in tegmentum portion of brain stem (between dorsal and ventral portions):

- Midbrain—nuclei of CN III, IV
- Pons—nuclei of CN V, VI, VII, VIII
- Medulla—nuclei of CN IX, X, XII
- Spinal cord—nucleus of CN XI

Lateral nuclei = sensory (aLar plate).
—Sulcus limitans—
Medial nuclei = Motor (basal plate).

Cranial nerve reflexes

REFLEX	AFFERENT	EFFERENT
Corneal	V_1 ophthalmic (nasociliary branch)	VII (temporal branch: orbicularis oculi)
Lacrimation	V_1 (loss of reflex does not preclude emotional tears)	VII
Jaw jerk	V_3 (sensory—muscle spindle from masseter)	V_3 (motor—masseter)
Pupillary	II	III
Gag	IX	X

Vagal nuclei

Nucleus Solitarius	Visceral Sensory information (e.g., taste, baroreceptors, gut distention).	VII, IX, X.
Nucleus aMbiguus	Motor innervation of pharynx, larynx, and upper esophagus (e.g., swallowing, palate elevation).	IX, X, XI (cranial portion)
Dorsal motor nucleus	Sends autonomic (parasympathetic) fibers to heart, lungs, and upper GI.	X.

Cranial nerve and vessel pathways	Cribriform plate (CN I). Middle cranial fossa (CN II–VI)—through sphenoid bone: ▪ Optic canal (CN II, ophthalmic artery, central retinal vein) ▪ Superior orbital fissure (CN III, IV, V_1, VI, ophthalmic vein, sympathetic fibers) ▪ Foramen Rotundum (CN V_2) ▪ Foramen Ovale (CN V_3) ▪ Foramen spinosum (middle meningeal artery) Posterior cranial fossa (CN VII–XII)—through temporal or occipital bone: ▪ Internal auditory meatus (CN VII, VIII) ▪ Jugular foramen (CN IX, X, XI, jugular vein) ▪ Hypoglossal canal (CN XII) ▪ Foramen magnum (spinal roots of CN XI, brain stem, vertebral arteries)	Divisions of CN V exit owing to Standing Room Only.

Cavernous sinus

A collection of venous sinuses on either side of the pituitary. Blood from eye and superficial cortex → cavernous sinus → internal jugular vein.

CN III, IV, V₁, V₂, and VI and postganglionic sympathetic fibers en route to the orbit all pass through the cavernous sinus. Cavernous portion of internal carotid artery is also here.

The nerves that control extraocular muscles (plus V_1 and V_2) pass through the cavernous sinus.

Cavernous sinus syndrome (e.g., due to mass effect, fistula, thrombosis)—ophthalmoplegia and ↓ corneal and maxillary sensation with normal visual acuity. CN VI commonly affected.

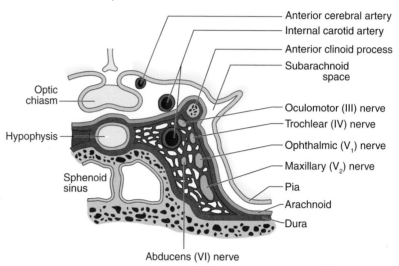

Common cranial nerve lesions

CN V motor lesion	Jaw deviates **toward** side of lesion due to unopposed force from the opposite pterygoid muscle.
CN X lesion	Uvula deviates **away** from side of lesion. Weak side collapses and uvula points away.
CN XI lesion	Weakness turning head to contralateral side of lesion (SCM). Shoulder droop on side of lesion (trapezius). The left SCM contracts to help turn the head to the right.
CN XII lesion (LMN)	Tongue deviates **toward** side of lesion ("lick your wounds") due to weakened tongue muscles on the affected side.

Auditory physiology

Outer ear	Visible portion of ear (pinna), includes auditory canal and eardrum. Transfers sound waves via vibration of eardrum.
Middle ear	Air-filled space with three bones called the ossicles (malleus, incus, stapes). Ossicles conduct and amplify sound from eardrum to inner ear.
Inner ear	Snail-shaped, fluid-filled cochlea. Contains basilar membrane that vibrates 2° to sound waves. Vibration transduced via specialized hair cells → auditory nerve signaling → brainstem. Each frequency leads to vibration at specific location on the basilar membrane (tonotopy): ▪ Low frequency heard at apex near helicotrema (wide and flexible). ▪ High frequency heard best at base of cochlea (thin and rigid).

Hearing loss

	RINNE TEST	WEBER TEST
Conductive	Abnormal (bone > air)	Localizes to affected ear
Sensorineural	Normal (air > bone)	Localizes to unaffected ear
Noise-induced	Damage to stereocilliated cells in organ of Corti; loss of high-frequency hearing 1st; sudden extremely loud noises can produce hearing loss due to tympanic membrane rupture.	

Facial lesions

UMN lesion	Lesion of motor cortex or connection between cortex and facial nucleus. Contralateral paralysis of lower face; forehead spared due to bilateral UMN innervation.	
LMN lesion	Ipsilateral paralysis of upper **and** lower face.	
Facial nerve palsy 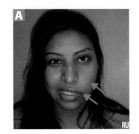	Complete destruction of the facial nucleus itself or its branchial efferent fibers (facial nerve proper). Peripheral ipsilateral facial paralysis (drooping smile 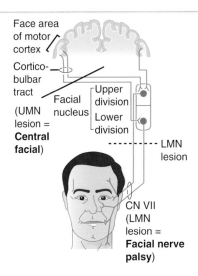) with inability to close eye on involved side. Can occur idiopathically (called **Bell palsy** [A]); gradual recovery in most cases. Associated with Lyme disease, herpes simplex and (less common) herpes zoster, sarcoidosis, tumors, and diabetes. Treatment includes corticosteroids.	

| **Mastication muscles** | 3 muscles close jaw: **M**asseter, te**M**poralis, **M**edial pterygoid. 1 opens: lateral pterygoid. All are innervated by the trigeminal nerve (V$_3$). | **M**'s Munch. **L**ateral **L**owers (when speaking of pterygoids with respect to jaw motion). "It takes more muscle to keep your mouth shut." |

Eye and retina

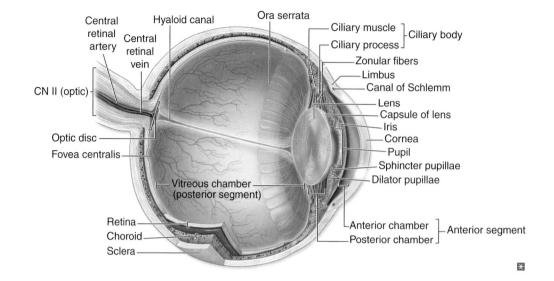

Common eye conditions

Refractive errors	Impaired vision that improves with glasses.
Hyperopia	Eye too short for refractive power of cornea and lens → light focused behind retina.
Myopia	Eye too long for refractive power of cornea and lens → light focused in front of retina.
Astigmatism	Abnormal curvature of cornea resulting in different refractive power at different axes.
Presbyopia	Decrease in focusing ability during accommodation due to sclerosis and ↓ elasticity.
Uveitis	Inflammation of anterior uvea and iris, with hypopyon (sterile pus), accompanied by conjunctival redness 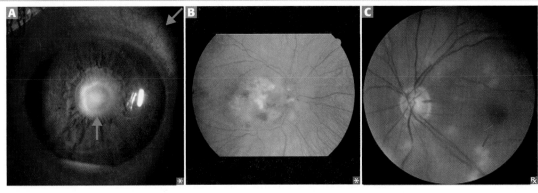A. Often associated with systemic inflammatory disorders (e.g., sarcoid, rheumatoid arthritis, juvenile idiopathic arthritis, TB, HLA-B27–associated conditions).
Retinitis	Retinal edema and necrosis leading to scar B. Often viral (CMV, HSV, HZV). Associated with immunosuppression.
Central retinal artery occlusion	Acute, painless monocular vision loss. Retina cloudy with attenuated vessels and "cherry-red" spot at the fovea C.
Retinal vein occlusion	Blockage of central or branch retinal vein due to compression from nearby arterial atherosclerosis. Retinal hemorrhage and edema in affected area.
Diabetic retinopathy	Retinal damage due to chronic hyperglycemia. Two types: Non-proliferative—damaged capillaries leak blood → lipids and fluid seep into retina → hemorrhages and macular edema. Treatment: blood sugar control, macular laser. Proliferative—chronic hypoxia results in new blood vessel formation with resultant traction on retina. Treatment: peripheral retinal photocoagulation, anti-VEGF injections.

Aqueous humor pathway

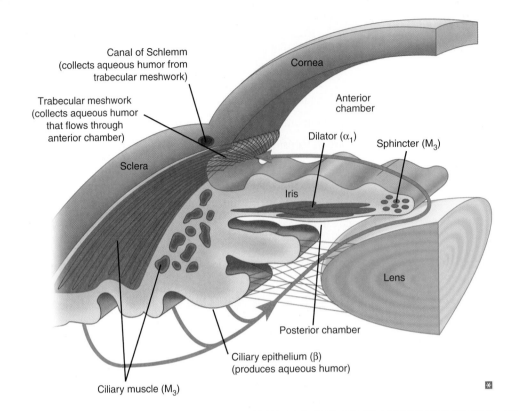

Glaucoma	Optic disc atrophy with characteristic cupping, usually with ↑ intraocular pressure (IOP) and progressive peripheral visual field loss.
Open angle	Associated with ↑ age, African-American race, family history. Painless, more common in U.S. Primary—cause unclear. Secondary—blocked trabecular meshwork from WBCs (e.g., uveitis), RBCs (e.g., vitreous hemorrhage), retinal elements (e.g., retinal detachment).
Closed/narrow angle	Primary—enlargement or forward movement of lens against central iris (pupil margin) leads to obstruction of normal aqueous flow through pupil → fluid builds up behind iris, pushing peripheral iris against cornea and impeding flow through trabecular meshwork. Secondary—hypoxia from retinal disease (e.g., diabetes, vein occlusion) induces vasoproliferation in iris that contracts angle. **Chronic closure**—often asymptomatic with damage to optic nerve and peripheral vision. **Acute closure**—true ophthalmic emergency. ↑ IOP pushes iris forward → angle closes abruptly. Very painful, sudden vision loss, halos around lights, rock-hard eye, frontal headache. Do not give epinephrine because of its mydriatic effect.

Cataract 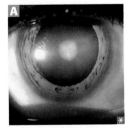	Painless, often bilateral, opacification of lens **A** → ↓ in vision. Risk factors: ↑ age, smoking, EtOH, excessive sunlight, prolonged corticosteroid use, classic galactosemia, galactokinase deficiency, diabetes (sorbitol), trauma, infection.

Papilledema

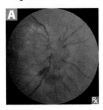

Optic disc swelling (usually bilateral) due to ↑ intracranial pressure (e.g., 2° to mass effect). Enlarged blind spot and elevated optic disc with blurred margins seen on fundoscopic exam **A**.

Extraocular muscles and nerves

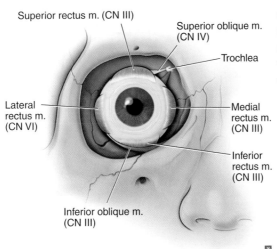

Superior rectus m. (CN III)
Superior oblique m. (CN IV)
Trochlea
Lateral rectus m. (CN VI)
Medial rectus m. (CN III)
Inferior rectus m. (CN III)
Inferior oblique m. (CN III)

CN VI innervates the Lateral Rectus.
CN IV innervates the Superior Oblique.
CN III innervates the Rest.
The "chemical formula" $LR_6SO_4R_3$.
The superior oblique abducts, intorts, and depresses while adducted.

CN III damage—eye looks down and out; ptosis, pupillary dilation, loss of accommodation.
CN IV damage—eye moves upward, particularly with contralateral gaze and head tilt toward the side of the lesion (problems going down stairs, may present with compensatory head tilt in the opposite direction).
CN VI damage—medially directed eye that cannot abduct.

Testing extraocular muscles

To test the function of each muscle, have the patient look in the following directions (e.g., to test SO, have patient depress eye from adducted position):

IOU: to test Inferior Oblique, have patient look Up.
Obliques move the eye in the Opposite direction.

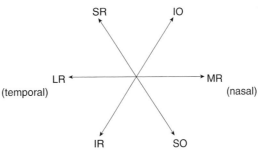

SR   IO

LR ◀━━━━━━━━━▶ MR
(temporal)   (nasal)

IR   SO

Pupillary control

Miosis (constriction, parasympathetic):
- 1st neuron: Edinger-Westphal nucleus to ciliary ganglion via CN III
- 2nd neuron: short ciliary nerves to pupillary sphincter muscles

Mydriasis (dilation, sympathetic)
- 1st neuron: hypothalamus to ciliospinal center of Budge (C8–T2)
- 2nd neuron: exit at T1 to superior cervical ganglion (travels along cervical sympathetic chain near lung apex, subclavian vessels)
- 3rd neuron: plexus along internal carotid, through cavernous sinus; enters orbit as long ciliary nerve to pupillary dilator muscles

---

Pupillary light reflex

Light in either retina sends a signal via CN II to pretectal nuclei (dashed lines) in midbrain that activates bilateral Edinger-Westphal nuclei; pupils contract bilaterally (consensual reflex).

Result: illumination of 1 eye results in bilateral pupillary constriction.

Marcus Gunn pupil (afferent pupillary defect)—due to optic nerve damage or severe retinal injury.
↓ bilateral pupillary constriction when light is shone in affected eye relative to unaffected eye. Tested with the "swinging flashlight test."

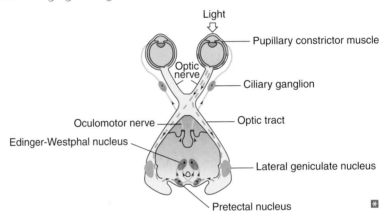

Cranial nerve III

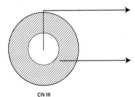

CN III has both motor (central) and parasympathetic (peripheral) components.

Motor output to ocular muscles—affected primarily by vascular disease (e.g., diabetes: glucose → sorbitol) due to ↓ diffusion of oxygen and nutrients to the interior fibers from compromised vasculature that resides on outside of nerve. Signs: ptosis, "down and out" gaze.

Parasympathetic output—fibers on the periphery are 1st affected by compression (e.g., posterior communicating artery aneurysm, uncal herniation). Signs: diminished or absent pupillary light reflex, "blown pupil" often with "down-and-out" gaze.

Retinal detachment

Separation of neurosensory layer of retina (photoreceptor layer with rods and cones) from outermost pigmented epithelium (normally shields excess light, supports retina) → degeneration of photoreceptors → vision loss. May be 2° to retinal breaks, diabetic traction, inflammatory effusions.

Breaks more common in patients with high myopia and are often preceded by posterior vitreous detachment (flashes and floaters) and eventual monocular loss of vision like a "curtain drawn down." Surgical emergency.

Age-related macular degeneration

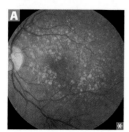

Degeneration of macula (central area of retina). Causes distortion (metamorphopsia) and eventual loss of central vision (scotomas).

- Dry (nonexudative, > 80%)—deposition of yellowish extracellular material in and beneath Bruch membrane and retinal pigment epithelium ("drusen") with gradual ↓ in vision. Prevent progression with multivitamin and antioxidant supplements.
- Wet (exudative, 10–15%)—rapid loss of vision due to bleeding 2° to choroidal neovascularization. Treat with anti-vascular endothelial growth factor injections (anti-VEGF) or laser.

Visual field defects

1. Right anopia
2. Bitemporal hemianopia (pituitary lesion, chiasm)
3. Left homonymous hemianopia
4. Left upper quadrantic anopia (right temporal lesion, MCA)
5. Left lower quadrantic anopia (right parietal lesion, MCA)
6. Left hemianopia with macular sparing (PCA infarct), macula → bilateral projection to occiput
7. Central scotoma (macular degeneration)

Meyer loop—inferior retina; loops around inferior horn of lateral ventricle.
Dorsal optic radiation—superior retina; takes shortest path via internal capsule.

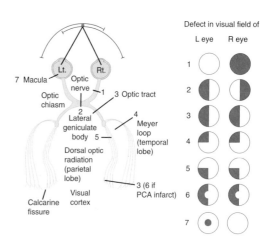

Note: When an image hits 1° visual cortex, it is upside down and left-right reversed.

Internuclear ophthalmoplegia (INO)

Medial longitudinal fasciculus (MLF): pair of tracts that allows for crosstalk between CN VI and CN III nuclei. Coordinates both eyes to move in same horizontal direction. Highly myelinated (must communicate quickly so eyes move at same time). Lesions seen in patients with demyelination (e.g., multiple sclerosis).

Lesion in MLF = INO: lack of communication such that when CN VI nucleus activates ipsilateral lateral rectus, contralateral CN III nucleus does not stimulate medial rectus to fire. Abducting eye gets nystagmus (CN VI overfires to stimulate CN III). Convergence normal.

MLF in MS.

When looking left, the left nucleus of CN VI fires, which contracts the left lateral rectus and stimulates the contralateral (right) nucleus of CN III via the right MLF to contract the right medial rectus.

Directional term (e.g., right INO, left INO) refers to which eye is paralyzed.

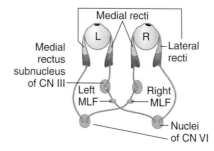

Medial recti

Medial rectus subnucleus of CN III

Lateral recti

Left MLF

Right MLF

Nuclei of CN VI

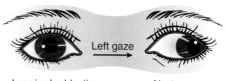

Right INO (right MLF lesion)

Left gaze

Impaired adduction

Nystagmus

▸ NEUROLOGY–PATHOLOGY

Dementia	A ↓ in cognitive ability, memory, or function with intact consciousness.	
DISEASE	**DESCRIPTION**	**HISTOLOGIC/GROSS FINDINGS**
Alzheimer disease	Most common cause in elderly. Down syndrome patients have an ↑ risk of developing Alzheimer. Familial form (10%) associated with the following altered proteins (respective chromosomes in parentheses): ▪ Early onset: APP (Chr 21), presenilin-1 (Chr 14), presenilin-2 (Chr 1) ▪ Late onset: ApoE4 (Chr 19) ApoE2 (Chr 19) is protective.	Widespread cortical atrophy. Narrowing of gyri and widening of sulci ↓ ACh Senile plaques **A**: extracellular β-amyloid core; may cause amyloid angiopathy → intracranial hemorrhage; Aβ (amyloid-β) synthesized by cleaving amyloid precursor protein (APP) Neurofibrillary tangles: intracellular, hyperphosphorylated tau protein = insoluble cytoskeletal elements; tangles correlate with degree of dementia
Pick disease (frontotemporal dementia)	Dementia, aphasia, parkinsonian aspects; change in personality. Spares parietal lobe and posterior ⅔ of superior temporal gyrus.	Pick bodies: spherical tau protein aggregates Frontotemporal atrophy
Lewy body dementia	Initially dementia and visual hallucinations followed by parkinsonian features.	α-synuclein defect
Creutzfeldt-Jakob disease	Rapidly progressive (weeks to months) dementia with myoclonus ("startle myoclonus").	Spongiform cortex Prions (PrP^c → PrP^{sc} sheet [β-pleated sheet resistant to proteases])
Other causes	Multi-infarct (2nd most common cause of dementia in elderly); syphilis; HIV; vitamins B_1, B_3, or B_{12} deficiency; Wilson disease; and NPH.	

Multiple sclerosis

Autoimmune inflammation and demyelination of CNS (brain and spinal cord). Patients can present with optic neuritis (sudden loss of vision resulting in Marcus Gunn pupils) internuclear ophthalmoplegia, hemiparesis, hemisensory symptoms, or bladder/bowel incontinence. Relapsing and remitting course. Most often affects women in their 20s and 30s; more common in whites.

Charcot classic triad of MS is a SIN:
- Scanning speech
- Intention tremor (also Incontinence and Internuclear ophthalmoplegia)
- Nystagmus

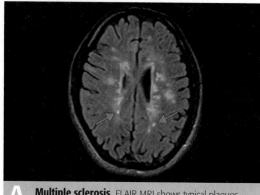

A **Multiple sclerosis.** FLAIR MRI shows typical plaques (arrows). �҂

FINDINGS

↑ protein (IgG) in CSF. Oligoclonal bands are diagnostic. MRI is gold standard. Periventricular plaques **A** (areas of oligodendrocyte loss and reactive gliosis) with destruction of axons. Multiple white matter lesions separated in space and time.

TREATMENT

β-interferon, immunosuppression, natalizumab. Symptomatic treatment for neurogenic bladder (catheterization, muscarinic antagonists), spasticity (baclofen, GABA receptor agonist), pain (opioids).

Acute inflammatory demyelinating polyradiculopathy

Most common variant of Guillain-Barré syndrome. Autoimmune condition that destroys Schwann cells → inflammation and demyelination of peripheral nerves and motor fibers. Results in symmetric ascending muscle weakness/paralysis beginning in lower extremities. Facial paralysis in 50% of cases. Autonomic function may be severely affected (e.g., cardiac irregularities, hypertension, or hypotension). Almost all patients survive; the majority recover completely after weeks to months.

Findings: ↑ CSF protein with normal cell count (albuminocytologic dissociation). ↑ protein → papilledema.

Associated with infections (*Campylobacter jejuni* and CMV) → autoimmune attack of peripheral myelin due to molecular mimicry, inoculations, and stress, but no definitive link to pathogens.

Respiratory support is critical until recovery. Additional treatment: plasmapheresis, IV immune globulins.

Other demyelinating and dysmyelinating diseases

Progressive multifocal leukoencephalopathy	Demyelination of CNS due to destruction of oligodendrocytes. Associated with JC virus. Seen in 2–4% of AIDS patients (reactivation of latent viral infection). Rapidly progressive, usually fatal. ↑ risk associated wtih natalizumab.
Acute disseminated (postinfectious) encephalomyelitis	Multifocal perivenular inflammation and demyelination after infection (commonly measles or VZV) or certain vaccinations (e.g., rabies, smallpox).
Metachromatic leukodystrophy	Autosomal recessive lysosomal storage disease, most commonly due to arylsulfatase A deficiency. Buildup of sulfatides → impaired production of myelin sheath. Findings: central and peripheral demyelination with ataxia, dementia.
Charcot-Marie-Tooth disease	Also known as hereditary motor and sensory neuropathy (HMSN). Group of progressive hereditary nerve disorders related to the defective production of proteins involved in the structure and function of peripheral nerves or the myelin sheath. Typically autosomal dominant inheritance pattern and associated with scoliosis and foot deformities (high or flat arches).
Krabbe disease	Autosomal recessive lysosomal storage disease due to deficiency of galactocerebrosidase. Buildup of galactocerebroside and psychosine destroys myelin sheath. Findings: peripheral neuropathy, developmental delay, optic atrophy, globoid cells.
Adrenoleukodystrophy	X-linked genetic disorder typically affecting males. Disrupts metabolism of very-long-chain fatty acids → excessive buildup in nervous system, adrenal gland, and testes. Progressive disease that can lead to long-term coma/death and adrenal gland crisis.

Seizures

	Characterized by synchronized, high-frequency neuronal firing. Variety of forms.
Partial (focal) seizures	Affect 1 area of the brain. Most commonly originate in medial temporal lobe. Often preceded by seizure aura; can secondarily generalize. Types: ▪ **Simple partial** (consciousness intact)—motor, sensory, autonomic, psychic ▪ **Complex partial** (impaired consciousness)
Generalized seizures	Diffuse. Types: ▪ **Absence** (petit mal)—3 Hz, no postictal confusion, blank stare ▪ **Myoclonic**—quick, repetitive jerks ▪ **Tonic-clonic** (grand mal)—alternating stiffening and movement ▪ **Tonic**—stiffening ▪ **Atonic**—"drop" seizures (falls to floor); commonly mistaken for fainting

Epilepsy—a disorder of recurrent seizures (febrile seizures are not epilepsy).

Status epilepticus—continuous seizure for > 30 min or recurrent seizures without regaining consciousness between seizures for > 30 min. Medical emergency.

Causes of seizures by age:
- Children—genetic, infection (febrile), trauma, congenital, metabolic
- Adults—tumors, trauma, stroke, infection
- Elderly—stroke, tumor, trauma, metabolic, infection

Differentiating headaches   Pain due to irritation of structures such as the dura, cranial nerves, or extracranial structures.

CLASSIFICATION	LOCALIZATION	DURATION	DESCRIPTION	TREATMENT
Cluster[a]	Unilateral	15 min–3 hr; repetitive	Repetitive brief headaches. Excruciating periorbital pain with lacrimation and rhinorrhea. May induce Horner syndrome. More common in males.	Inhaled oxygen, sumatriptan
Tension	Bilateral	> 30 min (typically 4–6 hr); constant	Steady pain. No photophobia or phonophobia. No aura.	Analgesics, NSAIDs, acetaminophen; amitriptyline for chronic pain
Migraine	Unilateral	4–72 hr	Pulsating pain with nausea, photophobia, or phonophobia. May have "aura." Due to irritation of CN V, meninges, or blood vessels (release of substance P, CGRP, vasoactive peptides).	Abortive therapies (e.g., triptans, NSAIDs) and prophylactic (propranolol, topiramate, calcium channel blockers, amitriptyline). POUND–Pulsatile, One-day duration, Unilateral, Nausea, Disabling

Other causes of headache include subarachnoid hemorrhage ("worst headache of life"), meningitis, hydrocephalus, neoplasia, and arteritis.

[a]Cluster headaches can be differentiated from trigeminal neuralgia based on duration. Trigeminal neuralgia produces repetitive shooting pain in the distribution of CN V that lasts (typically) for < 1 minute. The pain from cluster headaches lasts considerably longer (> 15 minutes).

Vertigo	Sensation of spinning while actually stationary. Subtype of "dizziness," but distinct from "lightheadedness."
Peripheral vertigo	More common. Inner ear etiology (e.g., semicircular canal debris, vestibular nerve infection, Ménière disease). Positional testing → delayed horizontal nystagmus.
Central vertigo	Brain stem or cerebellar lesion (e.g., stroke affecting vestibular nuclei or posterior fossa tumor). Findings: directional change of nystagmus, skew deviation, diplopia, dysmetria. Positional testing → immediate nystagmus in any direction; may change directions. Focal neurological findings.

Neurocutaneous disorders

Sturge-Weber syndrome	Congenital, non-inherited (somatic), developmental anomaly of neural crest derivatives (mesoderm/ectoderm) due to activating mutation of GNAQ gene. Affects small (capillary-sized) blood vessels → port-wine stain of the face **A** (non-neoplastic "birthmark" in CN V_1/V_2 distribution); ipsilateral leptomeningeal angioma **B** → seizures/epilepsy; intellectual disability; and episcleral hemangioma → ↑ IOP → early-onset glaucoma. **STURGE**-Weber: Sporadic, port-wine Stain; Tram track Ca^{2+} (opposing gyri); Unilateral; Retardation, Glaucoma, GNAQ gene; Epilepsy.
Tuberous sclerosis	**HAMARTOMAS**: Hamartomas in CNS and skin; Angiofibromas **C**; Mitral regurgitation; Ash-leaf spots; cardiac Rhabdomyoma; (Tuberous sclerosis); autosomal dOminant; Mental retardation; renal Angiomyolipoma **D**; Seizures, Shagreen patches. ↑ incidence of subependymal astrocytomas and ungual fibromas.
Neurofibromatosis type I (von Recklinghausen disease)	Café-au-lait spots **E**, Lisch nodules (pigmented iris hamartomas **F**), neurofibromas in skin, optic gliomas, pheochromocytomas. Mutated *NF1* tumor suppressor gene (neurofibromin, a negative regulator of Ras) on chromosome 17. Skin tumors of NF-1 are derived from neural crest cells.
von Hippel-Lindau disease	Cavernous hemangiomas in skin, mucosa, organs; bilateral renal cell carcinomas; hemangioblastoma (high vascularity with hyperchromatic nuclei **G**) in retina, brain stem, cerebellum **H**; and pheochromocytomas. Autosomal dominant; mutated *VHL* tumor suppressor gene on chromosome 3, which results in constitutive expression of HIF (transcription factor) and activation of angiogenic growth factors.

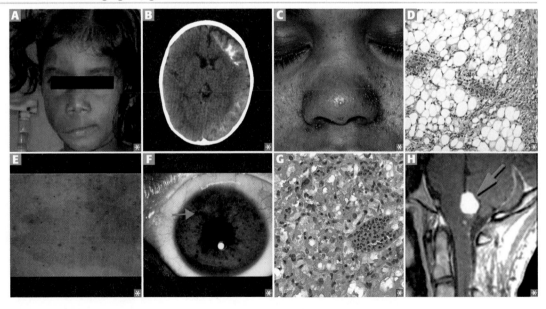

Adult primary brain tumors

Glioblastoma multiforme (grade IV astrocytoma)	Common, highly malignant 1° brain tumor with ~ 1-year median survival. Found in cerebral hemispheres **A**. Can cross corpus callosum ("butterfly glioma"). Stain astrocytes for GFAP. "Pseudopalisading" **B** pleomorphic tumor cells—border central areas of necrosis and hemorrhage.
Meningioma	Common, typically benign 1° brain tumor. Most often occurs in convexities of hemispheres (near surfaces of brain) and parasagittal region. Arises from arachnoid cells, is extra-axial (external to brain parenchyma), and may have a dural attachment ("tail" **C**). Often asymptomatic; may present with seizures or focal neurological signs. Resection and/or radiosurgery. Spindle cells concentrically arranged in a whorled pattern; psammoma bodies (laminated calcifications **D**).
Hemangioblastoma	Most often cerebellar **E**. Associated with von Hippel-Lindau syndrome when found with retinal angiomas. Can produce erythropoietin → 2° polycythemia. Closely arranged, thin-walled capillaries with minimal interleaving parenchyma **F**.
Schwannoma	Usually found at cerebellopontine angle **G**. Schwann cell origin **H**, S-100 ⊕; often localized to CN VIII → acoustic schwannoma (aka acoustic neuroma). Resectable or treated with stereotactic radiosurgery. Bilateral acoustic schwannomas found in NF-2.
Oligodendroglioma	Relatively rare, slow growing. Most often in frontal lobes **I**. Chicken-wire capillary pattern. Oligodendrocytes = "fried egg" cells—round nuclei with clear cytoplasm **J**. Often calcified in oligodendroglioma.
Pituitary adenoma	Most commonly prolactinoma **K**. Bitemporal hemianopia (**L** shows normal visual field above, patient's perspective below) due to pressure on optic chiasm. Hyper- or hypopituitarism are sequelae.

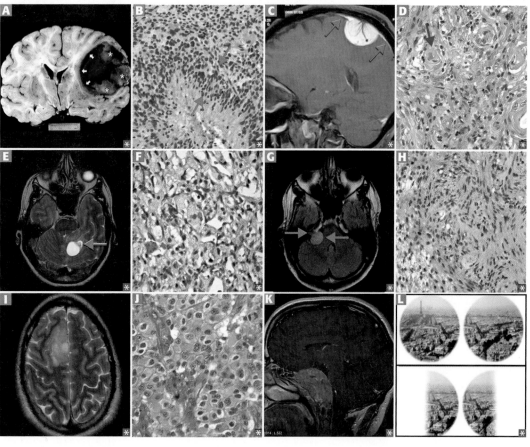

Childhood primary brain tumors

Pilocytic (low-grade) astrocytoma	Usually well circumscribed. In children, most often found in posterior fossa **A** (e.g., cerebellum). May be supratentorial. GFAP ⊕. Benign; good prognosis.	Rosenthal fibers—eosinophilic, corkscrew fibers **B**. Cystic + solid (gross).
Medulloblastoma	Highly malignant cerebellar tumor **C**. A form of primitive neuroectodermal tumor. Can compress 4th ventricle, causing hydrocephalus. Can send "drop metastases" to spinal cord.	Homer-Wright rosettes. Solid (gross), small blue cells **D** (histology).
Ependymoma	Ependymal cell tumors most commonly found in 4th ventricle **E**. Can cause hydrocephalus. Poor prognosis.	Characteristic perivascular rosettes **F**. Rod-shaped blepharoplasts (basal ciliary bodies) found near nucleus.
Craniopharyngioma	Benign childhood tumor, may be confused with pituitary adenoma (both can cause bitemporal hemianopia). Most common childhood supratentorial tumor.	Derived from remnants of Rathke pouch. Calcification is common **G**, **H** (tooth enamel–like).

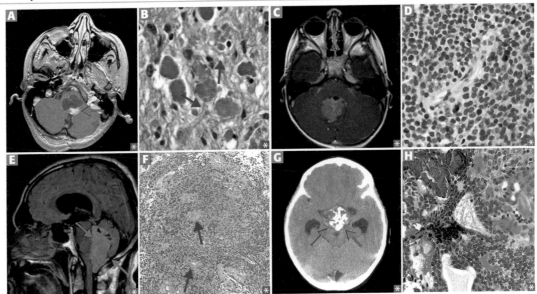

Herniation syndromes

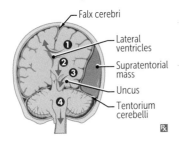

Falx cerebri
Lateral ventricles
Supratentorial mass
Uncus
Tentorium cerebelli

❶ Cingulate (subfalcine) herniation under falx cerebri		Can compress anterior cerebral artery.
❷ Downward transtentorial (central) herniation		
❸ Uncal herniation		Uncus = medial temporal lobe. Compresses ipsilateral CN III (blown pupil, "down-and-out" gaze), ipsilateral PCA (contralateral homonymous hemianopsia), contralateral crus cerebri (ipsilateral paralysis, "false localization" sign).
❹ Cerebellar tonsillar herniation into the foramen magnum		Coma and death result when these herniations compress the brain stem (and inhibit respiration).

▶ NEUROLOGY–PHARMACOLOGY

Glaucoma drugs	↓ IOP via ↓ amount of aqueous humor (inhibit synthesis/secretion or ↑ drainage).	
DRUG	MECHANISM	SIDE EFFECTS
α-agonists		
Epinephrine	↓ aqueous humor synthesis via vasoconstriction	Mydriasis; do not use in closed-angle glaucoma
Brimonidine (α_2)	↓ aqueous humor synthesis	Blurry vision, ocular hyperemia, foreign body sensation, ocular allergic reactions, ocular pruritus
β-blockers		
Timolol, betaxolol, carteolol	↓ aqueous humor synthesis	No pupillary or vision changes
Diuretics		
Acetazolamide	↓ aqueous humor synthesis via inhibition of carbonic anhydrase	No pupillary or vision changes
Cholinomimetics		
Direct (pilocarpine, carbachol) **Indirect (physostigmine, echothiophate)**	↑ outflow of aqueous humor via contraction of ciliary muscle and opening of trabecular meshwork Use pilocarpine in emergencies—very effective at opening meshwork into canal of Schlemm	Miosis and cyclospasm (contraction of ciliary muscle)
Prostaglandin		
Latanoprost ($PGF_{2\alpha}$)	↑ outflow of aqueous humor	Darkens color of iris (browning)

Opioid analgesics	Morphine, fentanyl, codeine, loperamide, methadone, meperidine, dextromethorphan, diphenoxylate.
MECHANISM	Act as agonists at opioid receptors (mu = morphine, delta = enkephalin, kappa = dynorphin) to modulate synaptic transmission—open K^+ channels, close Ca^{2+} channels → ↓ synaptic transmission. Inhibit release of ACh, norepinephrine, 5-HT, glutamate, substance P.
CLINICAL USE	Pain, cough suppression (dextromethorphan), diarrhea (loperamide and diphenoxylate), acute pulmonary edema, maintenance programs for heroin addicts (methadone).
TOXICITY	Addiction, respiratory depression, constipation, miosis (pinpoint pupils), additive CNS depression with other drugs. Tolerance does not develop to miosis and constipation. Toxicity treated with naloxone or naltrexone (opioid receptor antagonist).

Butorphanol

MECHANISM	Mu-opioid receptor **partial** agonist and kappa-opioid receptor agonist; produces analgesia.
CLINICAL USE	Severe pain (migraine, labor, etc.). Causes less respiratory depression than full opioid agonists.
TOXICITY	Can cause opioid withdrawal symptoms if patient is also taking full opioid agonist (competition for opioid receptors). Overdose not easily reversed with naloxone.

Tramadol

MECHANISM	Very weak opioid agonist; also inhibits serotonin and norepinephrine reuptake (works on multiple neurotransmitters—"**tram it all**" in with **tramadol**).
CLINICAL USE	Chronic pain.
TOXICITY	Similar to opioids. Decreases seizure threshold. Serotonin syndrome.

Epilepsy drugs

	PARTIAL (FOCAL)		GENERALIZED			MECHANISM	SIDE EFFECTS	NOTES
	SIMPLE	COMPLEX	TONIC-CLONIC	ABSENCE	STATUS EPILEPTICUS			
Ethosuximide				* ✓		Blocks thalamic T-type Ca^{2+} channels	GI, fatigue, headache, urticaria, Steven-Johnson syndrome. EFGHIJ—Ethosuximide causes Fatigue, GI distress, Headache, Itching, and Stevens-Johnson syndrome	Sucks to have Silent (absence) Seizures
Benzodiazepines (diazepam, lorazepam)					** ✓	↑ $GABA_A$ action	Sedation, tolerance, dependence, respiratory depression	Also for eclampsia seizures (1st line is $MgSO_4$)
Phenytoin	✓	✓	* ✓		*** ✓	↑ Na^+ channel inactivation; zero-order kinetics	Nystagmus, diplopia, ataxia, sedation, gingival hyperplasia, hirsutism, peripheral neuropathy, megaloblastic anemia, teratogenesis (fetal hydantoin syndrome) SLE-like syndrome, induction of cytochrome P-450, lymphadenopathy, Stevens-Johnson syndrome, osteopenia	Fosphenytoin for parenteral use
Carbamazepine	* ✓	* ✓	* ✓			↑ Na^+ channel inactivation	Diplopia, ataxia, blood dyscrasias (agranulocytosis, aplastic anemia), liver toxicity, teratogenesis, induction of cytochrome P-450, SIADH, Stevens-Johnson syndrome	1st line for trigeminal neuralgia
Valproic acid	✓	✓	* ✓	✓		↑ Na^+ channel inactivation, ↑ GABA concentration by inhibiting GABA transaminase	GI, distress, rare but fatal hepatotoxicity (measure LFTs), neural tube defects in fetus (spina bifida), tremor, weight gain, contraindicated in pregnancy	Also used for myoclonic seizures, bipolar disorder
Gabapentin	✓	✓	✓			Primarily inhibits high-voltage-activated Ca^{2+} channels; designed as GABA analog	Sedation, ataxia	Also used for peripheral neuropathy, postherpetic neuralgia, migraine prophylaxis, bipolar disorder
Phenobarbital	✓	✓	✓			↑ $GABA_A$ action	Sedation, tolerance, dependence, induction of cytochrome P-450, cardiorespiratory depression	1st line in neonates
Topiramate	✓	✓	✓			Blocks Na^+ channels, ↑ GABA action	Sedation, mental dulling, kidney stones, weight loss	Also used for migraine prevention
Lamotrigine	✓	✓	✓	✓		Blocks voltage-gated Na^+ channels	Stevens-Johnson syndrome (must be titrated slowly)	
Levetiracetam	✓	✓	✓			Unknown; may modulate GABA and glutamate release		
Tiagabine	✓	✓				↑ GABA by inhibiting re-uptake		
Vigabatrin	✓	✓				↑ GABA by irreversibly inhibiting GABA transaminase		
Stevens-Johnson syndrome	Prodrome of malaise and fever followed by rapid onset of erythematous/purpuric macules (oral, ocular, genital). Skin lesions progress to epidermal necrosis and sloughing.							

* = 1st line; ** = 1st line for acute; *** = 1st line for prophylaxis.

Barbiturates	Phenobarbital, pentobarbital, thiopental, secobarbital.
MECHANISM	Facilitate $GABA_A$ action by ↑ **duration** of Cl^- channel opening, thus ↓ neuron firing (barbi**dur**ates ↑ **dur**ation). Contraindicated in porphyria.
CLINICAL USE	Sedative for anxiety, seizures, insomnia, induction of anesthesia (thiopental).
TOXICITY	Respiratory and cardiovascular depression (can be fatal); CNS depression (can be exacerbated by EtOH use); dependence; drug interactions (induces cytochrome P-450). Overdose treatment is supportive (assist respiration and maintain BP).

Benzodiazepines	Diazepam, lorazepam, triazolam, temazepam, oxazepam, midazolam, chlordiazepoxide, alprazolam.	
MECHANISM	Facilitate $GABA_A$ action by ↑ **frequency** of Cl^- channel opening. ↓ REM sleep. Most have long half-lives and active metabolites (exceptions: triazolam, oxazepam, and midazolam are short acting → higher addictive potential).	"**Fren**zodiazepines" ↑ **frequency**. Benzos, barbs, and EtOH all bind the $GABA_A$ receptor, which is a ligand-gated Cl^- channel.
CLINICAL USE	Anxiety, spasticity, status epilepticus (lorazepam and diazepam), detoxification (especially alcohol withdrawal–DTs), night terrors, sleepwalking, general anesthetic (amnesia, muscle relaxation), hypnotic (insomnia).	
TOXICITY	Dependence, additive CNS depression effects with alcohol. Less risk of respiratory depression and coma than with barbiturates. Treat overdose with flumazenil (competitive antagonist at GABA benzodiazepine receptor).	

Nonbenzodiazepine hypnotics	**Z**olpidem (Ambien), **Z**aleplon, es**Z**opiclone. "All **ZZZ**s put you to sleep."
MECHANISM	Act via the BZ1 subtype of the GABA receptor. Effects reversed by flumazenil.
CLINICAL USE	Insomnia.
TOXICITY	Ataxia, headaches, confusion. Short duration because of rapid metabolism by liver enzymes. Unlike older sedative-hypnotics, cause only modest day-after psychomotor depression and few amnestic effects. ↓ dependence risk than benzodiazepines.

Anesthetics—general principles	CNS drugs must be lipid soluble (cross the blood-brain barrier) or be actively transported. Drugs with ↓ solubility in blood = rapid induction and recovery times. Drugs with ↑ solubility in lipids = ↑ potency = $\dfrac{1}{MAC}$
	MAC = Minimal Alveolar Concentration (of inhaled anesthetic) required to prevent 50% of subjects from moving in response to noxious stimulus (e.g., skin incision). Examples: N_2O has ↓ blood and lipid solubility, and thus fast induction and low potency. Halothane, in contrast, has ↑ lipid and blood solubility, and thus high potency and slow induction.

Inhaled anesthetics	Halothane, enflurane, isoflurane, sevoflurane, methoxyflurane, nitrous oxide.
MECHANISM	Mechanism unknown.
EFFECTS	Myocardial depression, respiratory depression, nausea/emesis, ↑ cerebral blood flow (↓ cerebral metabolic demand).
TOXICITY	Hepatotoxicity (halothane), nephrotoxicity (methoxyflurane), proconvulsant (enflurane), expansion of trapped gas in a body cavity (nitrous oxide). Can cause **malignant hyperthermia**—rare, life-threatening hereditary condition in which inhaled anesthetics (except nitrous oxide) and succinylcholine induce fever and severe muscle contractions. Treatment: dantrolene.

Intravenous anesthetics

Barbiturates	Thiopental—high potency, high lipid solubility, rapid entry into brain. Used for induction of anesthesia and short surgical procedures. Effect terminated by rapid redistribution into tissue (i.e., skeletal muscle) and fat. ↓ cerebral blood flow.	B. B. King on OPIOIDS PROPOses FOOLishly.
Benzodiazepines	Midazolam most common drug used for endoscopy; used adjunctively with gaseous anesthetics and narcotics. May cause severe postoperative respiratory depression, ↓ BP (treat overdose with flumazenil), and anterograde amnesia.	
Arylcyclohexylamines (Ketamine)	PCP analogs that act as dissociative anesthetics. Block NMDA receptors. Cardiovascular stimulants. Cause disorientation, hallucination, and bad dreams. ↑ cerebral blood flow.	
Opioids	Morphine, fentanyl used with other CNS depressants during general anesthesia.	
Propofol	Used for sedation in ICU, rapid anesthesia induction, and short procedures. Less postoperative nausea than thiopental. Potentiates $GABA_A$.	

Local anesthetics	Esters—procaine, cocaine, tetracaine. Amides—lIdocaIne, mepIvacaIne, bupIvacaIne (amIdes have 2 I's in name).
MECHANISM	Block Na^+ channels by binding to specific receptors on inner portion of channel. Preferentially bind to activated Na^+ channels, so most effective in rapidly firing neurons. 3° amine local anesthetics penetrate membrane in uncharged form, then bind to ion channels as charged form.
PRINCIPLE	Can be given with vasoconstrictors (usually epinephrine) to enhance local action—↓ bleeding, ↑ anesthesia by ↓ systemic concentration. In infected (acidic) tissue, alkaline anesthetics are charged and cannot penetrate membrane effectively → need more anesthetic. Order of nerve blockade: small-diameter fibers > large diameter. Myelinated fibers > unmyelinated fibers. Overall, size factor predominates over myelination such that small myelinated fibers > small unmyelinated fibers > large myelinated fibers > large unmyelinated fibers. Order of loss: (1) pain, (2) temperature, (3) touch, (4) pressure.
CLINICAL USE	Minor surgical procedures, spinal anesthesia. If allergic to esters, give amides.
TOXICITY	CNS excitation, severe cardiovascular toxicity (bupivacaine), hypertension, hypotension, and arrhythmias (cocaine).

Neuromuscular blocking drugs	Used for muscle paralysis in surgery or mechanical ventilation. Selective for motor (vs. autonomic) nicotinic receptor.
Depolarizing	Succinylcholine—strong ACh receptor agonist; produces sustained depolarization and prevents muscle contraction. Reversal of blockade: ▪ Phase I (prolonged depolarization)—no antidote. Block potentiated by cholinesterase inhibitors. ▪ Phase II (repolarized but blocked; ACh receptors are available, but desensitized)—antidote consists of cholinesterase inhibitors. Complications include hypercalcemia, hyperkalemia, and malignant hyperthermia.
Nondepolarizing	Tubocurarine, atracurium, mivacurium, pancuronium, vecuronium, rocuronium—competitive antagonists—compete with ACh for receptors. Reversal of blockade—neostigmine (must be given with atropine to prevent muscarinic effects such as bradycardia), edrophonium, and other cholinesterase inhibitors.

Dantrolene	
MECHANISM	Prevents the release of Ca^{2+} from the sarcoplasmic reticulum of skeletal muscle.
CLINICAL USE	Used to treat malignant hyperthermia and neuroleptic malignant syndrome (a toxicity of antipsychotic drugs).

Parkinson disease drugs

Parkinsonism is due to loss of dopaminergic neurons and excess cholinergic activity.

STRATEGY	AGENTS	
Dopamine agonists	Bromocriptine (ergot), pramipexole, ropinirole (non-ergot); non-ergots are preferred	**BALSA:** Bromocriptine
↑ dopamine	Amantadine (may ↑ dopamine release); also used as an antiviral against influenza A and rubella; toxicity = ataxia L-dopa/carbidopa (converted to dopamine in CNS)	Amantadine Levodopa (with carbidopa) Selegiline (and COMT inhibitors) Antimuscarinics For essential or familial tremors, use a β-blocker (e.g., propranolol).
Prevent dopamine breakdown	Selegiline (selective MAO type B inhibitor); entacapone, tolcapone (COMT inhibitors— prevent L-dopa degradation → ↑ dopamine availability)	
Curb excess cholinergic activity	Benztropine (Antimuscarinic; improves tremor and rigidity but has little effect on bradykinesia)	**Park** your Mercedes-**Benz.**

L-dopa (levodopa)/carbidopa

MECHANISM	↑ level of dopamine in brain. Unlike dopamine, L-dopa can cross blood-brain barrier and is converted by dopa decarboxylase in the CNS to dopamine. Carbidopa, a peripheral decarboxylase inhibitor, is given with L-dopa to ↑ the bioavailability of L-dopa in the brain and to limit peripheral side effects.
CLINICAL USE	Parkinson disease.
TOXICITY	Arrhythmias from ↑ peripheral formation of catecholamines. Long-term use can lead to dyskinesia following administration ("on-off" phenomenon), akinesia between doses.

Selegiline

MECHANISM	Selectively inhibits MAO-B, which preferentially metabolizes dopamine over norepinephrine and 5-HT, thereby ↑ the availability of dopamine.
CLINICAL USE	Adjunctive agent to L-dopa in treatment of Parkinson disease.
TOXICITY	May enhance adverse effects of L-dopa.

Alzheimer drugs

Memantine

MECHANISM	NMDA receptor antagonist; helps prevent excitotoxicity (mediated by Ca^{2+}).
TOXICITY	Dizziness, confusion, hallucinations.

Donepezil, galantamine, rivastigmine

MECHANISM	AChE inhibitors.
TOXICITY	Nausea, dizziness, insomnia.

Huntington drugs

Neurotransmitter changes in Huntington disease: ↓ GABA, ↓ ACh, ↑ dopamine.
Treatments:
- Tetrabenazine and reserpine—inhibit vesicular monoamine transporter (VMAT); limit dopamine vesicle packaging and release.
- Haloperidol—dopamine receptor antagonist.

Sumatriptan

MECHANISM	5-HT$_{1B/1D}$ agonist. Inhibits trigeminal nerve activation; prevents vasoactive peptide release; induces vasoconstriction. Half-life < 2 hours.	A **SUM**o wrestler **TRIP**s **AN**d falls on your head.
CLINICAL USE	Acute migraine, cluster headache attacks.	
TOXICITY	Coronary vasospasm (contraindicated in patients with CAD or Prinzmetal angina), mild tingling.	

▶ NOTES

Psychiatry

"A *Freudian slip is when you say one thing but mean your mother.*"

—Anonymous

"*Men will always be mad, and those who think they can cure them are the maddest of all.*"

—Voltaire

"*Anyone who goes to a psychiatrist ought to have his head examined.*"

—Samuel Goldwyn

The DSM-5 was released by the American Psychiatric Association in 2013, reclassifying several psychiatric conditions and updating diagnostic criteria. We have updated this chapter to reflect certain DSM-5 revisions.

▶ PSYCHIATRY—PSYCHOLOGY

Classical conditioning	Learning in which a natural response (salivation) is elicited by a conditioned, or learned, stimulus (bell) that previously was presented in conjunction with an unconditioned stimulus (food).	Usually deals with **involuntary** responses. Pavlov's classical experiments with dogs—ringing the bell provoked salivation.

Operant conditioning	Learning in which a particular action is elicited because it produces a punishment or reward. Usually deals with **voluntary** responses.
Positive reinforcement	Desired reward produces action (mouse presses button to get food).
Negative reinforcement	Target behavior (response) is followed by removal of aversive stimulus (mouse presses button to turn off continuous loud noise).
Punishment	Repeated application of aversive stimulus extinguishes unwanted behavior.
Extinction	Discontinuation of reinforcement (positive or negative) eventually eliminates behavior. Can occur in operant or classical conditioning.

Transference and countertransference

Transference	Patient projects feelings about formative or other important persons onto physician (e.g., psychiatrist is seen as parent).
Countertransference	Doctor projects feelings about formative or other important persons onto patient (e.g., patient reminds physician of younger sibling).

Ego defenses	Unconscious mental processes used to resolve conflict and prevent undesirable feelings (e.g., anxiety, depression).

IMMATURE DEFENSES	DESCRIPTION	EXAMPLE
Acting out	Expressing unacceptable feelings and thoughts through actions.	Tantrums.
Dissociation	Temporary, drastic change in personality, memory, consciousness, or motor behavior to avoid emotional stress.	Extreme forms can result in dissociative identity disorder (multiple personality disorder).
Denial	Avoiding the awareness of some painful reality.	A common reaction in newly diagnosed AIDS and cancer patients.
Displacement	Transferring avoided ideas and feelings to some neutral person or object (vs. projection).	Mother yells at her child, because her husband yelled at her.
Fixation	Partially remaining at a more childish level of development (vs. regression).	Men fixating on sports games.
Identification	Modeling behavior after another person who is more powerful (though not necessarily admired).	Abused child identifies with an abuser.
Isolation (of affect)	Separating feelings from ideas and events.	Describing murder in graphic detail with no emotional response.

Ego defenses *(continued)*

IMMATURE DEFENSES	DESCRIPTION	EXAMPLE
Projection	Attributing an unacceptable internal impulse to an external source (vs. displacement).	A man who wants another woman thinks his wife is cheating on him.
Rationalization	Proclaiming logical reasons for actions actually performed for other reasons, usually to avoid self-blame.	After getting fired, claiming that the job was not important anyway.
Reaction formation	Replacing a warded-off idea or feeling by an (unconsciously derived) emphasis on its opposite (vs. sublimation).	A patient with libidinous thoughts enters a monastery.
Regression	Turning back the maturational clock and going back to earlier modes of dealing with the world (vs. fixation).	Seen in children under stress such as illness, punishment, or birth of a new sibling (e.g., bedwetting in a previously toilet-trained child when hospitalized).
Repression	Involuntary withholding an idea or feeling from conscious awareness (vs. suppression).	Not remembering a conflictual or traumatic experience; pressing bad thoughts into the unconscious.
Splitting	Believing that people are either all good or all bad at different times due to intolerance of ambiguity. Commonly seen in borderline personality disorder.	A patient says that all the nurses are cold and insensitive but that the doctors are warm and friendly.
MATURE DEFENSES		
Altruism	Alleviating guilty feelings by unsolicited generosity toward others.	Mafia boss makes large donation to charity.
Humor	Appreciating the amusing nature of an anxiety-provoking or adverse situation.	Nervous medical student jokes about the boards.
Sublimation	Replacing an unacceptable wish with a course of action that is similar to the wish but does not conflict with one's value system (vs. reaction formation).	Teenager's aggression toward his father is redirected to perform well in sports.
Suppression	Intentional withholding of an idea or feeling from conscious awareness (vs. repression).	Choosing to not worry about the big game until it is time to play.

Mature adults wear a **SASH**: Sublimation, Altruism, Suppression, Humor.

▶ PSYCHIATRY–PATHOLOGY

Infant deprivation effects	Long-term deprivation of affection results in: ▪ ↓ muscle tone ▪ Poor language skills ▪ Poor socialization skills ▪ Lack of basic trust ▪ Anaclitic depression (infant withdrawn/ unresponsive) ▪ Weight loss ▪ Physical illness	The 4 W's: **W**eak, **W**ordless, **W**anting (socially), **W**ary. Deprivation for > 6 months can lead to irreversible changes. Severe deprivation can result in infant death.

Child abuse

	Physical abuse	Sexual abuse
EVIDENCE	Healed fractures on x-ray (e.g., spiral fractures are highly suggestive of abuse), burns (e.g., cigarette, scalding), subdural hematomas, pattern marks/bruising (e.g., belts, electrical cords), rib fractures, retinal hemorrhage or detachment	Genital, anal, or oral trauma; STDs; UTIs
ABUSER	Usually biological mother	Known to victim, usually male
EPIDEMIOLOGY	~3000 deaths/yr in U.S., 80% < 3 yr old	Peak incidence 9–12 years old

Child neglect

Failure to provide a child with adequate food, shelter, supervision, education, and/or affection. Most common form of child maltreatment. Evidence: poor hygiene, malnutrition, withdrawal, impaired social/emotional development, failure to thrive.

As with child abuse, child neglect must be reported to local child protective services.

Childhood and early-onset disorders

Attention-deficit hyperactivity disorder	Onset before age 12. Limited attention span and poor impulse control. Characterized by hyperactivity, impulsivity, and/or inattention in multiple settings (school, home, places of worship, etc.). Normal intelligence, but commonly coexists with difficulties in school. Continues into adulthood in as many as 50% of individuals. Associated with ↓ frontal lobe volume/metabolism. Treatment: methylphenidate, amphetamines, atomoxetine, behavioral interventions (reinforcement, reward).
Conduct disorder	Repetitive and pervasive behavior violating the basic rights of others (e.g., physical aggression, destruction of property, theft). After age 18, many of these patients will meet criteria for diagnosis of antisocial personality disorder.
Oppositional defiant disorder	Enduring pattern of hostile, defiant behavior toward authority figures in the absence of serious violations of social norms.
Tourette syndrome	Onset before age 18. Characterized by sudden, rapid, recurrent, nonrhythmic, stereotyped motor and vocal tics that persist for > 1 year. Lifetime prevalence of 0.1–1.0% in the general population. Coprolalia (involuntary obscene speech) found in only 10–20% of patients. Associated with OCD and ADHD. Treatment: antipsychotics and behavioral therapy.
Separation anxiety disorder	Common onset at 7–9 years. Overwhelming fear of separation from home or loss of attachment figure. May lead to factitious physical complaints to avoid going to or staying at school. Treatment: SSRIs and relaxation techniques/behavioral interventions.

Pervasive developmental disorders	Characterized by difficulties with language and failure to acquire or early loss of social skills.
Autism spectrum disorder	Characterized by poor social interactions, communication deficits, repetitive/ritualized behaviors, and restricted interests. Must present in early childhood. May or may not be accompanied by intellectual disability; rarely accompanied by unusual abilities (savants). More common in boys.
Rett disorder	X-linked disorder seen almost exclusively in girls (affected males die in utero or shortly after birth). Symptoms usually become apparent around ages 1–4, including regression characterized by loss of development, loss of verbal abilities, intellectual disability, ataxia, and stereotyped hand-wringing.

Neurotransmitter changes with disease

DISORDER	NEUROTRANSMITTER CHANGES
Alzheimer disease	↓ ACh
Anxiety	↑ norepinephrine, ↓ GABA, ↓ 5-HT
Depression	↓ norepinephrine, ↓ 5-HT, ↓ dopamine
Huntington disease	↓ GABA, ↓ ACh, ↑ dopamine
Parkinson disease	↓ dopamine, ↑ 5-HT, ↑ ACh
Schizophrenia	↑ dopamine

Understanding these changes can help guide pharmacologic treatment choice.

Orientation	Patient's ability to know who he or she is, where he or she is, and the date and time. Common causes of loss of orientation: alcohol, drugs, fluid/electrolyte imbalance, head trauma, hypoglycemia, infection, nutritional deficiencies.	Order of loss: 1st—time; 2nd—place; last—person. Often abbreviated in the medical chart as "alert and oriented × 3" (AO×3).

Amnesias

Retrograde amnesia	Inability to remember things that occurred before a CNS insult.
Anterograde amnesia	Inability to remember things that occurred after a CNS insult (no new memory).
Korsakoff amnesia	Classic anterograde amnesia caused by thiamine deficiency and the associated destruction of mammillary bodies. May also include some retrograde amnesia. Seen in alcoholics, and associated with confabulations.
Dissociative amnesia	Inability to recall important personal information, usually subsequent to severe trauma or stress. May be accompanied by **dissociative fugue** (abrupt travel or wandering during a period of dissociative amnesia, associated with traumatic circumstances).

Cognitive disorder	Significant change in cognition (memory, attention, language, judgment) from previous level of functioning. Associated with abnormalities in CNS, a general medical condition, medications, or substance use. Includes delirium and dementia.	

Delirium	"Waxing and waning" level of consciousness with acute onset; rapid ↓ in attention span and level of arousal. Characterized by disorganized thinking, hallucinations (often visual), illusions, misperceptions, disturbance in sleep-wake cycle, cognitive dysfunction.
	Usually 2° to other illness (e.g., CNS disease, infection, trauma, substance abuse/withdrawal, metabolic/electrolyte disturbances, hemorrhage, urinary/fecal retention).
	Most common presentation of altered mental status in inpatient setting. Abnormal EEG.
	Treatment:
	  ▪ Identify and address underlying cause.
	  ▪ Optimize brain condition (O_2, hydration, pain, etc.).
	  ▪ Antipsychotics (mainly haloperidol).
		Delirium = changes in senso**rium**.
		Check for drugs with anticholinergic effects.
		Often reversible.
		
		T-A-DA approach (**T**olerate, **A**nticipate, **D**on't **A**gitate) helpful for management.

Dementia	Gradual ↓ in intellectual ability or "cognition" without affecting level of consciousness. Characterized by memory deficits, aphasia, apraxia, agnosia, loss of abstract thought, behavioral/personality changes, impaired judgment. A patient with dementia can develop delirium (e.g., patient with Alzheimer disease who develops pneumonia is at ↑ risk for delirium). Irreversible causes: Alzheimer disease, Lewy body dementia, Huntington disease, Pick disease, cerebral infarcts, Creutzfeldt-Jakob disease, chronic substance abuse (due to neurotoxicity of drugs). Reversible causes: NPH, vitamin B_{12} deficiency, hypothyroidism, neurosyphilis, HIV (partially). ↑ incidence with age. EEG usually normal.	"De**mem**tia" is characterized by **mem**ory loss. Usually irreversible. In elderly patients, depression may present like dementia (pseudodementia).

Psychosis	A distorted perception of reality (psychosis) characterized by delusions, hallucinations, and/or disorganized thinking. Psychosis can occur in patients with medical illness, psychiatric illness, or both.
Hallucinations	Perceptions in the absence of external stimuli (e.g., seeing a light that is not actually present).
Delusions	Unique, false beliefs about oneself or others that persist despite the facts (e.g., thinking aliens are communicating with you).
Disorganized speech	Words and ideas are strung together based on sounds, puns, or "loose associations."

Hallucination types

Visual	More commonly a feature of medical illness (e.g., drug intoxication) than psychiatric illness.
Auditory	More commonly a feature of psychiatric illness (e.g., schizophrenia) than medical illness.
Olfactory	Often occur as an aura of psychomotor epilepsy and in brain tumors.
Gustatory	Rare.
Tactile	Common in alcohol withdrawal (e.g., formication—the sensation of bugs crawling on one's skin). Also seen in cocaine abusers ("cocaine crawlies").
HypnaGOgic	Occurs while GOing to sleep.
HypnoPOMPic	Occurs while waking from sleep ("POMPous upon awakening").

Schizophrenia	Chronic mental disorder with periods of psychosis, disturbed behavior and thought, and decline in functioning that lasts > 6 months. Associated with ↑ dopaminergic activity, ↓ dendritic branching. Diagnosis requires 2 or more of the following (first 4 in this list are "positive symptoms"): <ul><li>Delusions</li><li>Hallucinations—often auditory</li><li>Disorganized speech (loose associations)</li><li>Disorganized or catatonic behavior</li><li>"Negative symptoms"—flat affect, social withdrawal, lack of motivation, lack of speech or thought</li></ul>**Brief psychotic disorder**—< 1 month, usually stress related. **Schizophreniform disorder**—1–6 months. **Schizoaffective disorder**—at least 2 weeks of stable mood with psychotic symptoms, plus a major depressive, manic, or mixed (both) episode. 2 subtypes: bipolar or depressive.	Genetics and environment contribute to the etiology of schizophrenia. Frequent cannabis use is associated with psychosis/schizophrenia in teens. Lifetime prevalence—1.5% (males = females, blacks = whites). Presents earlier in men (late teens to early 20s vs. late 20s to early 30s in women). Patients are at ↑ risk for suicide.

Delusional disorder	Fixed, persistent, untrue belief system **lasting > 1 month**. Functioning otherwise not impaired. Example: a woman who genuinely believes she is married to a celebrity when, in fact, she is not.

Dissociative disorders

Dissociative identity disorder	Formerly known as multiple personality disorder. Presence of 2 or more distinct identities or personality states. More common in women. Associated with history of sexual abuse, PTSD, depression, substance abuse, borderline personality, and somatoform conditions.
Depersonalization/ derealization disorder	Persistent feelings of detachment or estrangement from one's own body, thoughts, perceptions, and actions (depersonalization) or one's environment (derealization).

Mood disorder	Characterized by an abnormal range of moods or internal emotional states and loss of control over them. Severity of moods causes distress and impairment in social and occupational functioning. Includes major depressive disorder, bipolar disorder, dysthymic disorder, and cyclothymic disorder. Psychotic features (delusions or hallucinations) may be present.

Manic episode	Distinct period of abnormally and persistently elevated, expansive, or irritable mood and abnormally and persistently increased activity or energy **lasting at least 1 week**. Often disturbing to patient. Diagnosis requires hospitalization or at least 3 of the following (manics **DIG FAST**): <ul><li>Distractibility</li><li>Irresponsibility—seeks pleasure without regard to consequences (hedonistic)</li><li>Grandiosity—inflated self-esteem</li></ul><ul><li>Flight of ideas—racing thoughts</li><li>↑ in goal-directed Activity/psychomotor Agitation</li><li>↓ need for Sleep</li><li>Talkativeness or pressured speech</li></ul>

Hypomanic episode	Like manic episode except mood disturbance is not severe enough to cause marked impairment in social and/or occupational functioning or to necessitate hospitalization. No psychotic features. Lasts at least 4 consecutive days.

Bipolar disorder	Bipolar I defined by the presence of at least 1 manic episode with or without a hypomanic or depressive episode. Bipolar II defined by the presence of a hypomanic and a depressive episode. Patient's mood and functioning usually return to normal between episodes. Use of antidepressants can lead to ↑ mania. High suicide risk. Treatment: mood stabilizers (e.g., lithium, valproic acid, carbamazepine), atypical antipsychotics. **Cyclothymic disorder**—dysthymia and hypomania; milder form of bipolar disorder **lasting at least 2 years**.

Major depressive disorder	May be self-limited disorder, with major depressive episodes usually **lasting 6–12 months**. Episodes characterized by **at least 5 of the following 9 symptoms for 2 or more weeks** (symptoms must include patient-reported depressed mood or anhedonia and occur more frequently as the disorder progresses).	SIG E CAPS:

SIG E CAPS:
- Sleep disturbance
- Loss of Interest (anhedonia)
- Guilt or feelings of worthlessness
- Energy loss and fatigue
- Concentration problems
- Appetite/weight changes
- Psychomotor retardation or agitation
- Suicidal ideations
- Depressed mood

Persistent depressive disorder (dysthymia)— depression, often milder, **lasting at least 2 years**.

Seasonal affective disorder—symptoms usually associated with winter season; improves in response to full-spectrum bright-light exposure.

Patients with depression typically have the following changes in their sleep stages:
- ↓ slow-wave sleep
- ↓ REM latency
- ↑ REM early in sleep cycle
- ↑ total REM sleep
- Repeated nighttime awakenings
- Early-morning awakening (important screening question)

Atypical depression	Differs from classical forms of depression. Characterized by mood reactivity (being able to experience improved mood in response to positive events, albeit briefly), "reversed" vegetative symptoms (hypersomnia and weight gain), leaden paralysis (heavy feeling in arms and legs), and long-standing interpersonal rejection sensitivity. Most common subtype of depression. Treatment: MAO inhibitors, SSRIs.

Postpartum mood disturbances	Onset within 4 weeks of delivery.
Maternal (postpartum) "blues"	50–85% incidence rate. Characterized by depressed affect, tearfulness, and fatigue starting 2–3 days after delivery. **Usually resolves within 10 days**. Treatment: supportive. Follow-up to assess for possible postpartum depression.
Postpartum depression	10–15% incidence rate. Characterized by depressed affect, anxiety, and poor concentration starting within 4 weeks after delivery. **Lasts 2 weeks to a year or more**. Treatment: antidepressants, psychotherapy.
Postpartum psychosis	0.1–0.2% incidence rate. Characterized by delusions, hallucinations, confusion, unusual behavior, and possible homicidal/suicidal ideations or attempts. Usually **lasts days to 4–6 weeks**. Treatment: antipsychotics, antidepressants, possible inpatient hospitalization, assessment of child safety.

Pathologic grief	Normal bereavement characterized by shock, denial, guilt, and somatic symptoms. Duration varies widely, up to 6–12 months. May experience simple hallucinations (e.g., hearing name called). Pathologic grief includes excessively intense grief; prolonged grief lasting > 6–12 months; or grief that is delayed, inhibited, or denied. May experience depressive symptoms, delusions, and hallucinations.
Electroconvulsive therapy	Treatment option for major depressive disorder refractory to other treatment and for pregnant women with major depressive disorder. Also considered when immediate response is necessary (acute suicidality), in depression with psychotic features, and for catatonia. Produces a relatively painless seizure in an anesthetized patient. Adverse effects include disorientation, temporary headache, and partial anterograde/retrograde amnesia usually fully resolving in 6 months.

Risk factors for suicide completion

Sex (male), Age (teenager or elderly), Depression, Previous attempt, Ethanol or drug use, loss of Rational thinking, Sickness (medical illness, 3 or more prescription medications), Organized plan, No spouse (divorced, widowed, or single, especially if childless), Social support lacking.
Women try more often; men succeed more often.

SAD PERSONS are more likely to complete suicide.

Anxiety disorder

Inappropriate experience of fear/worry and its physical manifestations (anxiety) when the source of the fear/worry is either not real or insufficient to account for the severity of the symptoms. Symptoms interfere with daily functioning. Lifetime prevalence of 30% in women and 19% in men. Includes panic disorder, phobias, and generalized anxiety disorder.

Panic disorder

Defined by the presence of recurrent panic attacks (periods of intense fear and discomfort peaking in 10 minutes with at least 4 of the following): Palpitations, Paresthesias, Abdominal distress, Nausea, Intense fear of dying or losing control, lIght-headedness, Chest pain, Chills, Choking, disConnectedness, Sweating, Shaking, Shortness of breath. Strong genetic component. Treatment: cognitive behavioral therapy, SSRIs, venlafaxine, benzodiazepines (risk of tolerance, physical dependence).

PANICS.
Diagnosis requires attack followed by 1 month (or more) of 1 (or more) of the following: persistent concern of additional attacks, worrying about consequences of the attack, or behavioral change related to attacks.
Symptoms are the systemic manifestations of fear.

Specific phobia	Fear that is excessive or unreasonable and interferes with normal function. Cued by presence or anticipation of a specific object or situation. Person recognizes fear is excessive. Can treat with systematic desensitization.
	Social anxiety disorder—exaggerated fear of embarrassment in social situations (e.g., public speaking, using public restrooms). Treatment: SSRIs.
	Agoraphobia—exaggerated fear of open or enclosed places, using public transportation, being in line or in crowds, or leaving home alone.
Generalized anxiety disorder	Pattern of uncontrollable anxiety for **at least 6 months** that is unrelated to a specific person, situation, or event. Associated with sleep disturbance, fatigue, GI disturbance, and difficulty concentrating. Treatment: SSRIs, SNRIs, buspirone, cognitive behavioral therapy.
	Adjustment disorder—emotional symptoms (anxiety, depression) causing impairment following an identifiable psychosocial stressor (e.g., divorce, illness) and **lasting < 6 months** (> 6 months in presence of chronic stressor).
Obsessive-compulsive disorder	Recurring intrusive thoughts, feelings, or sensations (obsessions) that cause severe distress; relieved in part by the performance of repetitive actions (compulsions). Ego dystonic: behavior inconsistent with one's own beliefs and attitudes (vs. obsessive-compulsive personality disorder). Associated with Tourette disorder. Treatment: SSRIs, clomipramine.
	Body dysmorphic disorder—preoccupation with minor or imagined defect in appearance, leading to significant emotional distress or impaired functioning; patients often repeatedly seek cosmetic surgery.
Post-traumatic stress disorder	Persistent reexperiencing of a previous traumatic event (e.g., war, rape, robbery, serious accident, fire). May involve nightmares or flashbacks, intense fear, helplessness, or horror. Leads to avoidance of stimuli associated with the trauma and persistently ↑ arousal. **Disturbance lasts > 1 month,** with onset of symptoms beginning anytime after event, and causes significant distress, negative cognitive alterations, and/or impaired functioning. Treatment: psychotherapy, SSRIs.
	Acute stress disorder—lasts between 3 days and 1 month.

Malingering	Patient **consciously** fakes, profoundly exaggerates, or claims to have a disorder in order to attain a specific 2° (**external**) **gain** (e.g., avoiding work, obtaining compensation). Poor compliance with treatment or follow-up of diagnostic tests. Complaints cease after gain (vs. factitious disorder).

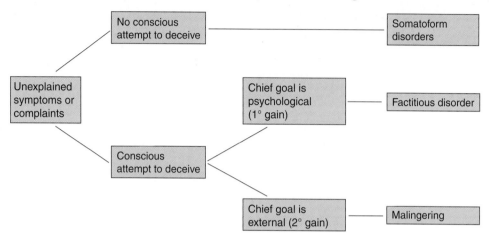

Factitious disorders	Patient **consciously** creates physical and/or psychological symptoms in order to assume "sick role" and to get medical attention (1° [**internal**] **gain**).
Munchausen syndrome	**Chronic** factitious disorder with predominantly physical signs and symptoms. Characterized by a history of multiple hospital admissions and willingness to receive invasive procedures.
Munchausen syndrome by proxy	When illness in a child or elderly patient is caused by the caregiver. Motivation is to assume a sick role by proxy. Form of child/elder abuse.

Somatic symptom and related disorders	Category of disorders characterized by physical symptoms with no identifiable physical cause. Both illness production and motivation are **unconscious** drives. Symptoms not intentionally produced or feigned. More common in women.
Somatic symptom disorder	Variety of complaints in one or more organ systems lasting for months to years. Associated with excessive, persistent thoughts and anxiety about symptoms. May co-occur with medical illness.
Conversion disorder	Sudden loss of sensory or motor function (e.g., paralysis, blindness, mutism), often following an acute stressor; patient is aware of but sometimes indifferent toward symptoms ("la belle indifférence"); more common in females, adolescents, and young adults.
Illness anxiety disorder (hypochondriasis)	Preoccupation with and fear of having a serious illness despite medical evaluation and reassurance.

Personality	
Personality trait	An enduring, repetitive pattern of perceiving, relating to, and thinking about the environment and oneself.
Personality disorder	Inflexible, maladaptive, and rigidly pervasive pattern of behavior causing subjective distress and/or impaired functioning; person is usually not aware of problem. Usually presents by early adulthood. Three clusters, A, B, and C; remember as **Weird**, **Wild**, and **Worried** based on symptoms.

Cluster A personality disorders	Odd or eccentric; inability to develop meaningful social relationships. No psychosis; genetic association with schizophrenia.	"**Weird**" (**A**ccusatory, **A**loof, **A**wkward).
Paranoid	Pervasive distrust and suspiciousness; projection is the major defense mechanism.	
Schizoid	Voluntary social withdrawal, limited emotional expression, content with social isolation (vs. avoidant).	Schizoi**d** = **d**istant.
Schizotypal	Eccentric appearance, odd beliefs or magical thinking, interpersonal awkwardness.	Schizo**typal** = magical **t**hinking.
Cluster B personality disorders	Dramatic, emotional, or erratic; genetic association with mood disorders and substance abuse.	"**Wild**" (**B**ad to the **B**one).
Antisocial	Disregard for and violation of rights of others, criminality, impulsivity; males > females; must be > 18 years old and have history of conduct disorder before age 15. Conduct disorder if < 18 years old.	Antisocial = **s**ociopath.
Borderline	Unstable mood and interpersonal relationships, impulsiveness, self-mutilation, boredom, sense of emptiness; females > males; splitting is a major defense mechanism.	
Histrionic	Excessive emotionality and excitability, attention seeking, sexually provocative, overly concerned with appearance.	
Narcissistic	Grandiosity, sense of entitlement; lacks empathy and requires excessive admiration; often demands the "best" and reacts to criticism with rage.	
Cluster C personality disorders	Anxious or fearful; genetic association with anxiety disorders.	"**Worried**" (**C**owardly, **C**ompulsive, **C**lingy).
Avoidant	Hypersensitive to rejection, socially inhibited, timid, feelings of inadequacy, desires relationships with others (vs. schizoid).	
Obsessive-compulsive	Preoccupation with order, perfectionism, and control; ego-syntonic: behavior consistent with one's own beliefs and attitudes (vs. OCD).	
Dependent	Submissive and clinging, excessive need to be taken care of, low self-confidence.	

Keeping "schizo-" straight	**Schizoid**	<	**Schizotypal**	<	**Schizophrenic**	<	**Schizoaffective**
			(schizoid + odd thinking)		(greater odd thinking than schizotypal)		(schizophrenic psychotic symptoms + bipolar or depressive mood disorder)

Schizophrenia time course:

    < 1 mo—brief psychotic disorder, usually stress related

    1–6 mo—schizophreniform disorder

    > 6 mo—schizophrenia

Eating disorders

Anorexia nervosa	Excessive dieting +/− purging; intense fear of gaining weight, body image distortion, and ↑ exercise, leading to a body weight well below ideal (≈ BMI < 17 kg/m^2). Associated with ↓ bone density. Severe weight loss, metatarsal stress fractures, amenorrhea, lanugo (fine body hair), anemia, and electrolyte disturbances. Osteoporosis caused in part by ↓ estrogen over time. Seen primarily in adolescent girls. Commonly coexists with depression.
Bulimia nervosa	Binge eating +/− purging; often followed by self-induced vomiting or use of laxatives, diuretics, or emetics. Body weight often maintained within normal range. Associated with parotitis, enamel erosion, electrolyte disturbances, alkalosis, dorsal hand calluses from induced vomiting (Russell sign). Seen predominantly in adolescent girls.

Gender dysphoria	Strong, persistent cross-gender identification. Characterized by persistent discomfort with one's sex assigned at birth, causing significant distress and/or impaired functioning. Affected individuals are often referred to as transgender.
	Transsexualism—desire to live as the opposite **sex**, often through surgery or hormone treatment.
	Transvestism—paraphilia, not gender dysphoria. Wearing clothes (e.g., **vest**) of the opposite sex (cross-dressing).

Sexual dysfunction	Includes sexual desire disorders (hypoactive sexual desire or sexual aversion), sexual arousal disorders (erectile dysfunction), orgasmic disorders (anorgasmia and premature ejaculation), and sexual pain disorders (dyspareunia and vaginismus). Differential diagnosis includes:

- Drugs (e.g., antihypertensives, neuroleptics, SSRIs, ethanol)
- Diseases (e.g., depression, diabetes, STDs)
- Psychological (e.g., performance anxiety)

Sleep terror disorder	Periods of terror with screaming in the middle of the night; occurs during slow-wave sleep. Most common in children. Occurs during non-REM sleep (no memory of arousal) as opposed to nightmares that occur during REM sleep (memory of a scary dream). Cause unknown, but triggers may include emotional stress, fever, or lack of sleep. Usually self limited.

Narcolepsy

Disordered regulation of sleep-wake cycles; 1° characteristic is excessive daytime sleepiness.

Caused by ↓ orexin production in lateral hypothalamus.

Also associated with:

- Hypnagogic (just before sleep) or hypnopompic (just before awakening) hallucinations.
- Nocturnal and narcoleptic sleep episodes that start off with REM sleep.
- Cataplexy (loss of all muscle tone following a strong emotional stimulus, such as laughter) in some patients.

Strong genetic component. Treatment: daytime stimulants (e.g., amphetamines, modafinil) and nighttime sodium oxybate (GHB).

Hypnagogic—going to sleep
Hypnopompic—post-sleep

Substance use disorder

Maladaptive pattern of substance use defined as 2 or more of the following signs in 1 year:

- Tolerance—need more to achieve same effect
- Withdrawal
- Substance taken in larger amounts, or over longer time, than desired
- Persistent desire or unsuccessful attempts to cut down
- Significant energy spent obtaining, using, or recovering from substance
- Important social, occupational, or recreational activities reduced because of substance use
- Continued use in spite of knowing the problems that it causes
- Craving
- Recurrent use in physically dangerous situations
- Failure to fulfill major obligations at work, school, or home due to use
- Social or interpersonal conflicts related to substance use

Stages of change in overcoming substance addiction

1. **Precontemplation**—not yet acknowledging that there is a problem
2. **Contemplation**—acknowledging that there is a problem, but not yet ready or willing to make a change
3. **Preparation/determination**—getting ready to change behavior
4. **Action/willpower**—changing behaviors
5. **Maintenance**—maintaining the behavior change
6. **Relapse**—returning to old behaviors and abandoning new changes

Psychoactive drug intoxication and withdrawal

DRUG	INTOXICATION	WITHDRAWAL
Depressants		
	Nonspecific: mood elevation, ↓ anxiety, sedation, behavioral disinhibition, respiratory depression.	Nonspecific: anxiety, tremor, seizures, insomnia.
Alcohol	Emotional lability, slurred speech, ataxia, coma, blackouts. Serum γ-glutamyltransferase (GGT)—sensitive indicator of alcohol use. Lab AST value is twice ALT value.	Mild alcohol withdrawal: symptoms similar to other depressants. Severe alcohol withdrawal can cause autonomic hyperactivity and DTs (5–15% mortality rate). Treatment for DTs: benzodiazepines.
Opioids (e.g., morphine, heroin, methadone)	Euphoria, respiratory and CNS depression, ↓ gag reflex, pupillary constriction (pinpoint pupils), seizures (overdose). Treatment: naloxone, naltrexone.	Sweating, dilated pupils, piloerection ("cold turkey"), fever, rhinorrhea, yawning, nausea, stomach cramps, diarrhea ("flu-like" symptoms). Treatment: long-term support, methadone, buprenorphine.
Barbiturates	Low safety margin, marked respiratory depression. Treatment: symptom management (assist respiration, ↑ BP).	Delirium, life-threatening cardiovascular collapse.
Benzodiazepines	Greater safety margin. Ataxia, minor respiratory depression. Treatment: supportive care; consider flumazenil (competitive benzodiazepine antagonist).	Sleep disturbance, depression, rebound anxiety, seizure (can be triggered by reversal with flumazenil).
Stimulants		
	Nonspecific: mood elevation, psychomotor agitation, insomnia, cardiac arrhythmias, tachycardia, anxiety.	Nonspecific: post-use "crash," including depression, lethargy, weight gain, headache.
Amphetamines	Euphoria, grandiosity, pupillary dilation, prolonged wakefulness and attention, hypertension, tachycardia, anorexia, paranoia, fever. Severe: cardiac arrest, seizure.	Anhedonia, ↑ appetite, hypersomnolence, existential crisis.
Cocaine	Impaired judgment, pupillary dilation, hallucinations (including tactile), paranoid ideations, angina, sudden cardiac death. Treatment: benzodiazepines.	Hypersomnolence, malaise, severe psychological craving, depression/suicidality.
Caffeine	Restlessness, ↑ diuresis, muscle twitching.	Lack of concentration, headache.
Nicotine	Restlessness.	Irritability, anxiety, craving. Treatment: nicotine patch, gum, or lozenges; bupropion/varenicline.

Psychoactive drug intoxication and withdrawal *(continued)*

DRUG	INTOXICATION	WITHDRAWAL
Hallucinogens		
PCP	Belligerence, impulsiveness, fever, psychomotor agitation, analgesia, vertical and horizontal nystagmus, tachycardia, homicidality, psychosis, delirium, seizures. Treatment: benzodiazepines, rapid-acting antipsychotic.	Depression, anxiety, irritability, restlessness, anergia, disturbances of thought and sleep.
LSD	Perceptual distortion (visual, auditory), depersonalization, anxiety, paranoia, psychosis, possible flashbacks.	
Marijuana (cannabinoid)	Euphoria, anxiety, paranoid delusions, perception of slowed time, impaired judgment, social withdrawal, ↑ appetite, dry mouth, conjunctival injection, hallucinations. Prescription form is dronabinol (tetrahydrocannabinol isomer): used as antiemetic (chemotherapy) and appetite stimulant (in AIDS).	Irritability, depression, insomnia, nausea, anorexia. Most symptoms peak in 48 hours and last for 5–7 days. Generally detectable in urine for 4–10 days.

Heroin addiction	Users at ↑ risk for hepatitis, abscesses, overdose, hemorrhoids, AIDS, and right-sided endocarditis. Look for track marks (needle sticks in veins). Treatments described below.	
Methadone	Long-acting oral opiate; used for heroin detoxification or long-term maintenance.	
Naloxone + buprenorphine	Partial agonist; long acting with fewer withdrawal symptoms than methadone. Naloxone is not active when taken orally, so withdrawal symptoms occur only if injected (lower abuse potential).	
Naltrexone	Long-acting opioid antagonist used for relapse prevention once detoxified.	

Alcoholism	Physiologic tolerance and dependence with symptoms of withdrawal (tremor, tachycardia, hypertension, malaise, nausea, DTs) when intake is interrupted. Complications: alcoholic cirrhosis, hepatitis, pancreatitis, peripheral neuropathy, testicular atrophy. Treatment: disulfiram (to condition the patient to abstain from alcohol use), naltrexone, supportive care. Alcoholics Anonymous and other peer support groups are helpful in sustaining abstinence.	
Wernicke-Korsakoff syndrome	Caused by thiamine deficiency. Triad of confusion, ophthalmoplegia, and ataxia (**Wernicke encephalopathy**). May progress to irreversible memory loss, confabulation, personality change (**Korsakoff psychosis**). Associated with periventricular hemorrhage/necrosis of mammillary bodies. Treatment: IV vitamin B_1 (thiamine).	
Mallory-Weiss syndrome	Longitudinal partial thickness tear at the gastroesophageal junction caused by excessive vomiting. Often presents with hematemesis. Associated with pain (vs. esophageal varices).	

Delirium tremens (DTs)	Life-threatening alcohol withdrawal syndrome that peaks 2–5 days after last drink. Symptoms in order of appearance: autonomic system hyperactivity (tachycardia, tremors, anxiety, seizures), psychotic symptoms (hallucinations, delusions), confusion. Treatment: benzodiazepines.	

▶ **PSYCHIATRY–PHARMACOLOGY**

Treatment for selected psychiatric conditions

PSYCHIATRIC CONDITION	PREFERRED DRUGS
ADHD	Methylphenidate
Alcohol withdrawal	Benzodiazepines
Anxiety	SSRIs, SNRIs, buspirone
Bipolar disorder	"Mood stabilizers" (e.g., lithium, valproic acid, carbamazepine), atypical antipsychotics
Bulimia	SSRIs
Depression	SSRIs, SNRIs, TCAs, bupropion, mirtazapine (especially with insomnia)
Obsessive-compulsive disorder	SSRIs, clomipramine
Panic disorder	SSRIs, venlafaxine, benzodiazepines
PTSD	SSRIs
Schizophrenia	Antipsychotics
Social phobias	SSRIs, β-blockers
Tourette syndrome	Antipsychotics (e.g., haloperidol, risperidone)

CNS stimulants	Methylphenidate, dextroamphetamine, methamphetamine, phentermine.
MECHANISM	↑ catecholamines at the synaptic cleft, especially norepinephrine and dopamine.
CLINICAL USE	ADHD, narcolepsy, appetite control.

Antipsychotics (neuroleptics)	Haloperidol, trifluoperazine, fluphenazine, thioridazine, chlorpromazine (haloperidol + "-azines").	
MECHANISM	All typical antipsychotics block dopamine D_2 receptors ($\uparrow$ [cAMP]).	High potency: Trifluoperazine, Fluphenazine, Haloperidol (Try to Fly High)—neurologic side effects (EPS symptoms).
CLINICAL USE	Schizophrenia (primarily positive symptoms), psychosis, acute mania, Tourette syndrome.	Low potency: Chlorpromazine, Thioridazine (Cheating Thieves are low)—non-neurologic side effects (anticholinergic, antihistamine, and α_1-blockade effects).
TOXICITY	Highly lipid soluble and stored in body fat; thus, very slow to be removed from body. Extrapyramidal system side effects (e.g., dyskinesias). Treatment: benztropine or diphenhydramine. Endocrine side effects (e.g., dopamine receptor antagonism $\rightarrow$ hyperprolactinemia $\rightarrow$ galactorrhea). Side effects arising from blocking muscarinic (dry mouth, constipation), α_1 (hypotension), and histamine (sedation) receptors.	Chlorpromazine—Corneal deposits; Thioridazine—reTinal deposits; haloperidol—NMS, tardive dyskinesia. Evolution of EPS side effects: • 4 hr acute dystonia (muscle spasm, stiffness, oculogyric crisis) • 4 day akathisia (restlessness) • 4 wk bradykinesia (parkinsonism) • 4 mo tardive dyskinesia
OTHER TOXICITIES	**Neuroleptic malignant syndrome (NMS)**—rigidity, myoglobinuria, autonomic instability, hyperpyrexia. Treatment: dantrolene, D_2 agonists (e.g., bromocriptine). **Tardive dyskinesia**—stereotypic oral-facial movements as a result of long-term antipsychotic use. Potentially irreversible.	For NMS, think **FEVER**: Fever Encephalopathy Vitals unstable Enzymes $\uparrow$ Rigidity of muscles

Atypical antipsychotics	Olanzapine, clozapine, quetiapine, risperidone, aripiprazole, ziprasidone.	It's atypical for old closets to quietly risper from A to Z.
MECHANISM	Not completely understood. Varied effects on $5\text{-}HT_2$, dopamine, and α- and H_1-receptors.	
CLINICAL USE	Schizophrenia—both positive and negative symptoms. Also used for bipolar disorder, OCD, anxiety disorder, depression, mania, Tourette syndrome.	
TOXICITY	Fewer extrapyramidal and anticholinergic side effects than traditional antipsychotics. Olanzapine/clozapine may cause significant weight gain. Clozapine may cause agranulocytosis (requires weekly WBC monitoring) and seizure. Risperidone may increase prolactin (causing lactation and gynecomastia) $\rightarrow$ $\downarrow$ GnRH, LH, and FSH (causing irregular menstruation and fertility issues). Ziprasidone may prolong the QT interval.	Must watch clozapine clozely!

Lithium

MECHANISM	Not established; possibly related to inhibition of phosphoinositol cascade.	**LMNOP:**
CLINICAL USE	Mood stabilizer for bipolar disorder; blocks relapse and acute manic events. Also SIADH.	Lithium side effects— **M**ovement (tremor) **N**ephrogenic diabetes insipidus
TOXICITY	Tremor, sedation, edema, heart block, hypothyroidism, polyuria (ADH antagonist causing nephrogenic diabetes insipidus), teratogenesis. Fetal cardiac defects include Ebstein anomaly and malformation of the great vessels. Narrow therapeutic window requires close monitoring of serum levels. Almost exclusively excreted by the kidneys; most is reabsorbed at the proximal convoluted tubules following Na^+ reabsorption.	Hyp**O**thyroidism **P**regnancy problems

Buspirone

MECHANISM	Stimulates 5-HT$_{1A}$ receptors.	I'm always anxious if the **bus** will be on time, so I take **bus**pirone.
CLINICAL USE	Generalized anxiety disorder. Does not cause sedation, addiction, or tolerance. Takes 1–2 weeks to take effect. Does not interact with alcohol (vs. barbiturates, benzodiazepines).	

Antidepressants

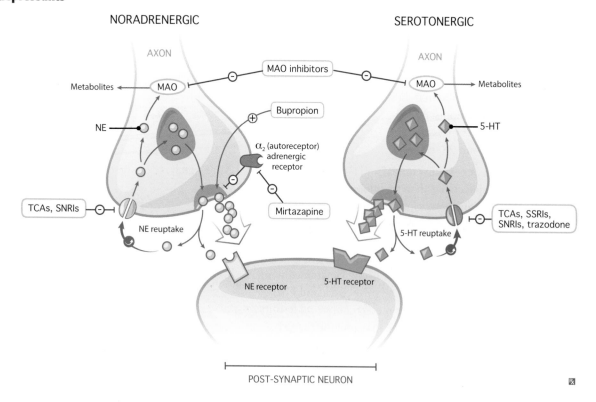

SSRIs	Fluoxetine, paroxetine, sertraline, citalopram.	Flashbacks paralyze senior citizens.
MECHANISM	5-HT–specific reuptake inhibitors.	It normally takes 4–8 weeks for antidepressants to have an effect.
CLINICAL USE	Depression, generalized anxiety disorder, panic disorder, OCD, bulimia, social phobias, PTSD.	
TOXICITY	Fewer than TCAs. GI distress, sexual dysfunction (anorgasmia and ↓ libido). **Serotonin syndrome** with any drug that ↑ 5-HT (e.g., MAO inhibitors, SNRIs, TCAs)—hyperthermia, confusion, myoclonus, cardiovascular collapse, flushing, diarrhea, seizures. Treatment: cyproheptadine (5-HT$_2$ receptor antagonist).	

SNRIs	Venlafaxine, duloxetine.
MECHANISM	Inhibit 5-HT and norepinephrine reuptake.
CLINICAL USE	Depression. Venlafaxine is also used in generalized anxiety and panic disorders; duloxetine is also indicated for diabetic peripheral neuropathy.
TOXICITY	↑ BP most common; also stimulant effects, sedation, nausea.

Tricyclic antidepressants	Amitriptyline, nortriptyline, imipramine, desipramine, clomipramine, doxepin, amoxapine (all TCAs end in -iptyline or -ipramine except doxepin and amoxapine).
MECHANISM	Block reuptake of norepinephrine and 5-HT.
CLINICAL USE	Major depression, OCD (clomipramine), fibromyalgia.
TOXICITY	Sedation, α_1-blocking effects including postural hypotension, and atropine-like (anticholinergic) side effects (tachycardia, urinary retention, dry mouth). 3° TCAs (amitriptyline) have more anticholinergic effects than 2° TCAs (nortriptyline) have. Desipramine is less sedating, but has a higher seizure incidence. Tri-C's: Convulsions, Coma, Cardiotoxicity (arrhythmias); also respiratory depression, hyperpyrexia. Confusion and hallucinations in elderly due to anticholinergic side effects (use nortriptyline). Treatment: NaHCO$_3$ for cardiovascular toxicity.

Monoamine oxidase (MAO) inhibitors	Tranylcypromine, Phenelzine, Isocarboxazid, Selegiline (selective MAO-B inhibitor). (MAO Takes Pride In Shanghai).
MECHANISM	Nonselective MAO inhibition ↑ levels of amine neurotransmitters (norepinephrine, 5-HT, dopamine).
CLINICAL USE	Atypical depression, anxiety, hypochondriasis.
TOXICITY	Hypertensive crisis (most notably with ingestion of tyramine, which is found in many foods such as wine and cheese); CNS stimulation. Contraindicated with SSRIs, TCAs, St. John's wort, meperidine, and dextromethorphan (to prevent serotonin syndrome).

Atypical antidepressants

Bupropion	Also used for smoking cessation. ↑ norepinephrine and dopamine via unknown mechanism. Toxicity: stimulant effects (tachycardia, insomnia), headache, seizure in bulimic patients. No sexual side effects.	
Mirtazapine	α_2-antagonist (↑ release of norepinephrine and 5-HT) and potent $5\text{-}HT_2$ and $5\text{-}HT_3$ receptor antagonist. Toxicity: sedation (which may be desirable in depressed patients with insomnia), ↑ appetite, weight gain (which may be desirable in elderly or anorexic patients), dry mouth.	
Trazodone	Primarily blocks $5\text{-}HT_2$ and α_1-adrenergic receptors. Used primarily for insomnia, as high doses are needed for antidepressant effects. Toxicity: sedation, nausea, priapism, postural hypotension.	Called trazobone due to male-specific side effects.

Renal

"But I know all about love already. I know precious little still about kidneys."

—Aldous Huxley, *Antic Hay*

"This too shall pass. Just like a kidney stone."

—Hunter Madsen

"I drink too much. The last time I gave a urine sample it had an olive in it."

—Rodney Dangerfield

▸ RENAL–EMBRYOLOGY

Kidney embryology

Pronephros—week 4; then degenerates.

Mesonephros—functions as interim kidney for 1st trimester; later contributes to male genital system.

Metanephros—permanent; first appears in 5th week of gestation; nephrogenesis continues through 32–36 weeks of gestation.

- ▪ Ureteric bud—derived from caudal end of mesonephric duct; gives rise to ureter, pelvises, calyces, and collecting ducts; fully canalized by 10th week
- ▪ Metanephric mesenchyme—ureteric bud interacts with this tissue; interaction induces differentiation and formation of glomerulus through to distal convoluted tubule
- ▪ Aberrant interaction between these 2 tissues may result in several congenital malformations of the kidney

Ureteropelvic junction—last to canalize → most common site of obstruction (hydronephrosis) in fetus.

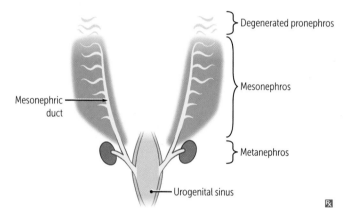

Degenerated pronephros

Mesonephros

Mesonephric duct

Metanephros

Urogenital sinus

Potter sequence (syndrome)

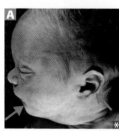

Oligohydramnios → compression of developing fetus → limb deformities, facial anomalies (low-set ears and retrognathia [arrows in **A**]), and compression of chest → pulmonary hypoplasia (cause of death).

Causes include ARPKD, posterior urethral valves, bilateral renal agenesis.

Babies who can't "Pee" in utero develop Potter syndrome.

POTTER syndrome associated with:
   Pulmonary hypoplasia
   Oligohydramnios (trigger)
   Twisted face
   Twisted skin
   Extremity defects
   Renal failure (in utero)

Horseshoe kidney

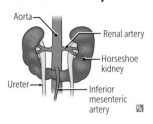

Aorta
Renal artery
Horseshoe kidney
Ureter
Inferior mesenteric artery

Inferior poles of both kidneys fuse 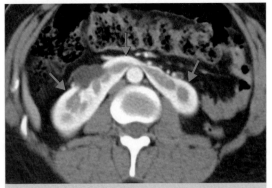. As they ascend from pelvis during fetal development, horseshoe kidneys get trapped under inferior mesenteric artery and remain low in the abdomen. Kidney functions normally. ↑ risk for ureteropelvic junction obstruction, hydronephrosis, renal stones, and rarely renal cancer (Wilms tumor). Associated with Turner syndrome.

A **Horseshoe kidney.** Axial CT of abdomen with contrast shows enhancing midline fused kidney (arrows).

Multicystic dysplastic kidney

Due to abnormal interaction between ureteric bud and metanephric mesenchyme. This leads to a nonfunctional kidney consisting of cysts and connective tissue. If unilateral (most common), generally asymptomatic with compensatory hypertrophy of contralateral kidney. Often diagnosed prenatally via ultrasound.

▶ RENAL–ANATOMY

Kidney anatomy and glomerular structure

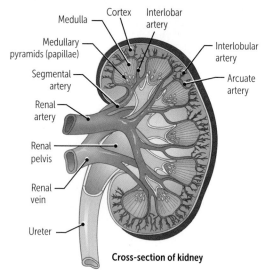

Medulla
Cortex
Interlobar artery
Medullary pyramids (papillae)
Interlobular artery
Segmental artery
Arcuate artery
Renal artery
Renal pelvis
Renal vein
Ureter

Cross-section of kidney

The left kidney is taken during living donor transplantation because it has a longer renal vein.

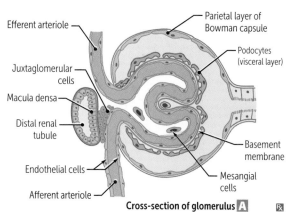

Efferent arteriole
Parietal layer of Bowman capsule
Juxtaglomerular cells
Podocytes (visceral layer)
Macula densa
Distal renal tubule
Endothelial cells
Basement membrane
Afferent arteriole
Mesangial cells

Cross-section of glomerulus A ℞

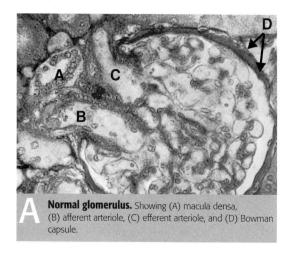

A **Normal glomerulus.** Showing (A) macula densa, (B) afferent arteriole, (C) efferent arteriole, and (D) Bowman capsule.

Ureters: course

Ureters pass **under** uterine artery and **under** ductus deferens (retroperitoneal).

"Water (ureters) **under** the bridge (uterine artery, vas deferens)."

Gynecologic procedures involving ligation of the uterine vessels may damage the ureter → ureteral obstruction or ureteral leak.

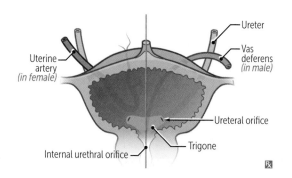

Ureter
Uterine artery (in female)
Vas deferens (in male)
Ureteral orifice
Internal urethral orifice
Trigone

℞

▸ RENAL–PHYSIOLOGY

Fluid compartments

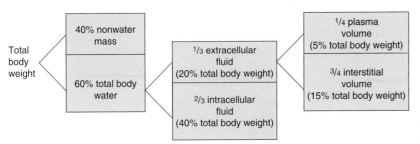

HIKIN': **HI**gh **K** **IN**tracellular.
60–40–20 rule (% of body weight):
- 60% total body water
- 40% ICF
- 20% ECF

Plasma volume measured by radiolabeled albumin.
Extracellular volume measured by inulin.
Osmolarity = 290 mOsm/L.

Glomerular filtration barrier

Responsible for filtration of plasma according to size and net charge.
Composed of:
- Fenestrated capillary endothelium (size barrier)
- Fused basement membrane with heparan sulfate (negative charge barrier)
- Epithelial layer consisting of podocyte foot processes

The charge barrier is lost in nephrotic syndrome, resulting in albuminuria, hypoproteinemia, generalized edema, and hyperlipidemia.

Renal clearance

$C_x = U_x V/P_x$ = volume of plasma from which the substance is completely cleared per unit time.
$C_x <$ GFR: net tubular reabsorption of X.
$C_x >$ GFR: net tubular secretion of X.
$C_x =$ GFR: no net secretion or reabsorption.

Be familiar with calculations.
C_x = clearance of X (mL/min).
U_x = urine concentration of X (mg/mL).
P_x = plasma concentration of X (mg/mL).
V = urine flow rate (mL/min).

Glomerular filtration rate

Inulin clearance can be used to calculate GFR because it is freely filtered and is neither reabsorbed nor secreted.
$$GFR = U_{inulin} \times V/P_{inulin} = C_{inulin}$$
$$= K_f [(P_{GC} - P_{BS}) - (\pi_{GC} - \pi_{BS})].$$
(GC = glomerular capillary; BS = Bowman space.) π_{BS} normally equals zero.

Normal GFR ≈ 100 mL/min.
Creatinine clearance is an approximate measure of GFR. Slightly overestimates GFR because creatinine is moderately secreted by the renal tubules.
Incremental reductions in GFR define the stages of chronic kidney disease.

Effective renal plasma flow

Effective renal plasma flow (ERPF) can be estimated using *para*-aminohippuric acid (PAH) clearance because it is both filtered and actively secreted in the proximal tubule. Nearly all PAH entering the kidney is excreted.
$$ERPF = U_{PAH} \times V/P_{PAH} = C_{PAH}.$$
$$RBF = RPF/(1 - Hct).$$
ERPF underestimates true renal plasma flow (RPF) by ~10%.

Filtration

Filtration fraction (FF) = GFR/RPF.
Normal FF = 20%.
Filtered load (mg/min) = GFR (mL/min)
  × plasma concentration (mg/mL).

GFR can be estimated with creatinine
  clearance.
RPF is best estimated with PAH clearance.

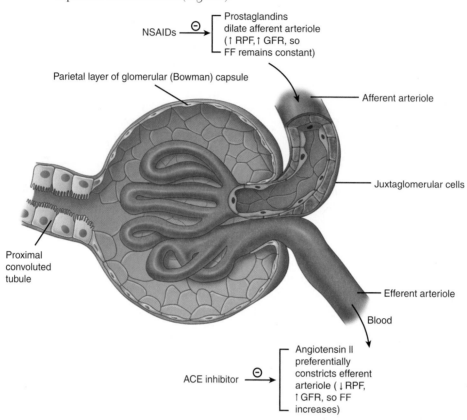

NSAIDs ⊖→ Prostaglandins
dilate afferent arteriole
(↑ RPF, ↑ GFR, so
FF remains constant)

Parietal layer of glomerular (Bowman) capsule

Afferent arteriole

Juxtaglomerular cells

Proximal
convoluted
tubule

Efferent arteriole

Blood

ACE inhibitor ⊖→ Angiotensin II
preferentially
constricts efferent
arteriole (↓ RPF,
↑ GFR, so FF
increases)

Changes in glomerular dynamics

Effect	RPF	GFR	FF (GFR/RPF)
Afferent arteriole constriction	↓	↓	—
Efferent arteriole constriction	↓	↑	↑
↑ plasma protein concentration	—	↓	↓
↓ plasma protein concentration	—	↑	↑
Constriction of ureter	—	↓	↓

Calculation of reabsorption and secretion rate

Filtered load = GFR × P_x.
Excretion rate = V × U_x.
Reabsorption = filtered − excreted.
Secretion = excreted − filtered.

Glucose clearance

Glucose at a normal plasma level is completely reabsorbed in proximal tubule by Na^+/glucose cotransport.

At plasma glucose of ~200 mg/dL, glucosuria begins (threshold). At ~375 mg/dL, all transporters are fully saturated (T_m).

Glucosuria is an important clinical clue to diabetes mellitus.

Normal pregnancy ↓ reabsorption of glucose and amino acids in the proximal tubule → glucosuria and aminoaciduria.

Amino acid clearance

Sodium-dependent transporters in proximal tubule reabsorb amino acids.

Hartnup disease—autosomal recessive disorder. Deficiency of neutral amino acid (e.g., tryptophan) transporters in proximal renal tubular cells and on enterocytes. Leads to neutral aminoaciduria and ↓ absorption from the gut; results in pellagra-like symptoms; treat with high-protein diet and nicotinic acid.

Nephron physiology

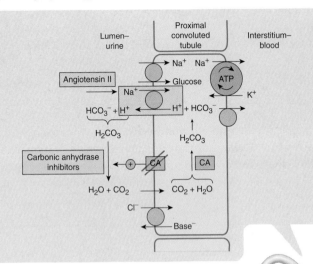

Early proximal convoluted tubule (PCT)—contains brush border. Reabsorbs all of the glucose and amino acids and most of the HCO_3^-, Na^+, Cl^-, PO_4^{3-}, K^+, and H_2O. Isotonic absorption. Generates and secretes NH_3, which acts as a buffer for secreted H^+.
PTH—inhibits Na^+/PO_4^{3-} cotransport $\rightarrow PO_4^{3-}$ excretion.
AT II—stimulates Na^+/H^+ exchange $\rightarrow \uparrow Na^+$, H_2O, and HCO_3^- reabsorption (permitting contraction alkalosis).
65–80% Na^+ reabsorbed.

Thin descending loop of Henle—passively reabsorbs H_2O via medullary hypertonicity (impermeable to Na^+). Concentrating segment. Makes urine hypertonic.

Loop of Henle

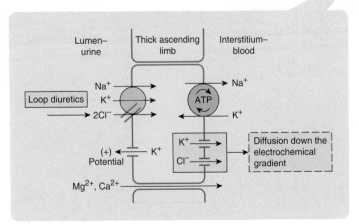

Thick ascending loop of Henle—actively reabsorbs Na^+, K^+, and Cl^-. Indirectly induces the paracellular reabsorption of Mg^{2+} and Ca^{2+} through (+) lumen potential generated by K^+ backleak. Impermeable to H_2O. Makes urine less concentrated as it ascends.
10–20% Na^+ reabsorbed.

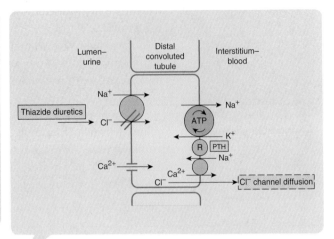

Early distal convoluted tubule (DCT)—actively reabsorbs Na^+, Cl^-. Makes urine hypotonic.
PTH—$\uparrow Ca^{2+}/Na^+$ exchange $\rightarrow Ca^{2+}$ reabsorption.
5–10% Na^+ reabsorbed.

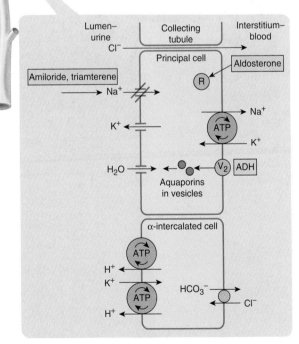

Collecting tubule—reabsorbs Na^+ in exchange for secreting K^+ and H^+ (regulated by aldosterone).
Aldosterone—acts on mineralocorticoid receptor $\rightarrow$ insertion of Na^+ channel on luminal side.
ADH—acts at V_2 receptor $\rightarrow$ insertion of aquaporin H_2O channels on luminal side.
3–5% Na^+ reabsorbed.

Renal tubular defects

Fanconi syndrome	Reabsorptive defect in PCT. Associated with ↑ excretion of nearly all amino acids, glucose, HCO_3^-, and PO_4^{3-}. May result in metabolic acidosis (proximal renal tubular acidosis). Causes include hereditary defects (e.g., Wilson disease), ischemia, and nephrotoxins/drugs.	The kidneys put out **FAB**ulous **G**littering **L**iquid: **FA**nconi syndrome is the 1st defect (PCT) **B**artter syndrome is next (thick ascending loop of Henle) **G**itelman syndrome is after Bartter (DCT) **L**iddle syndrome is last (collecting tubule)
Bartter syndrome	Reabsorptive defect in thick ascending loop of Henle. Autosomal recessive, affects Na^+/K^+/$2Cl^-$ cotransporter. Results in hypokalemia and metabolic alkalosis with hypercalciuria.	
Gitelman syndrome	Reabsorptive defect of NaCl in DCT. Autosomal recessive. Less severe than Bartter syndrome. Leads to hypokalemia and metabolic alkalosis, but without hypercalciuria.	
Liddle syndrome	↑ Na^+ reabsorption in distal and collecting tubules (↑ activity of epithelial Na^+ channel). Autosomal dominant. Results in hypertension, hypokalemia, metabolic alkalosis, ↓ aldosterone. Treatment: Amiloride.	

Relative concentrations along proximal tubules

TF/P > 1 when: Solute is reabsorbed less quickly than water

TF/P = 1 when: Solute and water are reabsorbed at same rate

TF/P < 1 when: Solute is reabsorbed more quickly than water

$$\frac{TF}{P} = \frac{[\text{Tubular fluid}]}{[\text{Plasma}]}$$

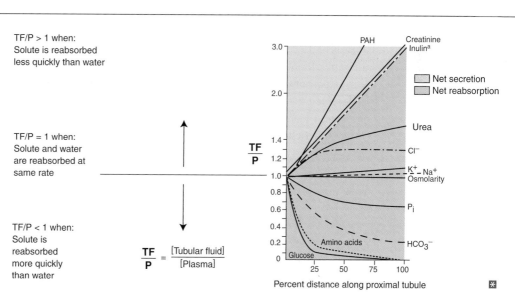

[a]Neither secreted nor reabsorbed; concentration increases as water is reabsorbed.

Tubular inulin ↑ in concentration (but not amount) along the proximal tubule as a result of water reabsorption.

Cl^- reabsorption occurs at a slower rate than Na^+ in early proximal tubule and then matches the rate of Na^+ reabsorption more distally. Thus, its relative concentration ↑ before it plateaus.

Renin-angiotensin-aldosterone system

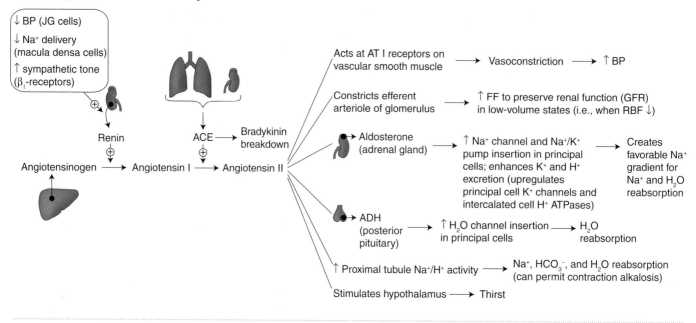

AT II	Affects baroreceptor function; limits reflex bradycardia, which would normally accompany its pressor effects. Helps maintain blood volume and blood pressure.
ANP	Released from atria in response to ↑ volume; may act as a "check" on renin-angiotensin-aldosterone system; relaxes vascular smooth muscle via cGMP, causing ↑ GFR, ↓ renin.
ADH	Primarily regulates osmolarity; also responds to low blood volume states.
Aldosterone	Primarily regulates ECF Na^+ content and volume; responds to low blood volume states.

| Juxtaglomerular apparatus | Consists of JG cells (modified smooth muscle of afferent arteriole) and the macula densa (NaCl sensor, part of the distal convoluted tubule). JG cells secrete renin in response to ↓ renal blood pressure, ↓ NaCl delivery to distal tubule, and ↑ sympathetic tone (β_1). | JGA defends GFR via renin-angiotensin-aldosterone system. β-blockers can decrease BP by inhibiting β_1-receptors of the JGA, causing ↓ renin release. *Juxta* = close by. |

Kidney endocrine functions

Erythropoietin	Released by interstitial cells in the peritubular capillary bed in response to hypoxia.
1,25-(OH)$_2$ vitamin D	Proximal tubule cells convert 25-OH vitamin D to 1,25-(OH)$_2$ vitamin D (active form).
Renin	Secreted by JG cells in response to ↓ renal arterial pressure and ↑ renal sympathetic discharge (β$_1$ effect).
Prostaglandins	Paracrine secretion vasodilates the afferent arterioles to ↑ RBF.

For 1,25-(OH)$_2$ vitamin D:

25-OH vitamin D ——— 1α-hydroxylase ———→ 1,25-(OH)$_2$ vitamin D

⊕

PTH

For Prostaglandins:

NSAIDs block renal-protective prostaglandin synthesis → constriction of the afferent arteriole and ↓ GFR; this may result in acute renal failure.

Hormones acting on kidney

Angiotensin II (AT II)
Synthesized in response to ↓ BP. Causes efferent arteriole constriction → ↑ GFR and ↑ FF but with compensatory Na$^+$ reabsorption in proximal and distal nephron. Net effect: preservation of renal function in low-volume state (↑ FF) with simultaneous Na$^+$ reabsorption (both proximal and distal) to maintain circulating volume.

Atrial natriuretic peptide (ANP)
Secreted in response to ↑ atrial pressure. Causes ↑ GFR and ↑ Na$^+$ filtration **with no compensatory Na$^+$ reabsorption** in distal nephron. Net effect: Na$^+$ loss and volume loss.

Parathyroid hormone (PTH)
Secreted in response to ↓ plasma [Ca^{2+}], ↑ plasma [PO$_4^{3-}$], or ↓ plasma 1,25-(OH)$_2$ vitamin D. Causes ↑ [Ca^{2+}] reabsorption (DCT), ↓ [PO$_4^{3-}$] reabsorption (PCT), and ↑ 1,25-(OH)$_2$ vitamin D production (↑ Ca^{2+} and PO$_4^{3-}$ absorption from gut via vitamin D).

Aldosterone
Secreted in response to ↓ blood volume (via AT II) and ↑ plasma [K$^+$]; causes ↑ Na$^+$ reabsorption, ↑ K$^+$ secretion, ↑ H$^+$ secretion.

ADH (vasopressin)
Secreted in response to ↑ plasma osmolarity and ↓ blood volume. Binds to receptors on principal cells, causing ↑ number of water channels and ↑ H$_2$O reabsorption.

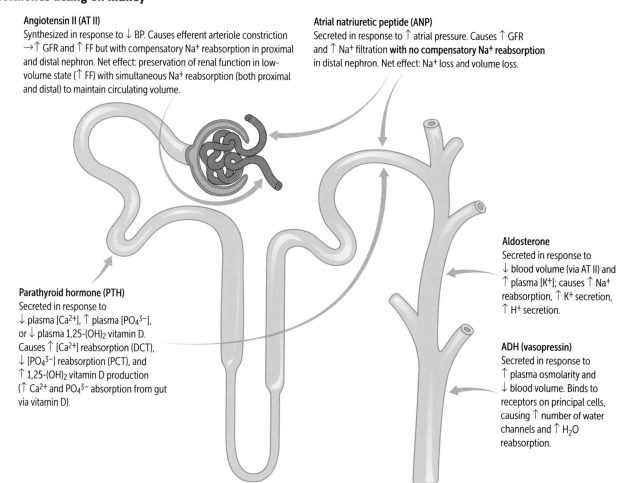

Potassium shifts

SHIFTS K⁺ OUT OF CELL (CAUSING HYPERKALEMIA)	SHIFTS K⁺ INTO CELL (CAUSING HYPOKALEMIA)
Digitalis	
HyperOsmolarity	Hypo-osmolarity
Insulin deficiency	Insulin ($\uparrow$ Na⁺/K⁺ ATPase)
Lysis of cells	
Acidosis	Alkalosis
β-adrenergic antagonist	β-adrenergic agonist ($\uparrow$ Na⁺/K⁺ ATPase)
Patient with hyperkalemia? DO Insulin LAβ work.	Insulin shifts K⁺ into cells

Electrolyte disturbances

ELECTROLYTE	LOW SERUM CONCENTRATION	HIGH SERUM CONCENTRATION
Na⁺	Nausea and malaise, stupor, coma	Irritability, stupor, coma
K⁺	U waves on ECG, flattened T waves, arrhythmias, muscle weakness	Wide QRS and peaked T waves on ECG, arrhythmias, muscle weakness
Ca²⁺	Tetany, seizures, QT prolongation	**Stones** (renal), **bones** (pain), **groans** (abdominal pain), **psychiatric overtones** (anxiety, altered mental status), but not necessarily calciuria
Mg²⁺	Tetany, torsades de pointes	$\downarrow$ DTRs, lethargy, bradycardia, hypotension, cardiac arrest, hypocalcemia
PO₄³⁻	Bone loss, osteomalacia	Renal stones, metastatic calcifications, hypocalcemia

Acid-base physiology

	pH	P$_{CO_2}$	[HCO₃⁻]	COMPENSATORY RESPONSE
Metabolic acidosis	$\downarrow$	$\downarrow$	$\downarrow$	Hyperventilation (immediate)
Metabolic alkalosis	$\uparrow$	$\uparrow$	$\uparrow$	Hypoventilation (immediate)
Respiratory acidosis	$\downarrow$	$\uparrow$	$\uparrow$	$\uparrow$ renal [HCO₃⁻] reabsorption (delayed)
Respiratory alkalosis	$\uparrow$	$\downarrow$	$\downarrow$	$\downarrow$ renal [HCO₃⁻] reabsorption (delayed)

Key: $\uparrow \downarrow$ = 1° disturbance; $\downarrow \uparrow$ = compensatory response.

Henderson-Hasselbalch equation: $pH = 6.1 + \log \dfrac{[HCO_3^-]}{0.03 \, P_{CO_2}}$

The predicted respiratory compensation for a simple metabolic acidosis can be calculated using the Winters formula. If the measured P$_{CO_2}$ differs significantly from the predicted P$_{CO_2}$, then a mixed acid-base disorder is likely present:

$$P_{CO_2} = 1.5 \, [HCO_3^-] + 8 \pm 2$$

Acidosis/alkalosis

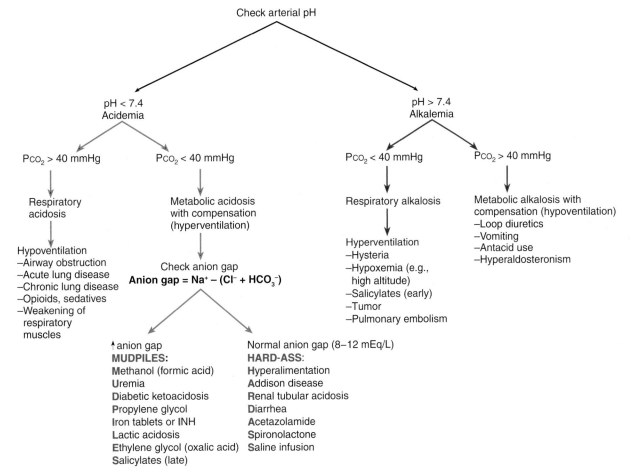

Check arterial pH

pH < 7.4
Acidemia

P_{CO_2} > 40 mmHg

Respiratory
acidosis

Hypoventilation
–Airway obstruction
–Acute lung disease
–Chronic lung disease
–Opioids, sedatives
–Weakening of
 respiratory
 muscles

P_{CO_2} < 40 mmHg

Metabolic acidosis
with compensation
(hyperventilation)

Check anion gap
Anion gap = Na$^+$ – (Cl$^-$ + HCO$_3^-$)

↑ anion gap
MUDPILES:
Methanol (formic acid)
Uremia
Diabetic ketoacidosis
Propylene glycol
Iron tablets or INH
Lactic acidosis
Ethylene glycol (oxalic acid)
Salicylates (late)

Normal anion gap (8–12 mEq/L)
HARD-ASS:
Hyperalimentation
Addison disease
Renal tubular acidosis
Diarrhea
Acetazolamide
Spironolactone
Saline infusion

pH > 7.4
Alkalemia

P_{CO_2} < 40 mmHg

Respiratory alkalosis

Hyperventilation
–Hysteria
–Hypoxemia (e.g.,
 high altitude)
–Salicylates (early)
–Tumor
–Pulmonary embolism

P_{CO_2} > 40 mmHg

Metabolic alkalosis with
compensation (hypoventilation)
–Loop diuretics
–Vomiting
–Antacid use
–Hyperaldosteronism

Renal tubular acidosis	A disorder of the renal tubules which leads to non-anion gap hyperchloremic metabolic acidosis.
RTA TYPE	NOTES
Type 1 **(distal, pH > 5.5)**	Defect in ability of α intercalated cells to secrete H⁺. Thus, new HCO_3^- is not generated → metabolic acidosis. Associated with **hypokalemia**, ↑ risk for calcium phosphate kidney stones (due to ↑ urine pH and ↑ bone turnover). Causes—amphotericin B toxicity, analgesic nephropathy, multiple myeloma (light chains), and congenital anomalies (obstruction) of the urinary tract.
Type 2 **(proximal, pH < 5.5)**	Defect in proximal tubule HCO_3^- reabsorption results in ↑ excretion of HCO_3^- in urine and subsequent metabolic acidosis. Urine is acidified by α intercalated cells in collecting tubule. Associated with **hypokalemia**, ↑ risk for hypophosphatemic rickets. Causes—Fanconi syndrome (e.g., Wilson disease), chemicals toxic to proximal tubule (e.g., lead, aminoglycosides), and carbonic anhydrase inhibitors.
Type 4 **(hyperkalemic, pH < 5.5)**	Hypoaldosteronism, aldosterone resistance, or K⁺-sparing diuretics. The resulting hyperkalemia impairs ammoniagenesis in the proximal tubule → ↓ buffering capacity and ↓ H⁺ excretion into urine.

▶ RENAL–PATHOLOGY

Casts in urine	Presence of casts indicates that hematuria/pyuria is of renal (vs. bladder) origin.	
RBC casts	Glomerulonephritis, ischemia, or malignant hypertension.	Bladder cancer, kidney stones → hematuria, no casts. Acute cystitis → pyuria, no casts.
WBC casts	Tubulointerstitial inflammation, acute pyelonephritis, transplant rejection.	
Fatty casts ("oval fat bodies")	Nephrotic syndrome.	
Granular ("muddy brown") casts	Acute tubular necrosis.	
Waxy casts	Advanced renal disease/chronic renal failure.	
Hyaline casts	Nonspecific, can be a normal finding, often seen in concentrated urine samples.	

Nomenclature of glomerular disorders

TYPE	CHARACTERISTICS	EXAMPLE
Focal	< 50% of glomeruli are involved	Focal segmental glomerulosclerosis
Diffuse	> 50% of glomeruli are involved	Diffuse proliferative glomerulonephritis
Proliferative	Hypercellular glomeruli	Mesangial proliferative
Membranous	Thickening of glomerular basement membrane	Membranous nephropathy
1° glomerular disease	Involves only glomeruli, thus a 1° disease of the kidney	Minimal change disease
2° glomerular disease	Involves glomeruli and other organs, thus a disease of another organ system, or a systemic disease that has impact on the kidney	SLE, diabetic nephropathy

Glomerular diseases

Nephritic syndrome*

Acute poststreptococcal glomerulonephritis

Rapidly progressive glomerulonephritis

Berger disease (IgA glomerulonephropathy)

Alport syndrome

Both

Diffuse proliferative glomerulonephritis

Membranoproliferative glomerulonephritis

Nephrotic syndrome

Focal segmental glomerulosclerosis

Membranous nephropathy

Minimal change disease

Amyloidosis

Diabetic glomerulonephropathy

*Note that classic nephritic disorders can exhibit nephrotic features.

Nephrotic syndrome

NephrOtic syndrome presents with massive prOteinuria (> 3.5 g/day, frothy urine), hyperlipidemia, fatty casts, edema. Associated with thromboembolism (hypercoagulable state due to AT III loss in urine) and ↑ risk of infection (loss of immunoglobulins).

Focal segmental glomerulosclerosis	LM—segmental sclerosis and hyalinosis **A**. IF ⊖. EM—effacement of foot process similar to minimal change disease. Most common cause of nephrotic syndrome in African Americans and Hispanics. Can be idiopathic or associated with HIV infection, sickle cell disease, heroin abuse, massive obesity, interferon treatment, and chronic kidney disease due to congenital absence or surgical removal. Inconsistent response to steroid therapy and may progress to chronic renal disease.

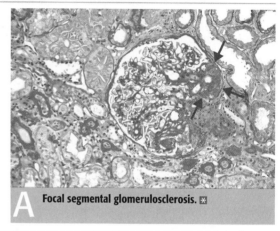
A Focal segmental glomerulosclerosis. ▣

Membranous nephropathy	LM—diffuse capillary and GBM thickening **B**. IF—granular as a result of immune complex deposition. Nephrotic presentation of SLE. EM—"spike and dome" appearance with subepithelial deposits. Most common cause of 1° nephrotic syndrome in Caucasian adults. Can be idiopathic or associated with antibody to phospholipase A_2 receptor, drugs (e.g., NSAIDs, penicillamine), infections (e.g., HBV, HCV), SLE, or solid tumors. Poor response to steroid therapy and may progress to chronic renal disease.

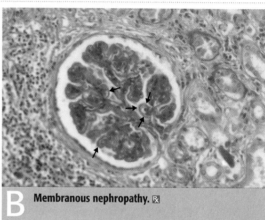
B Membranous nephropathy. ℞

Minimal change disease (lipoid nephrosis)	LM—normal glomeruli (lipid may be seen in PCT cells). IF ⊖. EM—effacement of foot processes **C**. Most common in children. May be triggered by recent infection, immunization, or immune stimulus. May be associated with Hodgkin lymphoma (e.g., cytokine-mediated damage). Excellent response to corticosteroids.

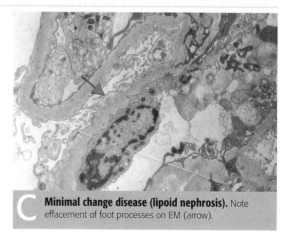
C Minimal change disease (lipoid nephrosis). Note effacement of foot processes on EM (arrow).

Amyloidosis	LM—Congo red stain shows apple-green birefringence under polarized light. Kidney is the most commonly involved organ (systemic amyloidosis). Associated with chronic conditions (e.g., multiple myeloma, TB, rheumatoid arthritis).

Nephrotic syndrome *(continued)*

Membrano-proliferative glomerulonephritis	Type I—subendothelial immune complex (IC) deposits with granular IF; "tram-track" appearance due to GBM splitting caused by mesangial ingrowth 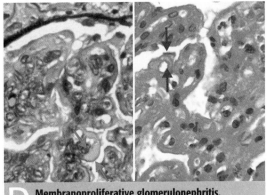. Type II—intramembranous IC deposits; "dense deposits." MPGN is a nephritic syndrome that can also present with nephrotic syndrome. Type I is associated with HBV, HCV. May also be idiopathic. Type II is associated with C3 nephritic factor (stabilizes C3 convertase → ↓ serum C3 levels).	**D** **Membranoproliferative glomerulonephritis.** H&E (right) and PAS (left) stain showing thickened "tram tracks." ℞
Diabetic glomerulo-nephropathy	LM—mesangial expansion, GBM thickening, eosinophilic nodular glomerulosclerosis (Kimmelstiel-Wilson lesion) 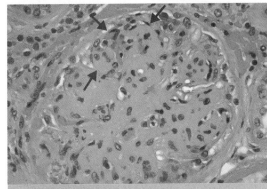. Nonenzymatic glycosylation of GBM → ↑ permeability, thickening. Nonenzymatic glycosylation of efferent arterioles → ↑ GFR → mesangial expansion.	**E** **Diabetic glomerulosclerosis.** Arrows point to one of several Kimmelstiel-Wilson lesions. Note the light pink diffuse mesangial expansion. ℞

LM = light microscopy; EM = electron microscopy; IF = immunofluorescence.

Nephritic syndrome	NephrItic syndrome = an Inflammatory process. When it involves glomeruli, it leads to hematuria and RBC casts in urine. Associated with azotemia, oliguria, hypertension (due to salt retention), and proteinuria (< 3.5 g/day).	
Acute poststreptococcal glomerulonephritis	LM—glomeruli enlarged and hypercellular. IF—("starry sky") granular appearance ("lumpy-bumpy") due to IgG, IgM, and C3 deposition along GBM and mesangium. EM—subepithelial immune complex (IC) humps.	Most frequently seen in children. Occurs ~2 weeks after group A streptococcal infection of the pharynx or skin. Resolves spontaneously. Type III hypersensitivity reaction. Presents with peripheral and periorbital edema, dark urine (cola-colored), and hypertension. ↑ anti-DNase B titers and ↓ complement levels.
Rapidly progressive (crescentic) glomerulonephritis (RPGN)	LM and IF—crescent-moon shape ▣. Crescents consist of fibrin and plasma proteins (e.g., C3b) with glomerular parietal cells, monocytes, and macrophages. Several disease processes may result in this pattern, including: ▪ **Goodpasture syndrome**—type II hypersensitivity; antibodies to GBM and alveolar basement membrane → linear IF ▪ Granulomatosis with polyangiitis (Wegener) ▪ Microscopic polyangiitis	Poor prognosis. Rapidly deteriorating renal function (days to weeks). Hematuria/hemoptysis. PR3-ANCA/c-ANCA. MPO-ANCA/p-ANCA.
Diffuse proliferative glomerulonephritis (DPGN)	Due to SLE or MPGN. LM—"wire looping" of capillaries. EM—subendothelial and sometimes intramembranous IgG-based ICs often with C3 deposition. IF—granular.	Most common cause of death in SLE. DPGN and MPGN can present as nephrotic syndrome and nephritic syndrome concurrently.
IgA nephropathy (Berger disease)	LM—mesangial proliferation. EM—mesangial IC deposits. IF—IgA-based IC deposits in mesangium. Seen with Henoch-Schönlein purpura.	Often presents/flares with a URI or acute gastroenteritis. Episodic hematuria with RBC casts.
Alport syndrome	Mutation in type IV collagen → thinning and splitting of the glomerular basement membrane. Most commonly X-linked.	Glomerulonephritis, deafness, and, less commonly, eye problems.

Kidney stones   Can lead to severe complications, such as hydronephrosis and pyelonephritis. Presents with unilateral flank tenderness, colicky pain radiating to groin, and hematuria. Treat and prevent by encouraging fluid intake.

CONTENT	PRECIPITATES AT	X-RAY FINDINGS	URINE CRYSTAL	NOTES
Calcium (80%)	↑ pH (calcium phosphate) ↓ pH (calcium oxalate)	Radiopaque	Envelope **A** or dumbbell shaped	Calcium oxalate, calcium phosphate, or both. Promoted by hypercalciuria (idiopathic or 2° to conditions that cause hypercalcemia, such as cancer and ↑ PTH). Oxalate crystals can result from ethylene glycol (antifreeze), vitamin C abuse, or Crohn disease. Treatments for recurrent stones include thiazides and citrate. Most common kidney stone presentation: calcium oxalate stone in a patient with hypercalciuria and normocalcemia.
Ammonium magnesium phosphate (15%)	↑ pH	Radiopaque	Coffin lid **B**	Also known as struvite. Caused by infection with urease ⊕ bugs (*Proteus mirabilis, Staphylococcus, Klebsiella*) that hydrolyze urea to ammonia → urine alkalinization. Can form staghorn calculi **C** that can be a nidus for UTIs. Treatment: eradication of underlying infection and surgical removal of stone.
Uric acid (5%)	↓ pH	RadiolUcent	Rhomboid or rosettes **D**	Risk factors: ↓ urine volume, arid climates, and acidic pH. Visible on CT and ultrasound, but not x-ray. Strong association with hyperuricemia (e.g., gout). Often seen in diseases with ↑ cell turnover, such as leukemia. Treatment: alkalinization of urine.
Cystine (1%)	↓ pH	Radiopaque	Hexagonal **E**	Mostly seen in children, 2° to cystinuria. Can form staghorn calculi. Sodium nitroprusside test ⊕. Treatment: alkalinization of urine and hydration.

Hydronephrosis

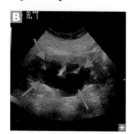

Distention/dilation of the renal pelvis and calyces A B. Usually caused by urinary tract obstruction (e.g., renal stones, BPH, cervical cancer, injury to ureter); other causes include retroperitoneal fibrosis and vesicoureteral reflux. Dilation occurs proximal to site of pathology. Only impairs renal function if bilateral or patient only has one kidney. Leads to compression atrophy of renal cortex and medulla.

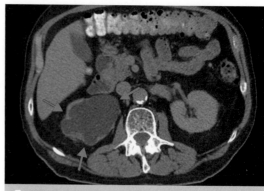

A **Hydronephrosis.** Markedly dilated right renal collecting system with cortical atrophy (chronic hydronephrosis, arrows). ✱

Renal cell carcinoma

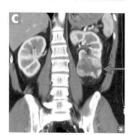

Originates from proximal tubule cells → polygonal clear cells A filled with accumulated lipids and carbohydrates. Most common in men 50–70 years old. ↑ incidence with smoking and obesity. Manifests clinically with hematuria, palpable mass B C, 2° polycythemia, flank pain, fever, and weight loss. Invades renal vein then IVC and spreads hematogenously; metastasizes to lung and bone.

Most common 1° renal malignancy.
Associated with gene deletion on chromosome 3 (sporadic or inherited as von Hippel-Lindau syndrome). RCC = 3 letters = chromosome 3.
Associated with paraneoplastic syndromes (ectopic EPO, ACTH, PTHrP).
"Silent" cancer because commonly presents as a metastatic neoplasm.
Treatment: resection if localized disease. Immunotherapy or targeted therapy for advanced/metastatic disease. Resistant to chemotherapy and radiation therapy.

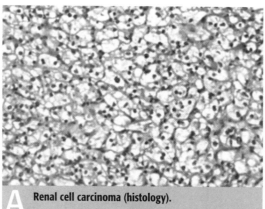

A **Renal cell carcinoma (histology).**

B **Renal cell carcinoma (gross).** Large, aggressive tumor with peripheral rim of displaced renal parenchyma (arrows). ✱

Renal oncocytoma

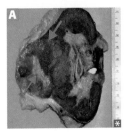

Benign epithelial cell tumor (arrows in 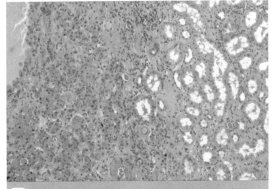 point to a well-circumscribed mass with a central scar). Large eosinophilic cells with abundant mitochondria without perinuclear clearing B (vs. chromophobe renal cell carcinoma). Presents with painless hematuria, flank pain, and abdominal mass.
Treatment: nephrectomy.

Renal oncocytoma. H&E stain shows round to polygonal cells with granular eosinophilic cytoplasm and round nuclei.

Wilms tumor (nephroblastoma)

Most common renal malignancy of early childhood (ages 2–4). Contains embryonic glomerular structures. Presents with huge, palpable flank mass and/or hematuria.

"Loss of function" mutations of tumor suppressor genes *WT1* or *WT2* on chromosome 11. May be part of Beckwith-Wiedemann syndrome or **WAGR** complex: **W**ilms tumor, **A**niridia, **G**enitourinary malformation, and mental **R**etardation (intellectual disability).

Transitional cell carcinoma

Most common tumor of urinary tract system (can occur in renal calyces, renal pelvis, ureters, and bladder) A. Painless hematuria (no casts) suggests bladder cancer.
Associated with problems in your Pee SAC: **P**henacetin, **S**moking, **A**niline dyes, and **C**yclophosphamide.

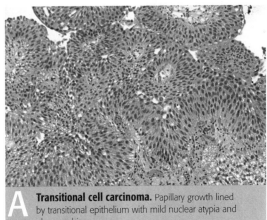

Transitional cell carcinoma. Papillary growth lined by transitional epithelium with mild nuclear atypia and pleomorphism.

Squamous cell carcinoma of the bladder

Chronic irritation of urinary bladder → squamous metaplasia → dysplasia and squamous cell carcinoma.
Risk factors include *Schistosoma haematobium* infection (Middle East), chronic cystitis, smoking, and chronic nephrolithiasis. Presents with painless hematuria.

Acute infectious cystitis

Inflammation of urinary bladder. Presents as suprapubic pain, dysuria, urinary frequency, and urgency. Systemic signs (e.g., fever, chills) are usually absent.

Risk factors include female gender (short urethra), sexual intercourse ("honeymoon cystitis"), and indwelling catheters.

Causes:

- *E. coli* (most common).
- *Staphylococcus saprophyticus*—seen in sexually active young women (*E. coli* is still more common in this group).
- *Klebsiella*.
- *Proteus mirabilis*—urine has ammonia scent.
- Adenovirus—hemorrhagic cystitis.

Lab findings—positive for leukocyte esterase ⊕. Nitrites appear for gram-negative organisms (especially *E. coli*). Sterile pyuria and ⊖ urine cultures suggest urethritis by *Neisseria gonorrhoeae* or *Chlamydia trachomatis*.

Pyelonephritis

Acute

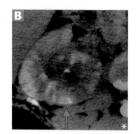

Affects cortex with relative sparing of glomeruli/vessels **A**. Presents with dysuria, fever, costovertebral angle tenderness, nausea, and vomiting.

Causes include ascending UTI (*E. coli* is most common), vesicoureteral reflux, and hematogenous spread to kidney. Often presents with white cell casts in urine. CT shows striated parenchymal enhancement (arrow in **B**).

Risk factors include indwelling urinary catheter, urinary tract obstruction, diabetes mellitus, and pregnancy.

Complications include chronic pyelonephritis, renal papillary necrosis, and perinephric abscess.

Treatment: antibiotics.

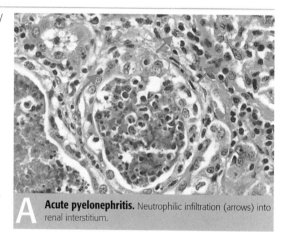

A **Acute pyelonephritis.** Neutrophilic infiltration (arrows) into renal interstitium.

Chronic

The result of recurrent episodes of acute pyelonephritis. Typically requires predisposition to infection such as vesicoureteral reflux or chronically obstructing kidney stones.

Coarse, asymmetric corticomedullary scarring, blunted calyx. Tubules can contain eosinophilic casts resembling thyroid tissue **C** (thyroidization of kidney).

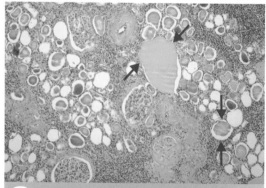

C **Chronic pyelonephritis.** Lymphocytic infiltrate (tiny purple debris); arrows indicate eosinophilic casts within the tubules (thyroidization). ℞

Drug-induced interstitial nephritis (tubulointerstitial nephritis)	Acute interstitial renal inflammation. Pyuria (classically eosinophils) and azotemia occurring after administration of drugs that act as haptens, inducing hypersensitivity. Nephritis typically occurs 1–2 weeks after certain drugs (e.g., diuretics, penicillin derivatives, sulfonamides, rifampin), but can occur months after starting NSAIDs.	Associated with fever, rash, hematuria, and costovertebral angle tenderness, but can be asymptomatic.
Diffuse cortical necrosis	Acute generalized cortical infarction of both kidneys. Likely due to a combination of vasospasm and DIC.	Associated with obstetric catastrophes (e.g., abruptio placentae) and septic shock.

Acute tubular necrosis

Most common cause of intrinsic renal failure. Self-reversible in some cases, but can be fatal if left untreated. Death most often occurs during initial oliguric phase.

Key finding: granular ("muddy brown") casts 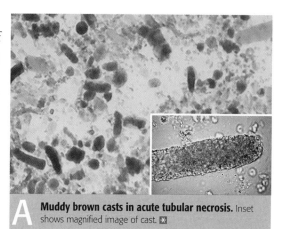. 3 stages:

1. Inciting event
2. Maintenance phase—oliguric; lasts 1–3 weeks; risk of hyperkalemia, metabolic acidosis
3. Recovery phase—polyuric; BUN and serum creatinine fall; risk of hypokalemia

Can be caused by ischemic or nephrotoxic injury:

- Ischemic—2° to ↓ renal blood flow (e.g., hypotension, shock, sepsis, hemorrhage, CHF). Results in death of tubular cells that may slough into tubular lumen 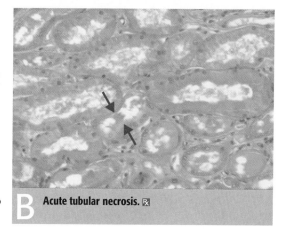 (proximal tubule and thick ascending limb are highly susceptible to injury).
- Nephrotoxic—2° to injury resulting from toxic substances (e.g., aminoglycosides, radiocontrast agents, lead, cisplatin), crush injury (myoglobinuria), hemoglobinuria. Proximal tubule is particularly susceptible to injury.

A **Muddy brown casts in acute tubular necrosis.** Inset shows magnified image of cast.

B **Acute tubular necrosis.**

Renal papillary necrosis

Sloughing of renal papillae → gross hematuria and proteinuria. May be triggered by a recent infection or immune stimulus. Associated with:

- Diabetes mellitus
- Acute pyelonephritis
- Chronic phenacetin use (acetaminophen is phenacetin derivative)
- Sickle cell anemia and trait

Acute kidney injury (acute renal failure)	In normal nephron, BUN is reabsorbed (for countercurrent multiplication), but creatinine is not. Acute kidney injury is defined as an abrupt decline in renal function with ↑ creatinine and ↑ BUN over a period of several days.
Prerenal azotemia	As a result of ↓ RBF (e.g., hypotension) → ↓ GFR. Na^+/H_2O and urea retained by kidney in an attempt to conserve volume, so BUN/creatinine ratio ↑.
Intrinsic renal failure	Generally due to acute tubular necrosis or ischemia/toxins; less commonly due to acute glomerulonephritis (e.g., RPGN). Patchy necrosis leads to debris obstructing tubule and fluid backflow across necrotic tubule → ↓ GFR. Urine has epithelial/granular casts. BUN reabsorption is impaired → ↓ BUN/creatinine ratio.
Postrenal azotemia	Due to outflow obstruction (stones, BPH, neoplasia, congenital anomalies). Develops only with bilateral obstruction.

Variable	Prerenal	Intrinsic Renal	Postrenal
Urine osmolality (mOsm/kg)	> 500	< 350	< 350
Urine Na^+ (mEq/L)	< 20	> 40	> 40
FENa	< 1%	> 2%	> 1% (mild) > 2% (severe)
Serum BUN/Cr	> 20	< 15	> 15

Consequences of renal failure	Inability to make urine and excrete nitrogenous wastes.
	
	Consequences (**MAD HUNGER**):
	■ Metabolic Acidosis
	■ Dyslipidemia (especially ↑ triglycerides)
	■ Hyperkalemia
	■ Uremia—clinical syndrome marked by ↑ BUN and ↑ creatinine
	  ■ Nausea and anorexia
	  ■ Pericarditis
	  ■ Asterixis
	  ■ Encephalopathy
	  ■ Platelet dysfunction
	■ Na^+/H_2O retention (CHF, pulmonary edema, hypertension)
	■ Growth retardation and developmental delay (in children)
	■ Erythropoietin failure (anemia)
	■ Renal osteodystrophy
		2 forms of renal failure—acute (e.g., ATN) and chronic (e.g., hypertension, diabetes, congenital anomalies).

Renal osteodystrophy	Failure of vitamin D hydroxylation, hypocalcemia, and hyperphosphatemia → 2° hyperparathyroidism. Hyperphosphatemia also independently ↓ serum Ca^{2+} by causing tissue calcifications, whereas ↓ $1,25\text{-}(OH)_2$ vitamin D → ↓ intestinal Ca^{2+} absorption. Causes subperiosteal thinning of bones.

Renal cyst disorders

ADPKD	Formerly adult polycystic kidney disease. Innumerable cysts 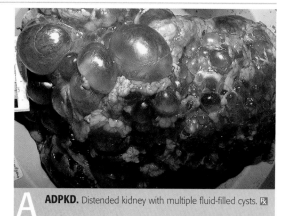 causing bilateral enlarged kidneys (arrows in **B**), ultimately destroy the kidney parenchyma. Presents with flank pain, hematuria, hypertension, urinary infection, progressive renal failure. Autosomal **D**ominant; mutation in *PKD1* (85% of cases, chromosome 16) or *PKD2* (15% of cases, chromosome 4). Death from complications of chronic kidney disease or hypertension (caused by ↑ renin production). Associated with berry aneurysms, mitral valve prolapse, benign hepatic cysts.	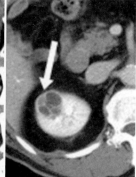 **ADPKD.** Distended kidney with multiple fluid-filled cysts. ℞

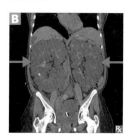

ARPKD	Formerly infantile polycystic kidney disease. Infantile presentation in parenchyma. Autosomal **R**ecessive. Associated with congenital hepatic fibrosis. Significant renal failure in utero can lead to Potter sequence. Concerns beyond neonatal period include hypertension, portal hypertension, and progressive renal insufficiency.

Medullary cystic disease	Inherited disease causing tubulointerstitial fibrosis **C** and progressive renal insufficiency with inability to concentrate urine. Medullary cysts usually not visualized; shrunken kidneys on ultrasound. Poor prognosis.

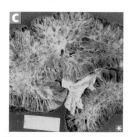

Simple vs. complex renal cyst	Simple cysts usually found in outer cortex filled with ultrafiltrate **D**. Very common, and account for majority of all renal masses. Found incidentally and typically asymptomatic. Complex cysts, including those that are septated, enhanced, or have solid components as seen on CT, require follow-up or removal due to risk of renal cell carcinoma.	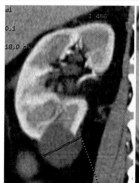 **Simple vs complex renal cyst.** Coronal CT on the left shows 2-cm, low-density, non-enhancing, homogeneous simple cyst on the lower pole. ⊞ Axial CT on the right shows multi-septated complex cyst with nodule (white arrow) that requires follow-up. ⊞

▶ RENAL–PHARMACOLOGY

Diuretics: site of action

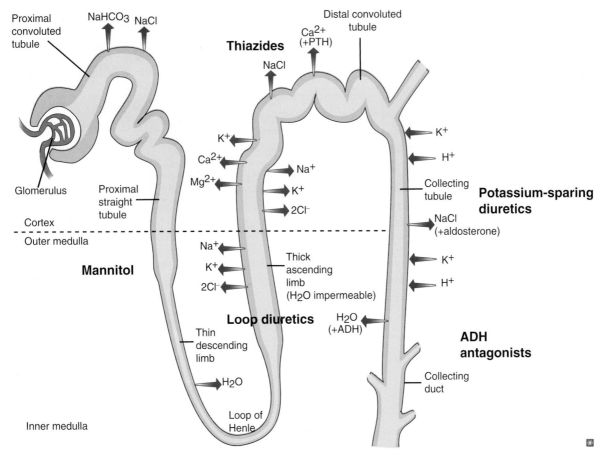

Mannitol

MECHANISM	Osmotic diuretic, ↑ tubular fluid osmolarity, producing ↑ urine flow, ↓ intracranial/intraocular pressure.
CLINICAL USE	Drug overdose, ↑ intracranial/intraocular pressure.
TOXICITY	Pulmonary edema, dehydration. Contraindicated in anuria, CHF.

Acetazolamide

MECHANISM	Carbonic anhydrase inhibitor. Causes self-limited $NaHCO_3$ diuresis and ↓ total-body HCO_3^- stores.
CLINICAL USE	Glaucoma, urinary alkalinization, metabolic alkalosis, altitude sickness, pseudotumor cerebri.
TOXICITY	Hyperchloremic metabolic acidosis, paresthesias, NH_3 toxicity, sulfa allergy.

"ACID"azolamide causes ACIDosis.

Loop diuretics

Furosemide

MECHANISM	Sulfonamide loop diuretic. Inhibits cotransport system ($Na^+/K^+/2\ Cl^-$) of thick ascending limb of loop of Henle. Abolishes hypertonicity of medulla, preventing concentration of urine. Stimulates PGE release (vasodilatory effect on afferent arteriole); inhibited by NSAIDs. ↑ Ca^{2+} excretion. Loops Lose calcium.
CLINICAL USE	Edematous states (CHF, cirrhosis, nephrotic syndrome, pulmonary edema), hypertension, hypercalcemia.
TOXICITY	Ototoxicity, Hypokalemia, Dehydration, Allergy (sulfa), Nephritis (interstitial), Gout.

OH DANG!

Ethacrynic acid

MECHANISM	Phenoxyacetic acid derivative (not a sulfonamide). Essentially same action as furosemide.
CLINICAL USE	Diuresis in patients allergic to sulfa drugs.
TOXICITY	Similar to furosemide; can cause hyperuricemia; never use to treat gout.

Hydrochlorothiazide

MECHANISM	Thiazide diuretic. Inhibits NaCl reabsorption in early distal tubule, ↓ diluting capacity of the nephron. ↓ Ca^{2+} excretion.
CLINICAL USE	Hypertension, CHF, idiopathic hypercalciuria, nephrogenic diabetes insipidus, osteoporosis.
TOXICITY	Hypokalemic metabolic alkalosis, hyponatremia, hyperGlycemia, hyperLipidemia, hyperUricemia, and hyperCalcemia. Sulfa allergy.

HyperGLUC.

K⁺-sparing diuretics

	Spironolactone and eplerenone; Triamterene, and Amiloride.
MECHANISM	Spironolactone and eplerenone are competitive aldosterone receptor antagonists in the cortical collecting tubule. Triamterene and amiloride act at the same part of the tubule by blocking Na^+ channels in the CCT.
CLINICAL USE	Hyperaldosteronism, K⁺ depletion, CHF.
TOXICITY	Hyperkalemia (can lead to arrhythmias), endocrine effects with spironolactone (e.g., gynecomastia, antiandrogen effects).

The K⁺ STAys.

Diuretics: electrolyte changes

Urine NaCl	↑ (all diuretics except acetazolamide). Serum NaCl may ↓ as a result.
Urine K⁺	↑ with loop and thiazide diuretics. Serum K⁺ may ↓ as a result.
Blood pH	↓ (**acidemia**): carbonic anhydrase inhibitors— ↓ HCO_3^- reabsorption. K⁺ sparing—aldosterone blockade prevents K⁺ secretion and H⁺ secretion. Additionally, hyperkalemia leads to K⁺ entering all cells (via H⁺/K⁺ exchanger) in exchange for H⁺ exiting cells.
	↑ (**alkalemia**): loop diuretics and thiazides cause alkalemia through several mechanisms:
	▪ Volume contraction → ↑ AT II → ↑ Na^+/H⁺ exchange in proximal tubule → ↑ HCO_3^- reabsorption ("contraction alkalosis")
	▪ K⁺ loss leads to K⁺ exiting all cells (via H⁺/K⁺ exchanger) in exchange for H⁺ entering cells
	▪ In low K⁺ state, H⁺ (rather than K⁺) is exchanged for Na^+ in cortical collecting tubule, → alkalosis and "paradoxical aciduria"
Urine Ca²⁺	↑ with loop diuretics: ↓ paracellular Ca^{2+} reabsorption → hypocalcemia.
	↓ with **thiazides**: Enhanced paracellular Ca^{2+} reabsorption in distal tubule.

ACE inhibitors	Captopril, enalapril, lisinopril.	
MECHANISM	Inhibit ACE → ↓ angiotensin II → ↓ GFR by preventing constriction of efferent arterioles. Levels of renin ↑ as a result of loss of feedback inhibition. Inhibition of ACE also prevents inactivation of bradykinin, a potent vasodilator.	Angiotensin II receptor blockers (-sartans) have effects similar to ACE inhibitors but do not ↑ bradykinin → ↓ risk of cough or angioedema.
CLINICAL USE	Hypertension, CHF, proteinuria, diabetic nephropathy. Prevent unfavorable heart remodeling as a result of chronic hypertension.	
TOXICITY	Cough, Angioedema (contraindicated in C1 esterase inhibitor deficiency), Teratogen (fetal renal malformations), ↑ Creatinine (↓ GFR), Hyperkalemia, and Hypotension. Avoid in bilateral renal artery stenosis, because ACE inhibitors will further ↓ GFR → renal failure.	Captopril's CATCHH.

Reproductive

"Artificial insemination is when the farmer does it to the cow instead of the bull."

—Student essay

"Whoever called it necking was a poor judge of anatomy."

—Groucho Marx

"See, the problem is that God gives men a brain and a penis, and only enough blood to run one at a time."

—Robin Williams

▶ REPRODUCTIVE–EMBRYOLOGY

Important genes of embryogenesis

Sonic hedgehog gene	Produced at base of limbs in zone of polarizing activity. Involved in patterning along anterior-posterior axis. Involved in CNS development; mutation can cause holoprosencephaly.
Wnt-7 gene	Produced at apical ectodermal ridge (thickened ectoderm at distal end of each developing limb). Necessary for proper organization along dorsal-ventral axis.
FGF gene	Produced at apical ectodermal ridge. Stimulates mitosis of underlying mesoderm, providing for lengthening of limbs.
Homeobox (Hox) genes	Involved in segmental organization of embryo in a craniocaudal direction. Hox mutations → appendages in wrong locations.

Early fetal development

DAY 0	Fertilization by sperm, forming zygote, initiating embryogenesis.	
WITHIN WEEK 1	hCG secretion begins around the time of implantation of blastocyst.	
WITHIN WEEK 2	Bilaminar disc (epiblast, hypoblast). 2 weeks = 2 layers.	
WITHIN WEEK 3	Trilaminar disc. 3 weeks = 3 layers. Gastrulation. Primitive streak, notochord, mesoderm and its organization, and neural plate begin to form.	
WEEKS 3–8 (EMBRYONIC PERIOD)	Neural tube formed by neuroectoderm and closes by week 4. Organogenesis. Extremely susceptible to teratogens.	
WEEK 4	Heart begins to beat. Upper and lower limb buds begin to form. 4 weeks = 4 limbs.	
WEEK 6	Fetal cardiac activity visible by transvaginal ultrasound.	
WEEK 10	Genitalia have male/female characteristics.	

Gastrulation	Process that forms the trilaminar embryonic disc. Establishes the ectoderm, mesoderm, and endoderm germ layers. Starts with the epiblast invaginating to form the primitive streak.

Embryologic derivatives

Ectoderm

Surface ectoderm	Adenohypophysis (from Rathke pouch); lens of eye; epithelial linings of oral cavity, sensory organs of ear, and olfactory epithelium; epidermis; anal canal below the pectinate line; parotid, sweat, and mammary glands.	**Craniopharyngioma**—benign Rathke pouch tumor with cholesterol crystals, calcifications.
Neuroectoderm	Brain (neurohypophysis, CNS neurons, oligodendrocytes, astrocytes, ependymal cells, pineal gland), retina and optic nerve, spinal cord.	Neuroectoderm—think CNS.
Neural crest	PNS (dorsal root ganglia, cranial nerves, celiac ganglion, Schwann cells, ANS), melanocytes, chromaffin cells of adrenal medulla, parafollicular (C) cells of thyroid, pia and arachnoid, bones of the skull, odontoblasts, aorticopulmonary septum.	Neural crest—think PNS and non-neural structures nearby.

Mesoderm	Muscle, bone, connective tissue, serous linings of body cavities (e.g., peritoneum), spleen (derived from foregut mesentery), cardiovascular structures, lymphatics, blood, wall of gut tube, vagina, kidneys, adrenal cortex, dermis, testes, ovaries.
	Notochord induces ectoderm to form neuroectoderm (neural plate). Its only postnatal derivative is the nucleus pulposus of the intervertebral disc.
		Mesodermal defects = VACTERL:
		  Vertebral defects
		  Anal atresia
		  Cardiac defects
		  Tracheo-Esophageal fistula
		  Renal defects
		  Limb defects (bone and muscle)

Endoderm	Gut tube epithelium (including anal canal above the pectinate line), most of urethra (derived from urogenital sinus), luminal epithelial derivatives (e.g., lungs, liver, gallbladder, pancreas, eustachian tube, thymus, parathyroid, thyroid follicular cells).	

Types of errors in organ morphogenesis

Agenesis	Absent organ due to absent primordial tissue.
Aplasia	Absent organ despite presence of primordial tissue.
Hypoplasia	Incomplete organ development; primordial tissue present.
Deformation	Extrinsic disruption; occurs after the embryonic period.
Disruption	2° breakdown of a previously normal tissue or structure (e.g., amniotic band syndrome).
Malformation	Intrinsic disruption; occurs during the embryonic period (weeks 3–8).
Sequence	Abnormalities result from a single 1° embryological event (e.g., oligohydramnios → Potter sequence).

Teratogens

Most susceptible in 3rd–8th weeks (embryonic period—organogenesis) of pregnancy. Before week 3: all-or-none effects. After week 8: growth and function affected.

TERATOGEN	EFFECTS ON FETUS	NOTES
Medications		
ACE inhibitors	Renal damage	
Alkylating agents	Absence of digits, multiple anomalies	
Aminoglycosides	CN VIII toxicity	A mean guy hit the baby in the ear.
Carbamazepine	Neural tube defects, craniofacial defects, fingernail hypoplasia, developmental delay, IUGR	
Diethylstilbestrol (DES)	Vaginal clear cell adenocarcinoma, congenital Müllerian anomalies	
Folate antagonists	Neural tube defects	
Lithium	Ebstein anomaly (atrialized right ventricle)	
Methimazole	Aplasia cutis congenita	
Phenytoin	Fetal hydantoin syndrome: microcephaly, dysmorphic craniofacial features, hypoplastic nails and distal phalanges, cardiac defects, IUGR, intellectual disability	
Tetracyclines	Discolored teeth	"Teethracyclines"
Thalidomide	Limb defects (phocomelia, micromelia— "flipper" limbs)	Limb defects with "tha-limb-domide."
Valproate	Inhibition of maternal folate absorption → neural tube defects	Valproate inhibits folate absorption
Warfarin	Bone deformities, fetal hemorrhage, abortion, ophthalmologic abnormalities	Do not wage warfare on the baby; keep it heppy with heparin (does not cross placenta).
Substance abuse		
Alcohol	Common cause of birth defects and intellectual disability; fetal alcohol syndrome	
Cocaine	Abnormal fetal growth and fetal addiction; placental abruption	
Smoking (nicotine, CO)	A leading cause of low birth weight in developed countries; associated with preterm labor, placental problems, IUGR, ADHD	
Other		
Iodine (lack or excess)	Congenital goiter or hypothyroidism (cretinism)	
Maternal diabetes	Caudal regression syndrome (anal atresia to sirenomelia), congenital heart defects, neural tube defects	
Vitamin A (excess)	Extremely high risk for spontaneous abortions and birth defects (cleft palate, cardiac abnormalities)	
X-rays	Microcephaly, intellectual disability	

Fetal infections and certain antibiotics can also cause congenital malformations (see the Microbiology chapter).

Fetal alcohol syndrome

One of the leading causes of congenital malformations in the United States. Newborns of mothers who consumed significant amounts of alcohol during pregnancy have an ↑ incidence of congenital abnormalities, including intellectual disability, pre- and postnatal developmental retardation, microcephaly, holoprosencephaly, facial abnormalities, (smooth philtrum, thin upper lip, small palpebral fissures, hypertelorism), limb dislocation, and heart defects.

Twinning

Dizygotic twins arise from 2 eggs that are separately fertilized by 2 different sperm (always 2 zygotes), and will have 2 separate amniotic sacs and 2 separate placentas (chorions). Monozygotic twins arise from 1 fertilized egg (1 egg + 1 sperm) that splits into 2 zygotes in early pregnancy. The degree of separation between monozygotic twins depends on when the fertilized egg splits into 2 zygotes. The timing of this separation determines the number of chorions and the number of amnions.

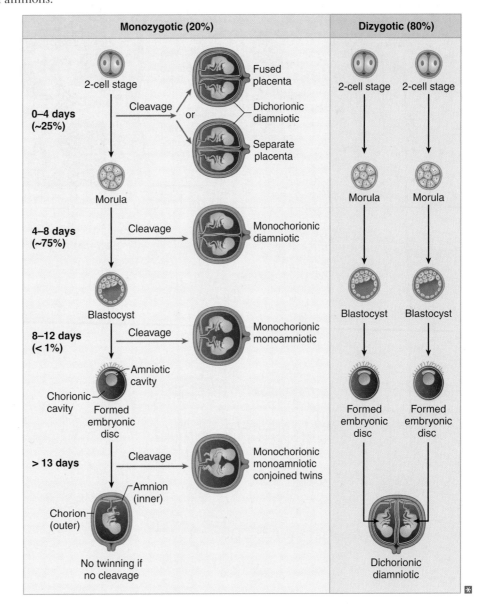

Placental development   1° site of nutrient and gas exchange between mother and fetus.

Fetal component

Cytotrophoblast	Inner layer of chorionic villi.	Cytotrophoblast makes Cells.
Syncytiotrophoblast	Outer layer of chorionic villi; secretes hCG (structurally similar to LH; stimulates corpus luteum to secrete progesterone during first trimester).	

Maternal component

Decidua basalis	Derived from the endometrium. Maternal blood in lacunae.

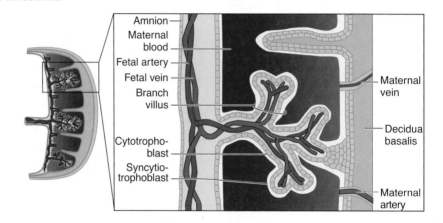

Umbilical cord	Umbilical arteries (2)—return deoxygenated blood from fetal internal iliac arteries to placenta 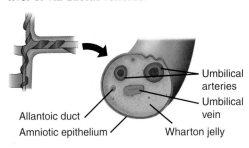. Umbilical vein (1)—supplies oxygenated blood from placenta to fetus; drains into IVC via liver or via ductus venosus.	Single umbilical artery is associated with congenital and chromosomal anomalies. Umbilical arteries and veins are derived from allantois.

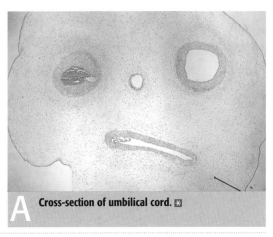

A **Cross-section of umbilical cord.**

Urachus	In the 3rd week the yolk sac forms the allantois, which extends into the urogenital sinus. Allantois becomes the urachus, a duct between fetal bladder and yolk sac. Failure of urachus to obliterate results in: ▪ **Patent urachus**—urine discharge from umbilicus. ▪ **Urachal cyst**—partial failure of urachus to obliterate; fluid-filled cavity lined with uroepithelium, between umbilicus and bladder. Can lead to infection, adenocarcinoma. ▪ **Vesicourachal diverticulum**—outpouching of bladder.
Vitelline duct	7th week—obliteration of vitelline duct (omphalo-mesenteric duct), which connects yolk sac to midgut lumen. Failure of vitelline duct to close results in: ▪ **Vitelline fistula** → meconium discharge from umbilicus. ▪ **Meckel diverticulum**—partial closure, with patent portion attached to ileum (true diverticulum). May have ectopic gastric mucosa and/or pancreatic tissue → melena, periumbilical pain, and ulcers.

Aortic arch derivatives	Develop into the arterial system.	
1st	Part of **ma**xillary artery (branch of external carotid).	1st arch is **ma**ximal.
2nd	**S**tapedial artery and hyoid artery.	**S**econd = **S**tapedial.
3rd	Common **C**arotid artery and proximal part of internal **C**arotid artery.	**C** is 3rd letter of alphabet.
4th	On left, aortic arch; on right, proximal part of right subclavian artery.	4th arch (4 limbs) = systemic.
6th	Proximal part of pulmonary arteries and (on left only) ductus arteriosus.	6th arch = pulmonary and the pulmonary-to-systemic shunt (ductus arteriosus).

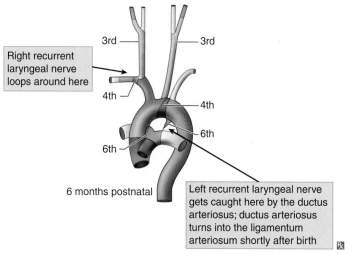

Right recurrent laryngeal nerve loops around here

3rd   3rd

4th   4th

6th   6th

6 months postnatal

Left recurrent laryngeal nerve gets caught here by the ductus arteriosus; ductus arteriosus turns into the ligamentum arteriosum shortly after birth

Branchial apparatus	Also called pharyngeal apparatus. Composed of branchial clefts, arches, and pouches. Branchial clefts—derived from ectoderm. Also called branchial grooves. Branchial arches—derived from mesoderm (muscles, arteries) and neural crest (bones, cartilage). Branchial pouches—derived from endoderm.	**CAP** covers outside to inside: **C**lefts = ectoderm **A**rches = mesoderm **P**ouches = endoderm

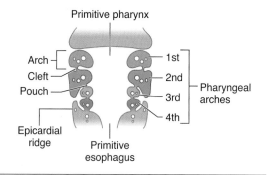

Primitive pharynx

Arch
Cleft
Pouch

1st
2nd
3rd
4th

Pharyngeal arches

Epicardial ridge

Primitive esophagus

Branchial cleft derivatives	1st cleft develops into external auditory meatus. 2nd through 4th clefts form temporary cervical sinuses, which are obliterated by proliferation of 2nd arch mesenchyme. Persistent cervical sinus → branchial cleft cyst within lateral neck.

Branchial arch derivatives

ARCH	CARTILAGE	MUSCLES	NERVES[a]	ABNORMALITIES/COMMENTS
1st arch	Meckel cartilage: Mandible, Malleus, incus, spheno-Mandibular ligament	Muscles of Mastication (temporalis, Masseter, lateral and Medial pterygoids), Mylohyoid, anterior belly of digastric, tensor tympani, tensor veli palatini	CN V_2 and V_3 chew	Treacher Collins syndrome: 1st-arch neural crest fails to migrate → mandibular hypoplasia, facial abnormalities
2nd arch	Reichert cartilage: Stapes, Styloid process, lesser horn of hyoid, Stylohyoid ligament	Muscles of facial expression, Stapedius, Stylohyoid, platySma, belly of digastric	CN VII (facial expression) smile	Congenital pharyngo-cutaneous fistula: persistence of cleft and pouch → fistula between tonsillar area and lateral neck
3rd arch	Cartilage: greater horn of hyoid	Stylopharyngeus (think of stylopharyngeus innervated by glossopharyngeal nerve)	CN IX (stylo-pharyngeus) swallow stylishly	
4th–6th arches	Cartilages: thyroid, cricoid, arytenoids, corniculate, cuneiform	4th arch: most pharyngeal constrictors; cricothyroid, levator veli palatini 6th arch: all intrinsic muscles of larynx except cricothyroid	4th arch: CN X (superior laryngeal branch) simply swallow 6th arch: CN X (recurrent laryngeal branch) speak	Arches 3 and 4 form posterior ⅓ of tongue; arch 5 makes no major developmental contributions

[a]These are the only CNs with both motor and sensory components (except V_2, which is sensory only).

When at the restaurant of the golden **arches**, children tend to first **chew** (1), then **smile** (2), then **swallow styl**ishly (3) or **simply swallow** (4), and then **speak** (6).

Branchial pouch derivatives

1st pouch	Develops into middle ear cavity, eustachian tube, mastoid air cells.	1st pouch contributes to endoderm-lined structures of ear.	Ear, tonsils, bottom-to-top: 1 (ear), 2 (tonsils), 3 dorsal (**bottom** for inferior parathyroids), 3 ventral (**to** = thymus), 4 (**top** = superior parathyroids).
2nd pouch	Develops into epithelial lining of palatine tonsil.		
3rd pouch	Dorsal wings—develops into **inferior** parathyroids. Ventral wings—develops into thymus.	3rd pouch contributes to 3 structures (thymus, left and right inferior parathyroids). 3rd-pouch structures end up **below** 4th-pouch structures.	
4th pouch	Dorsal wings—develops into **superior** parathyroids.		
DiGeorge syndrome	Aberrant development of 3rd and 4th pouches → T-cell deficiency (thymic aplasia) and hypocalcemia (failure of parathyroid development). Associated with cardiac defects (conotruncal anomalies).		
MEN 2A	Mutation of germline *RET* (neural crest cells): <ul><li>Adrenal medulla (pheochromocytoma).</li><li>Parathyroid (tumor): 3rd/4th pharyngeal pouch.</li><li>Parafollicular cells (medullary thyroid cancer): derived from neural crest cells; associated with the 4th/5th pharyngeal pouches.</li></ul>		

Cleft lip and cleft palate

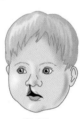

Cleft lip

Cleft lip—failure of fusion of the maxillary and medial nasal processes (formation of 1° palate).

Cleft palate—failure of fusion of the two lateral palatine processes or failure of fusion of lateral palatine processes with the nasal septum and/or median palatine process (formation of 2° palate).

Cleft lip and cleft palate have two distinct etiologies, but often occur together.

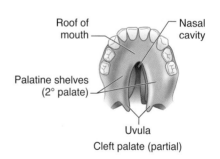

Cleft palate (partial)

Genital embryology

Female	Default development. Mesonephric duct degenerates and paramesonephric duct develops.	
Male	SRY gene on Y chromosome—produces testis-determining factor (testes development). Sertoli cells secrete Müllerian inhibitory factor (MIF) that suppresses development of paramesonephric ducts. Leydig cells secrete androgens that stimulate the development of mesonephric ducts.	Gubernaculum Indifferent gonad Mesonephros Paramesonephric duct Mesonephric duct Urogenital sinus
Paramesonephric (Müllerian) duct	Develops into female internal structures—fallopian tubes, uterus, and upper portion of vagina (lower portion from urogenital sinus). Müllerian duct abnormalities result in anatomical defects that may present as 1° amenorrhea in females with fully developed 2° sexual characteristics (indicator of functional ovaries).	
Mesonephric (Wolffian) duct	Develops into male internal structures (except prostate)—Seminal vesicles, Epididymis, Ejaculatory duct, and Ductus deferens (SEED).	

Bicornuate uterus   Results from incomplete fusion of the paramesonephric ducts (vs. complete failure of fusion, resulting in double uterus and vagina). Can lead to anatomic defects → recurrent miscarriages.

SRY gene

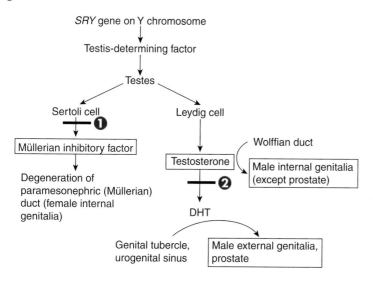

❶ No Sertoli cells or lack of Müllerian inhibitory factor: develop both male and female internal genitalia and male external genitalia

❷ 5α-reductase deficiency: inability to convert testosterone into DHT; male internal genitalia, ambiguous external genitalia until puberty (when ↑ testosterone levels cause masculinization)

Male/female genital homologs

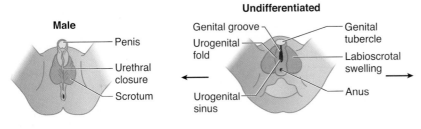

Dihydrotestosterone		Estrogen
Glans penis ←	Genital tubercle	→ Glans clitoris
Corpus cavernosum and spongiosum ←	Genital tubercle	→ Vestibular bulbs
Bulbourethral glands (of Cowper) ←	Urogenital sinus	→ Greater vestibular glands (of Bartholin)
Prostate gland ←	Urogenital sinus	→ Urethral and paraurethral glands (of Skene)
Ventral shaft of penis (penile urethra) ←	Urogenital folds	→ Labia minora
Scrotum ←	Labioscrotal swelling	→ Labia majora

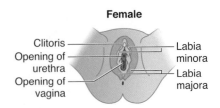

Congenital penile abnormalities

Hypospadias	Abnormal opening of penile urethra on **inferior** (ventral) side of penis due to failure of urethral folds to close.	Hypospadias is more common than epispadias. Fix hypospadias to prevent UTIs. **Hypo** is below.
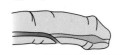		
Epispadias	Abnormal opening of penile urethra on **superior** (dorsal) side of penis due to faulty positioning of genital tubercle.	Exstrophy of the bladder is associated with Epispadias. When you have Epispadias, you hit your Eye when you pEE.
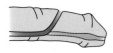		

Descent of testes and ovaries

	MALE REMNANT	FEMALE REMNANT
Gubernaculum (band of fibrous tissue)	Anchors testes within scrotum.	Ovarian ligament + round ligament of uterus.
Processus vaginalis (evagination of peritoneum)	Forms tunica vaginalis.	Obliterated.

▶ REPRODUCTIVE–ANATOMY

Gonadal drainage

Venous drainage	Left ovary/testis → left gonadal vein → left renal vein → IVC. Right ovary/testis → right gonadal vein → IVC.	"Left gonadal vein takes the Longest way." Because the left spermatic vein enters the left renal vein at a 90° angle, flow is less continuous on the left than on the right. → left venous pressure > right venous pressure → varicocele more common on the left.
Lymphatic drainage	Ovaries/testes → para-aortic lymph nodes. Distal vagina/vulva/scrotum → superficial inguinal nodes. Proximal vagina/uterus → obturator, external iliac and hypogastric nodes.	

Female reproductive anatomy

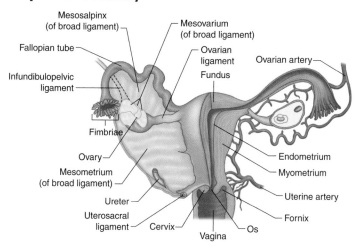
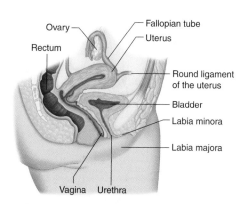

Posterior view

Sagittal view

LIGAMENT	CONNECTS	STRUCTURES CONTAINED	NOTES
Infundibulopelvic ligament (suspensory ligament of the ovaries)	Ovaries to lateral pelvic wall	Ovarian vessels	Ligate vessels during oophorectomy to avoid bleeding. Ureter courses retroperitoneally, close to gonadal vessels. At risk of injury during ligation of ovarian vessels.
Cardinal ligament (not labeled)	Cervix to side wall of pelvis	Uterine vessels	Ureter at risk of injury during ligation of uterine vessels in hysterectomy.
Round ligament of the uterus	Uterine fundus to labia majora		Derivative of gubernaculum. Travels through **round** inguinal canal; above the artery of Sampson.
Broad ligament	Uterus, fallopian tubes, and ovaries to pelvic side wall	Ovaries, fallopian tubes, and round ligaments of uterus	Mesosalpinx, mesometrium, and mesovarium are the components of the broad ligament.
Ovarian ligament	Medial pole of ovary to lateral uterus	—	A derivative of the gubernaculum. **O**varian **L**igament **L**atches to **L**ateral uterus.

Female reproductive epithelial histology

TISSUE	HISTOLOGY/NOTES
Vagina	Stratified squamous epithelium, nonkeratinized
Ectocervix	Stratified squamous epithelium, nonkeratinized
Endocervix	Simple columnar epithelium
Transformation zone	Squamocolumnar junction (most common area for cervical cancer)
Uterus	Simple columnar epithelium with long tubular glands
Fallopian tube	Simple columnar epithelium, many ciliated cells, a few secretory (peg) cells
Ovary, outer surface	Simple cuboidal epithelium (germinal epithelium covering surface of ovary)

Female sexual response cycle

Most commonly described as phase of excitement (uterus elevates, vaginal lubrication), plateau (expansion of inner vagina), orgasm (contraction of uterus), and resolution; mediated by autonomic nervous system. Also causes tachycardia and skin flushing.

Male reproductive anatomy

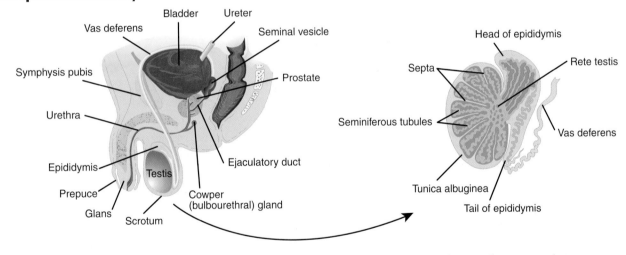

Pathway of sperm during ejaculation—
    SEVEN UP:
    Seminiferous tubules
    Epididymis
    Vas deferens
    Ejaculatory ducts
    (Nothing)
    Urethra
    Penis

Autonomic innervation of the male sexual response

Erection—Parasympathetic nervous system (pelvic nerve):
- NO → ↑ cGMP → smooth muscle relaxation → vasodilation → proerectile.
- Norepinephrine → ↑ $[Ca^{2+}]_{in}$ → smooth muscle contraction → vasoconstriction → antierectile.

Emission—Sympathetic nervous system (hypogastric nerve).

Ejaculation—visceral and somatic nerves (pudendal nerve).

Point and Shoot.

Sildenafil and vardenafil inhibit cGMP breakdown.

Seminiferous tubules

CELL	FUNCTION	LOCATION/NOTES
Spermatogonia (germ cells)	Maintain germ pool and produce 1° spermatocytes	Line seminiferous tubules 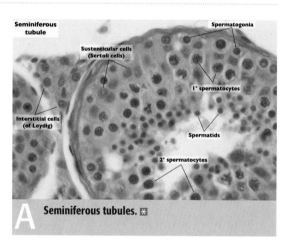
Sertoli cells (non–germ cells)	Secrete inhibin → inhibit FSH Secrete androgen-binding protein → maintain local levels of testosterone Tight junctions between adjacent Sertoli cells form blood-testis barrier → isolate gametes from autoimmune attack Support and nourish developing spermatozoa Regulate spermatogenesis Produce MIF	Line seminiferous tubules Convert testosterone and androstenedione to estrogen via aromatase Sertoli cells Support Sperm Synthesis
	Temperature sensitive; ↓ sperm production and ↓ inhibin with ↑ temperature	↑ temperature seen in varicocele, cryptorchidism
Leydig cells (endocrine cells)	Secrete testosterone in the presence of LH; testosterone production unaffected by temperature	Interstitium Also contain aromatase

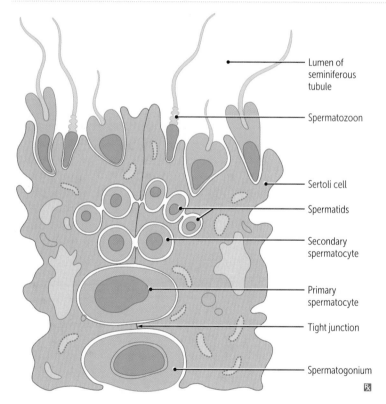

Lumen of seminiferous tubule

Spermatozoon

Sertoli cell

Spermatids

Secondary spermatocyte

Primary spermatocyte

Tight junction

Spermatogonium

A Seminiferous tubules.

Seminiferous tubule

Spermatogonia

Sustenticular cells (Sertoli cells)

1° spermatocytes

Interstitial cells (of Leydig)

Spermatids

2° spermatocytes

▶ REPRODUCTIVE–PHYSIOLOGY

Estrogen

SOURCE	Ovary (17β-estradiol), placenta (estriol), adipose tissue (estrone via aromatization)	Potency: estradiol > estrone > estriol
FUNCTION	Development of genitalia and breast, female fat distribution Growth of follicle, endometrial proliferation, ↑ myometrial excitability Upregulation of estrogen, LH, and progesterone receptors; feedback inhibition of FSH and LH, then LH surge; stimulation of prolactin secretion ↑ transport proteins, SHBG; ↑ HDL; ↓ LDL	Pregnancy: ▪ 50-fold ↑ in estradiol and estrone ▪ 1000-fold ↑ in estriol (indicator of fetal well-being) Estrogen receptors expressed in the cytoplasm; translocate to the nucleus when bound by ligand

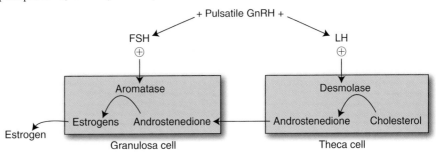

Progesterone

SOURCE	Corpus luteum, placenta, adrenal cortex, testes	Fall in progesterone after delivery disinhibits prolactin → lactation. ↑ progesterone is indicative of ovulation. **Progesterone is pro-gestation.** **Prolactin is pro-lactation.**
FUNCTION	Stimulation of endometrial glandular secretions and spiral artery development Maintenance of pregnancy ↓ myometrial excitability Production of thick cervical mucus, which inhibits sperm entry into the uterus ↑ body temperature Inhibition of gonadotropins (LH, FSH) Uterine smooth muscle relaxation (preventing contractions) ↓ estrogen receptor expressivity Prevents endometrial hyperplasia	

Tanner stages of sexual development

A Tanner stage is assigned independently to genitalia, pubic hair, and breast (e.g., a person can have Tanner stage 2 genitalia, Tanner stage 3 pubic hair).

  I. Childhood (prepubertal)

  II. Pubic hair appears (pubarche); breast buds form (thelarche)

  III. Pubic hair darkens and becomes curly; penis size/length ↑; breasts enlarge

  IV. Penis width ↑, darker scrotal skin, development of glans; raised areolae

  V. Adult; areolae are no longer raised

Menstrual cycle

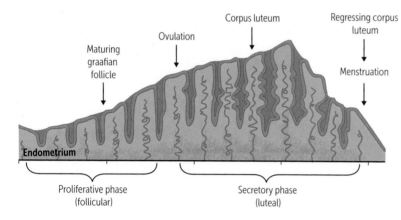

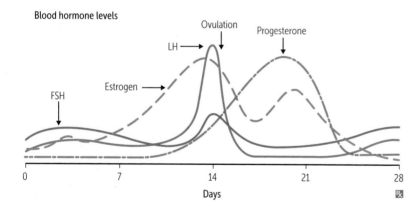

Follicular phase can vary in length. Luteal phase is usually a constant 14 days. Ovulation day + 14 days = menstruation.

Follicular growth is fastest during 2nd week of proliferative phase.

Estrogen stimulates endometrial proliferation.

Progesterone maintains endometrium to support implantation.

↓ progesterone → ↓ fertility.

Oligomenorrhea: > 35-day cycle.

Polymenorrhea: < 21-day cycle.

Metrorrhagia (intermenstrual bleeding): frequent but irregular menstruation.

Menorrhagia (heavy menstrual bleeding): > 80 mL blood loss or > 7 days of menses.

Menometrorrhagia: heavy, irregular menstruation at irregular intervals.

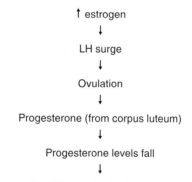

↑ estrogen
↓
LH surge
↓
Ovulation
↓
Progesterone (from corpus luteum)
↓
Progesterone levels fall
↓
Menstruation (via apoptosis of endometrial cells)

Oogenesis

1° oocytes begin meiosis I during fetal life and complete meiosis I just prior to ovulation.

Meiosis I is arrested in prOphase I for years until Ovulation (1° oocytes).

Meiosis II is arrested in metaphase II until fertilization (2° oocytes).

An egg met a sperm.

If fertilization does not occur within 1 day, the 2° oocyte degenerates.

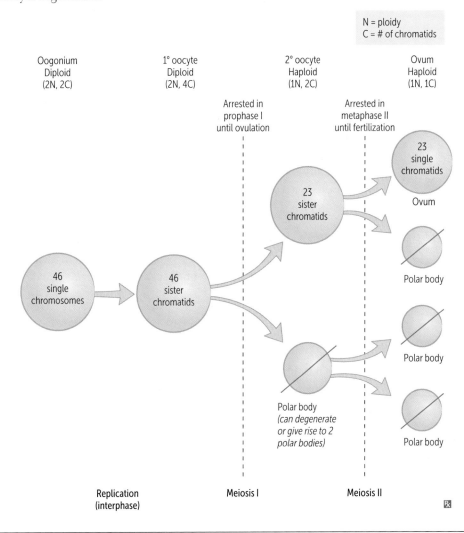

Ovulation	↑ estrogen, ↑ GnRH receptors on anterior pituitary. Estrogen surge then stimulates LH release → ovulation (rupture of follicle). ↑ temperature (progesterone induced).	Mittelschmerz refers to transient mid-cycle ovulatory pain; classically associated with peritoneal irritation (e.g., follicular swelling/rupture, fallopian tube contraction). Can mimic appendicitis.

Pregnancy

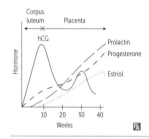

Fertilization most commonly occurs in upper end of fallopian tube (the ampulla). Occurs within 1 day of ovulation.

Implantation within the wall of the uterus occurs 6 days after fertilization. Syncytiotrophoblasts secrete hCG, which is detectable in blood 1 week after conception and on home test in urine 2 weeks after conception.

Lactation

After labor, the ↓ in progesterone and estrogen disinhibits lactation. Suckling is required to maintain milk production, since ↑ nerve stimulation ↑ oxytocin and prolactin.
Prolactin—induces and maintains lactation and ↓ reproductive function.
Oxytocin—assists in milk letdown; also promotes uterine contractions.
Breastmilk is the ideal nutrition for infants < 6 months old. Contains maternal immunoglobulins (conferring passive immunity; mostly IgA), macrophages, and lymphocytes. Breastmilk reduces infant infections and is associated with ↓ risk for the child to develop asthma, allergies, diabetes mellitus, and obesity. Exclusively breastfed infants require vitamin D supplementation.
Breastfeeding ↓ maternal risk of breast and ovarian cancer, and facilitates mother-child bonding.

hCG

SOURCE	Syncytiotrophoblast of placenta.
FUNCTION	Maintains the corpus luteum (and thus progesterone) for the 1st trimester by acting like LH (otherwise no luteal cell stimulation, and abortion results). In the 2nd and 3rd trimesters, the placenta synthesizes its own estriol and progesterone and the corpus luteum degenerates. Used to detect pregnancy because it appears early in the urine (see above). α subunit structurally identical to α subunits of LH, FSH, and TSH. β subunit is unique (pregnancy tests detect β subunit). hCG is ↑ in multiple gestations and pathologic states (e.g., hydatidiform mole, choriocarcinoma).

Menopause

↓ estrogen production due to age-linked decline in number of ovarian follicles. Average age at onset is 51 years (earlier in smokers).

Usually preceded by 4–5 years of abnormal menstrual cycles. Source of estrogen (estrone) after menopause becomes peripheral conversion of androgens, ↑ androgens → hirsutism.

↑↑ FSH is specific for menopause (loss of negative feedback on FSH due to ↓ estrogen).

Hormonal changes: ↓ estrogen, ↑↑ FSH, ↑ LH (no surge), ↑ GnRH.

Menopause causes **HAVOCS**: Hot flashes, Atrophy of the Vagina, Osteoporosis, Coronary artery disease, Sleep disturbances.

Menopause before age 40 can indicate premature ovarian failure.

Spermatogenesis

Spermatogenesis begins at puberty with spermatogonia. Full development takes 2 months. Occurs in seminiferous tubules. Produces spermatids that undergo spermiogenesis (loss of cytoplasmic contents, gain of acrosomal cap) to form mature spermatozoon.

"Gonium" is going to be a sperm; "Zoon" is "Zooming" to egg.

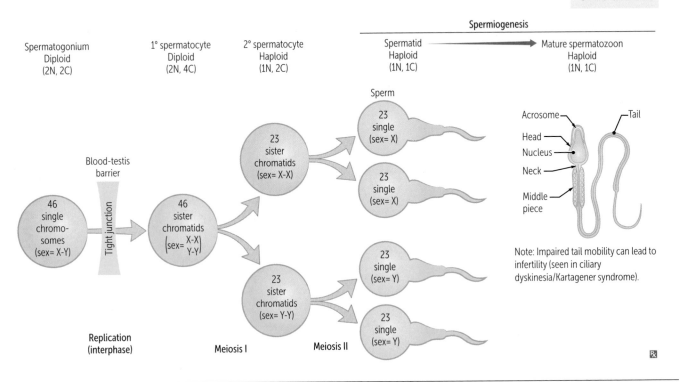

N = ploidy
C = # of chromatids

Note: Impaired tail mobility can lead to infertility (seen in ciliary dyskinesia/Kartagener syndrome).

Androgens	Testosterone, dihydrotestosterone (DHT), androstenedione.	
SOURCE	DHT and testosterone (testis), **AnD**rostenedione (**AD**renal)	Potency: DHT > testosterone > androstenedione.
FUNCTION	Testosterone: ■ Differentiation of epididymis, vas deferens, seminal vesicles (genitalia, except prostate) ■ Growth spurt: penis, seminal vesicles, sperm, muscle, RBCs ■ Deepening of voice ■ Closing of epiphyseal plates (via estrogen converted from testosterone) ■ Libido DHT: ■ Early—differentiation of penis, scrotum, prostate ■ Late—prostate growth, balding, sebaceous gland activity	Testosterone is converted to DHT by the enzyme 5α-reductase, which is inhibited by finasteride. In the male, androgens are converted to estrogen by cytochrome P-450 aromatase (primarily in adipose tissue and the testis). Aromatase is the key enzyme in the conversion of androgens to estrogen. Exogenous testosterone → inhibition of hypothalamic–pituitary–gonadal axis → ↓ intratesticular testosterone → ↓ testicular size → azoospermia.

▶ REPRODUCTIVE–PATHOLOGY

Sex chromosome disorders of sexual development

Klinefelter syndrome [male] (XXY), 1:850 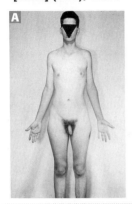	Testicular atrophy, eunuchoid body shape, tall, long extremities, gynecomastia, female hair distribution A. May present with developmental delay. Presence of inactivated X chromosome (Barr body). Common cause of hypogonadism seen in infertility work-up.	Dysgenesis of seminiferous tubules → ↓ inhibin → ↑ FSH. Abnormal Leydig cell function → ↓ testosterone → ↑ LH → ↑ estrogen.
Turner syndrome [female] (XO) 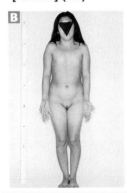	Short stature (if untreated), ovarian dysgenesis (streak ovary), shield chest, bicuspid aortic valve, preductal coarctation (femoral < brachial pulse, notched ribs), lymphatic defects (result in webbed neck or cystic hygroma; lymphedema in feet, hands), horseshoe kidney B. Most common cause of 1° amenorrhea. No Barr body.	"Hugs and kisses" (XO) from Tina Turner. Menopause before menarche. ↓ estrogen leads to ↑ LH, FSH. Can result from mitotic or meiotic error. Can be complete monosomy (45,XO) or mosaicism (e.g., 45,XO/46,XX). Pregnancy is possible in some cases (oocyte donation, exogenous estradiol-17β and progesterone).
Double Y males [male] (XYY), 1:1000	Phenotypically normal, very tall, severe acne, antisocial behavior (seen in 1–2% of XYY males). Normal fertility. Small percentage diagnosed with autism spectrum disorders.	
True hermaphroditism (46,XX or 47,XXY)	Also called ovotesticular disorder of sex development. Both ovary and testicular tissue present (ovotestis); ambiguous genitalia. Very rare.	

Diagnosing disorders of sex hormones	Testosterone	LH	Diagnosis
	↑	↑	Defective androgen receptor
	↑	↓	Testosterone-secreting tumor, exogenous steroids
	↓	↑	1° hypogonadism
	↓	↓	Hypogonadotropic hypogonadism

Other disorders of sex development	Include terms pseudohermaphrodite, hermaphrodite, and intersex. Disagreement between the phenotypic (external genitalia) and gonadal (testes vs. ovaries) sex.
Female pseudo-hermaphrodite (XX)	Ovaries present, but external genitalia are virilized or ambiguous. Due to excessive and inappropriate exposure to androgenic steroids during early gestation (e.g., congenital adrenal hyperplasia or exogenous administration of androgens during pregnancy).
Male pseudo-hermaphrodite (XY)	Testes present, but external genitalia are female or ambiguous. Most common form is androgen insensitivity syndrome (testicular feminization).

Aromatase deficiency	Inability to synthesize estrogens from androgens. Masculinization of female (46,XX) infants (ambiguous genitalia), and ↑ serum testosterone and androstenedione. Can present with maternal virilization during pregnancy (fetal androgens cross the placenta).

Androgen insensitivity syndrome (46,XY)	Defect in androgen receptor resulting in normal-appearing female; female external genitalia with rudimentary vagina; uterus and fallopian tubes generally absent; presents with scant sexual hair; develops testes (often found in labia majora; surgically removed to prevent malignancy). ↑ testosterone, estrogen, LH (vs. sex chromosome disorders).

5α-reductase deficiency	Autosomal recessive; sex limited to genetic males (46,XY). Inability to convert testosterone to DHT. Ambiguous genitalia until puberty, when ↑ testosterone causes masculinization/↑ growth of external genitalia. Testosterone/estrogen levels are normal; LH is normal or ↑. Internal genitalia are normal.

Kallmann syndrome	Failure to complete puberty; a form of hypogonadotropic hypogonadism. Defective migration of GnRH cells and formation of olfactory bulb; ↓ synthesis of GnRH in the hypothalamus; anosmia; ↓ GnRH, FSH, LH, testosterone, and infertility (low sperm count in males; amenorrhea in females).

Hydatidiform mole

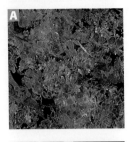

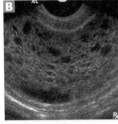

Cystic swelling of chorionic villi and proliferation of chorionic epithelium (only trophoblast). Treatment—dilation and curettage and methotrexate. Monitor β-hCG.

	Complete mole	Partial mole
KARYOTYPE	46,XX; 46,XY	69,XXX; 69,XXY; 69,XYY
hCG	↑↑↑↑	↑
UTERINE SIZE	↑	—
CONVERT TO CHORIOCARCINOMA	2%	Rare
FETAL PARTS	No	Yes (partial = fetal parts)
COMPONENTS	Enucleated egg + single sperm (subsequently duplicates paternal DNA); empty egg + 2 sperm is rare	2 sperm + 1 egg
RISK OF COMPLICATIONS	15–20% malignant trophoblastic disease	Low risk of malignancy (< 5%)
SYMPTOMS	Vaginal bleeding, enlarged uterus, hyperemesis, pre-eclampsia, hyperthyroidism	Vaginal bleeding, abdominal pain
IMAGING	Honeycombed uterus or "clusters of grapes" A, "snowstorm" on ultrasound B	Fetal parts

Hypertension in pregnancy

Gestational hypertension (pregnancy-induced hypertension)	BP > 140/90 mmHg after the 20th week of gestation. No pre-existing hypertension. No proteinuria or end-organ damage.	Treatment: antihypertensives (α-methyldopa, labetalol, hydralazine, nifedipine), deliver at 39 weeks.
Preeclampsia	Defined as hypertension (> 140/90 mmHg) and proteinuria (> 300 mg/24 hr) after 20th week of gestation to 6 weeks postpartum (< 20 weeks suggests molar pregnancy). Severe features include BP > 160/110 mmHg with or without end-organ damage, e.g., headache, scotoma, oliguria, ↑ AST/ALT, thrombocytopenia. Caused by abnormal placental spiral arteries, results in maternal endothelial dysfunction, vasoconstriction, or hyperreflexia. Incidence ↑ in patients with preexisting hypertension, diabetes, chronic renal disease, or autoimmune disorders. Complications: placental abruption, coagulopathy, renal failure, uteroplacental insufficiency, or eclampsia.	Treatment: antihypertensives, deliver at 34 weeks (severe) or 37 weeks (mild), IV magnesium sulfate to prevent seizure.
Eclampsia	Preeclampsia + maternal seizures. Maternal death due to stroke → intracranial hemorrhage or ARDS.	Treatment: antihypertensives, IV magnesium sulfate, immediate delivery.
HELLP syndrome	Hemolysis, Elevated Liver enzymes, Low Platelets. A manifestation of severe preeclampsia, although may occur without hypertension.	Treatment: immediate delivery.

Pregnancy complications

Placental abruption (abruptio placentae)	Premature separation (partial or complete) of placenta from uterine wall before delivery of infant. Risk factors: trauma (e.g., motor vehicle accident), smoking, hypertension, preeclampsia, cocaine abuse. Presentation: **abrupt**, painful bleeding (concealed or apparent) in third trimester; possible DIC, maternal shock, fetal distress. Life threatening for mother and fetus.

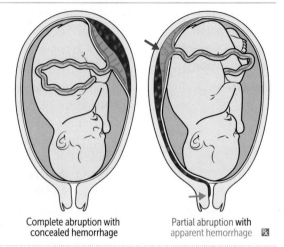

Complete abruption with concealed hemorrhage

Partial abruption with apparent hemorrhage

Placenta accreta/ increta/percreta	Defective decidual layer → abnormal attachment and separation after delivery. Risk factors: prior C-section, inflammation, placenta previa. Three types distinguishable by the depth of penetration: **Placenta** accreta—placenta **attaches** to myometrium without penetrating it; most common type. **Placenta** increta—placenta penetrates **into** myometrium. **Placenta** percreta—placenta penetrates ("**perforates**") through the myometrium and into uterine serosa (invades entire uterine wall); can result in placental attachment to rectum or bladder. Presentation: no separation of placenta after delivery → massive bleeding. Life threatening for mother.

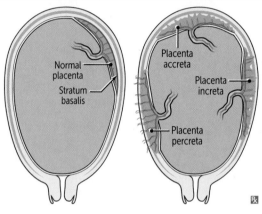

Normal placenta
Stratum basalis
Placenta accreta
Placenta increta
Placenta percreta

Placenta previa	Attachment of placenta to lower uterine segment. Lies near (marginal, not shown), partially covers (partial), or completely covers internal cervical os. Risk factors: multiparity, prior C-section.

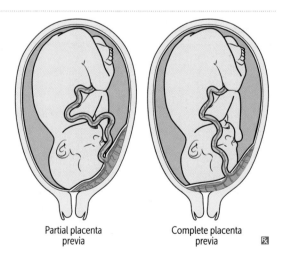

Partial placenta previa

Complete placenta previa

Pregnancy complications *(continued)*

Retained placental tissue	May cause postpartum hemorrhage, ↑ risk of infection.

Ectopic pregnancy

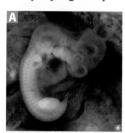

Most often in ampulla of fallopian tube (**A** shows 10-mm embryo within oviduct at 7 weeks' gestation). Suspect with history of amenorrhea, lower-than-expected rise in hCG based on dates, and sudden lower abdominal pain; confirm with ultrasound. Often clinically mistaken for appendicitis.

Pain with or without bleeding.
Risk factors:
- History of infertility
- Salpingitis (PID)
- Ruptured appendix
- Prior tubal surgery

Amniotic fluid abnormalities

Polyhydramnios	> 1.5–2 L of amniotic fluid; associated with fetal malformations (e.g., esophageal/duodenal atresia, anencephaly; both result in inability to swallow amniotic fluid), maternal diabetes, fetal anemia, multiple gestations.
Oligohydramnios	< 0.5 L of amniotic fluid; associated with placental insufficiency, bilateral renal agenesis, or posterior urethral valves (in males) and resultant inability to excrete urine. Any profound oligohydramnios can cause Potter sequence.

Cervical pathology

Dysplasia and carcinoma in situ

Disordered epithelial growth; begins at basal layer of squamocolumnar junction (transition zone) and extends outward. Classified as CIN 1, CIN 2, or CIN 3 (severe dysplasia or carcinoma in situ), depending on extent of dysplasia. Associated with HPV 16 and HPV 18, which produce both the E6 gene product (inhibits $p53$ suppressor gene) and E7 gene product (inhibits RB suppressor gene). May progress slowly to invasive carcinoma if left untreated. Typically asymptomatic (detected with Pap smear) or presents as abnormal vaginal bleeding (often postcoital).
Risk factors: multiple sexual partners (#1), smoking, early sexual intercourse, HIV infection.

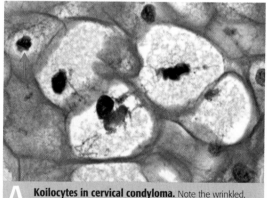

Koilocytes in cervical condyloma. Note the wrinkled, "raisinoid" nuclei, some of which have clearing or a perinuclear halo (arrow). ℞

Invasive carcinoma

Often squamous cell carcinoma. Pap smear can catch cervical dysplasia (koilocytes **A**) before it progresses to invasive carcinoma. Lateral invasion can block ureters, causing renal failure.

Endometritis 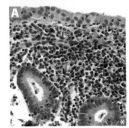	Inflammation of the endometrium (with plasma cells and lymphocytes) 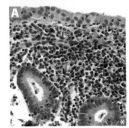 associated with retained products of conception following delivery (vaginal/C-section)/miscarriage/abortion or foreign body such as an IUD. Retained material in uterus promotes infection by bacterial flora from vagina or intestinal tract. Treatment: gentamicin + clindamycin with or without ampicillin.

Endometriosis

Non-neoplastic endometrial glands/stroma outside of the endometrial cavity 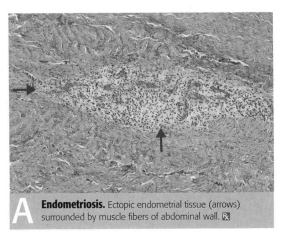. Can be found anywhere; most common sites are ovary, pelvis, and peritoneum. In the ovary, appears as an endometrioma (blood-filled "chocolate cyst").

Can be due to retrograde flow, metaplastic transformation of multipotent cells, or transportation of endometrial tissue via the lymphatic system.

Characterized by cyclic pelvic pain, bleeding, dysmenorrhea, dyspareunia, dyschezia (pain with defecation), infertility; **normal-sized** uterus.

Treatment: NSAIDs, OCPs, progestins, GnRH agonists, surgery.

Endometriosis. Ectopic endometrial tissue (arrows) surrounded by muscle fibers of abdominal wall. ℞

Adenomyosis	Extension of endometrial tissue (glandular) into the uterine myometrium. Caused by hyperplasia of the basalis layer of the endometrium.	Dysmenorrhea, menorrhagia. Uniformly **enlarged**, **soft**, globular uterus. Treatment: hysterectomy

Adenomyoma (polyp)	Well-circumscribed collection of endometrial tissue within the uterine wall. May contain smooth muscle cells. Can extend into the endometrial cavity in the form of a polyp.

Endometrial proliferation

Endometrial hyperplasia	Abnormal endometrial gland proliferation usually caused by excess estrogen stimulation. ↑ risk for endometrial carcinoma. Clinically manifests as postmenopausal vaginal bleeding. Risk factors include anovulatory cycles, hormone replacement therapy, polycystic ovarian syndrome, and granulosa cell tumor.
Endometrial carcinoma	Most common gynecologic malignancy. Peak occurrence at 55–65 years old. Clinically presents with vaginal bleeding. Typically preceded by endometrial hyperplasia. Risk factors include prolonged use of estrogen without progestins, obesity, diabetes, hypertension, nulliparity, and late menopause. ↑ myometrial invasion → ↓ prognosis.

Leiomyoma (fibroid)

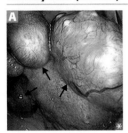

Most common tumor in females. Often presents with multiple discrete tumors **A**. ↑ incidence in blacks. Benign smooth muscle tumor; malignant transformation is rare. Estrogen sensitive—tumor size ↑ with pregnancy and ↓ with menopause. Peak occurrence at 20–40 years old. May be asymptomatic, cause abnormal uterine bleeding, or result in miscarriage. Severe bleeding may lead to iron deficiency anemia. Does not progress to leiomyosarcoma. Whorled pattern of smooth muscle bundles with well-demarcated borders.

Gynecologic tumor epidemiology

Incidence—endometrial > ovarian > cervical (data pertain to the United States; cervical cancer is most common worldwide).
Worst prognosis—ovarian > cervical > endometrial.

Premature ovarian failure

Premature atresia of ovarian follicles in women of reproductive age. Patients present with signs of menopause after puberty but before age 40.

↓ estrogen, ↑ LH, FSH.

Most common causes of anovulation

Pregnancy, polycystic ovarian syndrome, obesity, HPO axis abnormalities, premature ovarian failure, hyperprolactinemia, thyroid disorders, eating disorders, female athletes, Cushing syndrome, adrenal insufficiency.

Polycystic ovarian syndrome (Stein-Leventhal syndrome)

Hyperandrogenism due to deranged steroid synthesis by theca cells, hyperinsulinemia. Estrogen ↑ steroid hormone–binding globulin (SHBG) and ↓ LH, ultimately resulting in ↓ free testosterone; insulin and testosterone ↓ SHBG → ↑ free testosterone. ↑ LH due to pituitary/hypothalamus dysfunction. Results in enlarged, bilateral cystic ovaries **A**; presents with amenorrhea/oligomenorrhea, hirsutism, acne, infertility. Associated with obesity. ↑ risk of endometrial cancer 2° to ↑ estrogens from the aromatization of testosterone and absence of progesterone.

Treatment for hirsutism, acne: weight reduction, OCPs (estrogen ↑ SHBG and ↓ LH → ↓ free testosterone), antiandrogens; for infertility: clomiphene citrate (blocks negative feedback of circulating estrogen, ↓ FSH, LH), metformin (↑ insulin sensitivity, ↓ insulin levels, results in ↓ testosterone; enables LH surge); for endometrial protection: cyclic progesterones (antagonizes endometrial proliferation).

↑ LH, ↑ FSH (LH:FSH, 3:1), ↑ testosterone, ↑ estrogen (from aromatization).
Most common cause of infertility in women.

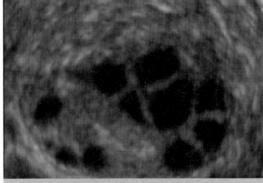

A Polycystic ovarian syndrome. Ultrasound shows multiple follicles in ovary. ✱

Ovarian cysts

Follicular cyst	Distention of unruptured graafian follicle. May be associated with hyperestrogenism and endometrial hyperplasia. Most common ovarian mass in young women.
Corpus luteum cyst	Hemorrhage into persistent corpus luteum. Commonly regresses spontaneously.
Theca-lutein cyst	Often bilateral/multiple. Due to gonadotropin stimulation. Associated with choriocarcinoma and moles.
Hemorrhagic cyst	Blood vessel rupture in cyst wall. Cyst grows with ↑ blood retention; usually self-resolves.
Dermoid cyst	Mature teratoma. Cystic growths filled with various types of tissue such as fat, hair, teeth, bits of bone, and cartilage.
Endometrioid cyst	Endometriosis within ovary with cyst formation. Varies with menstrual cycle. When filled with dark, reddish-brown blood it is called a "chocolate cyst."

Ovarian neoplasms	Most common adnexal mass in women > 55 years old. Can be benign or malignant. Arise from surface epithelium, germ cells, and sex cord stromal tissue.
	Majority of malignant tumors arise from epithelial cells. Majority (95%) are epithelial (serous cystadenocarcinoma most common). Risk ↑ with advanced age, infertility, endometriosis, PCOS, genetic predisposition (*BRCA-1* or *BRCA-2* mutation, HNPCC, strong family history). Risk ↓ with previous pregnancy, history of breastfeeding, OCPs, tubal ligation. Presents with adnexal mass, abdominal distension, bowel obstruction, pleural effusion. Diagnose surgically. Monitor progression by measuring CA-125 levels (not good for screening).

Benign ovarian neoplasms

Serous cystadenoma	Most common ovarian neoplasm. Thin-walled, uni- or multilocular. Lined with fallopian-like epithelium. Often bilateral.
Mucinous cystadenoma	Multiloculated, large. Lined by mucus-secreting epithelium **A**.
Endometrioma	Mass arising from growth of ectopic endometrial tissue. Complex mass on ultrasound. Presents with pelvic pain, dysmenorrhea, dyspareunia.
Mature cystic teratoma (dermoid cyst)	Germ cell tumor, most common ovarian tumor in women 20–30 years old. Can contain elements from all 3 germ layers; teeth, hair, sebum **B** are common components. Can present with pain 2° to ovarian enlargement or torsion. Can also contain functional thyroid tissue and present as hyperthyroidism (struma ovarii) **C**.
Brenner tumor	Looks like bladder. Solid tumor that is pale yellow-tan in color and appears encapsulated. "Coffee bean" nuclei on H&E stain.
Fibromas	Bundles of spindle-shaped fibroblasts. **Meigs syndrome**—triad of ovarian fibroma, ascites, and hydrothorax. Pulling sensation in groin.
Thecoma	Like granulosa cell tumors, may produce estrogen. Usually present as abnormal uterine bleeding in a postmenopausal woman.

Ovarian neoplasms (continued)

Malignant ovarian neoplasms

Immature teratoma	Aggressive, contains fetal tissue, neuroectoderm. Immature teratoma is most typically represented by immature/embryonic-like neural tissue. Mature teratoma are more likely to contain thyroid tissue.
Granulosa cell tumor	Most common sex cord stromal tumor. Predominantly women in their 50s. Often produce estrogen and/or progesterone and present with abnormal uterine bleeding, sexual precocity (in pre-adolescents), breast tenderness. Histology shows Call-Exner bodies (resemble primordial follicles).
Serous cystadenocarcinoma	Most common ovarian neoplasm, frequently bilateral. Psammoma bodies.
Mucinous cystadenocarcinoma	Pseudomyxoma peritonei–intraperitoneal accumulation of mucinous material from ovarian or appendiceal tumor.
Dysgerminoma	Most common in adolescents. Equivalent to male seminoma but rarer. 1% of all ovarian tumors; 30% of germ cell tumors. Sheets of uniform "fried egg" cells **D**. hCG, LDH = tumor markers.
Choriocarcinoma	Rare; can develop during or after pregnancy in mother or baby. Malignancy of trophoblastic tissue **E** (cytotrophoblasts, syncytiotrophoblasts); **no** chorionic villi present. ↑ frequency of theca-lutein cysts. Presents with abnormal β-hCG, shortness of breath, hemoptysis. Hematogenous spread to lungs. Very responsive to chemotherapy.
Yolk sac (endodermal sinus) tumor	Aggressive, in ovaries or testes (boys) and sacrococcygeal area in young children. Most common tumor in male infants. Yellow, friable (hemorrhagic), solid mass. 50% have Schiller-Duval bodies (resemble glomeruli) **F**. AFP = tumor marker.
Krukenberg tumor	GI malignancy that metastasizes to the ovaries, causing a mucin-secreting signet cell adenocarcinoma.

Vaginal tumors

Squamous cell carcinoma (SCC)	Usually 2° to cervical SCC; 1° vaginal carcinoma rare.
Clear cell adenocarcinoma	Affects women who had exposure to DES in utero.
Sarcoma botryoides (rhabdomyosarcoma variant)	Affects girls < 4 years old; spindle-shaped tumor cells that are desmin ⊕.

Breast pathology

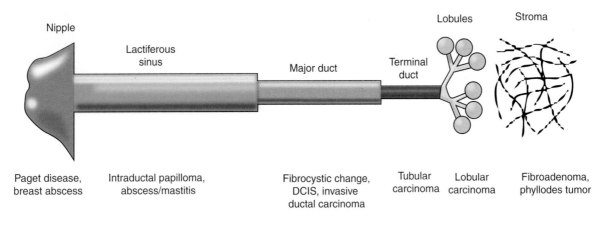

| Paget disease, breast abscess | Intraductal papilloma, abscess/mastitis | Fibrocystic change, DCIS, invasive ductal carcinoma | Tubular carcinoma | Lobular carcinoma | Fibroadenoma, phyllodes tumor |

Benign breast tumors

TYPE	CHARACTERISTICS	EPIDEMIOLOGY	NOTES
Fibroadenoma	**Small**, mobile, firm mass with sharp edges.	Most common tumor in those < 35 years old.	↑ size and tenderness with ↑ estrogen (e.g., pregnancy, prior to menstruation). Not a precursor to breast cancer.
Intraductal papilloma	Small tumor that grows in lactiferous ducts. Typically beneath areola.		Serous or bloody nipple discharge. Slight (1.5–2×) ↑ in risk for carcinoma.
Phyllodes tumor	**Large** bulky mass of connective tissue and cysts. "Leaf-like" projections.	Most common in 6th decade.	Some may become malignant.

Malignant breast tumors	Commonly postmenopausal. Usually arise from terminal duct lobular unit. Overexpression of estrogen/progesterone receptors or *c-erbB2* (HER-2, an EGF receptor) is common; triple negative (ER ⊖, PR ⊖, and Her2/Neu ⊖) more aggressive; type affects therapy and prognosis. Axillary lymph node involvement indicating metastasis is the single most important prognostic factor. Most often located in upper-outer quadrant of breast.	Risk factors: ↑ estrogen exposure, ↑ total number of menstrual cycles, older age at 1st live birth, obesity (↑ estrogen exposure as adipose tissue converts androstenedione to estrone), *BRCA1* and *BRCA2* gene mutations, African American ethnicity (↑ risk for triple ⊖ breast cancer).

TYPE	CHARACTERISTICS	NOTES
Noninvasive		
Ductal carcinoma in situ (DCIS)	Fills ductal lumen. Arises from ductal atypia **A**. Often seen early as microcalcifications on mammography.	Early malignancy without basement membrane penetration.
Comedocarcinoma	Ductal, caseous necrosis **B**. Subtype of DCIS.	

A **DCIS.** Note neoplastic cells confined to the duct (black arrow) and engorged blood vessel (blue arrow). ℞

B **Comedocarcinoma.** Note central necrosis (arrow) surrounded by cancer cells. ✳

Paget disease 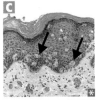	Results from underlying DCIS. Eczematous patches on nipple. Paget cells = large cells in epidermis with clear halo **C**.	Suggests underlying DCIS. Also seen on vulva, though does not suggest underlying malignancy.
Invasive		
Invasive ductal	Firm, fibrous, "rock-hard" mass with sharp margins and small, glandular, duct-like cells. Grossly, see classic "stellate" infiltration.	Worst and most invasive. Most common (76% of all breast cancers).
Invasive lobular	Orderly row of cells ("Indian file").	Often bilateral with multiple lesions in the same location.
Medullary	Fleshy, cellular, lymphocytic infiltrate.	Good prognosis.
Inflammatory	Dermal lymphatic invasion by breast carcinoma. Peau d'orange (breast skin resembles orange peel); neoplastic cells block lymphatic drainage.	50% survival at 5 years.

Common breast conditions

Proliferative breast disease	Most common cause of "breast lumps" from age 25 to menopause. Presents with premenstrual breast pain and multiple lesions, often bilateral. Fluctuation in size of mass. Usually does not indicate ↑ risk of carcinoma. Histologic types: ▪ **Fibrosis**—hyperplasia of breast stroma. ▪ **Cystic**—fluid filled, blue dome. Ductal dilation. ▪ **Sclerosing adenosis**—↑ acini and intralobular fibrosis. Associated with calcifications. Often confused with cancer. ↑ risk (1.5–2×) of developing cancer. ▪ **Epithelial hyperplasia**—↑ in number of epithelial cell layers in terminal duct lobule. ↑ risk of carcinoma with atypical cells. Occurs in women > 30 years old.
Acute mastitis	Breast abscess; during breast-feeding, ↑ risk of bacterial infection through cracks in the nipple; *S. aureus* is the most common pathogen. Treat with dicloxacillin and continued breast-feeding.
Fat necrosis	A benign, usually painless lump; forms as a result of injury to breast tissue. Abnormal calcification on mammography; biopsy shows necrotic fat, giant cells. Up to 50% of patients may not report trauma.
Gynecomastia	Occurs in males 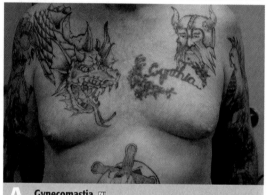. Results from hyperestrogenism (cirrhosis, testicular tumor, puberty, old age), Klinefelter syndrome, or drugs (**S**pironolactone, marijuana [**D**ope], **D**igitalis, **E**strogen, **C**imetidine, **A**lcohol, **H**eroin, **D**opamine D$_2$ antagonists, **K**etoconazole). ("**Some Dope Drugs E**asily **C**reate **A**wkward **H**airy **DD K**nockers.")

A **Gynecomastia.** RU

Prostate pathology

Prostate pathology	Prostatitis—dysuria, frequency, urgency, low back pain. Acute: bacterial (e.g., *E. coli*); chronic: bacterial or abacterial (most common).

Benign prostatic hyperplasia	Common in men > 50 years old. Hyperplasia (not hypertrophy) of the prostate gland. Characterized by a smooth, elastic, firm nodular enlargement of the periurethral (lateral and middle) lobes, which compress the urethra into a vertical slit. Not considered a premalignant lesion. Often presents with ↑ frequency of urination, nocturia, difficulty starting and stopping the stream of urine, and dysuria. May lead to distention and hypertrophy of the bladder, hydronephrosis, and UTIs. ↑ free prostate-specific antigen (PSA). Treatment: α$_1$-antagonists (terazosin, tamsulosin), which cause relaxation of smooth muscle; finasteride.

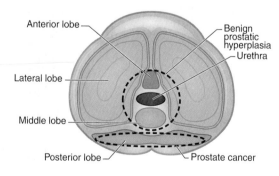

Anterior lobe — Benign prostatic hyperplasia — Urethra

Lateral lobe —

Middle lobe —

Posterior lobe — Prostate cancer

Prostatic adenocarcinoma	Common in men > 50 years old. Arises most often from the posterior lobe (peripheral zone) of the prostate gland 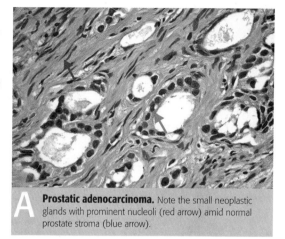 and is most frequently diagnosed by ↑ PSA and subsequent needle core biopsies. Prostatic acid phosphatase (PAP) and PSA are useful tumor markers (↑ total PSA, with ↓ fraction of free PSA). Osteoblastic metastases in bone may develop in late stages, as indicated by lower back pain and an ↑ in serum ALP and PSA.

A **Prostatic adenocarcinoma.** Note the small neoplastic glands with prominent nucleoli (red arrow) amid normal prostate stroma (blue arrow).

Cryptorchidism	Undescended testis (one or both); impaired spermatogenesis (since sperm develop best at temperatures < 37°C); can have normal testosterone levels (Leydig cells are unaffected by temperature); associated with ↑ risk of germ cell tumors. Prematurity ↑ the risk of cryptorchidism. ↓ inhibin, ↑ FSH, and ↑ LH; testosterone ↓ in bilateral cryptorchidism, normal in unilateral.

Varicocele	Dilated veins in pampiniform plexus as a result of ↑ venous pressure; most common cause of scrotal enlargement in adult males; most often on the left side because of ↑ resistance to flow from left gonadal vein drainage into the left renal vein; can cause infertility because of ↑ temperature; "bag of worms" appearance; diagnosed by ultrasound with Doppler 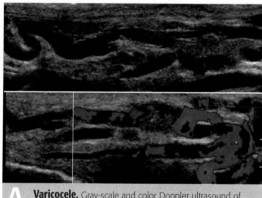. Treatment: varicocelectomy, embolization by interventional radiologist.

A **Varicocele.** Gray-scale and color Doppler ultrasound of dilated pampiniform veins. ✳

Testicular germ cell tumors	~95% of all testicular tumors. Most often occur in young men. Risk factors: cryptorchidism, Klinefelter syndrome. Can present as a mixed germ cell tumor. Differential diagnosis for testicular mass that does not transilluminate: cancer.
Seminoma	Malignant; painless, homogenous testicular enlargement; most common testicular tumor, most common in 3rd decade, never in infancy. Large cells in lobules with watery cytoplasm and a "fried egg" appearance. ↑ placental ALP. Radiosensitive. Late metastasis, excellent prognosis.
Yolk sac (endodermal sinus) tumor	Yellow, mucinous. Aggressive malignancy of testes, analogous to ovarian yolk sac tumor. Schiller-Duval bodies resemble primitive glomeruli. Most common testicular tumor in boys < 3 years old.
Choriocarcinoma	Malignant, ↑ hCG. Disordered syncytiotrophoblastic and cytotrophoblastic elements. Hematogenous metastases to lungs and brain (may present with "hemorrhagic stroke" due to bleeding into the metastasis. May produce gynecomastia or symptoms of hyperthyroidism (hCG is an LH and TSH analog).
Teratoma	Unlike in females, mature teratoma in adult males may be malignant. Benign in children. ↑ hCG and/or AFP in 50% of cases.
Embryonal carcinoma	Malignant, hemorrhagic mass with necrosis; painful; worse prognosis than seminoma. Often glandular/papillary morphology. "Pure" embryonal carcinoma is rare; most commonly mixed with other tumor types. May be associated with ↑ hCG and normal AFP levels when pure (↑ AFP when mixed).

Testicular non–germ cell tumors	5% of all testicular tumors. Mostly benign.
Leydig cell	Contains Reinke crystals; usually androgen producing, gynecomastia in men, precocious puberty in boys. Golden brown color.
Sertoli cell	Androblastoma from sex cord stroma.
Testicular lymphoma	Most common testicular cancer in older men. Not a primary cancer, arises from lymphoma metastases to testes. Aggressive.

Tunica vaginalis lesions	Lesions in the serous covering of testis present as testicular masses that can be transilluminated (vs. testicular tumors). Hydrocele—↑ fluid 2° to incomplete obliteration of processus vaginalis Spermatocele—dilated epididymal duct

Penile pathology

Squamous cell carcinoma	More common in Asia, Africa, and South America. Precursor in situ lesions: Bowen disease (in penile shaft, presents as leukoplakia), erythroplasia of Queyrat (cancer of glans, presents as erythroplakia), Bowenoid papulosis (presents as reddish papules). Associated with HPV, lack of circumcision.
Priapism	Painful sustained erection not associated with sexual stimulation or desire. Associated with trauma, sickle cell disease (sickled RBCs get trapped in vascular channels), medications (anticoagulants, PDE-5 inhibitors, antidepressants, α-blockers, cocaine).

▶ REPRODUCTIVE–PHARMACOLOGY

Control of reproductive hormones

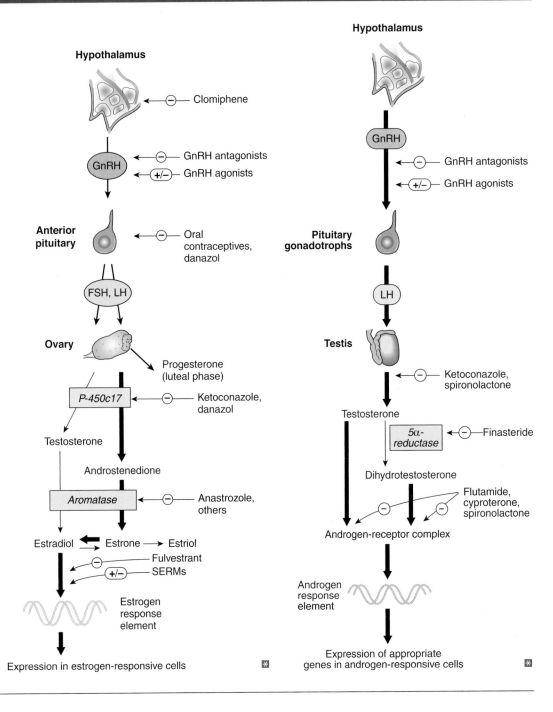

Leuprolide

MECHANISM	GnRH analog with agonist properties when used in pulsatile fashion; antagonist properties when used in continuous fashion (downregulates GnRH receptor in pituitary → ↓ FSH/LH).	Leuprolide can be used in lieu of GnRH.
CLINICAL USE	Infertility (pulsatile), prostate cancer (continuous—use with flutamide), uterine fibroids (continuous), precocious puberty (continuous).	
TOXICITY	Antiandrogen, nausea, vomiting.	

Estrogens (ethinyl estradiol, DES, mestranol)

MECHANISM	Bind estrogen receptors.
CLINICAL USE	Hypogonadism or ovarian failure, menstrual abnormalities, HRT in postmenopausal women; use in men with androgen-dependent prostate cancer.
TOXICITY	↑ risk of endometrial cancer, bleeding in postmenopausal women, clear cell adenocarcinoma of vagina in females exposed to DES in utero, ↑ risk of thrombi. Contraindications—ER ⊕ breast cancer, history of DVTs.

Selective estrogen receptor modulators—SERMs

Clomiphene	Antagonist at estrogen receptors in hypothalamus. Prevents normal feedback inhibition and ↑ release of LH and FSH from pituitary, which stimulates ovulation. Used to treat infertility due to anovulation (e.g., PCOS). May cause hot flashes, ovarian enlargement, multiple simultaneous pregnancies, and visual disturbances.
Tamoxifen	Antagonist on breast tissue; agonist at uterus, bone; associated with endometrial cancer, thromboembolic events. Primarily used to treat and prevent recurrence of ER ⊕ breast cancer.
Raloxifene	Agonist on bone; antagonist at uterus; also ↑ risk of thromboembolic events; ↓ resorption of bone → used to treat osteoporosis.

Hormone replacement therapy

Used for relief or prevention of menopausal symptoms (e.g., hot flashes, vaginal atrophy) and osteoporosis (↑ estrogen, ↓ osteoclast activity).

Unopposed estrogen replacement therapy (ERT) ↑ the risk of endometrial cancer, so progesterone is added. Possible increased cardiovascular risk.

Anastrozole/exemestane

Aromatase inhibitors used in postmenopausal women with breast cancer.

Progestins

MECHANISM	Bind progesterone receptors, ↓ growth and ↑ vascularization of endometrium.
CLINICAL USE	Used in oral contraceptives and in the treatment of endometrial cancer and abnormal uterine bleeding.

Mifepristone (RU-486)

MECHANISM	Competitive inhibitor of progestins at progesterone receptors.
CLINICAL USE	Termination of pregnancy. Administered with misoprostol (PGE_1).
TOXICITY	Heavy bleeding, GI effects (nausea, vomiting, anorexia), abdominal pain.

Oral contraception (synthetic progestins, estrogen)

Estrogen and progestins inhibit LH/FSH and thus prevent estrogen surge. No estrogen surge → no LH surge → no ovulation.

Progestins cause thickening of the cervical mucus, thereby limiting access of sperm to uterus. Progestins also inhibit endometrial proliferation, thus making endometrium less suitable for the implantation of an embryo.

Contraindications—smokers > 35 years old (↑ risk of cardiovascular events), patients with history of thromboembolism and stroke or history of estrogen-dependent tumor.

Terbutaline

β_2-agonist that relaxes the uterus; used to ↓ contraction frequency in women during labor.

Danazol

MECHANISM	Synthetic androgen that acts as partial agonist at androgen receptors.
CLINICAL USE	Endometriosis and hereditary angioedema.
TOXICITY	Weight gain, edema, acne, hirsutism, masculinization, ↓ HDL levels, hepatotoxicity.

Testosterone, methyltestosterone

MECHANISM	Agonist at androgen receptors.
CLINICAL USE	Treats hypogonadism and promotes development of 2° sex characteristics; stimulation of anabolism to promote recovery after burn or injury.
TOXICITY	Causes masculinization in females; ↓ intratesticular testosterone in males by inhibiting release of LH (via negative feedback) → gonadal atrophy. Premature closure of epiphyseal plates. ↑ LDL, ↓ HDL.

Antiandrogens

Testosterone $\xrightarrow{5\alpha\text{-reductase}}$ DHT (more potent).

Finasteride	A 5α-reductase inhibitor (↓ conversion of testosterone to DHT). Useful in BPH. Also promotes hair growth—used to treat male-pattern baldness.	To prevent male-pattern hair loss, give a drug that will encourage female breast growth.
Flutamide	A nonsteroidal competitive inhibitor of androgens at the testosterone receptor. Used in prostate carcinoma.	
Ketoconazole	Inhibits steroid synthesis (inhibits 17,20-desmolase).	Ketoconazole and spironolactone are used in the treatment of polycystic ovarian syndrome to prevent hirsutism. Both have side effects of gynecomastia and amenorrhea.
Spironolactone	Inhibits steroid binding, 17α-hydroxylase, and 17,20-desmolase.	

Tamsulosin	α_1-antagonist used to treat BPH by inhibiting smooth muscle contraction. Selective for $\alpha_{1A,D}$ receptors (found on prostate) vs. vascular α_{1B} receptors.

Sildenafil, vardenafil		
MECHANISM	Inhibit phosphodiesterase 5, causing ↑ cGMP, smooth muscle relaxation in the corpus cavernosum, ↑ blood flow, and penile erection.	Sildenafil and vardenafil fill the penis.
CLINICAL USE	Treatment of erectile dysfunction.	
TOXICITY	Headache, flushing, dyspepsia, impaired blue-green color vision. Risk of life-threatening hypotension in patients taking nitrates.	"Hot and sweaty," but then Headache, Heartburn, Hypotension.

Respiratory

"There's so much pollution in the air now that if it weren't for our lungs, there'd be no place to put it all."

—Robert Orben

"Mars is essentially in the same orbit. Somewhat the same distance from the Sun, which is very important. We have seen pictures where there are canals, we believe, and water. If there is water, that means there is oxygen. If there is oxygen, that means we can breathe."

—Former Vice President Dan Quayle

"None of us is different either as barbarian or as Greek; for we all breathe into the air with mouth and nostrils."

—Antiphon

"Life is not the amount of breaths you take; it's the moments that take your breath away."

—Hitch

▸ RESPIRATORY–ANATOMY

Respiratory tree

Conducting zone	Large airways consist of nose, pharynx, larynx, trachea, and bronchi. Small airways consist of bronchioles and terminal bronchioles (large numbers in parallel → least airway resistance). Warms, humidifies, and filters air but does not participate in gas exchange → "anatomic dead space." Cartilage and goblet cells extend to end of bronchi. Pseudostratified ciliated columnar cells (beat mucus up and out of lungs) extend to beginning of terminal bronchioles, then transition to cuboidal cells. Airway smooth muscles extend to end of terminal bronchioles (sparse beyond this point).
Respiratory zone	Lung parenchyma; consists of respiratory bronchioles, alveolar ducts, and alveoli. Participates in gas exchange. Mostly cuboidal cells in respiratory bronchioles, then simple squamous cells up to alveoli. No cilia. Alveolar macrophages clear debris and participate in immune response.

pseudostratified columnar epithelium
↓ (beginning of terminal bronchioles)
cuboidal epithelium
↓
squamous cells.

Pulmonary artery — Alveolar duct
Alveolar sacs
Pulmonary vein
Alveolar capillary beds
Alveoli

Pneumocytes

Type I cells	97% of alveolar surfaces. Line the alveoli. Squamous; thin for optimal gas diffusion.
Type II cells	Secrete pulmonary surfactant → ↓ alveolar surface tension and prevention of alveolar collapse (atelectasis). Cuboidal and clustered. Also serve as precursors to type I cells and other type II cells. Type II cells proliferate during lung damage.
Club (Clara) cells *Reserve cells.*	Nonciliated; low-columnar/cuboidal with secretory granules. Secrete component of surfactant; degrade toxins; act as reserve cells.

$$\text{Collapsing pressure } (P) = \frac{2 \text{ (surface tension)}}{\text{radius}}$$

Alveoli have ↑ tendency to collapse on expiration as radius ↓ (law of Laplace).

Pulmonary surfactant is a complex mix of lecithins, the most important of which is dipalmitoylphosphatidylcholine.

Surfactant synthesis begins around week 26 of gestation, but mature levels are not achieved until around week 35.

Lecithin-to-sphingomyelin ratio > 2.0 in amniotic fluid indicates fetal lung maturity.

Lung relations

Right lung has 3 lobes; Left has Less Lobes (2) and Lingula (homologue of right middle lobe). Right lung is more common site for inhaled foreign body because the <u>right</u> main stem <u>bronchus</u> is <u>wider</u> and <u>more vertical</u> than the left.

Aspirate a peanut:
- While upright—lower portion of right inferior lobe. *RLL .*
- While supine—superior portion of right inferior lobe.

supine = superior (portion). RLL .

Instead of a middle lobe, the left lung has a space occupied by the heart. The relation of the pulmonary artery to the bronchus at each lung hilus is described by **RALS**—Right Anterior; Left Superior.

ic: Right PA = in front of bronchus
Left PA = superior to bronchus

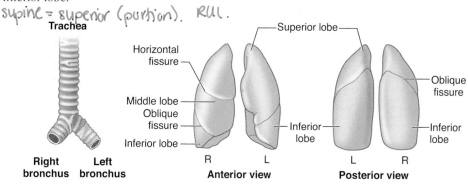

Trachea

Right bronchus   Left bronchus

Horizontal fissure

Middle lobe
Oblique fissure

Inferior lobe

Superior lobe

Oblique fissure

Inferior lobe

Inferior lobe

R   L
Anterior view

L   R
Posterior view

Diaphragm structures

Central tendon

Inferior vena cava (T8)

Esophagus (T10)

Rib   Aorta (T12)
Vertebrae

Inferior view

Structures perforating diaphragm:
- At T8: IVC
- At T10: esophagus, vagus (CN 10; 2 trunks) *✓ nerve*
- At T12: aorta (red), thoracic duct (white), azygos vein (blue) ("At **T-1-2** it's the **red**, **white**, and **blue**")

Diaphragm is innervated by **C3, 4,** and **5** (phrenic nerve). Pain from diaphragm irritation (e.g., air or blood in peritoneal cavity) can be referred to the shoulder (C5) and the trapezius ridge (C3, 4).

Number of letters = T level:
T8: vena cava
T10: "oesophagus"
T12: aortic hiatus

I (IVC) **ate** (8) **ten** (10) **eggs** (esophagus) at (aorta) **twelve** (12).

C3, 4, 5 keeps the diaphragm **alive**.

▶ RESPIRATORY–PHYSIOLOGY

Lung volumes

Inspiratory reserve volume (IRV)	Air that can still be breathed in after normal inspiration
Tidal volume (TV)	Air that moves into lung with each quiet inspiration, typically 500 mL
Expiratory reserve volume (ERV)	Air that can still be breathed out after normal expiration
Residual volume (RV)	Air in lung after maximal expiration; cannot be measured on spirometry
Inspiratory capacity (IC)	IRV + TV *how much you can inspire total*
Functional residual capacity (FRC)	RV + ERV (volume in lungs after normal expiration)
Vital capacity (VC)	TV + IRV + ERV ⟹ Maximum volume of gas that can be expired after a maximal inspiration
Total lung capacity (TLC)	IRV + TV + ERV + RV Volume of gas present in lungs after a maximal inspiration *EVERYTHING.*

Lung volumes (LITER):

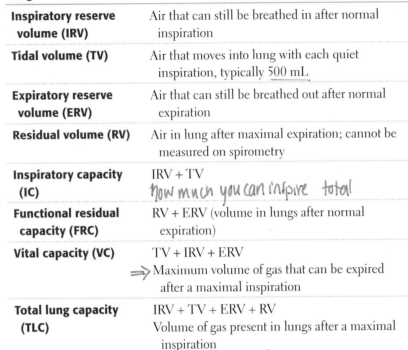
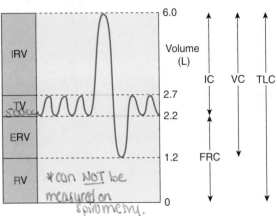

can NOT be measured on spirometry.

A capacity is a sum of ≥ 2 volumes.

| **Determination of physiologic dead space** | $V_D = V_T \times \dfrac{P_aCO_2 - P_ECO_2}{P_aCO_2}$ V_D = physiologic dead space = anatomic dead space of conducting airways plus functional dead space in alveoli; apex of healthy lung is largest contributor of functional dead space. Volume of inspired air that does not take part in gas exchange. V_T = tidal volume. *(@ breathing = ~500cc)* P_aCO_2 = arterial P_{CO_2}, P_ECO_2 = expired air P_{CO_2}. | Taco, Paco, Peco, Paco (refers to order of variables in equation) |

↳ *anatomic dead space + V/Q mismatch areas.*

Can see what was produced.

Ventilation

Minute ventilation (V_E)	Total volume of gas entering the lungs per minute $V_E = V_T \times$ respiratory rate (RR) *= TV × RR*
Alveolar ventilation (V_A)	Volume of gas per unit time that reaches the alveoli $V_A = (V_T - V_D) \times RR$

↳ *need to factor in the dead space.*

Lung and chest wall

Tendency for lungs to collapse inward and chest wall to spring outward.

At FRC, inward pull of lung is balanced by outward pull of chest wall, and system pressure is atmospheric.

Elastic properties of both chest wall and lungs determine their combined volume.

At FRC, airway and alveolar pressures are 0, and intrapleural pressure is negative (prevents pneumothorax). PVR is at minimum.

Compliance—change in lung volume for a given change in pressure; ↓ in pulmonary fibrosis, pneumonia, and pulmonary edema; ↑ in emphysema and normal aging.

FRC= Residual Volume + ERV (ie. air still lungs after breathing).

PVR= pulm. vascular resistance.

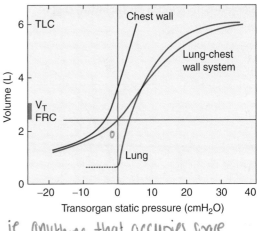

ie. anything that occupies space.

Hemoglobin

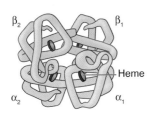

β₂ β₁
Heme
α₂ α₁

Hemoglobin (Hb) is composed of 4 polypeptide subunits (2 α and 2 β) and exists in 2 forms:
- T (taut) form has low affinity for O_2.
- R (relaxed) form has high affinity for O_2 (300×). Hb exhibits positive cooperativity and negative allostery.

↑ Cl^-, H^+, CO_2, 2,3-BPG, and temperature favor taut form over relaxed form (shifts dissociation curve to right, leading to ↑ O_2 unloading).

Fetal Hb (2 α and 2 γ subunits) has lower affinity for 2,3-BPG than adult Hb and thus has higher affinity for O_2.

Taut in **T**issues.
Relaxed in **R**espiratory tract.

Hemoglobin modifications

Lead to tissue hypoxia from ↓ O_2 saturation and ↓ O_2 content.

Methemoglobin

Oxidized form of Hb (ferric, Fe^{3+}) that does not bind O_2 as readily, but has ↑ affinity for cyanide.

Iron in Hb is normally in a reduced state (ferrous, Fe^{2+}).

Methemoglobinemia may present with cyanosis and chocolate-colored blood.

To treat cyanide poisoning, use nitrites to oxidize Hb to methemoglobin, which binds cyanide. Use thiosulfate to bind this cyanide, forming thiocyanate, which is renally excreted.

Methemoglobinemia can be treated with methylene blue.

Nitrites cause poisoning by oxidizing Fe^{2+} to Fe^{3+}.

Just the 2 of us: ferrous is Fe^{2+}.

Rx = methylene blue.

Carboxyhemoglobin

Form of Hb bound to CO in place of O_2.

Causes ↓ oxygen-binding capacity with a left shift in the oxygen-hemoglobin dissociation curve. ↓ O_2 unloading in tissues.

CO has 200× greater affinity than O_2 for Hb.

CO = carbon monoxide

+fetal Hgb

Oxygen-hemoglobin dissociation curve

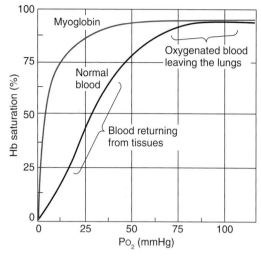

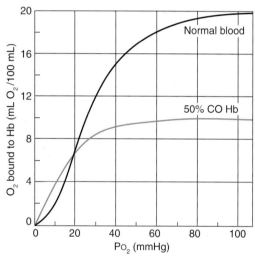

Sigmoidal shape due to positive cooperativity (i.e., tetrameric Hb molecule can bind 4 O_2 molecules and has higher affinity for each subsequent O_2 molecule bound). Myoglobin is monomeric and thus does not show positive cooperativity; curve lacks sigmoidal appearance.

When curve shifts to the right, ↓ affinity of Hb for O_2 (facilitates unloading of O_2 to tissue).

An ↑ in all factors (including H^+) causes a shift of the curve to the right.

A ↓ in all factors (including H^+) causes a shift of the curve to the left.

Fetal Hb has a higher affinity for O_2 than adult Hb, so its dissociation curve is shifted left.

Right shift—**BAT ACE**:
  BPG (2,3-BPG) (↑)
  Altitude → see p. 601.
  Temperature (↑)
  Acid (↑)
  CO_2 (↑)
  Exercise

NB. fetal Hgb not as responsive to 2,3. BPG.

Oxygen content of blood

(≈20.1 ccO_2/dL)

O_2 content = (O_2 binding capacity × % saturation) + dissolved O_2.

Normally 1 g Hb can bind 1.34 mL O_2; normal Hb amount in blood is 15 g/dL. Cyanosis results when deoxygenated Hb > 5 g/dL. (> ⅓)

O_2 binding capacity ≈ 20.1 mL O_2/dL.

→ amount dissolved in blood.

O_2 content of arterial blood ↓ as Hb falls, but O_2 saturation and arterial Po_2 do not.

O_2 delivery to tissues = cardiac output × O_2 content of blood.

	Hb level	% O₂ sat of Hb	Dissolved O₂ (Pao₂)	Total O₂ content
CO poisoning	Normal	↓ (CO competes with O₂)	Normal	↓
Anemia	↓	Normal	Normal	↓
Polycythemia	↑	Normal	Normal	↑

Pulmonary circulation

Normally a low-resistance, high-compliance system. PO_2 and PCO_2 exert opposite effects on pulmonary and systemic circulation. A ↓ in PAO_2 causes a hypoxic vasoconstriction that shifts blood away from poorly ventilated regions of lung to well-ventilated regions of lung.

Perfusion limited—O_2 (normal health), CO_2, N_2O. Gas equilibrates early along the length of the capillary. Diffusion can be ↑ only if blood flow ↑.

Diffusion limited—O_2 (emphysema, fibrosis), CO. Gas does not equilibrate by the time blood reaches the end of the capillary.

[handwritten: PAO₂ = pulm. art. O₂]

A consequence of pulmonary hypertension is cor pulmonale and subsequent right ventricular failure (jugular venous distention, edema, hepatomegaly).

Diffusion: $V_{gas} = A/T \times D_k(P_1 - P_2)$ where A = area, T = thickness, and $D_k(P_1 - P_2) \approx$ difference in partial pressures:

- A ↓ in emphysema.
- T ↑ in pulmonary fibrosis. *[handwritten: cannot diffuse as readily across the membrane.]*

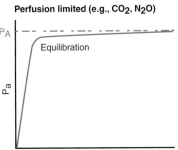

[handwritten below left graph: unless there is more flow, no further perfusion will take place. ↳exchange]

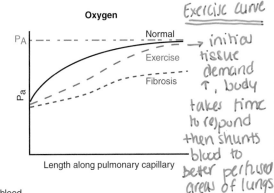

[handwritten right of Oxygen graph: Exercise curve → initial tissue demand ↑, body takes time to respond then shunts blood to better perfused areas of lungs.]

Perfusion limited (e.g., CO_2, N_2O) — Equilibration

Diffusion limited (e.g., CO) — Partial pressure difference between alveolar air and pulmonary capillary blood

Oxygen — Normal / Exercise / Fibrosis

Length along pulmonary capillary

P_a = partial pressure of gas in pulmonary capillary blood
P_A = partial pressure of gas in alveolar air

Pulmonary vascular resistance

$$PVR = \frac{P_{pulm\ artery} - P_{L\ atrium}}{cardiac\ output}$$

Remember: $\Delta P = Q \times R$, so $R = \Delta P / Q$

$R = 8\eta l / \pi r^4$

$P_{pulm\ artery}$ = pressure in pulmonary artery
$P_{L\ atrium}$ = pulmonary wedge pressure *[handwritten: ↳ what it is up against (returns to here).]*

η = viscosity of blood; l = vessel length;
r = vessel radius

Alveolar gas equation

$$PAO_2 = PIO_2 - \frac{PaCO_2}{R}$$

$$\approx 150 - \frac{PaCO_2}{0.8}$$

PAO_2 = alveolar PO_2 (mmHg).
PIO_2 = PO_2 in inspired air (mmHg).
$PaCO_2$ = arterial PCO_2 (mmHg).
R = respiratory quotient = CO_2 produced/O_2 consumed.

A-a gradient = $PAO_2 - PaO_2$ = 10–15 mmHg.
↑ A-a gradient may occur in hypoxemia; causes include shunting, V/Q mismatch, fibrosis (impairs diffusion).

Oxygen deprivation

Hypoxemia ($\downarrow Pao_2$)	Hypoxia ($\downarrow O_2$ delivery to tissue)	Ischemia (loss of blood flow)
Normal A-a gradient	$\downarrow$ cardiac output	Impeded arterial flow
▪ High altitude	Hypoxemia (↓O₂ content).	$\downarrow$ venous drainage
▪ Hypoventilation	Anemia (not enough Hgb to bind O₂)	
↑ A-a gradient	CO poisoning	
▪ V/Q mismatch		
▪ Diffusion limitation (eg. pulm. fibrosis)		
▪ Right-to-left shunt		

V/Q mismatch

Ideally, ventilation is matched to perfusion (i.e., V/Q = 1) in order for adequate gas exchange.
Lung zones:
- Apex of the lung—V/Q = 3 (wasted ventilation)
- Base of the lung—V/Q = 0.6 (wasted perfusion)

Both ventilation and perfusion are greater at the base of the lung than at the apex of the lung.

With exercise ($\uparrow$ cardiac output), there is vasodilation of apical capillaries, resulting in a V/Q ratio that approaches 1.

Certain organisms that thrive in high O_2 (e.g., TB) flourish in the apex.

V/Q → 0 = airway obstruction (shunt). In shunt, 100% O_2 does not improve Po_2.

V/Q → ∞ = blood flow obstruction (physiologic dead space). Assuming < 100% dead space, 100% O_2 improves Po_2.

c exercise get vaso-
dilation of arteries
in Apex so
. V/Q ~1 like
in lung base zone.

best matched
zone.

higher O₂ content
at end of expiration
b/c not utilised
2° to V/Q mismatch

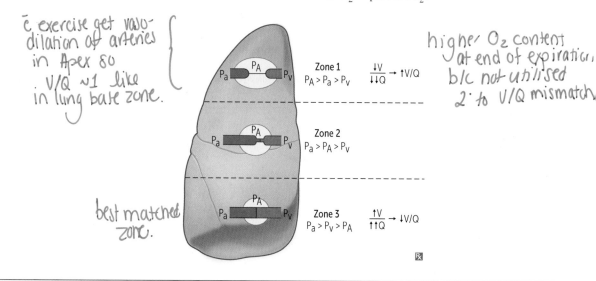

	Zone 1	$\dfrac{\downarrow V}{\downarrow\downarrow Q} \rightarrow \uparrow V/Q$
	$P_A > P_a > P_v$	
	Zone 2	
	$P_a > P_A > P_v$	
	Zone 3	$\dfrac{\uparrow V}{\uparrow\uparrow Q} \rightarrow \downarrow V/Q$
	$P_a > P_v > P_A$	

| **CO₂ transport** | CO_2 is transported from tissues to the lungs in 3 forms:
• HCO_3^- (90%).
• Carbaminohemoglobin or $HbCO_2$ (5%). CO_2 bound to Hb at N-terminus of globin (not heme). CO₂ binding favors taut form (O₂ unloaded).
• Dissolved CO_2 (5%). | In lungs, oxygenation of Hb promotes dissociation of H^+ from Hb. This shifts equilibrium toward CO_2 formation; therefore, CO_2 is released from RBCs (Haldane effect).
In peripheral tissue, ↑ H^+ from tissue metabolism shifts curve to right, unloading O_2 (Bohr effect).
Majority of blood CO_2 is carried as HCO_3^- in the plasma. |

NB. O₂ favors relaxed form
CO₂ favors taut form.

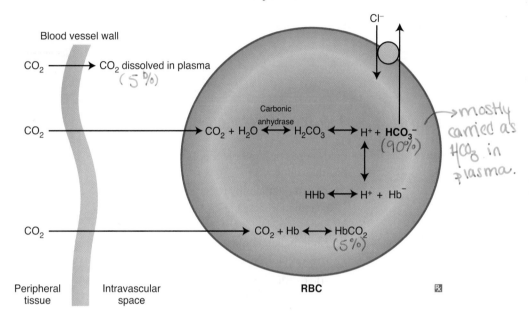

→ less dissolved in blood b/c less O₂ available in the air.

| **Response to high altitude** | ↓ atmospheric oxygen → ↓ PaO_2 → ↑ ventilation → ↓ $PaCO_2$.
Chronic ↑ in ventilation.
↑ erythropoietin → ↑ hematocrit and Hb (chronic hypoxia).
↑ 2,3-BPG (binds to Hb so that Hb releases more O_2). ✱
Cellular changes (↑ mitochondria).
↑ renal excretion of HCO_3^- (e.g., can augment by use of acetazolamide) to compensate for the respiratory alkalosis.
Chronic hypoxic pulmonary vasoconstriction results in RVH. |

↳ ® ventricular hypertrophy.

| **Response to exercise** | ↑ CO_2 production.
↑ O_2 consumption.
↑ ventilation rate to meet O_2 demand.
V/Q ratio from apex to base becomes more uniform. ~ V/Q = 1.
↑ pulmonary blood flow due to ↑ cardiac output.
↓ pH during strenuous exercise (2° to lactic acidosis). → causes more unloading of O₂ at tissues (® shift)
No change in PaO_2 and $PaCO_2$, but ↑ in venous CO_2 content and ↓ in venous O_2 content. |

arterial values of O₂ & CO₂.

▸ RESPIRATORY–PATHOLOGY

Rhinosinusitis

Obstruction of sinus drainage into nasal cavity → inflammation and pain over affected area (typically maxillary sinuses in adults 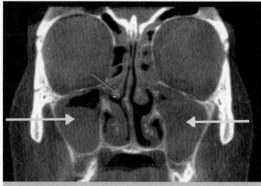). Most common acute cause is viral URI; may cause superimposed bacterial infection, most commonly *S. pneumoniae*, *H. influenzae*, and *M. catarrhalis*.

[handwritten] ⟶ ✳ Same organisms as seen in AOM.

A **Rhinosinusitis.** Coronal CT of the sinus shows bilateral maxillary sinusitis (yellow arrows) and unrelated nasal septal deviation (red arrow). ✳

[handwritten] → In Sinusitis & AOM → Involved organisms are S. pneumo, H. influenza & M. catarrhalis

Deep venous thrombosis

Predisposed by Virchow triad: *(predisposition)*
1. Stasis
2. Hypercoagulability (e.g., defect in coagulation cascade proteins, most commonly factor V Leiden)
3. Endothelial damage (exposed collagen triggers clotting cascade)
(need the trigger)

Approximately 95% of pulmonary emboli arise from deep leg veins.
Homan sign—dorsiflexion of foot → calf pain. *→ 50% accurate*
Use heparin for prevention and acute management; use warfarin for long-term prevention of DVT recurrence.

Pulmonary emboli

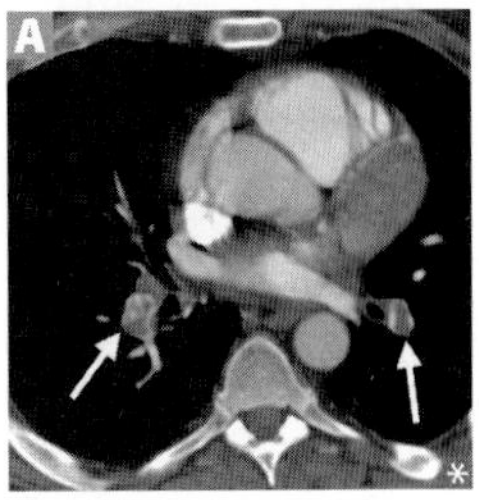

V/Q mismatch → hypoxemia → respiratory alkalosis. Sudden-onset dyspnea, chest pain, tachypnea. May present as sudden death.

Types: Fat, Air, Thrombus, Bacteria, Amniotic fluid, Tumor. Fat emboli—associated with long bone fractures and liposuction; classic triad of hypoxemia, neurologic abnormalities, and petechial rash.

(hematologic)

Amniotic fluid emboli—can lead to DIC, especially postpartum.

Gas emboli—nitrogen bubbles precipitate in ascending divers; treat with hyperbaric oxygen. → give 100% O_2

→ can sometimes also help resorb PE's. (if small)

An embolus moves like a FAT BAT.

CT pulmonary angiography is the imaging test of choice for a PE (look for filling defects) A B C.

DIC = disseminated intravascular coagulation.

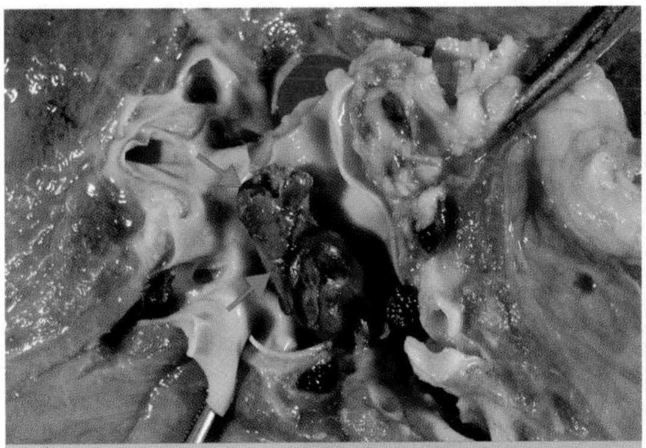

B **Pulmonary embolism.** Note large embolus (arrows) in the pulmonary artery.

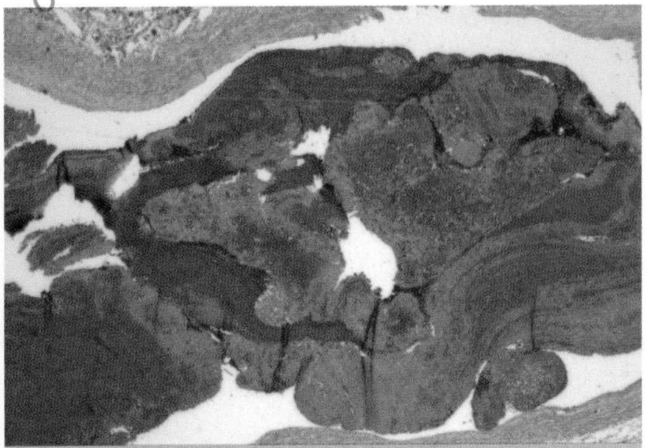

C **Pulmonary thromboembolus.** Lines of Zahn are interdigitating areas of pink (platelets, fibrin) and red (RBCs) found only in thrombi formed before death. Help distinguish pre- and postmortem thrombi.

pre-mortem thrombi = lines of Zahn.
↳ plts, fibrin & PRBC's.

FVC = forced vital capacity.

Obstructive lung diseases	Obstruction of air flow resulting in air trapping in the lungs. Airways close prematurely at high lung volumes → ↑ RV and ↓ FVC. PFTs: ↓↓ FEV_1, ↓ FVC → ↓ FEV_1/FVC ratio (hallmark), V/Q mismatch. Chronic, hypoxic pulmonary vasoconstriction can lead to cor pulmonale. *(like pulmonary hypertension).*	
TYPE	PATHOLOGY	OTHER
Chronic bronchitis ("blue bloater")	A form of COPD along with emphysema. Hyperplasia of mucus-secreting glands in the bronchi → Reid index (thickness of gland layer/total thickness of bronchial wall) > 50%.	Productive cough for > 3 months per year (not necessarily consecutive) for > 2 years. Disease of small airways. Findings: wheezing, crackles, cyanosis (early-onset hypoxemia due to shunting), late-onset dyspnea, CO_2 retention.
Emphysema ("pink puffer," barrel-shaped chest)	Enlargement of air spaces, ↓ recoil, ↑ compliance, ↓ DLCO resulting from destruction of alveolar walls **A**. Two types: <ul><li>Centriacinar—associated with smoking **B**.</li><li>Panacinar—associated with α_1-antitrypsin deficiency.</li></ul>	↑ elastase activity → loss of elastic fibers → ↑ lung compliance. Exhalation through pursed lips to ↑ airway pressure and prevent airway collapse during respiration. *(auto PEEP → like CPAP).*

A **Emphysema.** On microscopy, enlarged alveoli separated by thin septa seen on left. There is relative preservation of alveoli on right. ✦

B **Centriacinar emphysema.** Gross specimen shows multiple air-space cavities lined by heavy black carbon deposits. ✦

Asthma	Bronchial hyperresponsiveness causes reversible bronchoconstriction. Smooth muscle hypertrophy, Curschmann spirals (shed epithelium forms mucus plugs), and Charcot-Leyden crystals (formed from breakdown of eosinophils in sputum).	Can be triggered by viral URIs, allergens, and stress. Test with methacholine challenge. Findings: cough, wheezing, tachypnea, dyspnea, hypoxemia, ↓ I/E ratio, pulsus paradoxus, mucus plugging. ↳ *prolonged expiratory phase.*
Bronchiectasis	Chronic necrotizing infection of bronchi → permanently dilated airways, purulent sputum, recurrent infections, hemoptysis.	Associated with bronchial obstruction, poor ciliary motility (smoking), Kartagener syndrome, cystic fibrosis, allergic bronchopulmonary aspergillosis.

↳airways distal to foreign body obstruction if prolonged

Restrictive lung disease

Restricted lung expansion causes ↓ lung volumes (↓ FVC and TLC). PFTs: FEV_1/FVC ratio ≥ 80%. *→usually maintained ratio.*

Types:

- Poor breathing mechanics (extrapulmonary, peripheral hypoventilation, normal A-a gradient):
  - Poor muscular effort—polio, myasthenia gravis
  - Poor structural apparatus—scoliosis, morbid obesity

  } other than interstitium.
- Interstitial lung diseases (pulmonary ↓ diffusing capacity, ↑ A-a gradient):
  - Acute respiratory distress syndrome (ARDS)
  - Neonatal respiratory distress syndrome (hyaline membrane disease) *→ lacking surfactant.*
  - Pneumoconioses (anthracosis, silicosis, asbestosis)
  - Sarcoidosis: bilateral hilar lymphadenopathy, noncaseating granuloma; ↑ ACE and Ca^{2+}
  - Idiopathic pulmonary fibrosis (repeated cycles of lung injury and wound healing with ↑ collagen deposition)
  - Goodpasture syndrome
  - Granulomatosis with polyangiitis (Wegener)
  - Langerhans cell histiocytosis (eosinophilic granuloma)
  - Hypersensitivity pneumonitis
  - Drug toxicity (bleomycin, busulfan, amiodarone, methotrexate)

Hypersensitivity pneumonitis

Mixed type III/IV hypersensitivity reaction to environmental antigen → dyspnea, cough, chest tightness, headache. Often seen in farmers and those exposed to birds.

ppl who inspire particles that are # irritating to the lungs.

upper lobes affected   *lower lobes affected.*

Pneumoconioses	Coal workers' pneumoconiosis, silicosis, and asbestosis → ↑ risk of cor pulmonale and Caplan syndrome (rheumatoid arthritis and pneumoconioses with intrapulmonary nodules).	

Asbestosis

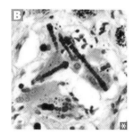

Associated with shipbuilding, roofing, and plumbing. "Ivory white," calcified pleural plaques **A** are pathognomonic of asbestos exposure, but are not precancerous. Associated with an ↑ incidence of bronchogenic carcinoma and mesothelioma.

Affects lower lobes.
Asbestos (ferruginous) bodies are golden-brown fusiform rods resembling dumbbells **B**.
Asbestos is from the roof (was common in insulation), but affects the base (lower lobes).
Silica and coal are from the base (earth), but affect the roof (upper lobes).

small particles penetrate deep into the distal airways causing irritation to the pleura ←

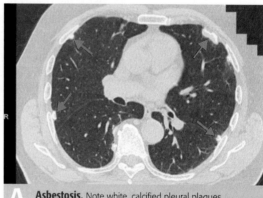

Asbestosis. Note white, calcified pleural plaques (arrows). ✼

Coal workers' pneumoconiosis	Prolonged coal dust exposure → macrophages laden with carbon → inflammation and fibrosis. Also known as black lung disease.	Affects upper lobes. **Anthracosis**—asymptomatic condition found in many urban dwellers exposed to sooty air.
Silicosis	Associated with foundries, sandblasting, and mines. Macrophages respond to silica and release fibrogenic factors, leading to fibrosis. It is thought that silica may disrupt phagolysosomes and impair macrophages, increasing susceptibility to TB. Also ↑ risk of bronchogenic carcinoma.	Affects upper lobes. ✻"Eggshell" calcification of hilar lymph nodes.

Neonatal respiratory distress syndrome	Surfactant deficiency → ↑ surface tension → alveolar collapse. A lecithin:sphingomyelin ratio < 1.5 in amniotic fluid is predictive of neonatal respiratory distress syndrome. Persistently low O_2 tension → risk of PDA. Therapeutic supplemental O_2 can result in retinopathy of prematurity and bronchopulmonary dysplasia. Risk factors: prematurity, maternal diabetes (due to ↑ fetal insulin), C-section delivery (↓ release of fetal glucocorticoids). *⌐ β-methasone.* Treatment: maternal steroids before birth; artificial surfactant for infant.

Need ↑ O_2 content in blood to close PDA (esp. 1ˢᵗ 24hrs)

Acute respiratory distress syndrome

May be caused by trauma, sepsis, shock, gastric aspiration, uremia, acute pancreatitis, or amniotic fluid embolism. Diffuse alveolar damage → ↑ alveolar capillary permeability → protein-rich leakage into alveoli and noncardiogenic pulmonary edema (normal PCWP) **A**. Results in formation of intra-alveolar hyaline membrane **B**. Initial damage due to release of neutrophilic substances toxic to alveolar wall, activation of coagulation cascade, and oxygen-derived free radicals.

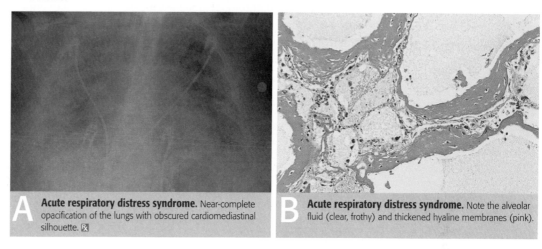

A Acute respiratory distress syndrome. Near-complete opacification of the lungs with obscured cardiomediastinal silhouette. ℞

B Acute respiratory distress syndrome. Note the alveolar fluid (clear, frothy) and thickened hyaline membranes (pink).

Obstructive vs. restrictive lung disease

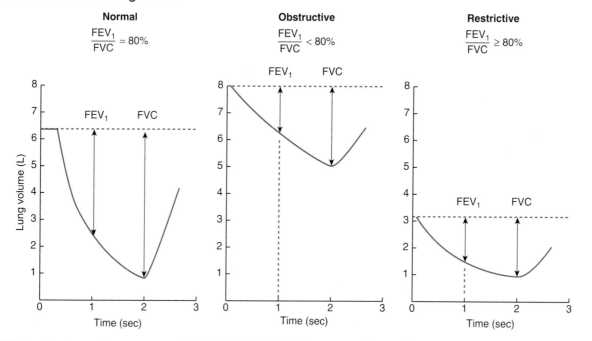

Normal

$$\frac{FEV_1}{FVC} = 80\%$$

Obstructive

$$\frac{FEV_1}{FVC} < 80\%$$

Restrictive

$$\frac{FEV_1}{FVC} \geq 80\%$$

Note: Obstructive lung volumes > normal (↑ TLC, ↑ FRC, ↑ RV); restrictive lung volumes < normal. In both obstructive and restrictive, FEV_1 and FVC are reduced. In obstructive, however, FEV_1 is more dramatically reduced compared to FVC, resulting in a ↓ FEV_1/FVC ratio.

Pulmonary hypertension	Normal pulmonary artery pressure = 10–14 mmHg; pulmonary hypertension ≥ 25 mmHg at rest. Results in arteriosclerosis, medial hypertrophy, and intimal fibrosis of pulmonary arteries.

Primary—due to an inactivating mutation in the *BMPR2* gene (normally functions to inhibit vascular smooth muscle proliferation); poor prognosis.

Secondary—due to COPD (destruction of lung parenchyma); mitral stenosis (↑ resistance → ↑ pressure); recurrent thromboemboli (↓ cross-sectional area of pulmonary vascular bed); autoimmune disease (e.g., systemic sclerosis; inflammation → intimal fibrosis → medial hypertrophy); left-to-right shunt (↑ shear stress → endothelial injury); sleep apnea or living at high altitude (hypoxic vasoconstriction).

Course: severe respiratory distress → cyanosis and RVH → death from decompensated cor pulmonale.

Sleep apnea	Repeated cessation of breathing > 10 seconds during sleep → disrupted sleep → daytime somnolence. Normal PaO_2 during the day.	Treatment: weight loss, CPAP, surgery. Hypoxia → ↑ EPO release → ↑ erythropoiesis.

Nocturnal hypoxia → systemic/pulmonary hypertension, arrhythmias (atrial fibrillation/flutter), and sudden death.

Central sleep apnea—no respiratory effort.

Obstructive sleep apnea—respiratory effort against airway obstruction. Associated with obesity, loud snoring.

Obesity hypoventilation syndrome—obesity (BMI ≥ 30 kg/m^2) → hypoventilation → ↓ PaO_2 and ↑ $PaCO_2$ during waking hours.

Lung–physical findings

ABNORMALITY	BREATH SOUNDS	PERCUSSION	FREMITUS	TRACHEAL DEVIATION
Pleural effusion	↓	Dull	↓	—
Atelectasis (bronchial obstruction)	↓	Dull	↓	Toward side of lesion
Spontaneous pneumothorax	↓	Hyperresonant	↓	—
Tension pneumothorax	↓	Hyperresonant	↓	Away from side of lesion
Consolidation (lobar pneumonia, pulmonary edema)	Bronchial breath sounds; late inspiratory crackles	Dull	↑	—

Lung cancer

Lung cancer is the leading cause of cancer death.
Presentation: cough, hemoptysis, bronchial obstruction, wheezing, pneumonic "coin" lesion on x-ray film or noncalcified nodule on CT.
In the lung, metastases (usually multiple lesions) are more common than 1° neoplasms. Most often from breast, colon, prostate, and bladder cancer.
Sites of metastases from lung cancer—adrenals, brain, bone (pathologic fracture), liver (jaundice, hepatomegaly).

SPHERE of complications:
  Superior vena cava syndrome
  Pancoast tumor
  Horner syndrome
  Endocrine (paraneoplastic)
  Recurrent laryngeal symptoms (hoarseness)
  Effusions (pleural or pericardial)
All lung cancer types except bronchial carcinoid are associated with smoking.
Squamous and Small cell carcinomas are Sentral (central).

TYPE	LOCATION	CHARACTERISTICS	HISTOLOGY
Adenocarcinoma	Peripheral	Most common lung cancer in nonsmokers and overall (except for metastases). Activating mutations include k-*ras*, *EGFR*, and *ALK*. Associated with hypertrophic osteoarthropathy (clubbing). Bronchioloalveolar subtype (adenocarcinoma in situ): CXR often shows hazy infiltrates similar to pneumonia; excellent prognosis.	Bronchioloalveolar subtype: grows along alveolar septa → apparent "thickening" of alveolar walls.
Squamous cell carcinoma	Central	Hilar mass arising from bronchus; Cavitation; Cigarettes; hyperCalcemia (produces PTHrP).	Keratin pearls and intercellular bridges **A**.
Small cell (oat cell) carcinoma	Central	Undifferentiated → very aggressive. May produce ACTH, ADH, or Antibodies against presynaptic Ca²⁺ channels (Lambert-Eaton myasthenic syndrome). Amplification of *myc* oncogenes common. Inoperable; treat with chemotherapy.	Neoplasm of neuroendocrine Kulchitsky cells → small dark blue cells **B**.
Large cell carcinoma	Peripheral	Highly anaplastic undifferentiated tumor; poor prognosis. Less responsive to chemotherapy; removed surgically.	Pleomorphic giant cells.
Bronchial carcinoid tumor	—	Excellent prognosis; metastasis rare. Symptoms usually due to mass effect; occasionally carcinoid syndrome (5-HT secretion → flushing, diarrhea, wheezing).	Nests of neuroendocrine cells; chromogranin A ⊕.

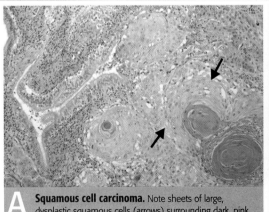

A **Squamous cell carcinoma.** Note sheets of large, dysplastic squamous cells (arrows) surrounding dark, pink keratin pearls (lower right).

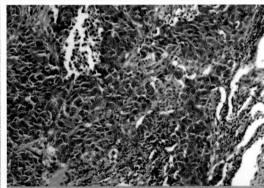

B **Small cell carcinoma.** Sheets of dark purple tumor cells with nuclear molding, high mitotic rate, necrosis, and "salt and pepper" neuroendocrine-type chromatin.

Mesothelioma

Malignancy of the pleura associated with asbestosis. Results in hemorrhagic pleural effusions and pleural thickening.

Psammoma bodies seen on histology.

Pancoast tumor

Carcinoma that occurs in apex of lung may affect cervical sympathetic plexus, causing Horner syndrome (ipsilateral ptosis, miosis, and anhidrosis), SVC syndrome, sensorimotor deficits, and hoarseness 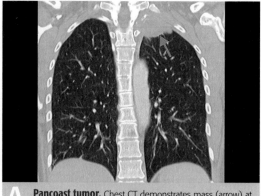.

A **Pancoast tumor.** Chest CT demonstrates mass (arrow) at the left lung apex. ✷

Superior vena cava syndrome

An obstruction of the SVC that impairs blood drainage from the head ("facial plethora"), neck (jugular venous distention), and upper extremities (edema). Commonly caused by malignancy and thrombosis from indwelling catheters. Medical emergency. Can raise intracranial pressure (if obstruction severe) → headaches, dizziness, and ↑ risk of aneurysm/rupture of intracranial arteries.

Pneumonia

TYPE	TYPICAL ORGANISMS	CHARACTERISTICS
Lobar	*S. pneumoniae* most frequently, also *Legionella*, *Klebsiella*	Intra-alveolar exudate → consolidation; may involve entire lung A B.
Bronchopneumonia	*S. pneumoniae, S. aureus, H. influenzae, Klebsiella*	Acute inflammatory infiltrates from bronchioles into adjacent alveoli; patchy distribution involving ≥ 1 lobe C.
Interstitial (atypical) pneumonia	Viruses (influenza, RSV, adenoviruses), *Mycoplasma, Legionella, Chlamydia*	Diffuse patchy inflammation localized to interstitial areas at alveolar walls; distribution involving ≥ 1 lobe D. Generally follows a more indolent course.

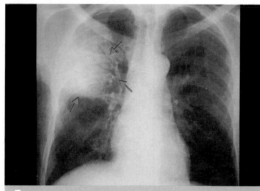

A **Lobar pneumonia.** Dense right upper lobe consolidation with branching air-bronchograms; sharp inferior margin represents the horizontal fissure.

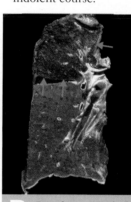

B **Bronchopneumonia (left) and lobar pneumonia (right).** Gross specimens show typical consolidation patterns. ✱, ✱

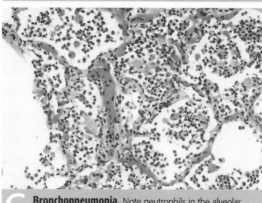

C **Bronchopneumonia.** Note neutrophils in the alveolar spaces. ✱

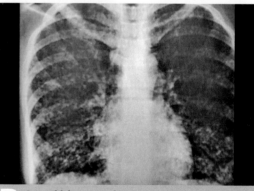

D **Interstitial pneumonia.** Coarse bilateral reticular opacities, worse on the right.

Lung abscess

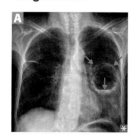

Localized collection of pus within parenchyma. Caused by: bronchial obstruction (e.g., cancer) or aspiration of oropharyngeal contents (especially in patients predisposed to loss of consciousness [e.g., alcoholics or epileptics]).

Air-fluid levels A often seen on CXR. Often due to *S. aureus* or anaerobes (*Bacteroides, Fusobacterium, Peptostreptococcus*).

Pleural effusions	Excess accumulation of fluid between the two pleural layers **A** → restricted lung expansion during inspiration.
Transudate	↓ protein content. Due to CHF, nephrotic syndrome, or hepatic cirrhosis.
Exudate	↑ protein content, cloudy. Due to malignancy, pneumonia, collagen vascular disease, trauma (occurs in states of ↑ vascular permeability). Must be drained in light of risk of infection.
Lymphatic	Also known as chylothorax. Due to thoracic duct injury from trauma, malignancy. Milky-appearing fluid; ↑ triglycerides.

A **Pleural effusion.** Blunting of the left costophrenic angle (arrow) due to fluid in the pleural space. ℞

Pneumothorax	Accumulation of air in the pleural space **A**. Unilateral chest pain and dyspnea, unilateral chest expansion, ↓ tactile fremitus, hyperresonance, diminished breath sounds, all on the affected side.
Spontaneous pneumothorax	Accumulation of air in the pleural space **A**. Occurs most frequently in tall, thin, young males because of rupture of apical blebs.
Tension pneumothorax	Usually occurs in setting of trauma or lung infection. Air is capable of entering pleural space but not exiting. Trachea deviates away from affected lung **B**.

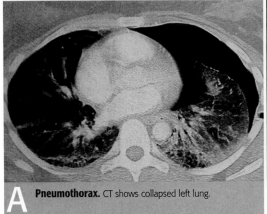

A **Pneumothorax.** CT shows collapsed left lung.

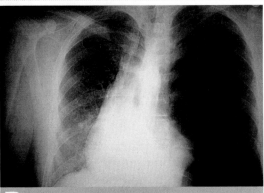

B **Tension pneumothorax.** Note the hyperlucent left lung field with low left hemidiaphragm (below the field of view) and rightward mediastinal shift.

▶ RESPIRATORY–PHARMACOLOGY

H₁ blockers	Reversible inhibitors of H_1 histamine receptors.	
1st generation	Diphenhydramine, dimenhydrinate, chlorpheniramine.	Names contain "-en/-ine" or "-en/-ate."
CLINICAL USES	Allergy, motion sickness, sleep aid.	
TOXICITY	Sedation, antimuscarinic, anti-α-adrenergic.	
2nd generation	Loratadine, fexofenadine, desloratadine, cetirizine.	Names usually end in "-adine."
CLINICAL USES	Allergy.	
TOXICITY	Far less sedating than 1st generation because of ↓ entry into CNS.	

Expectorants

Guaifenesin	Expectorant—thins respiratory secretions; does not suppress cough reflex.
***N*-acetylcysteine**	Mucolytic—can loosen mucous plugs in CF patients. Also used as an antidote for acetaminophen overdose.

Dextromethorphan	Antitussive (antagonizes NMDA glutamate receptors). Synthetic codeine analog. Has mild opioid effect when used in excess. Naloxone can be given for overdose. Mild abuse potential.

Pseudoephedrine, phenylephrine

MECHANISM	Sympathomimetic α-agonistic nonprescription nasal decongestants.
CLINICAL USE	Reduce hyperemia, edema, and nasal congestion; open obstructed eustachian tubes. Pseudoephedrine also illicitly used to make methamphetamine.
TOXICITY	Hypertension. Can also cause CNS stimulation/anxiety (pseudoephedrine).

Asthma drugs	Bronchoconstriction is mediated by (1) inflammatory processes and (2) parasympathetic tone; therapy is directed at these 2 pathways.
β₂-agonists	**Albuterol**—relaxes bronchial smooth muscle (β_2). Use during acute exacerbation.
	Salmeterol, formoterol—long-acting agents for prophylaxis. Adverse effects are tremor and arrhythmia.
Methylxanthines	**Theophylline**—likely causes bronchodilation by inhibiting phosphodiesterase → ↑ cAMP levels due to ↓ cAMP hydrolysis. Usage is limited because of narrow therapeutic index (cardiotoxicity, neurotoxicity); metabolized by cytochrome P-450. Blocks actions of adenosine.
Muscarinic antagonists	**Ipratropium**—competitive block of muscarinic receptors, preventing bronchoconstriction. Also used for COPD, as is tiotropium, a long-acting muscarinic antagonist.
Corticosteroids	**Beclomethasone, fluticasone**—inhibit the synthesis of virtually all cytokines. Inactivate NF-κB, the transcription factor that induces the production of TNF-α and other inflammatory agents. 1st-line therapy for chronic asthma.
Antileukotrienes	**Montelukast, zafirlukast**—block leukotriene receptors. Especially good for aspirin-induced asthma.
	Zileuton—a 5-lipoxygenase pathway inhibitor. Blocks conversion of arachidonic acid to leukotrienes.
Omalizumab	Monoclonal anti-IgE antibody. Binds mostly unbound serum IgE and blocks binding to FcεRI. Used in allergic asthma resistant to inhaled steroids and long-acting β₂-agonists.

Exposure to antigen
(dust, pollen, etc.)

⬜ Avoidance

Antigen and IgE ⊢−⊣ Omalizumab
on mast cells

⬜ Steroids

Mediators
(leukotrienes, histamine, etc.)

Steroids
Antileukotrienes ⬜

β-agonists
Theophylline
Muscarinic
antagonists ⬜

Late response:
inflammation

Early response:
bronchoconstriction

Bronchial
hyperreactivity

Symptoms

Treatment strategies in asthma

ATP

Bronchodilation

AC ← ⊕ **β-agonists**

⊕ ← cAMP

Bronchial tone

PDE ⊢−⊝ **Theophylline**

AMP

ACh ⊕ ⊕ Adenosine

Muscarinic antagonists ⊝

⊝ **Theophylline**

Bronchoconstriction

Methacholine	Muscarinic receptor agonist. Used in bronchial provocation challenge to help diagnose asthma.
Bosentan	Used to treat pulmonary arterial hypertension. Competitively antagonizes endothelin-1 receptors, ↓ pulmonary vascular resistance.

Rapid Review

"Study without thought is vain: thought without study is dangerous."
—Confucius

It is better, of course, to know useless things than to know nothing.
—Lucius Annaeus Seneca (ca. 4 BC–AD 65)

The following tables represent a collection of high-yield associations of diseases with their clinical findings, treatments, and pathophysiology. They serve as a quick review before the exam to tune your senses to commonly tested cases.

615

CLINICAL PRESENTATION	DIAGNOSIS/DISEASE
Abdominal pain, ascites, hepatomegaly	Budd-Chiari syndrome (posthepatic venous thrombosis)
Achilles tendon xanthoma	Familial hypercholesterolemia (↓ LDL receptor signaling)
Adrenal hemorrhage, hypotension, DIC	Waterhouse-Friderichsen syndrome (meningococcemia)
Anterior "drawer sign" ⊕	Anterior cruciate ligament injury
Arachnodactyly, lens dislocation, aortic dissection, hyperflexible joints	Marfan syndrome (fibrillin defect)
Athlete with polycythemia	2° to erythropoietin injection
Back pain, fever, night sweats, weight loss	Pott disease (vertebral TB)
Bilateral hilar adenopathy, uveitis	Sarcoidosis (noncaseating granulomas)
Blue sclera	Osteogenesis imperfecta (type I collagen defect)
Bluish line on gingiva	Burton line (lead poisoning)
Bone pain, bone enlargement, arthritis	Paget disease of bone (↑ osteoblastic and osteoclastic activity)
Bounding pulses, diastolic heart murmur, head bobbing	Aortic regurgitation
"Butterfly" facial rash and Raynaud phenomenon in a young female	Systemic lupus erythematosus
Café-au-lait spots, Lisch nodules (iris hamartoma)	Neurofibromatosis type I (+ pheochromocytoma, optic gliomas)
Café-au-lait spots, polyostotic fibrous dysplasia, precocious puberty, multiple endocrine abnormalities	McCune-Albright syndrome (mosaic G-protein signaling mutation)
Calf pseudohypertrophy	Muscular dystrophy (most commonly Duchenne): X-linked recessive deletion of dystrophin gene
"Cherry-red spots" on macula	Tay-Sachs (ganglioside accumulation) or Niemann-Pick (sphingomyelin accumulation), central retinal artery occlusion
Chest pain on exertion	Angina (stable: with moderate exertion; unstable: with minimal exertion)
Chest pain, pericardial effusion/friction rub, persistent fever following MI	Dressler syndrome (autoimmune-mediated post-MI fibrinous pericarditis, 1–12 weeks after acute episode)
Child uses arms to stand up from squat	Gowers sign (Duchenne muscular dystrophy)
Child with fever later develops red rash on face that spreads to body	"Slapped cheeks" (erythema infectiosum/fifth disease: parvovirus B19)
Chorea, dementia, caudate degeneration	Huntington disease (autosomal dominant CAG repeat expansion)
Chronic exercise intolerance with myalgia, fatigue, painful cramps, myoglobinuria	McArdle disease (muscle glycogen phosphorylase deficiency)
Cold intolerance	Hypothyroidism
Conjugate lateral gaze palsy, horizontal diplopia	Internuclear ophthalmoplegia (damage to MLF; bilateral [multiple sclerosis], unilateral [stroke])
Continuous "machine-like" heart murmur	PDA (close with indomethacin; open or maintain with misoprostol)
Cutaneous/dermal edema due to connective tissue deposition	Myxedema (caused by hypothyroidism, Graves disease [pretibial])

CLINICAL PRESENTATION	DIAGNOSIS/DISEASE
Dark purple skin/mouth nodules in a patient with AIDS	Kaposi sarcoma, associated with HHV-8
Deep, labored breathing/hyperventilation	Kussmaul respirations (diabetic ketoacidosis)
Dermatitis, dementia, diarrhea	Pellagra (niacin [vitamin B_3] deficiency)
Dilated cardiomyopathy, edema, alcoholism or malnutrition	Wet beriberi (thiamine [vitamin B_1] deficiency)
Dog or cat bite resulting in infection	*Pasteurella multocida* (cellulitis at inoculation site)
Dry eyes, dry mouth, arthritis	Sjögren syndrome (autoimmune destruction of exocrine glands)
Dysphagia (esophageal webs), glossitis, iron deficiency anemia	Plummer-Vinson syndrome (may progress to esophageal squamous cell carcinoma)
Elastic skin, hypermobility of joints	Ehlers-Danlos syndrome (type III collagen defect)
Enlarged, hard left supraclavicular node	Virchow node (abdominal metastasis)
Erythroderma, lymphadenopathy, hepatosplenomegaly, atypical T cells	Mycosis fungoides (cutaneous T-cell lymphoma) or Sézary syndrome (mycosis fungoides + malignant T cells in blood)
Facial muscle spasm upon tapping	Chvostek sign (hypocalcemia)
Fat, female, forty, and fertile	Cholelithiasis (gallstones)
Fever, chills, headache, myalgia following antibiotic treatment for syphilis	Jarisch-Herxheimer reaction (rapid lysis of spirochetes results in toxin release)
Fever, cough, conjunctivitis, coryza, diffuse rash	Measles
Fever, night sweats, weight loss	B symptoms (staging) of lymphoma
Fibrous plaques in soft tissue of penis	Peyronie disease (connective tissue disorder)
Gout, intellectual disability, self-mutilating behavior in a boy	Lesch-Nyhan syndrome (HGPRT deficiency, X-linked recessive)
Green-yellow rings around peripheral cornea	Kayser-Fleischer rings (copper accumulation from Wilson disease)
Hamartomatous GI polyps, hyperpigmentation of mouth/feet/hands	Peutz-Jeghers syndrome (inherited, benign polyposis can cause bowel obstruction; ↑ cancer risk, mainly GI)
Hepatosplenomegaly, osteoporosis, neurologic symptoms	Gaucher disease (glucocerebrosidase deficiency)
Hereditary nephritis, sensorineural hearing loss, cataracts	Alport syndrome (mutation in collagen IV)
Hyperphagia, hypersexuality, hyperorality, hyperdocility	Klüver-Bucy syndrome (bilateral amygdala lesion)
Hyperreflexia, hypertonia, Babinski sign present	UMN damage
Hyporeflexia, hypotonia, atrophy, fasciculations	LMN damage
Hypoxemia, polycythemia, hypercapnia	"Blue bloater" (chronic bronchitis: hyperplasia of mucous cells)
Indurated, ulcerated genital lesion	Nonpainful: chancre (1° syphilis, *Treponema pallidum*) Painful, with exudate: chancroid (*Haemophilus ducreyi*)
Infant with cleft lip/palate, microcephaly or holoprosencephaly, polydactyly, cutis aplasia	Patau syndrome (trisomy 13)
Infant with failure to thrive, hepatosplenomegaly, and neurodegeneration	Niemann-Pick disease (genetic sphingomyelinase deficiency)

CLINICAL PRESENTATION	DIAGNOSIS/DISEASE
Infant with hypoglycemia, failure to thrive, and hepatomegaly	Cori disease (debranching enzyme deficiency) or Von Gierke disease (glucose-6-phosphatase deficiency, more severe)
Infant with microcephaly, rocker-bottom feet, clenched hands, and structural heart defect	Edwards syndrome (trisomy 18)
Jaundice, palpable distended non-tender gallbladder	Courvoisier sign (distal obstruction of biliary tree)
Large rash with bull's-eye appearance	Erythema chronicum migrans from *Ixodes* tick bite (Lyme disease: *Borrelia*)
Lucid interval after traumatic brain injury	Epidural hematoma (middle meningeal artery rupture)
Male child, recurrent infections, no mature B cells	Bruton disease (X-linked agammaglobulinemia)
Mucosal bleeding and prolonged bleeding time	Glanzmann thrombasthenia (defect in platelet aggregation due to lack of GpIIb/IIIa)
Muffled heart sounds, distended neck veins, hypotension	Beck triad of cardiac tamponade
Multiple colon polyps, osteomas/soft tissue tumors, impacted/supernumerary teeth	Gardner syndrome (subtype of FAP)
Myopathy (infantile hypertrophic cardiomyopathy), exercise intolerance	Pompe disease (lysosomal α-1,4-glucosidase deficiency)
Neonate with arm paralysis following difficult birth	Erb-Duchenne palsy (superior trunk [C5–C6] brachial plexus injury: "waiter's tip")
No lactation postpartum, absent menstruation, cold intolerance	Sheehan syndrome (pituitary infarction)
Nystagmus, intention tremor, scanning speech, bilateral internuclear ophthalmoplegia	Multiple sclerosis
Oscillating slow/fast breathing	Cheyne-Stokes respirations (central apnea in CHF or ↑ intracranial pressure)
Painful blue fingers/toes, hemolytic anemia	Cold agglutinin disease (autoimmune hemolytic anemia caused by *Mycoplasma pneumoniae*, infectious mononucleosis)
Painful, pale, cold fingers/toes	Raynaud phenomenon (vasospasm in extremities)
Painful, raised red lesions on pad of fingers/toes	Osler nodes (infective endocarditis, immune complex deposition)
Painless erythematous lesions on palms and soles	Janeway lesions (infective endocarditis, septic emboli/microabscesses)
Painless jaundice	Cancer of the pancreatic head obstructing bile duct
Palpable purpura on buttocks/legs, joint pain, abdominal pain (child), hematuria	Henoch-Schönlein purpura (IgA vasculitis affecting skin and kidneys)
Pancreatic, pituitary, parathyroid tumors	MEN 1 (autosomal dominant)
Periorbital and/or peripheral edema, proteinuria, hypoalbuminemia, hypercholesterolemia	Nephrotic syndrome
Pink complexion, dyspnea, hyperventilation	"Pink puffer" (emphysema: centriacinar [smoking], panacinar [α_1-antitrypsin deficiency])
Polyuria, renal tubular acidosis type II, growth failure, electrolyte imbalances, hypophosphatemic rickets	Fanconi syndrome (proximal tubular reabsorption defect)

CLINICAL PRESENTATION	DIAGNOSIS/DISEASE
Pruritic, purple, polygonal planar papules and plaques (6 P's)	Lichen planus
Ptosis, miosis, anhidrosis	Horner syndrome (sympathetic chain lesion)
Pupil accommodates but doesn't react	Argyll Robertson pupil (neurosyphilis)
Rapidly progressive leg weakness that ascends following GI/ upper respiratory infection	Guillain-Barré syndrome (acute autoimmune inflammatory demyelinating polyneuropathy)
Rash on palms and soles	Coxsackie A, 2° syphilis, Rocky Mountain spotted fever
Recurrent colds, unusual eczema, high serum IgE	Hyper-IgE syndrome (Job syndrome: neutrophil chemotaxis abnormality)
Red "currant jelly" sputum in alcoholic or diabetic patients	*Klebsiella pneumoniae*
Red "currant jelly" stools	Acute mesenteric ischemia (adults), intussusception (infants)
Red, itchy, swollen rash of nipple/areola	Paget disease of the breast (sign of underlying neoplasm)
Red urine in the morning, fragile RBCs	Paroxysmal nocturnal hemoglobinuria
Renal cell carcinoma (bilateral), hemangioblastomas, angiomatosis, pheochromocytoma	von Hippel-Lindau disease (dominant tumor suppressor gene mutation)
Resting tremor, rigidity, akinesia, postural instability	Parkinson disease (nigrostriatal dopamine depletion)
Retinal hemorrhages with pale centers	Roth spots (bacterial endocarditis)
Severe jaundice in neonate	Crigler-Najjar syndrome (congenital unconjugated hyperbilirubinemia)
Severe RLQ pain with palpation of LLQ	Rovsing sign (acute appendicitis)
Severe RLQ pain with rebound tenderness	McBurney sign (acute appendicitis)
Short stature, ↑ incidence of tumors/leukemia, aplastic anemia	Fanconi anemia (genetic loss of DNA crosslink repair; often progresses to AML)
Single palmar crease	Down syndrome
Situs inversus, chronic sinusitis, bronchiectasis, infertility	Kartagener syndrome (dynein arm defect affecting cilia)
Skin hyperpigmentation, hypotension, fatigue	Addison disease (1° adrenocortical insufficiency causes ↑ ACTH and ↑ α-MSH production)
Slow, progressive muscle weakness in boys	Becker muscular dystrophy (X-linked missense mutation in dystrophin; less severe than Duchenne)
Small, irregular red spots on buccal/lingual mucosa with blue-white centers	Koplik spots (measles; rubeola virus)
Smooth, flat, moist, painless white lesions on genitals	Condylomata lata (2° syphilis)
Splinter hemorrhages in fingernails	Bacterial endocarditis
"Strawberry tongue"	Scarlet fever, Kawasaki disease, toxic shock syndrome
Streak ovaries, congenital heart disease, horseshoe kidney, cystic hygroma at birth, short stature, webbed neck, lymphedema	Turner syndrome (45,XO)
Sudden swollen/painful big toe joint, tophi	Gout/podagra (hyperuricemia)
Swollen gums, mucosal bleeding, poor wound healing, petechiae	Scurvy (vitamin C deficiency: can't hydroxylate proline/lysine for collagen synthesis)
Swollen, hard, painful finger joints	Osteoarthritis (osteophytes on PIP [Bouchard nodes], DIP [Heberden nodes])
Systolic ejection murmur (crescendo-decrescendo)	Aortic valve stenosis

CLINICAL PRESENTATION	DIAGNOSIS/DISEASE
Thyroid and parathyroid tumors, pheochromocytoma	MEN 2A (autosomal dominant *ret* mutation)
Thyroid tumors, pheochromocytoma, ganglioneuromatosis	MEN 2B (autosomal dominant *ret* mutation)
Toe extension/fanning upon plantar scrape	Babinski sign (UMN lesion)
Unilateral facial drooping involving forehead	Facial nerve (LMN CN VII palsy)
Urethritis, conjunctivitis, arthritis in a male	Reactive arthritis associated with HLA-B27
Vascular birthmark (port-wine stain)	Hemangioma (benign, but associated with Sturge-Weber syndrome)
Vomiting blood following gastroesophageal lacerations	Mallory-Weiss syndrome (alcoholic and bulimic patients)
Weight loss, diarrhea, arthritis, fever, adenopathy	Whipple disease (*Tropheryma whipplei*)
"Worst headache of my life"	Subarachnoid hemorrhage

▶ CLASSIC LABS/FINDINGS

LAB/DIAGNOSTIC FINDING	DIAGNOSIS/DISEASE
Anticentromere antibodies	Scleroderma (CREST)
Antidesmoglein (epithelial) antibodies	Pemphigus vulgaris (blistering)
Anti–glomerular basement membrane antibodies	Goodpasture syndrome (glomerulonephritis and hemoptysis)
Antihistone antibodies	Drug-induced SLE (hydralazine, INH, phenytoin, procainamide)
Anti-IgG antibodies	Rheumatoid arthritis (systemic inflammation, joint pannus, boutonnière deformity)
Antimitochondrial antibodies (AMAs)	1° biliary cirrhosis (female, cholestasis, portal hypertension)
Antineutrophil cytoplasmic antibodies (ANCAs)	Microscopic polyangiitis and Churg-Strauss syndrome (MPO-ANCA/p-ANCA); granulomatosis with polyangiitis (Wegener; PR3-ANCA/c-ANCA)
Antinuclear antibodies (ANAs: anti-Smith and anti-dsDNA)	SLE (type III hypersensitivity)
Antiplatelet antibodies	Idiopathic thrombocytopenic purpura
Anti-topoisomerase antibodies	Diffuse systemic scleroderma
Anti-transglutaminase/anti-gliadin/anti-endomysial antibodies	Celiac disease (diarrhea, distention, weight loss)
"Apple core" lesion on abdominal x-ray	Colorectal cancer (usually left-sided)
Azurophilic peroxidase ⊕ granular inclusions in granulocytes and myeloblasts	Auer rods (AML, especially the promyelocytic [M3] type)
Bacitracin response	Sensitive: *Streptococcus pyogenes* (group A); resistant: *Streptococcus agalactiae* (group B)
"Bamboo spine" on x-ray	Ankylosing spondylitis (chronic inflammatory arthritis: HLA-B27)
Basophilic nuclear remnants in RBCs	Howell-Jolly bodies (due to splenectomy or nonfunctional spleen)

LAB/DIAGNOSTIC FINDING	DIAGNOSIS/DISEASE
Basophilic stippling of RBCs	Lead poisoning or sideroblastic anemia
Bloody tap on LP	Subarachnoid hemorrhage
"Boot-shaped" heart on x-ray	Tetralogy of Fallot, RVH
Branching gram-positive rods with sulfur granules	*Actinomyces israelii*
Bronchogenic apical lung tumor on imaging	Pancoast tumor (can compress sympathetic ganglion and cause Horner syndrome)
"Brown" tumor of bone	Hyperparathyroidism or osteitis fibrosa cystica (deposited hemosiderin from hemorrhage gives brown color)
Cardiomegaly with apical atrophy	Chagas disease (*Trypanosoma cruzi*)
Cellular crescents in Bowman capsule	Rapidly progressive crescentic glomerulonephritis
"Chocolate cyst" of ovary	Endometriosis (frequently involves both ovaries)
Circular grouping of dark tumor cells surrounding pale neurofibrils	Homer-Wright rosettes (neuroblastoma, medulloblastoma, retinoblastoma)
Colonies of mucoid *Pseudomonas* in lungs	Cystic fibrosis (autosomal recessive mutation in *CFTR* gene → fat-soluble vitamin deficiency and mucous plugs)
↓ AFP in amniotic fluid/maternal serum	Down syndrome or other chromosomal abnormality
Degeneration of dorsal column nerves	Tabes dorsalis (3° syphilis), subacute combined degeneration (dorsal columns and lateral corticospinal tracts affected)
Depigmentation of neurons in substantia nigra	Parkinson disease (basal ganglia disorder: rigidity, resting tremor, bradykinesia)
Desquamated epithelium casts in sputum	Curschmann spirals (bronchial asthma; can result in whorled mucous plugs)
Disarrayed granulosa cells in eosinophilic fluid	Call-Exner bodies (granulosa-theca cell tumor of the ovary)
Dysplastic squamous cervical cells with nuclear enlargement and hyperchromasia	Koilocytes (HPV: predisposes to cervical cancer)
Enlarged cells with intranuclear inclusion bodies	"Owl eye" appearance of CMV
Enlarged thyroid cells with ground-glass nuclei	"Orphan Annie" eyes nuclei (papillary carcinoma of the thyroid)
Eosinophilic cytoplasmic inclusion in liver cell	Mallory body (alcoholic liver disease)
Eosinophilic cytoplasmic inclusion in nerve cell	Lewy body (Parkinson disease)
Eosinophilic globule in liver	Councilman body (toxic or viral hepatitis, often yellow fever)
Eosinophilic inclusion bodies in cytoplasm of hippocampal and cerebellar nerve cells	Negri bodies of rabies
Extracellular amyloid deposition in gray matter of brain	Senile plaques (Alzheimer disease)
Giant B cells with bilobed nuclei with prominent inclusions ("owl's eye")	Reed-Sternberg cells (Hodgkin lymphoma)
Glomerulus-like structure surrounding vessel in germ cells	Schiller-Duval bodies (yolk sac tumor)
"Hair on end" (crew-cut) appearance on x-ray	β-thalassemia, sickle cell anemia (marrow expansion)
hCG elevated	Choriocarcinoma, hydatidiform mole (occurs with and without embryo, and multiple pregnancy)
Heart nodules (granulomatous)	Aschoff bodies (rheumatic fever)

LAB/DIAGNOSTIC FINDING	DIAGNOSIS/DISEASE
Heterophile antibodies	Infectious mononucleosis (EBV)
Hexagonal, double-pointed, needle-like crystals in bronchial secretions	Bronchial asthma (Charcot-Leyden crystals: eosinophilic granules)
High level of D-dimers	DVT, PE, DIC
Hilar lymphadenopathy, peripheral granulomatous lesion in middle or lower lung lobes (can calcify)	Ghon complex (1° TB: *Mycobacterium* bacilli)
"Honeycomb lung" on x-ray or CT	Interstitial pulmonary fibrosis
Hypercoagulability (leading to migrating DVTs and vasculitis)	Trousseau syndrome (adenocarcinoma of pancreas or lung)
Hypersegmented neutrophils	Megaloblastic anemia (B_{12} deficiency: neurologic symptoms; folate deficiency: no neurologic symptoms)
Hypertension, hypokalemia, metabolic alkalosis	Conn syndrome
Hypochromic, microcytic anemia	Iron deficiency anemia, lead poisoning, thalassemia (fetal hemoglobin sometimes present)
Increased AFP in amniotic fluid/maternal serum	Dating error, anencephaly, spina bifida (neural tube defects)
Increased uric acid levels	Gout, Lesch-Nyhan syndrome, tumor lysis syndrome, loop and thiazide diuretics
Intranuclear eosinophilic droplet-like bodies	Cowdry type A bodies (HSV or CMV)
Iron-containing nodules in alveolar septum	Ferruginous bodies (asbestosis: ↑ chance of mesothelioma)
Keratin pearls on a skin biopsy	Squamous cell carcinoma
Large lysosomal vesicles in phagocytes, immunodeficiency	Chédiak-Higashi disease (congenital failure of phagolysosome formation)
"Lead pipe" appearance of colon on barium enema x-ray	Ulcerative colitis (loss of haustra)
Linear appearance of IgG deposition on glomerular basement membrane	Goodpasture syndrome
Low serum ceruloplasmin	Wilson disease (hepatolenticular degeneration)
"Lumpy bumpy" appearance of glomeruli on immunofluorescence	Poststreptococcal glomerulonephritis (immune complex deposition of IgG and C3b)
Lytic ("hole punched") bone lesions on x-ray	Multiple myeloma
Mammary gland ("blue domed") cyst	Fibrocystic change of the breast
Monoclonal antibody spike	▪ Multiple myeloma (usually IgG or IgA) ▪ Monoclonal gammopathy of undetermined significance (MGUS consequence of aging) ▪ Waldenström (M protein = IgM) macroglobulinemia ▪ Primary amyloidosis
Mucin-filled cell with peripheral nucleus	"Signet ring" (gastric carcinoma)
Narrowing of bowel lumen on barium x-ray	"String sign" (Crohn disease)
Necrotizing vasculitis (lungs) and necrotizing glomerulonephritis	Granulomatosis with polyangiitis (Wegener; PR3-ANCA/ c-ANCA) and Goodpasture syndrome (anti–basement membrane antibodies)
Needle-shaped, negatively birefringent crystals	Gout (monosodium urate crystals)
Nodular hyaline deposits in glomeruli	Kimmelstiel-Wilson nodules (diabetic nephropathy)
Novobiocin response	Sensitive: *Staphylococcus epidermidis*; resistant: *Staphylococcus saprophyticus*
"Nutmeg" appearance of liver	Chronic passive congestion of liver due to right heart failure

LAB/DIAGNOSTIC FINDING	DIAGNOSIS/DISEASE
"Onion skin" periosteal reaction	Ewing sarcoma (malignant round-cell tumor)
Optochin response	Sensitive: *Streptococcus pneumoniae*; resistant: viridans streptococci
Periosteum raised from bone, creating triangular area	Codman triangle on x-ray (osteosarcoma, Ewing sarcoma, pyogenic osteomyelitis)
Podocyte fusion or "effacement" on electron microscopy	Minimal change disease (child with nephrotic syndrome)
Polished, "ivory-like" appearance of bone at cartilage erosion	Eburnation (osteoarthritis resulting in bony sclerosis)
Protein aggregates in neurons from hyperphosphorylation of tau protein	Neurofibrillary tangles (Alzheimer disease) and Pick bodies (Pick disease)
Psammoma bodies	Meningiomas, papillary thyroid carcinoma, mesothelioma, papillary serous carcinoma of the endometrium and ovary
Pseudopalisading tumor cells on brain biopsy	Glioblastoma multiforme
RBC casts in urine	Acute glomerulonephritis
Rectangular, crystal-like, cytoplasmic inclusions in Leydig cells	Reinke crystals (Leydig cell tumor)
Renal epithelial casts in urine	Acute toxic/viral renal injury
Rhomboid crystals, positively birefringent	Pseudogout (calcium pyrophosphate dihydrate crystals)
Rib notching	Coarctation of the aorta
Ring-enhancing brain lesion in AIDS	*Toxoplasma gondii*, CNS lymphoma
Sheets of medium-sized lymphoid cells with scattered pale, tingible body–laden macrophages ("starry sky" histology)	Burkitt lymphoma (t[8:14] c-*myc* activation, associated with EBV; "black sky" made up of malignant cells)
Silver-staining spherical aggregation of tau proteins in neurons	Pick bodies (Pick disease: progressive dementia, changes in personality)
"Soap bubble" in femur or tibia on x-ray	Giant cell tumor of bone (generally benign)
"Spikes" on basement membrane, "dome-like" subepithelial deposits	Membranous glomerulonephritis (may progress to nephrotic syndrome)
Stacks of RBCs	Rouleaux formation (high ESR, multiple myeloma)
Stippled vaginal epithelial cells	"Clue cells" (*Gardnerella vaginalis*)
"Tennis racket"-shaped cytoplasmic organelles (EM) in Langerhans cells	Birbeck granules (Langerhans cell histiocytosis or histiocytosis X: eosinophilic granuloma)
Thrombi made of white/red layers	Lines of Zahn (arterial thrombus, layers of platelets/RBCs)
"Thumb sign" on lateral x-ray	Epiglottitis (*Haemophilus influenzae*)
Thyroid-like appearance of kidney	Chronic bacterial pyelonephritis
"Tram-track" appearance of capillary loops of glomerular basement membranes on light microscopy	Membranoproliferative glomerulonephritis
Triglyceride accumulation in liver cell vacuoles	Fatty liver disease (alcoholic or metabolic syndrome)
"Waxy" casts with very low urine flow	Chronic end-stage renal disease
WBC casts in urine	Acute pyelonephritis
WBCs that look "smudged"	CLL (almost always B cell)
"Wire loop" glomerular capillary appearance on light microscopy	Lupus nephropathy
Yellowish CSF	Xanthochromia (e.g., due to subarachnoid hemorrhage)

▶ CLASSIC/RELEVANT TREATMENTS

CONDITION	COMMON TREATMENT(S)
Absence seizures	Ethosuximide
Acute gout attack	NSAIDs, colchicine
Acute promyelocytic leukemia (M3)	All-*trans* retinoic acid
ADHD	Methylphenidate, amphetamines
Alcohol use disorder	AA + disulfiram, naltrexone, or acamprosate for patient. Al-Anon for patient's family
Alcohol withdrawal	Benzodiazepines
Anorexia	Nutrition, psychotherapy
Anticoagulation during pregnancy	Heparin
Arrhythmia in damaged cardiac tissue	Class IB antiarrhythmic (lidocaine, mexiletine, tocainide)
B_{12} deficiency	Vitamin B_{12} supplementation (work up cause with Schilling test)
Benign prostatic hyperplasia	Tamsulosin, finasteride
Bipolar disorder	Lithium, valproate, carbamazepine, lamotrigine (mood stabilizers)
Breast cancer in postmenopausal woman	Aromatase inhibitor (anastrozole)
Buerger disease	Smoking cessation
Bulimia nervosa	SSRIs
Candida albicans	Amphotericin B (systemic), nystatin (oral thrush), azoles (vaginitis)
Carcinoid syndrome	Octreotide
Chlamydia trachomatis	Doxycycline (+ ceftriaxone for gonorrhea coinfection), erythromycin eye drops (prophylaxis in infants)
Chronic gout	Probenecid (underexcretor), allopurinol (overproducer), febuxostat
Chronic hepatitis	IFN-α
Chronic myelogenous leukemia	Imatinib
Clostridium botulinum	Antitoxin
Clostridium difficile	Oral metronidazole; if refractory, oral vancomycin
Clostridium tetani	Antitoxin + vaccine booster + diazepam
CMV	Ganciclovir
Crohn disease	Corticosteroids, infliximab, methotrexate, azathioprine
Cryptococcus neoformans	Fluconazole (prophylaxis in AIDS patients)
Cyclophosphamide-induced hemorrhagic cystitis	Mesna
Depression	SSRIs (first-line)
Diabetes insipidus	DDAVP (central); hydrochlorothiazide, indomethacin, amiloride (nephrogenic)
Diabetes mellitus type 1	Dietary intervention (low sugar) + insulin replacement
Diabetes mellitus type 2	Dietary intervention, oral hypoglycemics, and insulin (if refractory)

CONDITION	COMMON TREATMENT(S)
Diabetic ketoacidosis	Fluids, insulin, K^+
Enterococci	Vancomycin/ampicillin + aminoglycoside
Erectile dysfunction	Sildenafil, vardenafil
ER ⊕ breast cancer	Tamoxifen
Ethylene glycol/methanol intoxication	Fomepizole (alcohol dehydrogenase inhibitor)
Haemophilus influenzae (B)	Rifampin (prophylaxis)
Generalized anxiety disorder	Buspirone
Granulomatosis with polyangiitis (Wegener)	Cyclophosphamide, corticosteroids
Heparin toxicity (acute)	Protamine sulfate
HER2/neu ⊕ breast cancer	Trastuzumab
Hyperaldosteronism	Spironolactone
Hypercholesterolemia	Statin (first-line)
Hypertriglyceridemia	Fibrate
Immediate anticoagulation	Heparin
Infertility	Leuprolide, GnRH (pulsatile), clomiphene
Influenza	Rimantadine, oseltamivir
Legionella pneumophila	Erythromycin
Long-term anticoagulation	Warfarin
Malaria	Chloroquine/mefloquine (for blood schizont), primaquine (for liver hypnozoite)
Malignant hyperthermia	Dantrolene
Medical abortion	Mifepristone
Migraine	Sumatriptan
MRSA	Vancomycin
Multiple sclerosis	β-interferon, immunosuppression, natalizumab
Mycobacterium tuberculosis	RIPE (rifampin, INH, pyrazinamide, ethambutol)
Neisseria gonorrhoeae	Ceftriaxone (add doxycycline to cover likely concurrent *Chlamydia*)
Neisseria meningitidis	Penicillin/ceftriaxone, rifampin (prophylaxis)
Neural tube defect prevention	Prenatal folic acid
Osteomalacia/rickets	Vitamin D supplementation
Osteoporosis	Bisphosphonates; calcium and vitamin D supplementation
Patent ductus arteriosus	Indomethacin
Pheochromocytoma	α-antagonists (e.g., phenoxybenzamine)
Pneumocystis jirovecii	TMP-SMX (prophylaxis in AIDS patient)
Prolactinoma	Bromocriptine (dopamine agonists)
Prostate cancer/uterine fibroids	Leuprolide, GnRH (continuous)
Prostate carcinoma	Flutamide

CONDITION	COMMON TREATMENT(S)
Pseudomonas aeruginosa	Antipseudomonal penicillin + aminoglycoside
Pulmonary arterial hypertension (idiopathic)	Sildenafil, bosentan, epoprostenol
Rickettsia rickettsii	Doxycycline, chloramphenicol (associated with aplastic anemia)
Ringworm infections	Terbinafine, griseofulvin, imidazole
Schizophrenia (negative symptoms)	5-HT_{2A} antagonists (e.g., 2nd-generation antipsychotics)
Schizophrenia (positive symptoms)	D_2 receptor antagonists (e.g., 1st- and 2nd-generation antipsychotics)
SIADH	Demeclocycline, lithium, vasopressin receptor antagonists
Sickle cell anemia	Hydroxyurea (↑ fetal hemoglobin)
Sporothrix schenckii	Oral potassium iodide
Stable angina	Sublingual nitroglycerin
Staphylococcus aureus	MSSA: nafcillin, oxacillin, dicloxacillin (antistaphylococcal penicillins); MRSA: vancomycin
Streptococcus bovis	Penicillin prophylaxis; evaluation for colon cancer if linked to endocarditis
Streptococcus pneumoniae	Penicillin/cephalosporin (systemic infection, pneumonia), vancomycin (meningitis)
Streptococcus pyogenes	Penicillin prophylaxis
Temporal arteritis	High-dose steroids
Tonic-clonic seizures	Phenytoin, valproate, carbamazepine
Toxoplasma gondii	Sulfadiazine + pyrimethamine
Treponema pallidum	Penicillin
Trichomonas vaginalis	Metronidazole (patient and partner)
Trigeminal neuralgia (tic douloureux)	Carbamazepine
Ulcerative colitis	5-ASA, infliximab, colectomy
UTI prophylaxis	TMP-SMX
Warfarin toxicity	Fresh frozen plasma (acute), vitamin K (chronic)

▶ KEY ASSOCIATIONS

DISEASE/FINDING	MOST COMMON/IMPORTANT ASSOCIATIONS
Actinic (solar) keratosis	Precursor to squamous cell carcinoma
Acute gastric ulcer associated with CNS injury	Cushing ulcer (↑ intracranial pressure stimulates vagal gastric secretion)
Acute gastric ulcer associated with severe burns	Curling ulcer (greatly reduced plasma volume results in sloughing of gastric mucosa)
Alternating areas of transmural inflammation and normal colon	Skip lesions (Crohn disease)
Aneurysm, dissecting	Hypertension

DISEASE/FINDING	MOST COMMON/IMPORTANT ASSOCIATIONS
Aortic aneurysm, abdominal and descending aorta	Atherosclerosis
Aortic aneurysm, arch	3° syphilis (syphilitic aortitis), vasa vasorum destruction
Aortic aneurysm, ascending	Marfan syndrome (idiopathic cystic medial degeneration)
Atrophy of the mammillary bodies	Wernicke encephalopathy (thiamine deficiency causing ataxia, ophthalmoplegia, and confusion)
Autosplenectomy (fibrosis and shrinkage)	Sickle cell anemia (hemoglobin S)
Bacteria associated with gastritis, peptic ulcer disease, and stomach cancer	*H. pylori*
Bacterial meningitis (adults and elderly)	*Streptococcus pneumoniae*
Bacterial meningitis (newborns and kids)	Group B streptococcus/*E.coli* (newborns), *S. pneumoniae*/ *Neisseria meningitidis* (kids)
Benign melanocytic nevus	Spitz nevus (most common in 1st two decades)
Bleeding disorder with GpIb deficiency	Bernard-Soulier syndrome (defect in platelet adhesion to von Willebrand factor)
Brain tumor (adults)	Supratentorial: metastasis > astrocytoma (including glioblastoma multiforme) > meningioma > schwannoma
Brain tumor (kids)	Infratentorial: medulloblastoma (cerebellum) or supratentorial: craniopharyngioma
Breast cancer	Infiltrating ductal carcinoma
Breast mass	Fibrocystic change, carcinoma (in postmenopausal women)
Breast tumor (benign)	Fibroadenoma
Cardiac 1° tumor (kids)	Rhabdomyoma, often seen in tuberous sclerosis
Cardiac manifestation of lupus	Libman-Sacks endocarditis (nonbacterial, affecting both sides of mitral valve)
Cardiac tumor (adults)	Metastasis, 1° myxoma (4:1 left to right atrium; "ball and valve")
Cerebellar tonsillar herniation	Chiari II malformation
Chronic arrhythmia	Atrial fibrillation (associated with high risk of emboli)
Chronic atrophic gastritis (autoimmune)	Predisposition to gastric carcinoma (can also cause pernicious anemia)
Clear cell adenocarcinoma of the vagina	DES exposure in utero
Compression fracture	Osteoporosis (type I: postmenopausal woman; type II: elderly man or woman)
Congenital adrenal hyperplasia, hypotension	21-hydroxylase deficiency
Congenital cardiac anomaly	VSD
Congenital conjugated hyperbilirubinemia (black liver)	Dubin-Johnson syndrome (inability of hepatocytes to secrete conjugated bilirubin into bile)
Constrictive pericarditis	TB (developing world); SLE (developed world)
Coronary artery involved in thrombosis	LAD > RCA > LCA
Cretinism	Iodine deficit/hypothyroidism

DISEASE/FINDING	MOST COMMON/IMPORTANT ASSOCIATIONS
Cushing syndrome	▪ Iatrogenic Cushing (from corticosteroid therapy) ▪ Adrenocortical adenoma (secretes excess cortisol) ▪ ACTH-secreting pituitary adenoma ▪ Paraneoplastic Cushing (due to ACTH secretion by tumors)
Cyanosis (early; less common)	Tetralogy of Fallot, transposition of great vessels, truncus arteriosus
Cyanosis (late; more common)	VSD, ASD, PDA
Death in CML	Blast crisis
Death in SLE	Lupus nephropathy
Dementia	Alzheimer disease, multiple infarcts
Demyelinating disease in young women	Multiple sclerosis
DIC	Severe sepsis, obstetric complications, cancer, burns, trauma, major surgery
Dietary deficit	Iron
Diverticulum in pharynx	Zenker diverticulum (diagnosed by barium swallow)
Ejection click	Aortic/pulmonic stenosis
Esophageal cancer	Squamous cell carcinoma (worldwide); adenocarcinoma (U.S.)
Food poisoning (exotoxin mediated)	*S. aureus*, *B. cereus*
Glomerulonephritis (adults)	Berger disease (IgA nephropathy)
Gynecologic malignancy	Endometrial carcinoma (most common in U.S.); cervical carcinoma (most common worldwide)
Heart murmur, congenital	Mitral valve prolapse
Heart valve in bacterial endocarditis	Mitral > aortic (rheumatic fever), tricuspid (IV drug abuse)
Helminth infection (U.S.)	*Enterobius vermicularis*, *Ascaris lumbricoides*
Hematoma—epidural	Rupture of middle meningeal artery (trauma; lentiform shaped)
Hematoma—subdural	Rupture of bridging veins (crescent shaped)
Hemochromatosis	Multiple blood transfusions or hereditary *HFE* mutation (can result in CHF, "bronze diabetes," and ↑ risk of hepatocellular carcinoma)
Hepatocellular carcinoma	Cirrhotic liver (associated with hepatitis B and C and with alcoholism)
Hereditary bleeding disorder	von Willebrand disease
Hereditary harmless jaundice	Gilbert syndrome (benign congenital unconjugated hyperbilirubinemia)
HLA-B27	Ankylosing spondylitis, reactive arthritis, ulcerative colitis, psoriatic arthritis
HLA-DR3 or -DR4	Diabetes mellitus type 1, rheumatoid arthritis, SLE

DISEASE/FINDING	MOST COMMON/IMPORTANT ASSOCIATIONS
Holosystolic murmur	VSD, tricuspid regurgitation, mitral regurgitation
Hypercoagulability, endothelial damage, blood stasis	Virchow triad (results in venous thrombosis)
Hypertension, 2°	Renal disease
Hypoparathyroidism	Accidental excision during thyroidectomy
Hypopituitarism	Pituitary adenoma (usually benign tumor)
Infection 2° to blood transfusion	Hepatitis C
Infections in chronic granulomatous disease	*Staphylococcus aureus, E. coli, Aspergillus* (catalase ⊕)
Intellectual disability	Down syndrome, fragile X syndrome
Kidney stones	<ul><li>Calcium = radiopaque</li><li>Struvite (ammonium) = radiopaque (formed by urease ⊕ organisms such as *Proteus vulgaris* or *Staphylococcus*)</li><li>Uric acid = radiolucent</li></ul>
Late cyanotic shunt (uncorrected left to right becomes right to left)	Eisenmenger syndrome (caused by ASD, VSD, PDA; results in pulmonary hypertension/polycythemia)
Liver disease	Alcoholic cirrhosis
Lysosomal storage disease	Gaucher disease
Male cancer	Prostatic carcinoma
Malignancy associated with noninfectious fever	Hodgkin lymphoma
Malignancy (kids)	ALL, medulloblastoma (cerebellum)
Metastases to bone	Prostate, breast > lung > thyroid
Metastases to brain	Lung > breast > genitourinary > melanoma > GI
Metastases to liver	Colon >> stomach, pancreas
Mitochondrial inheritance	Disease occurs in both males and females, inherited through females only
Mitral valve stenosis	Rheumatic heart disease
Mixed (UMN and LMN) motor neuron disease	Amyotrophic lateral sclerosis
Myocarditis	Coxsackie B
Nephrotic syndrome (adults)	Focal segmental glomerulosclerosis
Nephrotic syndrome (kids)	Minimal change disease
Neuron migration failure	Kallmann syndrome (hypogonadotropic hypogonadism and anosmia)
Nosocomial pneumonia	*Klebsiella, E. coli, Pseudomonas aeruginosa*
Obstruction of male urinary tract	BPH
Opening snap	Mitral stenosis
Opportunistic infection in AIDS	*Pneumocystis jirovecii* pneumonia
Osteomyelitis	*S. aureus*
Osteomyelitis in sickle cell disease	*Salmonella*
Osteomyelitis with IV drug use	*Pseudomonas, S. aureus*
Ovarian metastasis from gastric carcinoma or breast cancer	Krukenberg tumor (mucin-secreting signet-ring cells)
Ovarian tumor (benign, bilateral)	Serous cystadenoma

DISEASE/FINDING	MOST COMMON/IMPORTANT ASSOCIATIONS
Ovarian tumor (malignant)	Serous cystadenocarcinoma
Pancreatitis (acute)	Gallstones, alcohol
Pancreatitis (chronic)	Alcohol (adults), cystic fibrosis (kids)
Patient with ALL /CLL /AML /CML	ALL: child, CLL: adult > 60, AML: adult ~ 65, CML: adult 30–60
Pelvic inflammatory disease	*Chlamydia trachomatis*, *Neisseria gonorrhoeae*
Philadelphia chromosome t(9;22) (*bcr-abl*)	CML (may sometimes be associated with ALL/AML)
Pituitary tumor	Prolactinoma, somatotropic "acidophilic" adenoma
1° amenorrhea	Turner syndrome (45,XO)
1° bone tumor (adults)	Multiple myeloma
1° hyperaldosteronism	Adenoma of adrenal cortex
1° hyperparathyroidism	Adenomas, hyperplasia, carcinoma
1° liver cancer	Hepatocellular carcinoma (chronic hepatitis, cirrhosis, hemochromatosis, α_1-antitrypsin deficiency)
Pulmonary hypertension	COPD
Recurrent inflammation/thrombosis of small/medium vessels in extremities	Buerger disease (strongly associated with tobacco)
Renal tumor	Renal cell carcinoma: associated with von Hippel-Lindau and cigarette smoking; paraneoplastic syndromes (EPO, renin, PTH, ACTH)
Right heart failure due to a pulmonary cause	Cor pulmonale
S3 (protodiastolic gallop)	↑ ventricular filling (left-to-right shunt, mitral regurgitation, LV failure [CHF])
S4 (presystolic gallop)	Stiff/hypertrophic ventricle (aortic stenosis, restrictive cardiomyopathy)
2° hyperparathyroidism	Hypocalcemia of chronic kidney disease
Sexually transmitted disease	Chlamydia (usually coinfected with gonorrhea)
SIADH	Small cell carcinoma of the lung
Site of diverticula	Sigmoid colon
Sites of atherosclerosis	Abdominal aorta > coronary artery > popliteal artery > carotid artery
Stomach cancer	Adenocarcinoma
Stomach ulcerations and high gastrin levels	Zollinger-Ellison syndrome (gastrinoma of duodenum or pancreas)
t(14;18)	Follicular lymphomas (*bcl*-2 activation)
t(8;14)	Burkitt lymphoma (c-*myc* activation)
t(9;22)	Philadelphia chromosome, CML (*bcr-abl* fusion)
Temporal arteritis	Risk of ipsilateral blindness due to thrombosis of ophthalmic artery; polymyalgia rheumatica
Testicular tumor	Seminoma (malignant, radiosensitive)
Thyroid cancer	Papillary carcinoma

DISEASE/FINDING	MOST COMMON/IMPORTANT ASSOCIATIONS
Tumor in women	Leiomyoma (estrogen dependent, not precancerous)
Tumor of infancy	Hemangioma (usually regresses spontaneously by childhood)
Tumor of the adrenal medulla (adults)	Pheochromocytoma (usually benign)
Tumor of the adrenal medulla (kids)	Neuroblastoma (malignant)
Type of Hodgkin	Nodular sclerosis (vs. mixed cellularity, lymphocytic predominance, lymphocytic depletion)
Type of non-Hodgkin	Diffuse large cell
UTI	E. coli, Staphylococcus saprophyticus (young women)
Viral encephalitis affecting temporal lobe	HSV-1
Vitamin deficiency (U.S.)	Folate (pregnant women are at high risk; body stores only 3- to 4-month supply; prevents neural tube defects)

▶ EQUATION REVIEW

TOPIC	EQUATION	PAGE
Sensitivity	$\text{Sensitivity} = TP / (TP + FN)$	51
Specificity	$\text{Specificity} = TN / (TN + FP)$	51
Positive predictive value	$PPV = TP / (TP + FP)$	51
Negative predictive value	$NPV = TN / (FN + TN)$	51
Odds ratio (for case-control studies)	$\text{Odds ratio} = \dfrac{a/c}{b/d} = \dfrac{ad}{bc}$	53
Relative risk	$\text{Relative risk} = \dfrac{a/(a + b)}{c/(c + d)}$	53
Attributable risk	$\text{Attributable risk} = \dfrac{a}{a + b} - \dfrac{c}{c + d}$	53
Number needed to treat	1/absolute risk reduction	53
Number needed to harm	1/attributable risk	53
Hardy-Weinberg equilibrium	$p^2 + 2pq + q^2 = 1$ $p + q = 1$	85
Volume of distribution	$V_d = \dfrac{\text{amount of drug in the body}}{\text{plasma drug concentration}}$	239
Half-life	$t_{1/2} = \dfrac{0.693 \times V_d}{CL}$	239
Drug clearance	$CL = \dfrac{\text{rate of elimination of drug}}{\text{plasma drug concentration}} = V_d \times K_e \ (\text{elimination constant})$	239
Loading dose	$LD = \dfrac{C_p \times V_d}{F}$	239
Maintenance dose	$D = \dfrac{C_p \times CL \times \tau}{F}$	239

TOPIC	EQUATION	PAGE
Cardiac output	$$CO = \frac{\text{rate of } O_2 \text{ consumption}}{\text{arterial } O_2 \text{ content} - \text{venous } O_2 \text{ content}}$$	266
	$CO = \text{stroke volume} \times \text{heart rate}$	266
Mean arterial pressure	$MAP = \text{cardiac output} \times \text{total peripheral resistance}$	266
	$MAP = \frac{2}{3}\text{ diastolic} + \frac{1}{3}\text{ systolic}$	266
Stroke volume	$SV = EDV - ESV$	266
Ejection fraction	$$EF = \frac{SV}{EDV} = \frac{EDV - ESV}{EDV}$$	267
Resistance	$$\text{Resistance} = \frac{\text{driving pressure } (\Delta P)}{\text{flow } (Q)} = \frac{8\eta \text{ (viscosity)} \times \text{length}}{\pi r^4}$$	268
Net filtration pressure	$P_{net} = [(P_c - P_i) - (\pi_c - \pi_i)]$	281
	$J_v = \text{net fluid flow} = (K_f)(Pnet)$	281
Renal clearance	$C_x = U_x V / P_x$	525
Glomerular filtration rate	$GFR = U_{inulin} \times V / P_{inulin} = C_{inulin}$	525
	$GFR = K_f [(P_{GC} - P_{BS}) - (\pi_{GC} - \pi_{BS})]$	525
Effective renal plasma flow	$$ERPF = U_{PAH} \times \frac{V}{P_{PAH}} = C_{PAH}$$	525
Renal blood flow	$$RBF = \frac{RPF}{1 - Hct}$$	525
Filtration fraction	$$FF = \frac{GFR}{RPF}$$	526
Henderson-Hasselbalch equation (for extracellular pH)	$$pH = 6.1 + \log \frac{[HCO_3^-]}{0.03 \, P_{CO_2}}$$	532
Winters formula	$P_{CO_2} = 1.5 \, [HCO_3^-] + 8 \pm 2$	532
Physiologic dead space	$$V_D = V_T \times \frac{Pa_{CO_2} - Pe_{CO_2}}{Pa_{CO_2}}$$	596
Pulmonary vascular resistance	$$PVR = \frac{P_{\text{pulm artery}} - P_{\text{L atrium}}}{\text{cardiac output}}$$	599
Alveolar gas equation	$$PA_{O_2} = PI_{O_2} - \frac{Pa_{CO_2}}{R}$$	599

Top-Rated Review Resources

"Some books are to be tasted, others to be swallowed, and some few to be chewed and digested."

—Sir Francis Bacon

"Always read something that will make you look good if you die in the middle of it."

—P.J. O'Rourke

"So many books, so little time."

—Frank Zappa

"If one cannot enjoy reading a book over and over again, there is no use in reading it at all."

—Oscar Wilde

▶ HOW TO USE THE DATABASE

This section is a database of top-rated basic science review books, sample examination books, software, Web sites, and commercial review courses that have been marketed to medical students studying for the USMLE Step 1. At the end of the section is a list of publishers and independent bookstores with addresses and phone numbers. For each recommended resource, we list (where applicable) the **Title**, the **First Author** (or editor), the **Series Name** (where applicable), the **Current Publisher**, the **Copyright Year**, the **Number of Pages**, the **ISBN**, the **Approximate List Price**, the **Format** of the resource, and the **Number of Test Questions**. We also include **Summary Comments** that describe their style and overall utility for studying. Finally, each recommended resource receives a **Rating**. Within each section, resources are arranged first by Rating and then alphabetically by the first author within each Rating group.

A letter rating scale with six different grades reflects the detailed student evaluations for **Rated Resources.** Each rated resource receives a rating as follows:

A+	Excellent for boards review.
A A–	Very good for boards review; choose among the group.
B+ B	Good, but use only after exhausting better sources.
B–	Fair, but there are many better books in the discipline; or low-yield subject material.

The Rating is meant to reflect the overall usefulness of the resource in helping medical students prepare for the USMLE Step 1. This is based on a number of factors, including:

- The cost
- The readability of the text
- The appropriateness and accuracy of the material
- The quality and number of sample questions
- The quality of written answers to sample questions
- The quality and appropriateness of the illustrations (e.g., graphs, diagrams, photographs)
- The length of the text (longer is not necessarily better)
- The quality and number of other resources available in the same discipline
- The importance of the discipline for the USMLE Step 1

Please note that ratings do not reflect the quality of the resources for purposes other than reviewing for the USMLE Step 1. Many books with lower ratings are well written and informative but are not ideal for boards preparation. We have not listed or commented on general textbooks available in the basic sciences.

Evaluations are based on the cumulative results of formal and informal surveys of thousands of medical students at many medical schools across the country. The summary comments and overall ratings represent a consensus opinion, but there may have been a broad range of opinion or limited student feedback on any particular resource.

Please note that the data listed are subject to change in that:

- Publishers' prices change frequently.
- Bookstores often charge an additional markup.
- New editions come out frequently, and the quality of updating varies.
- The same book may be reissued through another publisher.

We actively encourage medical students and faculty to submit their opinions and ratings of these basic science review materials so that we may update our database. (See p. xvii, How to Contribute.) In addition, we ask that publishers and authors submit for evaluation review copies of basic science review books, including new editions and books not included in our database. We also solicit reviews of new books or suggestions for alternate modes of study that may be useful in preparing for the examination, such as flash cards, computer software, commercial review courses, and Web sites.

Disclaimer/Conflict of Interest Statement

No material in this book, including the ratings, reflects the opinion or influence of the publisher. All errors and omissions will gladly be corrected if brought to the attention of the authors through our blog at www.firstaidteam.com. Please note that USMLE-Rx and the entire *First Aid for the USMLE* series are publications by the senior authors of this book; their ratings are based solely on recommendations from the student authors of this book as well as data from the student survey and feedback forms.

A+   ***USMLEWorld Qbank***   *$119 - $399*   Test/2200 q
USMLEWORLD
www.usmleworld.com

An excellent bank of well-constructed questions that closely mirror those found on Step 1. Questions demand multistep reasoning and are often more difficult than those on the actual exam. Offers excellent, detailed explanations with figures and tables. Features a number of test customization and analysis options. Unfortunately, the program does not allow other application windows to be open for reference. Users can see cumulative results both over time and compared to other test takers. Another useful feature is that it gives a percentile score so the user can evaluate his or her performance compared to a large pool of other users who completed the same questions. Can be accessed through iPhone or Android mobile apps.

A   ***USMLE-Rx Qmax***   *$99–$199*   Test/2500 q
MEDIQ LEARNING
www.usmle-rx.com

A well-priced question bank that offers Step 1–style questions accompanied by thorough explanations. Some obscure material is omitted, making it more straightforward than other question banks. Each explanation includes high-yield facts and references from *First Aid*. However, the proportion of questions covering a given subject area does not always reflect the actual exam's relative emphasis. Question stems occasionally rely on "buzzwords." Most useful to help memorize *First Aid* facts. Provides detailed performance analyses. AMSA members are eligible for discounts.

A−   ***Kaplan Qbank***   *$99–$299*   Test/2200 q
KAPLAN
www.kaplanmedical.com

A high-quality question bank that covers most content found on Step 1, but sometimes emphasizes recall of overly specific details rather than integrative problem-solving skills. Test content and performance feedback can be organized by both organ system and discipline. Includes detailed explanations of all answer choices. Users can see cumulative results both over time and compared to other test takers. Can be accessed through iPhone or Android mobile apps.

B   ***USMLE Consult***   *$75–$395*   Test/2500 q
ELSEVIER
www.usmleconsult.com

A solid question bank that can be divided according to discipline and subject area. Questions are more straightforward than those on actual exam. Offers concise explanations with links to Student Consult and First Consult content. Users can see cumulative results both over time and compared to other test takers. Student Consult also offers a Robbins Pathology Test Bank (for an additional cost) featuring 500 USMLE-style questions. Purchase of any question bank includes use of the Scorrelator, a tool that predicts your USMLE Step 1 score from your performance on the question bank. Limited student feedback on Student Consult products.

A⁻

First Aid Q&A for the USMLE Step 1
LE

$44.95 Test/1000 q

McGraw-Hill, 2012, 765 pages, ISBN 9780071744027

A great source of approx. 1000 questions drawn from the USMLE-Rx Step 1 Qmax test bank, organized according to subject. Also features one full-length exam of 336 questions. Questions are easier than those found on Step 1, but provide representative coverage of the concepts typically tested. Includes brief but adequate explanations of both correct and incorrect answer choices.

B⁺

PreTest Clinical Vignettes for the USMLE Step 1
MCGRAW-HILL

$35.00 Test/322 q

McGraw-Hill, 2010, 318 pages, ISBN 9780071668064

Clinical vignette–style questions with detailed explanations, divided into seven blocks of 46 questions covering basic sciences. In general, questions are representative of the length and complexity of those on Step 1. Images (including pathology slides) are black and white and sometimes difficult to interpret. One of the better books in the PreTest series.

B

Kaplan USMLE Step 1 Qbook
KAPLAN

$44.99 Test/850 q

Kaplan, 2013, 456 pages, ISBN 9781419550478

A resource consisting of seventeen 50-question exams organized by the traditional basic science disciplines. Similar to the Kaplan Qbank, and offers good USMLE-style questions with clear, detailed explanations; however, lacks the classic images typically seen on the exam. Also includes a guide on test-taking strategies.

B

Lange Q&A: USMLE Step 1
KING

$51.00 Test/1200 q

McGraw-Hill, 2008, 528 pages, ISBN 9780071492195

Offers many questions organized by subject area along with three comprehensive practice exams. Questions are often challenging but are not always representative of Step 1 style—difficult concepts are tested, but multistep reasoning is not. Includes detailed explanations of both correct and incorrect answer choices. Black-and-white images only.

B

NMS Review for USMLE Step 1
LAZO

$54.99 Test/850 q

Lippincott Williams & Wilkins, 2005, 480 pages + CD-ROM, ISBN 9780781779210

A text and CD-ROM that offers 17 practice exams with answers. Some questions are too picky or difficult. Annotated explanations are well written but are sometimes unnecessarily detailed. The six pages of color plates are helpful. The CD-ROM attempts to simulate the computer-based testing format but is disorganized.

▶ INTERNET SITES

A⁻

Firecracker
FIRECRACKER INC.
www.firecracker.me

$25–$250 Review/
Test/1500 q

Learning platform divided into modules. The Step 1 module is divided into organ systems and in-cludes review of preclinical lecture material, periodic quizzes on flagged reviewed material, and USMLE-style questions in interface simulating real exam. Contains page references to *First Aid for the USMLE Step 1* and high-yield diagrams from assorted textbooks. You can grade how well you remem-ber the quiz answers (1–5), which allows the program to customize future quizzes. Features detailed performance analysis. Has a calendar for personalized study plan. Can be accessed on all smartphones and tablets. Very comprehensive, best if started early in preclinical years. Limited student feedback.

A⁻

WebPath: The Internet Pathology Laboratory
http://library.med.utah.edu/WebPath/

Free Review/
Test/1100 q

Features more than 2000 outstanding gross and microscopic images, clinical vignette questions, and case studies. Includes eight general pathology exams and 11 system-based exams with approximately 1000 questions. Also features 170 questions associated with images. Questions are useful for reviewing boards content but are typically easier and shorter. No multimedia practice questions. Tremendous resource, but in need of an update to retain Step 1 usefulness.

B+

The Pathology Guy
FRIEDLANDER
www.pathguy.com

Free Review

A free Web site containing extensive but poorly organized information on a variety of fundamental concepts in pathology. A high-yield summary intended for USMLE review can be found at www.path-guy.com/meltdown.txt, but the information given is limited by a lack of images and frequent digres-sions.

B

Lippincott's 350-Question Practice Test for USMLE Step 1
LIPPINCOTT WILLIAMS & WILKINS
www.lww.com/medstudent/usmle

Free Test/350 q

A free, full-length, seven-block, 350-question practice exam in a format similar to that of the real Step 1. Questions are easier than those on the actual exam, and the explanations provided are sparse. Users can bookmark questions and can choose between taking the test all at once or by section.

B

Radiopaedia.org
www.radiopaedia.org

Free Cases/Test

A user-friendly Web site with thousands of well-organized radiology cases and articles. Encyclopedia entries contain high-yield bullet points of anatomy and pathology. Images contain detailed descrip-tions but no arrows to demarcate findings. Quiz mode allows students to make a diagnosis based on radiographic findings. Content may be too broad for boards review but is a good complement to classes and clerkships.

B⁻   *The Whole Brain Atlas*   **Free**   Review

JOHNSON

http://www.med.harvard.edu/aanlib/

A collection of high-quality brain MR and CT images with views of normal and diseased brains. The interface is technologically impressive but complex, and many images are without explanations. Subject matter is overly specific, limiting its use as a boards review study tool. Useful adjunct to classes and clerkships.

B⁻   *Digital Anatomist Interactive Atlases*   **Free**   Review

UNIVERSITY OF WASHINGTON

www9.biostr.washington.edu/da.html

A good site containing an interactive neuroanatomy course along with a three-dimensional atlas of the brain, thorax, and knee. Atlases have computer-generated images and cadaver sections. Each atlas also has a quiz in which users identify structures in the slide images; however, questions do not focus on high-yield anatomy for Step 1.

▶ COMPREHENSIVE

A

First Aid Cases for the USMLE Step 1
LE   **$45.99** Review
McGraw-Hill, 2012, 411 pages, ISBN 9780071743976

A series of more than 400 high-yield cases divided into sections by organ system. Each case features a paragraph-long clinical vignette with relevant images, followed by questions and short, high-yield explanations. Offers great coverage of many frequently tested concepts, and integrates subject matter in the discussion of a single vignette. A good source of questions to review material outlined in *First Aid for the USMLE Step 1*.

A−

USMLE Step 1 Secrets
BROWN   **$39.95** Review
Elsevier, 2012, 880 pages, ISBN 9780323085144

Clarifies difficult concepts in a concise, easy-to-read manner. Employs a case-based format and integrates information well. Complements other boards study resources, with a focus on understanding preclinical fundamentals rather than on rote memorization. Slightly long for last-minute board cramming.

A−

First Aid for the Basic Sciences: General Principles
LE   **$72.00** Review
McGraw-Hill, 2012, 560 pages, ISBN 9780071743884

Excellent comprehensive review of the basic sciences covered in year 1 of medical school. Similar to the first part of *First Aid*, organized by discipline, and includes hundreds of full-color images and tables. Best if started with first-year coursework and then used as a reference during boards preparation.

A−

First Aid for the Basic Sciences: Organ Systems
LE   **$93.00** Review
McGraw-Hill, 2012, 858 pages, ISBN 9780071743952

A comprehensive review of the basic sciences covered in year 2 of medical school. Similar to the second part of *First Aid*, organized by organ system, and includes hundreds of full-color images and tables. Best if started with second-year coursework and then used as a reference during boards preparation. Each organ system contains discussion of embryology and anatomy, physiology, pathology, pharmacology, and a high-yield rapid review section.

A−

medEssentials for the USMLE Step 1
MANLEY   **$54.99** Review
Kaplan, 2012, 588 pages, ISBN 9781609780265

A comprehensive review divided into general principles and organ systems, and organized using high-yield tables and figures. Excellent for visual learners, but can be overly detailed and time consuming. Also includes color images in the back along with a monthly subscription to online interactive exercises, although these are of limited value for Step 1 preparation.

B+ **Cases & Concepts Step 1: Basic Science Review** $43.99 Review
CAUGHEY
Lippincott Williams & Wilkins, 2012, 400 pages

One hundred sixteen clinical cases integrating basic science with clinical data, followed by USMLE-style questions with answers and rationales. Thumbnail and key-concept boxes highlight key facts. Limited student feedback.

B+ **Step-Up to USMLE Step 1** $49.99 Review
JENKINS
Lippincott Williams & Wilkins, 2013, 432 pages, ISBN 9781451176940

An organ system–based review text with clinical vignettes that is useful for integrating the basic sciences covered in Step 1. The text is composed primarily of outlines, charts, tables, and diagrams, making the depth of material covered somewhat limited. Includes access to a sample online question bank.

B+ **USMLE Step 1 Recall: Buzzwords for the Boards** $50.99 Review
REINHEIMER
Lippincott Williams & Wilkins, 2007, 480 pages, ISBN 9780781770705

A review of core Step 1 topics presented in a two-column, quiz-yourself format. Best for a quick last-minute review before the exam. Covers many important subjects, but not comprehensive or tightly organized. Sometimes focuses on obscure details. Compare with the Déjà Review series. Includes all questions and answers in downloadable MP3 files so that files can be used on any digital audio playback device.

B+ **USMLE Images for the Boards: A Comprehensive Image-Based Review** $44.99 Review
TULLY
Elsevier, 2012, 296 pages, ISBN 1455709034

Contains over 400 images of content likely to be shown on the USMLE Step 1. Covers a wide variety of images including ECGs and radiological studies. Some images may be low yield for boards studying purposes, but still excellent as a supplement to preclinical courses.

B **USMLE Step 1 Made Ridiculously Simple** $29.95 Review
CARL
MedMaster, 2010, 400 pages, ISBN 9780940780910

A quick and easy read. Uses a table and chart format organized by subject, but some charts are poorly labeled. Consider as an adjunct to more comprehensive sources.

B **Déjà Review: USMLE Step 1** $27.00 Review
NAHEEDY
McGraw-Hill, 2010, 412 pages, ISBN 9780071627184

A comprehensive resource featuring questions and answers in a two-column, quiz-yourself format similar to that of the Recall series, divided according to discipline. Features a section of high-yield clinical vignettes along with useful mnemonics throughout. Contains a few mistakes, but remains a good alternative to flash cards as a last-minute review before the exam.

▶ ANATOMY, EMBRYOLOGY, AND NEUROSCIENCE

A⁻   **High-Yield Embryology**   **$35.99**   Review
DUDEK
Lippincott Williams & Wilkins, 2013, 176 pages, ISBN 9781451176100

A good review of a relatively low-yield subject. Offers excellent organization with clinical correlations.
Includes a high-yield list of embryologic origins of tissues.

A⁻   **High-Yield Neuroanatomy**   **$32.99**   Review/
FIX   Test/50 q
Lippincott Williams & Wilkins, 2008, 160 pages, ISBN 9780781779463

An easy-to-read, straightforward format with excellent diagrams and illustrations. Features a useful atlas
of brain section images, a glossary of important terms, an appendicized table of neurologic lesions, and
an expanded index. Overall, a great resource, but more detailed than what is required for Step 1.

A⁻   **Anatomy—An Essential Textbook**   **$44.99**   Review/
GILROY   Test/400 q
Thieme, 2013, 504 pages, ISBN 160406207X

A thorough, visually appealing approach to learning anatomy. Contains hundreds of colorful, helpful
illustrations. Presents material using a bullet-point format and in tables. Contains 400 USMLE-style
questions, with further opportunities to practice questions online.

A⁻   **Underground Clinical Vignettes: Anatomy**   **$31.99**   Review/
SWANSON   Test/20 q
Lippincott Williams & Wilkins, 2007, 256 pages, ISBN 9780781764759

Concise clinical cases illustrating approximately 100 frequently tested diseases with an anatomic basis. Cardinal signs, symptoms, and buzzwords are highlighted. Also includes 20 additional boards-style
questions. A useful source for isolating important anatomy concepts tested on Step 1.

A⁻   **USMLE Road Map: Gross Anatomy**   **$38.00**   Review/
WHITE   Test/150 q
McGraw-Hill, 2006, 240 pages, ISBN 9780071445160

An overview of high-yield gross anatomy with clinical correlations throughout. Also features numerous
effective charts and clinical problems with explanations at the end of each chapter. Features good integration of facts, but may be overly detailed and offers few illustrations. Lack of Step 1–related figures
limits usefulness. May require an anatomy reference text.

B⁺   **High-Yield Gross Anatomy**   **$35.99**   Review
DUDEK
Lippincott Williams & Wilkins, 2010, 320 pages, ISBN 9781605477633

A good review of gross anatomy with some clinical correlations. Contains well-labeled, high-yield radiographic images, but often goes into excessive detail that is beyond the scope of the boards.

B+ **Atlas of Anatomy** $79.99 Review
GILROY
Thieme, 2012, 704 pages, ISBN 9781604067453

A good atlas with more than 2200 high-quality, uncluttered illustrations. Includes clinical correlates and a brief introduction to new topics. Radiographs, MRIs, CT scans, and endoscopic views of the organs also included. Best if used as a reference or during coursework. Access to accompanying Web site with more than 600 illustrations, label on/off function, and timed self-tests also provided.

B+ **Clinical Anatomy Made Ridiculously Simple** $29.95 Review
GOLDBERG
MedMaster, 2010, 175 pages, ISBN 9780940780972

An easy-to-read text offering simple diagrams along with numerous mnemonics and amusing associations. The humorous style has variable appeal for students, so browse before buying. Offers good coverage of selected topics. Best if used during coursework. Includes more detail than typically tested on Step 1.

B+ **Rapid Review: Gross and Developmental Anatomy** $39.95 Review/
MOORE Test/450 q
Elsevier, 2010, 284 pages, ISBN 9780323072946

A detailed treatment of basic anatomy and embryology, presented in an outline format similar to that of other books in the series. More detailed than necessary for boards review. Contains high-yield charts and figures throughout, in color. Includes two 50-question tests with extensive explanations, with an additional 350 questions available online.

B+ **PreTest Neuroscience** $33.00 Test/500 q
SIEGEL
McGraw-Hill, 2013, 412 pages, ISBN 9780071791076

A high-yield introduction followed by 500 questions with detailed explanations. The question format has been improved to be more in-line with USMLE Step 1 questions. Sparse black and white images throughout the book

B+ **Crash Course: Anatomy** $39.95 Review
STERNHOUSE
Elsevier, 2012, 288 pages, ISBN 9780723436218

Part of the Crash Course review series for basic sciences, integrating clinical topics. Offers two-color illustrations, handy study tools, and Step 1 review questions. Includes online access. Provides a solid review of anatomy for Step 1. Best if started early.

B+ **Déjà Review: Neuroscience** $22.00 Review
TREMBLAY
McGraw-Hill, 2010, 247 pages, ISBN 9780071627276

A resource that features questions and answers in a two-column, quiz-yourself format similar to that of the Recall series. Includes several useful diagrams and CT images. A perfect length for Step 1 neurophysiology and anatomy review.

B+

USMLE Road Map: Neuroscience
WHITE

$36.00   Review/Test/300 q

McGraw-Hill, 2008, 224 pages, ISBN 9780071496230

An outline review of basic neuroanatomy and physiology with clinical correlations throughout. Also features high-yield facts in boldface along with numerous tables and figures. Clinical problems with explanations are given at the end of each chapter. May be overly detailed for Step 1 review, but a good tool to use as a reference.

B

Elsevier's Integrated Anatomy and Embryology
BOGART

$37.95   Review

Elsevier, 2007, 448 pages, ISBN 9781416031659

Part of the Integrated series that seeks to link basic science concepts across disciplines. Case-based and Step 1–style questions at the end of each chapter allow readers to gauge their comprehension of the material. Includes online access. Best if used during coursework. Limited student feedback.

B

BRS Embryology
DUDEK

$47.99   Review/Test

Lippincott Williams & Wilkins, 2010, 320 pages, ISBN 9781605479019

An outline-based review of embryology that is typical of the BRS series. Offers a good review, but has limited illustrations and includes much more detail than is required for Step 1. A discussion of congenital malformations is included at the end of each chapter along with relevant questions. The comprehensive exam at the end of the book is high yield.

B

Anatomy Flash Cards
GILROY

$34.95   Flash cards

Thieme, 2009, 376 flash cards, ISBN 9781604060720

High-quality illustrations with numbered labels on one side and answers on the other for self-testing. Occasional radiographic image. Best if used with coursework; too long for boards preparation. Limited student feedback.

B

Clinical Neuroanatomy Made Ridiculously Simple
GOLDBERG

$24.95   Review/Test/Few q

MedMaster, 2010, 87 pages + CD-ROM, ISBN 9780940780927

An easy-to-read, memorable, and simplified format with clever diagrams. Offers a quick, high-yield review of clinical neuroanatomy, but does not serve as a comprehensive resource for boards review. Places good emphasis on clinically relevant pathways, cranial nerves, and neurologic diseases. Includes a CD-ROM with CT and MR images as well as a tutorial on neurologic localization. Compare with *High-Yield Neuroanatomy*.

B

Netter's Anatomy Flash Cards
HANSEN

$39.95   Flash cards

Saunders, 2011, 676 flash cards, ISBN 9781437716757

Netter's illustrations with numbered labels on one side and answers on the other for self-testing. Each card includes a commentary on the structures and a clinical correlation. Best if used with coursework, but much too detailed for boards preparation. Lack of embryology correlates hurts Step 1 usefulness. Includes online access with additional bonus cards and more than 300 multiple-choice questions. Excellent iPhone app costs approximately the same and has additional functionality.

B   *Case Files: Gross Anatomy*   **$38.00**   Review
Toy
McGraw-Hill, 2008, 384 pages, ISBN 9780071489805

Review text that includes 53 well-chosen cases with discussion, comprehension questions, and a box of take-home pearls. Tables are good, but schematics are black and white and not representative of Step 1. A reasonable book to work through for those who benefit from problem-based learning.

B   *Rapid Review: Neuroscience*   **$38.95**   Review/
Weyhenmeyer   Test/350 q
Elsevier, 2006, 320 pages, ISBN 9780323022613

A detailed treatment of neuroscience, presented in an outline format similar to that of other books in the series. Should be started early given its extensive treatment of a relatively narrow topic. Contains high-yield charts and figures throughout. Includes two 50-question tests with extensive explanations as well as 250 additional questions online.

B−   *Gray's Anatomy for Students Flash Cards*   **$39.95**   Flash cards
Drake
Elsevier, 2010, 748 flash cards, ISBN 9780702031724

These flash cards feature renowned Gray's illustrations on the front and labels on the back for self-testing. Notes on clinical importance and reference to accompanying textbook given on back. Much too detailed information on a relatively low-yield subject for effective boards studying. Limited student feedback.

B−   *Case Files: Neuroscience*   **$38.00**   Review
Toy
McGraw-Hill, 2008, 408 pages, ISBN 9780071489218

Includes 48 clinical cases with lengthy discussion and 3–5 multiple-choice questions at the end of each case. Cases are well chosen, but the discussion is too lengthy. Questions are not the most representative of those seen on boards.

▸ BEHAVIORAL SCIENCE

A

High-Yield Behavioral Science   **$31.99**   Review
FADEM
Lippincott Williams & Wilkins, 2012, 144 pages, ISBN 9781451130300

An extremely concise yet comprehensive review of behavioral science for Step 1. Offers a logical presentation with charts, graphs, and tables, but lacks questions. Features brief but adequate coverage of statistics. Overall, an excellent, high-yield resource at an unrivaled price.

A–

BRS Behavioral Science   **$45.99**   Review/
FADEM   Test/500 q
Lippincott Williams & Wilkins, 2013, 336 pages, ISBN 9781451132106

An easy-to-read outline-format review of behavioral science. Offers good, detailed coverage of essential topics, but at a level of depth that often exceeds what is tested on Step 1. Incorporates excellent tables and charts as well as a short but complete statistics chapter. Features high-quality review questions, including a 100-question comprehensive exam.

A–

High-Yield Biostatistics, Epidemiology, and Public Health   **$36.99**   Review
GLASER
Lippincott Williams & Wilkins, 2013, 168 pages, ISBN 9781451130171

A well-written, easy-to-read text that offers extensive coverage of epidemiology and biostatistics. Includes good review questions and tables, but somewhat lengthy given the low-yield nature of the subject matter on Step 1.

A–

Clinical Biostatistics and Epidemiology Made Ridiculously Simple   **$22.95**   Review
WEAVER
MedMaster, 2011, 104 pages, ISBN 1935660020

An easy-to-read summary of all high-yield biostatistics and epidemiology. Contains highly relevant clinical examples and diagrams to enhance the learning experience. A good supplement for preclinical courses or boards studying.

B+

High-Yield Brain & Behavior   **$34.95**   Review
FADEM
Lippincott Williams & Wilkins, 2007, 256 pages, ISBN 9780781792288

Part of the new High-Yield Systems series that covers embryology, gross anatomy, radiology, histology, physiology, microbiology, and pharmacology as they relate to the nervous system. Written by the same author as the *High-Yield Behavioral Science* and *BRS Behavioral Science* texts. Overall, provides a good review of neuroscience and behavioral science but too much detail for most Step 1 takers.

B+

Jekel's Epidemiology, Biostatistics, Preventive Medicine, and Public Health   **$44.99**   Review
KATZ
Saunders, 2013, 420 pages, ISBN 1455706582

A solid, comprehensive review of the behavioral sciences to supplement preclinical coursework or boards studying. Strongest areas are biostatics and epidemiology. Emphasis on being succinct and teaching to high-yield points. May not cover all material tested on the boards. In-book questions were removed, but may still be accessed online.

B

USMLE Medical Ethics
FISCHER

$42.99 Review

Kaplan, 2012, 216 pages, ISBN 9781607149040

Includes 100 cases, each followed by a single question and a detailed explanation. Also offers guidelines on how Step 1 requires test takers to think about ethics and medicolegal questions. Unfortunately, a lengthy review for a low-yield subject.

B

Déjà Review: Behavioral Science
QUINN

$19.95 Review

McGraw-Hill, 2010, 226 pages, ISBN 9780071627283

Features questions and answers in a two-column, quiz-yourself format similar to that of the Recall series. Coverage of some topics is too lengthy for Step 1 review purposes, and order of information is nearly opposite that of *First Aid*. Limited student feedback.

B

Rapid Review: Behavioral Science
STEVENS

$39.95 Review/
Test/350 q

Elsevier, 2006, 320 pages, ISBN 9780323045711

Similar in style to other books in the Rapid Review series. Provides a good but low-yield review of a broad subject. Includes 100 questions and explanations along with an additional 250 questions online. Limited student feedback.

▶ BIOCHEMISTRY

Lange Flash Cards Biochemistry and Genetics
BARON

McGraw-Hill, 2012, 184 flash cards, ISBN 9780071765800

$35.00   Flash cards

Great flash cards featuring a clinical vignette on one side and concise discussion on the other. Each section contains 2–3 cards on biochemistry principles. Excellent resource for boards studying, but no carrying case included.

Rapid Review: Biochemistry
PELLEY

Elsevier, 2011, 208 pages, ISBN 9780323068871

$39.95   Review/ Test/350 q

A review of basic topics in biochemistry. Presented in outline format, but often goes beyond the level of detail tested on Step 1. High-yield disease correlation boxes are especially useful. Excellent tables and helpful figures are included throughout the text. Best if used as a reference to clarify topics. Offers 350 questions online.

Lippincott's Illustrated Reviews: Biochemistry
FERRIER

Lippincott Williams & Wilkins, 2012, 560 pages, ISBN 9781451175622

$69.99   Review/ Test/250 q

An excellent, integrative, and comprehensive review of biochemistry that includes good clinical correlations and highly effective color diagrams. Extremely detailed and requires significant time commitment, so it should be started with first-year coursework. High-yield summaries at the end of each chapter. Comes with access to the companion Web site with USMLE-style questions.

BRS Biochemistry, Molecular Biology, and Genetics
LIEBERMAN

Lippincott Williams & Wilkins, 2013, 432 pages, ISBN 9781451175622

$46.99   Review/Test

A highly detailed review featuring many excellent figures and clinical correlations highlighted in colored boxes. The biochemistry portion includes much more detail than required for Step 1, but may be useful for students without a strong biochemistry background or as a reference text. The molecular biology section is more focused and high yield. Also offers a chapter on laboratory techniques and a comprehensive, 120-question exam. Questions are clinically oriented.

USMLE Road Map: Biochemistry
MACDONALD

McGraw-Hill, 2007, 224 pages, ISBN 9780071442053

$36.00   Review

A clear, readable outline review of biochemistry with good four-color figures. High-yield references to important diseases of metabolism are scattered throughout, but coverage of clinical correlations is not comprehensive. Includes brief review questions at the end of each chapter. Lacks "big picture" integration of related pathways. Limited student feedback.

B+

Déjà Review: Biochemistry   **$22.00** Review
MANZOUL
McGraw-Hill, 2010, 206 pages, ISBN 9780071627177

Features questions and answers in a two-column, quiz-yourself format similar to that of the Recall series. Includes a helpful chapter on molecular biology and many good black-and-white diagrams. More detailed than is usually tested on Step 1.

B+

Medical Biochemistry—An Illustrated Review   **$39.99** Review
PANINI
Thieme, 2013, 441 pages, ISBN 1604063165

A comprehensive medical biochemistry study guide with an emphasis on images. Very detailed and may be better as a supplement to preclinical courses than as a review resource for the USMLE Step 1. Images and diagrams are helpful for solidifying knowledge. Online access available for additional content, including practice questions.

B+

Underground Clinical Vignettes: Biochemistry   **$31.99** Review/
SWANSON   Test/20 q
Lippincott Williams & Wilkins, 2007, 256 pages, ISBN 9780781764728

Concise clinical cases illustrating approximately 100 frequently tested diseases with a biochemical basis. Cardinal signs, symptoms, and buzzwords are highlighted. Also includes 20 additional boards-style questions. A nice review of "take-home" points for biochemistry and a useful supplement to other sources of review.

B+

PreTest Biochemistry and Genetics   **$33.00** Test/500 q
WILSON
McGraw-Hill, 2013, 570 pages, ISBN 9780071791441

500 questions with detailed, well-referenced explanations. Features a high-yield introduction and appendix, but may be overly detailed in some cases. A solid supplement to preclinical courses and board studying.

B

Clinical Biochemistry Made Ridiculously Simple   **$24.95** Review
GOLDBERG
MedMaster, 2010, 95 pages + foldout, ISBN 9780940780958

A conceptual approach to clinical biochemistry, presented with humor. The casual style does not appeal to all students. Offers a good overview and integration of all metabolic pathways. Includes a 23-page clinical review that is very high yield and crammable. Also contains a unique foldout "road map" of metabolism. For students who already have a solid grasp of biochemistry.

B

BRS Biochemistry and Molecular Biology Flash Cards   **$45.99** Flash cards
SWANSON
Lippincott Williams & Wilkins, 2007, 512 flash cards, ISBN 9780781779029

Quick-review flash cards covering a range of topics in biochemistry and molecular biology. Inadequate for learning purposes, as cards provide only snippets of isolated information and contain some inaccuracies.

B

High-Yield Biochemistry
WILCOX

$35.99   Review

Lippincott Williams & Wilkins, 2009, 128 pages, ISBN 9780781799249

A concise and crammable text in outline format with good clinical correlations at the end of each chapter. Features many diagrams and tables. Best used as a supplemental review, as explanations are scarce and details are limited.

B⁻

Case Files: Biochemistry
TOY

$37.00   Review

McGraw-Hill, 2008, 456 pages, ISBN 9780071486651

Includes 51 clinical cases with comprehensive discussion and summary box, but too much depth and not enough breadth for boards. Some cases will almost certainly *not* be tested. Questions at the end of each case are not representative of those seen on Step 1.

▶ **CELL BIOLOGY AND HISTOLOGY**

A− **High-Yield Cell and Molecular Biology** $29.95 Review
DUDEK
Lippincott Williams & Wilkins, 2010, 151 pages, ISBN 9781609135737

Cellular and molecular biology presented in an outline format, with good diagrams and clinical correlations. Includes USMLE-tested subjects that other review resources do not cover in detail, such as
laboratory techniques and second-messenger systems. Not all sections are equally useful; many students skim or read select chapters. Contains no questions or vignettes.

B+ **Rapid Review: Histology and Cell Biology** $39.95 Review/
BURNS   Test/350 q
Elsevier, 2006, 336 pages, ISBN 9780323044257

A resource whose format is similar to that of other books in the Rapid Review series. Features an outline of basic concepts with numerous charts, but histology images are limited. Two 50-question multiple-choice tests are presented with explanations, along with 250 more questions online.

B+ **Déjà Review: Histology and Cell Biology** $21.00 Review
SONG
McGraw-Hill, 2011, 300 pages, ISBN 9780071627269

Features questions and answers in a two-column, quiz-yourself format similar to that of the Recall series. Sections are divided by organ system and vary in quality. Histology images are few and are printed
in black and white. Good for a quick review, but some sections are lower yield than others.

B **Elsevier's Integrated Review: Genetics** $39.95 Review
ADKISON
Elsevier, 2011, 272 pages, ISBN 9780323074483

Part of the Integrated series that seeks to link basic science concepts across disciplines. Case-based and
Step 1–style questions at the end of each chapter allow readers to gauge their comprehension of the
material. Includes online access. Best if used during coursework; length and comprehensiveness make
this less useful as stand-alone Step 1 prep material.

B **High-Yield Genetics** $32.99 Review
DUDEK
Lippincott Williams & Wilkins, 2008, 134 pages, ISBN 9780781768771

A concise, clinically oriented summary of genetics in the popular outline format. Illustrated with schematic line drawings and photographs of the most clinically relevant diseases. By no means an exhaus-
tive resource.

B **USMLE Road Map: Genetics** $36.00 Review
SACK
McGraw-Hill, 2008, 224 pages, ISBN 9780071498203

Efficient review of genetics with an emphasis on clinical correlations. Includes a few questions at the
end of each chapter that are best suited to test comprehension and are not representative of Step 1.
Use only if genetics is a weak subject after reviewing *First Aid*; otherwise, too much depth for a quick
review.

B

USMLE Road Map: Histology
SHEEDLO

McGraw-Hill, 2005, 231 pages, ISBN 9780071440127

$38.00 Review

A concise review book with many clinical correlations. Questions at the end of each chapter are not in clinical vignette format but are suitable for testing comprehension. Black-and-white images. Good for a quick review of a low-yield subject.

B

Crash Course: Cell Biology and Genetics
STUBBS

Elsevier, 2013, 240 pages

$49.95 Review

Part of the Crash Course review series for basic sciences, integrating clinical topics. Offers two-color illustrations, handy study tools, and Step 1 review questions. Includes online access. Too much coverage for a low-yield subject.

B⁻

BRS Cell Biology and Histology
GARTNER

Lippincott Williams & Wilkins, 2010, 384 pages, ISBN 9781608313211

$42.99 Review/
Test/500 q

Covers concepts in cell biology and histology in an outline format. Can be used alone for cell biology study, but does not include enough histology images to be considered comprehensive on that subject. Includes more detail than is required for Step 1, and information is less high yield than that of other books in the BRS series.

B⁻

PreTest Anatomy, Histology, and Cell Biology
KLEIN

McGraw-Hill, 2010, 654 pages, ISBN 9780071623438

$35.00 Test/500 q

A resource containing difficult questions with detailed answers as well as some black-and-white images. Requires extensive time commitment, and much of the material is beyond what is required for Step 1. The most useful part of the book is the high-yield facts section at the beginning, which is divided according to discipline.

B⁻

Wheater's Functional Histology
YOUNG

Elsevier, 2006, 448 pages, ISBN 9780443068508

$79.95 Review

A color atlas with illustrations of normal histology with image captions and accompanying text. Far too detailed to use for boards studying given the low-yield nature of the material, but useful as a course-work text or boards reference. New edition expected December 2013.

▶ MICROBIOLOGY AND IMMUNOLOGY

A⁻ **_Basic Immunology_** $69.95 Review
ABBAS
Elsevier, 2012, 336 pages, ISBN 9781455707072

A useful text that offers clear explanations of complex topics in immunology. Best if used during the year in conjunction with coursework and later skimmed for quick Step 1 review. Includes colorful diagrams, images, tables, and a lengthy glossary for further study. Features online access.

A⁻ **_The Big Picture: Medical Microbiology_** $58.95 Review/
CHAMBERLAIN 100 q
McGraw-Hill, 2009, 456 pages, ISBN 9780071476614

Excellent full-color atlas of pathogens and clinical signs of infection. Discussion targets quick boards review. Especially good for visual learners. High-yield appendix. Includes 100 practice questions with discussion.

A⁻ **_Déjà Review: Microbiology & Immunology_** $19.95 Review
CHEN
McGraw-Hill, 2010, 424 pages, ISBN 9780071627153

Features questions and answers in a two-column, quiz-yourself format similar to that of the Recall series. Provides an excellent review of high-yield facts. Good mnemonics, but only a few images of pathogens in black and white. Good review text on a high-yield topic.

A⁻ **_Clinical Microbiology Made Ridiculously Simple_** $34.95 Review
GLADWIN
MedMaster, 2013, 400 pages, ISBN 9781935660156

An excellent, easy-to-read, detailed review of microbiology that includes clever and memorable mnemonics. The style of the series does not appeal to everyone, but it works extremely well for those who like the format. The sections on bacterial disease are most high yield, less emphasis placed on pharmacology. Recommended to read during coursework and review the concise charts at the end of each chapter during boards review. All images are cartoons; no microscopy images that appear on boards. Requires a supplemental source for immunology.

A⁻ **_Microcards Flash Cards_** $44.99 Flash cards
HARPAVAT
Lippincott Williams & Wilkins, 2011, 310 flash cards, ISBN 9781451112191

A well-organized and complete resource for students who like to use flash cards for review. Cards feature the clinical presentation, pathobiology, diagnosis, treatment, and high-yield facts for a particular organism. Some cards also include excellent flow charts organizing important classes of bacteria or viruses. Overall, a good review resource, but at times it is overly detailed, requiring a significant time commitment. Also useful as an aid with coursework.

A−   *High-Yield Microbiology and Infectious Diseases*   **$28.95**   Review/
HAWLEY   Test/200 q

Lippincott Williams & Wilkins, 2006, 240 pages, ISBN 9780781760324

A very concise review of central concepts and keywords, with chapters organized by microorganism. The last few sections contain brief questions and answers organized by organ system. Also offers a useful chapter on "microbial comparisons" that groups organisms by shared virulence factors, lab results, and the like. Some students may prefer alternative resources with more explanations.

A−   *Lange Review of Medical Microbiology and Immunology*   **$44.99**   Review/654 q
LEVINSON

McGraw-Hill, 2012, 710 pages, ISBN 9780071774345

A comprehensive review of all the microbiology and immunology that one needs to know for the USMLE Step 1. May also be easily used as a textbook for preclinical courses. Contains numerous color illustrations to help with studying. Includes practice questions and cases.

A−   *Review of Medical Microbiology*   **$46.95**   Test/550 q
MURRAY

Elsevier, 2005, 176 pages, ISBN 9780323033251

A resource that features Step 1–style questions divided into bacteriology, virology, mycology, and parasitology. All questions are accompanied by detailed explanations, and some are paired with high-quality images. Questions are similar to those on Step 1 and provide a nice review. Supplements Murray's *Medical Microbiology*.

A−   *Medical Microbiology and Immunology Flash Cards*   **$35.95**   Flash cards
ROSENTHAL

Elsevier, 2008, 414 flash cards, ISBN 9780323065337

Flash cards covering the microorganisms most commonly found on Step 1. Each card features full-color microscopic images and clinical presentations on one side and relevant bug information in conjunction with a short case on the other side. Also includes Student Consult online access for extra features. Overemphasizes "trigger words" related to each bug. Not a comprehensive resource.

A−   *Lange Microbiology & Infectious Diseases Flash Cards*   **$39.00**   Flash cards
SOMERS

McGraw-Hill, 2010, 200 flash cards, ISBN 9780071628792

Contains a clinical vignette on one side and discussion on the other. Excellent condensed summaries of pathogens, but limited by lack of images that will be tested on boards. Printed on thinner paper than the *Biochemistry & Genetics* component of the series, reducing durability.

A−   *Underground Clinical Vignettes: Microbiology Vol. I:*   **$34.99**   Review/
Virology, Immunology, Parasitology, Mycology   Test/20 q
SWANSON

Lippincott Williams & Wilkins, 2007, 256 pages, ISBN 9780781764704

A resource containing 100 concise clinical cases that illustrate frequently tested diseases in microbiology and immunology. Cardinal signs, symptoms, and buzzwords are highlighted. Also includes 20 additional boards-style questions. Best if used as a supplement to other review resources.

A-

Underground Clinical Vignettes: Microbiology Vol. II: Bacteriology
SWANSON

$32.99 Review/Test/20 q

Lippincott Williams & Wilkins, 2007, 256 pages, ISBN 9780781764711

A resource containing 100 concise clinical cases that illustrate frequently tested diseases in microbiology and immunology. Cardinal signs, symptoms, and buzzwords are highlighted. Also includes 20 additional boards-style questions. Best if used as a supplement to other review resources.

B+

Elsevier's Integrated Immunology and Microbiology
ACTOR

$39.95 Review

Elsevier, 2011, 192 pages, ISBN 9780323074476

Part of the Integrated series that seeks to link basic science concepts across disciplines. Case-based and Step 1–style questions at the end of each chapter allow users to gauge their comprehension of the material. Includes online access. Best if used during coursework. Limited student feedback.

B+

Case Studies in Immunology: Clinical Companion
GEHA

$59.00 Review

Garland Science, 2011, 363 pages, ISBN 9780815344414

A text that was originally designed as a clinical companion to *Janeway's Immunobiology*. Provides a great synopsis of the major disorders of immunity in a clinical vignette format. Integrates basic and clinical sciences. Features excellent images and illustrations from Janeway, as well as questions and discussions.

B+

Review of Medical Microbiology and Immunology
LEVINSON

$53.00 Review/Test/654 q

McGraw-Hill, 2012, 710 pages, ISBN 9780071774345

A clear, comprehensive text with outstanding diagrams and tables. Includes an excellent immunology section. The "Summary of Medically Important Organisms" (Part IX) is highly crammable. Can be detailed and dense at points, so best if started early with coursework. Includes practice questions of mixed quality and does not provide detailed explanation of answers. Compare with *Lippincott's Illustrated Reviews: Microbiology*.

B+

Rapid Review: Microbiology and Immunology
ROSENTHAL

$39.95 Review/Test/400 q

Elsevier, 2011, 240 pages, ISBN 9780323069380

A resource presented in a format similar to that of other books in the Rapid Review series. Contains many excellent tables and figures, but requires significant time commitment and is not as high yield as comparable review books. Includes access to companion Web site with more than 400 questions.

B

Lippincott's Illustrated Reviews: Immunology
DOAN

$52.99 Review/Test/Few q

Lippincott Williams & Wilkins, 2012, 384 pages, ISBN 9781451109375

A clearly written, highly detailed review of basic concepts in immunology. Features many useful tables and review questions at the end of each chapter. Offers abbreviated coverage of immune deficiencies and autoimmune disorders. Best if started with initial coursework and used as a reference during Step 1 study.

B

Lippincott's Illustrated Reviews: Microbiology
HARVEY

Lippincott Williams & Wilkins, 2012, 448 pages, ISBN 9781608317332

$59.99   Review/Test/
Few q

A comprehensive, highly illustrated review of microbiology that is similar in style to other titles in the Illustrated Reviews series. Includes a 50-page color section with more than 150 clinical and laboratory photographs. Compare with Levinson's *Review of Medical Microbiology and Immunology.*

B

High-Yield Immunology
JOHNSON

Lippincott Williams & Wilkins, 2006, 99 pages, ISBN 9780781774697

$32.99   Review

Accurately covers high-yield immunology concepts, although at times it includes more detail than necessary for Step 1 preparation. Good for quick review.

B

Pretest: Microbiology
KETTERING

McGraw-Hill, 2013, 462 pages, ISBN 9780071791045

$33.00   Review/
Test/500 q

Includes a short section on high-yield facts followed by 500 questions in a clinical vignette format. Questions are more difficult than encountered on the boards and some topics discussed are not likely to be tested. A good book to work through with coursework but too low yield for review purposes.

B

Crash Course: Immunology
NOVAK

Elsevier, 2006, 144 pages, ISBN 9781416030072

$57.95   Review

Part of the Crash Course review series for basic sciences, integrating clinical topics. Offers two-color illustrations, handy study tools, and Step 1 review questions. Includes online access. Good length and detail for boards review.

B

USMLE Road Map: Immunology
PARMELY

McGraw-Hill, 2006, 223 pages, ISBN 9780071452984

$31.95   Review

An outline review of immunology with a special focus on molecular mechanisms and laboratory techniques. Features abbreviated coverage of immunologic deficiency and autoimmune diseases that are emphasized on Step 1. Offers a collection of brief review questions at the end of each chapter. Limited student feedback.

B

Case Files: Microbiology
TOY

McGraw-Hill, 2008, 423 pages, ISBN 9780071492584

$37.00   Review

50 clinical microbiology cases followed by a clinical correlation, a discussion with boldfaced buzzwords, and questions. Cases are well chosen, but the text lacks the high-yield charts and tables found in other books in the Case Files series. Images are sparse and of poor black-and-white quality.

▶ PATHOLOGY

A+

Rapid Review: Pathology   **$49.95** Review/
GOLJAN   Test/350 q
Elsevier, 2013, 784 pages, ISBN 9780323087872

A comprehensive source for key concepts in pathology, presented in a bulleted outline format with
many high-yield tables and color figures. Features detailed explanations of disease mechanisms. Integrates concepts across disciplines with a strong clinical orientation. Lengthy, so best if started early
with coursework. Includes access to online Qbank.

A+

Pathoma   **$84.99 and up** Review/Lecture
SATTAR
Pathoma, 218 pages

Novel approach to pathology review, combining a focused textbook with 35 hours of online lectures.
Lectures combine "chalk talk" and slide formats to explain pathogenesis in an easy-to-understand manner. Excellent feedback from students.

A

The Big Picture: Pathology   **$55.00** Review/
KEMP   Test/130 q
McGraw-Hill, 2008, 512 pages, ISBN 9780071477482

Excellent full-color atlas of pathologic images with distilled notes on pathophysiology and treatment.
Good for quick review and especially good for visual learners. The 130 questions included at the end
are more straightforward than those seen on boards, but they emphasize important and tricky concepts.

A⁻

Pathophysiology for the Boards and Wards   **$46.99** Review/
AYALA   Test/75 q
Lippincott Williams & Wilkins, 2006, 430 pages, ISBN 9781405105101

A systems-based outline with a focus on pathology. Well organized with glossy color plates of relevant
pathology and excellent, concise tables. The appendix includes a helpful overview of neurology, immunology, unusual "zebra" syndromes, and high-yield pearls. Features good integration of Step 1–
relevant material from various subject areas. Compare with *Rapid Review: Pathology.*

A⁻

Lange Pathology Flash Cards   **$37.00** Flash cards
BARON
McGraw-Hill, 2013, 300 flash cards, ISBN 9780071793568

Flash cards with clinical vignette on one side and discussion including etiology, pathology, clinical
manifestations, and treatment on the other. Good tables to help organize diseases, but lack of images
limits its utility. Best if used in conjunction with another resource. Printed on thinner paper than the
Biochemistry & Genetics component of the series, reducing durability.

A⁻

Déjà Review: Pathology   **$22.00** Review
DAVIS
McGraw-Hill, 2010, 474 pages, ISBN 9780071627146

Features questions and answers in a two-column, quiz-yourself format similar to that of the Recall series. Integrates pathophysiology and pathology. Includes many vignette-style questions, but only a few
images in black and white. Limited student feedback.

A⁻   *Lippincott's Illustrated Q&A Review of Rubin's Pathology*
FENDERSON

$48.95   Review/Test/1100 q

Lippincott Williams & Wilkins, 2010, 336 pages, ISBN 9781608316403

A review book featuring more than 1100 multiple-choice questions that follow the Step 1 template. Questions frequently require multistep reasoning, probing the student's ability to integrate basic science knowledge in a clinical situation. Detailed rationales are linked to clinical vignettes and address incorrect answer choices. More than 300 full-color images link clinical and pathologic findings, with normal lab values provided for reference. Questions are presented both online and in print. Students can work through the online questions either in "quiz mode," which provides instant feedback, or in "test mode," which simulates the Step 1 experience. Overall, a resource that is similar in quality to *Robbins and Cotran Review of Pathology*.

A⁻   *Robbins and Cotran Review of Pathology*
KLATT

$49.95   Review/Test/1100 q

Elsevier, 2009, 451 pages, ISBN 9781416049302

A review question book that follows the main Robbins textbooks. Questions are more detailed, difficult, and arcane than those on the actual Step 1 exam, but the text offers a great review of pathology integrated with excellent images. Thorough answer explanations reinforce key points. Requires significant time commitment, so best if started with coursework.

A⁻   *BRS Pathology*
SCHNEIDER

$45.99   Review/Test/450 q

Lippincott Williams & Wilkins, 2013, 480 pages, ISBN 9781451115871

An excellent, concise review with appropriate content emphasis. Chapters are organized by organ system and feature an outline format with boldfacing of key facts. Includes good questions with explanations at the end of each chapter plus a comprehensive exam at the end of the book. Offers well-organized tables and diagrams as well as photographs representative of classic pathology. Contains a chapter on laboratory testing and "key associations" with each disease. The new edition contains excellent color images and access to an online test and interactive question bank. Most effective if started early in conjunction with coursework, as it does not discuss detailed mechanisms of disease pathology.

A⁻   *Underground Clinical Vignettes: Pathophysiology Vol. I: Pulmonary, Ob/Gyn, ENT, Hem/Onc*
SWANSON

$31.99   Review/Test/20 q

Lippincott Williams & Wilkins, 2007, 228 pages, ISBN 9780781764650

Concise clinical cases illustrating 100 frequently tested pathology and physiology concepts. Cardinal signs, symptoms, and buzzwords are highlighted. Also includes 20 additional boards-style questions. Best if used as a supplement to other sources of review.

A⁻   *Underground Clinical Vignettes: Pathophysiology Vol. II: GI, Neurology, Rheumatology, Endocrinology*
SWANSON

$32.99   Review/Test/20 q

Lippincott Williams & Wilkins, 2007, 256 pages, ISBN 9780781764667

Concise clinical cases illustrating 100 frequently tested pathology and physiology concepts. Cardinal signs, symptoms, and buzzwords are highlighted. Also includes 20 additional boards-style questions. Best if used as a supplement to other sources of review.

A− | *Underground Clinical Vignettes: Pathophysiology Vol. III: CV, Dermatology, GU, Orthopedics, General Surgery, Peds* | **$31.99** | Review/ Test/20 q

Swanson

Lippincott Williams & Wilkins, 2007, 256 pages, ISBN 9780781764681

Concise clinical cases illustrating 100 frequently tested pathology and physiology concepts. Cardinal signs, symptoms, and buzzwords are highlighted. Also includes 20 additional boards-style questions. Best if used as a supplement to other sources of review.

B+ | *MedMaps for Pathophysiology* | **$46.99** | Review

Agosti

Lippincott Williams & Wilkins, 2007, 259 pages, ISBN 9780781777551

A rapid review that contains 102 concept maps of disease processes and mechanisms organized by organ system, as well as classic diseases. Useful for both coursework and Step 1 preparation. Ample room is provided for notes. A good resource for looking up specific mechanisms, especially when used in conjunction with other primary review sources.

B+ | *Cases & Concepts Step 1: Pathophysiology Review* | **$42.95** | Review/ Test/150 q

Caughey

Lippincott Williams & Wilkins, 2009, 376 pages, ISBN 9780781782548

Eighty-eight clinical cases integrating basic science concepts with clinical data, followed by USMLE-style questions with answers and rationales. Thumbnail and key-concept boxes highlight key facts. Limited student feedback.

B+ | *Case Files: Pathology* | **$33.95** | Review

Toy

McGraw-Hill, 2008, 462 pages, ISBN 9780071486668

Includes 50 clinical cases followed by discussion, comprehension questions, and a pathology pearls box. Cases are well chosen and good for those who prefer problem-based learning; however, utility is limited by scarce and poor-quality black-and-white images.

B+ | *USMLE Road Map: Pathology* | **$38.00** | Test/500 q

Wettach

McGraw-Hill, 2009, 412 pages, ISBN 9780071482677

A concise yet thorough outline-format review of diseases that are tested on boards. Text is easy to read and includes a glossary of commonly used terms. Questions at the end of each chapter are useful only for testing comprehension. Black-and-white images.

B | *PreTest Pathology* | **$35.00** | Test/500 q

Brown

McGraw-Hill, 2010, 612 pages, ISBN 9780071623490

Difficult questions with detailed, complete answers. High-yield facts at the beginning are useful for concept summaries, but information can easily be obtained in better review books. Features high-quality black-and-white photographs and microscopy slides, making interpretation difficult. Best used as a supplement to other review books.

B

High-Yield Histopathology
DUDEK

$32.99 Review

Lippincott Williams & Wilkins, 2011, 328 pages, ISBN 9781609130152

A new book that reviews the relationship of basic histology to the pathology, physiology, and pharmacology of clinical conditions that are tested on Step 1. Includes case studies, numerous light and electron micrographs, and pathology photographs. Given its considerable length, should be started with coursework.

B

Pathophysiology of Disease: Introduction to Clinical Medicine
MCPHEE

$81.00 Review/Test/ Few q

McGraw-Hill, 2009, 768 pages, ISBN 9780071621670

An interdisciplinary text useful for understanding the pathophysiology of clinical symptoms. Effectively integrates the basic sciences with mechanisms of disease. Features great graphs, diagrams, and tables. In view of its length, most useful if started during coursework. Includes a few non–boards-style questions. The text's clinical emphasis nicely complements BRS Pathology.

B

Haematology at a Glance
MEHTA

$45.00 Review

Blackwell Science, 2014, 140 pages, ISBN 9781119969228

A resource that covers common hematologic issues. Includes color illustrations. Presented in a logical sequence that is easy to read. Good for use with coursework.

B

Pocket Companion to Robbins and Cotran Pathologic Basis of Disease
MITCHELL

$39.95 Review

Elsevier, 2012, 800 pages, ISBN 9781416054542

A resource that is good for reviewing keywords associated with most important diseases. Presented in a highly condensed format, but the text is complete and easy to understand. Contains no photographs or illustrations but does include tables. Useful as a quick reference.

B

PreTest Pathophysiology
MUFSON

$35.00 Test/500 q

McGraw-Hill, 2004, 480 pages, ISBN 9780071434928

Includes 500 questions and answers with explanations. Questions are often overly specific, and explanations vary in quality. Features a brief section of high-yield topics. Good economic value.

B

Color Atlas of Physiology
SILBERNAGL

$44.95 Review

Thieme, 2009, 456 pages, ISBN 9783135450063

A text containing more than 180 high-quality illustrations of disturbed physiologic processes that lead to dysfunction. An alternative to standard texts, but not high yield for boards review.

B

Crash Course: Pathology
XIU

$49.95 Review

Elsevier, 2012, 356 pages, ISBN 9780723436195

Part of the Crash Course review series for basic sciences, integrating clinical topics. Offers two-color illustrations, handy study tools, and Step 1 review questions. Includes online access. Best if started during coursework.

▶ **PHARMACOLOGY**

A

Déjà Review: Pharmacology
GLEASON

McGraw-Hill, 2010, 219 pages, ISBN 9780071627290

$19.95   Review

Features questions and answers in a two-column, quiz-yourself format similar to that of the Recall series. Covers most of the drugs needed for Step 1 succinctly. Includes clinical vignettes at the end of chapters for review.

A⁻

Lange Pharmacology Flash Cards
BARON

McGraw-Hill, 2013, 230 flash cards, ISBN 9780071792912

$37.00   Flash cards

A total of 230 pocket-sized flash cards featuring clinical vignettes involving relevant drugs, with high-yield information highlighted in bold. Information content of cards varies—too much information on some, not enough on others. Printed on less durable material.

A⁻

Pharm Cards: Review Cards for Medical Students
JOHANNSEN

Lippincott Williams & Wilkins, 2010, 240 flash cards, ISBN 9780781787413

$37.95   Flash cards

A series of flash cards that cover the mechanisms and side effects of major drugs and drug classes. Good for class review, but the level of detail is beyond what is necessary for Step 1. Lacks pharmacokinetics, but features good charts and diagrams. Well liked by students who enjoy flash card–based review. Compare with BRS Pharmacology Flash Cards.

A⁻

BRS Pharmacology Flash Cards
KIM

Lippincott Williams & Wilkins, 2004, 508 flash cards, ISBN 9780781747967

$45.99   Flash cards

A series of flash cards that facilitate memorization of the appropriate clinical use of drugs rather than describing mechanisms and toxicities in detail. Not a comprehensive review resource, but may be useful for those who find other pharm cards overwhelming. Considered by many to be an excellent resource for quick, last-minute review.

B⁺

Pharmacology for the Boards and Wards
AYALA

Lippincott Williams & Wilkins, 2006, 256 pages, ISBN 9781405105118

$43.99   Review/
Test/150 q

Like other books in the Boards and Wards series, the pharmacology volume is presented primarily in tabular format with bulleted key points. Review questions are in Step 1 style. At times can be too dense, but does a great job of focusing on the clinical aspects of drugs.

B⁺

Crash Course: Pharmacology
BATTISTA

Elsevier, 2012, 248 pages, ISBN 9780723436300

$39.95   Review

Part of the Crash Course review series for basic sciences, integrating clinical topics. Offers two-color illustrations, handy study tools, and Step 1–style review questions. Includes online access. Gives a solid, easy-to-follow overview of pharmacology. Limited student feedback.

B+ **Pharmacology Flash Cards**   **$37.95**   Flash cards
BRENNER
Elsevier, 2012, 616 flash cards, ISBN 9781455702817

Flash cards for more than 200 of the most commonly tested drugs. Cards include the name of the drug (both generic and brand) on the front and basic drug information on the back. Divided and color coded by class, and comes with a compact carrying case. Lacks figures and clinical vignettes.

B+ **Kaplan Medical USMLE Pharmacology**   **$44.99**   Flash cards
and Treatment Flashcards
FISCHER
Kaplan, 2011, 200 flash cards, ISBN 9781607148791

Excellent, easy-to-read flash cards with drug and questions on one side and discussion on the other, offering just the right amount of detail for the boards. Alternative to more traditional pharmacology textbooks.

B+ **Lippincott's Illustrated Reviews: Pharmacology**   **$66.99**   Review/
HARVEY   Test/200 q
Lippincott Williams & Wilkins, 2011, 608 pages, ISBN 978145111314

A resource presented in outline format with practice questions, many excellent illustrations, and comparison tables. Effectively integrates pharmacology and pathophysiology. The new edition has been updated to cover recent changes in pharmacotherapy. Best started with coursework, as it is highly detailed and requires significant time commitment.

B+ **Elsevier's Integrated Pharmacology**   **$39.95**   Review
KESTER
Elsevier, 2011, 264 pages, ISBN 9780323074452

Part of the Integrated series that seeks to link basic science concepts across disciplines. Case-based and Step 1–style questions at the end of each chapter allow readers to gauge their comprehension of the material. Includes online access. Best if used during coursework. Limited student feedback.

B+ **Rapid Review: Pharmacology**   **$39.95**   Review/
PAZDERNIK   450 q
Elsevier, 2010, 360 pages, ISBN 9780323068123

A detailed treatment of pharmacology, presented in an outline format similar to that of other books in the series. More detailed than necessary for Step 1 review. Contains high-yield charts and figures. Includes access to the companion Web site with 450 USMLE-style questions.

B+ **Pharmacology Recall**   **$34.95**   Review
RAMACHANDRAN
Lippincott Williams & Wilkins, 2008, 592 pages + audio, ISBN 9780781787307

A resource presented in the two-column, question-and-answer format typical of the Recall series. At times questions delve into more clinical detail than required for Step 1, but overall the breadth of coverage is appropriate. Includes a high-yield drug summary. Includes questions and answers that are recorded in MP3 format so that they can be used on any audio player.

B+ | **PreTest Pharmacology** | **$33.00** Test/500 q
SHLAFER
McGraw-Hill, 2013, 567 pages, ISBN 9780071791465

Good questions divided into sections by organ system and accompanied by detailed answers. Many questions have been rewritten to be more in line with the USMLE Step 1 question format. Others build graph-reading skills and multistep reasoning skills. Sections on general principles and autonomics are especially useful. This is a great resource for anyone looking for additional practice questions.

B+ | **Underground Clinical Vignettes Step 1: Pharmacology** | **$27.95** Review/
SWANSON | Test/20 q
Lippincott Williams & Wilkins, 2007, 256 pages, ISBN 9780781764858

Concise clinical cases illustrating approximately 100 frequently tested pharmacology concepts. Cardinal signs, symptoms, and buzzwords are highlighted. Also includes 20 additional boards-style questions. Omits some important drugs and lacks detail on mechanisms, so best used as a supplement to other sources of review.

B+ | **Katzung & Trevor's Pharmacology: Examination and Board Review** | **$52.00** Review/
TREVOR | Test/1000 q
McGraw-Hill, 2012, 640 pages, ISBN 9780071789233

A well-organized text with concise explanations. Features good charts and tables; the crammable list in Appendix I is especially high yield for Step 1 review. Also good for drug interactions and toxicities. Offers two practice exams but no explanations of the answers. Text includes many low-yield/obscure drugs. Compare with *Lippincott's Illustrated Reviews: Pharmacology*, both of which are better suited to complementing coursework than last-minute studying for boards.

B | **USMLE Road Map: Pharmacology** | **$38.00** Review
KATZUNG
McGraw-Hill, 2006, 178 pages, ISBN 9780071445818

An outline review of pharmacology divided either by organ system or by disease process. Includes a collection of brief review questions at the end of each chapter. The appendix has useful tables of common side effects and drug classes. Does not contain enough detail to serve as a comprehensive review. Limited student feedback.

B | **BRS Pharmacology** | **$46.99** Review/
ROSENFELD | Test/200 q
Lippincott Williams & Wilkins, 2013, 384 pages, ISBN 9781451175356

Features two-color tables and figures that summarize essential information for quick recall. A list of drugs organized by drug family is included in each chapter. Too detailed for boards review; best used as a reference. Also offers end-of-chapter review tests with Step 1–style questions and a comprehensive exam with explanations of answers. An additional question bank is available online.

B   ***Case Files: Pharmacology***   ***$35.00***   Review
        TOY

McGraw-Hill, 2013, 453 pages, ISBN 9780071790239

Includes 53 cases with detailed discussion, comprehension questions, and a box of clinical pearls. An appealing text for students who prefer problem-based learning, but lacks the level of detail typically tested on Step 1.

B   ***High-Yield Pharmacology***   ***$32.99***   Review
        WEISS

Lippincott Williams & Wilkins, 2009, 160 pages, ISBN 9780781792738

A succinct pharmacology review presented in an easy-to-follow outline format. Features a drug index, key points in bold, and summary tables of high-yield facts. Lacks details on mechanisms or drug specifics, so best used with a more comprehensive resource.

▶ PHYSIOLOGY

BRS Physiology
COSTANZO

$48.99 Review/Test/400 q

Lippincott Williams & Wilkins, 2010, 328 pages, ISBN 9780781798761

A clear, concise review of physiology that is both comprehensive and efficient, making for fast, easy reading. Includes excellent high-yield charts and tables, but lacks some figures from Costanzo's *Physiology*. Features high-quality practice questions with explanations in each chapter along with a clinically oriented final exam. An excellent boards review resource, but best if started early in combination with coursework. Respiratory and acid-base sections are comparatively weak.

BRS Physiology Cases and Problems
COSTANZO

$45.95 Review/Test/Many q

Lippincott Williams & Wilkins, 2012, 368 pages, ISBN 9781451120615

Sixty classic cases presented in vignette format with several questions per case. Includes exceptionally detailed explanations of answers. For students interested in an in-depth discussion of physiology concepts. May be useful for group review.

Physiology
COSTANZO

$59.95 Text

Saunders, 2013, 520 pages, ISBN 9781455708475

A comprehensive, clearly written text that covers concepts outlined in *BRS Physiology* in greater detail. Offers excellent color diagrams and charts. Each systems-based chapter features a detailed summary of objectives and a Step 1–relevant clinical case. Includes access to online interactive extras. Requires time commitment; best started with coursework.

The Big Picture: Medical Physiology
KIBBLE

$52.00 Review/Text/108 q

McGraw-Hill, 2009, 448 pages, ISBN 9780071485678

Well-written text supplemented by 450 illustrations. Chapters conclude with approximately 10 study questions/answers. Consistent organization facilitates relatively quick review. Includes a 108-question practice exam with answers. Best if started early with coursework.

Acid-Base, Fluids, and Electrolytes Made Ridiculously Simple
PRESTON

$22.95 Review

MedMaster, 2010, 156 pages, ISBN 9780940780989

A resource that covers major acid-base and renal physiology concepts. Provides information beyond the scope of Step 1, but remains a useful companion for studying kidney function, electrolyte disturbances, and fluid management. Includes scattered diagrams and questions at the end of each chapter. Consider using after exhausting more high-yield physiology review resources.

B+
Déjà Review: Physiology
GOULD

$19.95   Review

McGraw-Hill, 2010, 288 pages, ISBN 9780071627252

Features questions and answers in a two-column, quiz-yourself format similar to that of the Recall series. Includes helpful graphs and schematics. Contains clinical vignettes at the end of each organ system similar to those seen on the Step 1 exam.

B+
High-Yield Acid-Base Review
LONGENECKER

$30.99   Review

Lippincott Williams & Wilkins, 2006, 128 pages, ISBN 9780781796552

A concise and well-written description of acid-base disorders. Includes chapters discussing differential diagnoses and 12 clinical cases. Introduces a multistep approach to the material. A bookmark with useful factoids is included with the text. No index or questions.

B+
USMLE Road Map: Physiology
PASLEY

$38.00   Review/
Test/50 q

McGraw-Hill, 2006, 224 pages, ISBN 9780071445177

A text in outline format incorporating useful comparison charts and clear diagrams. Provides a concise approach to physiology. Clinical correlations are referenced to the text. Questions build on basic concepts and include detailed explanations. Limited student feedback.

B+
Appleton & Lange Review: Physiology
PENNEY

$43.95   Test/700 q

McGraw-Hill, 2003, 278 pages, ISBN 9780071377263

Step 1–style questions divided into subcategories under physiology. Good if subject-specific questions are desired, but may be too detailed for many students. Some diagrams are used to explain answers. A good way to test knowledge after coursework.

B
Rapid Review: Physiology
BROWN

$39.95   Review/
300 q

Elsevier, 2012, 288 pages, ISBN 9780323072601

A resource that offers a good review of physiology in a format typical of the Rapid Review series, albeit with more images. Includes online access to 350 questions along with other extras.

B
Elsevier's Integrated Physiology
CARROLL

$37.95   Review

Elsevier, 2006, 256 pages, ISBN 9780323043182

Part of the Integrated series that seeks to link basic science concepts across disciplines. A good text for initial coursework, but too long for Step 1 review. Case-based and Step 1–style questions are included at the end of each chapter. Limited student feedback.

B

High-Yield Physiology
DUDEK

$32.99   Review

Lippincott Williams & Wilkins, 2008, 240 pages, ISBN 9780781745871

An outline review of major concepts written at an appropriate level of depth for Step 1; includes especially detailed coverage of cardiovascular, respiratory, and renal physiology. Features many excellent diagrams and boxes highlighting important equations. Large blocks of dense text make it a slow and disorienting read at times. Limited student feedback.

B

Vander's Renal Physiology
EATON

$42.00   Text

McGraw-Hill, 2013, 240 pages, ISBN 9780071797481

Well-written text on renal physiology, with helpful but sparse diagrams and practice questions at the end of each chapter. May be too detailed for Step 1 review, however. Best if used with organ-based coursework to understand the principles of renal physiology.

B

PreTest Physiology
METTING

$33.00   Test/500 q

McGraw-Hill, 2013, 528 pages, ISBN 9780071791427

Contains questions with detailed, well-written explanations. One of the best of the PreTest series. Best for use by the motivated student after extensive review of other sources. Includes a high-yield facts section with useful diagrams and tables.

B

Endocrine Physiology
MOLINA

$45.95   Text

McGraw-Hill, 2013, 320 pages, ISBN 9780071796774

A review text on endocrine physiology. Questions at the end of each chapter are helpful to work through to solidify knowledge, but some are not representative of Step 1 questions. Provides more detailed explanations of endocrine physiology than Costanzo offers but much too lengthy for Step 1 review. May be useful as a coursework adjunct.

B

Netter's Physiology Flash Cards
MULRONEY

$35.95   Flash cards

Saunders, 2010, 200+ flash cards, ISBN 9781416046288

Flash cards contain a high-quality illustration on one side with question and commentary on the other. Good for self-testing, but too fragmented for learning purposes and not comprehensive enough for boards. Limited student feedback.

B

Case Files: Physiology
TOY

$37.00   Review

McGraw-Hill, 2009, 456 pages, ISBN 9780071493741

A review text divided into 51 clinical cases followed by clinical correlations, a discussion, and take-home pearls, presented in a format similar to that of other texts in the Case Files series. A few questions accompany each case. Too lengthy for rapid review; best for students who enjoy problem-based learning.

B

Pulmonary Pathophysiology: The Essentials
WEST

Lippincott Williams & Wilkins, 2012, 208 pages, ISBN 9781451107135

$47.99   Review/Test/50 q

A volume offering comprehensive coverage of respiratory physiology. Clearly organized with useful charts and diagrams. Review questions at the end of each chapter have letter answers only and no explanations. Best used as a course supplement during the second year.

B−

Clinical Physiology Made Ridiculously Simple
GOLDBERG

MedMaster, 2010, 160 pages, ISBN 9780940780941

$24.95   Review

An easy-to-read text with many amusing associations and memorable mnemonics. The style does not work for everyone. Not as well illustrated as the rest of the series, and lacks some important concepts. Best used as a supplement to other review books.

Commercial Review Courses

▶ COMMERCIAL REVIEW COURSES

Commercial preparation courses can be helpful for some students, but such courses are expensive and may leave limited time for independent study. They are usually an effective tool for students who feel overwhelmed by the volume of material they must review in preparation for the boards. Also note that while some commercial courses are designed for first-time test takers, others are geared toward students who are repeating the examination. Still other courses have been created for IMGs who want to take all three Steps in a limited amount of time. Finally, student experience and satisfaction with review courses are highly variable, and course content and structure can evolve rapidly. We thus suggest that you discuss options with recent graduates of review courses you are considering. Some student opinions can be found in discussion groups on the Internet.

Becker Healthcare

Becker Healthcare provides intensive and comprehensive live, online, and self-study review courses for students preparing for the USMLE and COMLEX. The 7-week Step 1 reviews are held throughout the year with small class sizes in order to increase student involvement and instructor accessibility. Becker Healthcare uses an active learning system that focuses on comprehension, retention, and application of concepts. Online program components include:

- Over 300 hours of live lectures
- Lecture notes (textbook and ebook format)
- USMLEWorld QBank for 3 months
- Clinical vignettes and case studies
- Daily question and answer sessions
- 2 NBME practice exams
- 0% financing available

Live programs are currently offered in Dallas, Texas. The fee range is $2599–$6499. The all-inclusive program tuition fee includes all of the above plus:

- Lodging
- Complimentary daily breakfast and lunch
- A full set of color textbooks
- Daily clinical vignettes
- Daily tutoring
- High-speed Internet service
- Local hotel shuttle service

Becker's Ultimate Live Online Step 1 Review Course includes:

- Lecture note textbooks
- Becker interactive ebook
- 2 NBME practice exams
- USMLEWorld Q Bank for 6 months
- 30 hours of integrated cases with Dr. Lionel Raymon

Becker's Self-Study USMLE Step 1 Review Course includes:

- "Until Your Exam" access
- Dual-degree MD and/or PhD instructors

- Full set of color textbooks
- On-screen PowerPoint slides
- 3-month USMLEWorld or 6-month USMLE Consult Qbank subscription
- Diagnostic exam
- Streaming video lectures

For more information, contact:

Becker Healthcare
3005 Highland Parkway
Downers Grove, IL 60515
Phone: (800) 683-8725
www.becker.com/health

Kaplan Medical

Kaplan Medical offers a wide range of options for USMLE preparation, including live lectures, center-based study, and online courses. All of its program offerings focus on providing the most exam-relevant information available.

Live Lectures. Kaplan's LivePrep offers a highly structured, interactive live lecture series led by expert faculty as 7-, 14-, or 16-week courses. This course's advantages include interaction with faculty and peers.

Kaplan also offers LivePrep Retreat, a 6-week course during which students stay and study in high-end hotel accommodations.

Center Study. Kaplan's CenterPrep, a center-based lecture course, is designed for medical students seeking flexibility. Essentially an independent study course, it is offered at Kaplan Centers across the United States for 3-, 6-, or 9-month periods. Students have access to more than 200 hours of video lecture review. CenterPrep features seven volumes of lecture notes and a full-length simulated exam with a complete performance analysis and detailed explanations. The course also includes a Personalized Learning System (PLS), which allows students to create a customized study schedule and track their performance.

Online Programs. Kaplan Medical provides online content- and question-based review. Classroom Anywhere, Kaplan's top-rated course, offers an interactive, online classroom experience with the benefit of live instruction delivered by expert faculty from wherever Internet access is available. Kaplan's OnlinePrep on-demand video lectures and Qbank are included in this course. This course is ideal for students who need a more comprehensive review option, but require a flexible study schedule or are unable to travel to one of Kaplan's live lecture locations.

Kaplan's popular Qbank allows students to create practice tests by discipline and organ system, difficulty, and yield; receive instant onscreen feedback; and track their cumulative performance. Kaplan offers Until Your Test access allowing students to get an immediate edge in school and repeat lectures as often as they like for the next 12 months. Kaplan's Qbank also includes a free integrated mobile app for iPhone and Android devices so students can practice questions on the go. Qbank demos are available at www.kaplanmedical.com.

For more information, call (800) 527-8378 or visit www.kaplanmedical.com.

Med School Tutors

Since 2007, Med School Tutors has helped students prepare for Step 1 by working with them one-on-one. Instead of offering courses, lectures, or videos, MST's approach is tailored to each student's weaknesses and strengths, according to their learning styles and schedules, and is guided by a personal coach who has scored high on Step 1.

Med School Tutors are medical students and residents who have excelled in their medical studies and training. Their minimum credentials include:

- Training at top medical schools and residency programs
- Superior standardized test scores (e.g., Step 1 > 245)
- Significant and verifiable teaching experience
- Interviewing and training with senior Step 1 coaches who have USMLE coaching experience

Med School Tutors assists students according to their needs. Comprehensive packages include:

- Personal day-by-day study schedule and plan
- Test-taking techniques and confidence-building exercises
- Assessment by question bank performance and NBME test analysis
- Selection and use of high-yield resources
- Integrated review of content with emphasis on student's weaknesses
- Emphasis on question/vignette-based learning
- Clinical reasoning skills training
- Holistic support throughout study period

Students start with a complimentary consultation and discussion of their needs and goals. This is followed by the tutor matching process and introduction to the tutor. Students then begin formal work with a trial session, the cost of which is discounted 2 hours for the price of 1. The trial session includes diagnostic assessment, teaching demonstration, Q&A, and the establishment of a personal study plan. Med School Tutors services are offered in person in Manhattan and near other select medical centers. Students also work with tutors seamlessly online via Web conferences.

For more information, visit www.medschooltutors.com or call (212) 327-0098.

Northwestern Medical Review

Northwestern Medical Review offers question bank services, live classes, online self-study review courses, and private tutoring in preparation for USMLE Step 1 and COMLEX Level I examinations. Duration of live courses is 5–16 days. Courses are taught by the authors of best-selling books and experienced Northwestern Medical Review lecturers. In addition to organized lecture notes and books for each subject, courses include Web-based question bank subscription, audio CDs, and a large pool of practice questions and simulated exams. The curriculum uses the unique built-in Adaptive-Flexi-Pass™ teaching methodology that progressively customizes content areas around the academic need of the student. In addition to customized onsite courses, public review sites are frequently offered in East Lansing, Mich.; Chicago; Philadelphia; and Hartford, Conn. Live courses are also globally available at international sites, including Puerto Rico, Mexico, India, China, Canada, Dubai, and other locations based on demand. Northwestern Medical Review offers a free retake option for all live courses as well as a liberal cancellation policy.

Tuition for each course is $465. Private tutoring, CBT question-bank access, and DVD materials are also available for purchase independent of the live-lecture plans.

For more information, contact:

Northwestern Medical Review
4800 Collins Rd. #22174
Lansing, MI 48909
Phone: (866) MedPass
Fax: (517) 347-7005
Email: contactus@northwesternmedicalreview.com
www.northwesternmedicalreview.com

PASS Program/PASS Program South

USMLE and COMLEX Review Program. The PASS Program offers a concept-based, clinically integrated curriculum to help students increase board scores, obtain residencies, and broaden their perspective of medicine. Helpful for a wide spectrum of students, including those trying to maximize scores on the first try and those struggling to stay in medical school. PASS accommodates all types of learners: auditory, visual, or kinesthetic, and, with the help of small class sizes, encourages students to interact and to ask questions.

Live Lectures. PASS offers 6-week, 8-week, 12-week, or extended-stay programs in Champaign, Ill., and St. Augustine, Fla. Facilities include computer labs, a state-of-the-art lecture hall, student lounges and study areas, and housing. Drill sessions and small study groups take place throughout the week. Tuition, which includes housing and security deposit, is $6775 for the 6-week course, $7600 for the 8-week course, and $12,350 for the 12-week course.

One-on-One Tutoring. Included with tuition, students receive one-on-one tutoring from an MD each week they attend the program. Six-week students receive two sessions per week and 8-week students receive three sessions in weeks 1–5 of the program and five sessions in weeks 6–8.

For more information, contact:

PASS Program
2302 Moreland Blvd.
Champaign, IL 61822
Phone: (217) 378-8018
Fax: (217) 378-7809
www.passprogram.net

PASS Program South
120 Sea Grove Main Street
St. Augustine, FL 32080
Phone: (904) 209-3140
www.passprogramsouth.com

The Princeton Review

The Princeton Review offers two flexible preparation options for the USMLE Step 1: the USMLE Online Course and the USMLE Online Workout.

USMLE Online Courses. The USMLE Online Courses offer the following:

- 75 hours of online review, including lessons, vignettes, and drills
- Complete review of all USMLE Step 1 subjects
- Three full-length CBTs
- Seven 1-hour subject-based tests
- Complete set of print materials
- 24/7 access to technical support
- Three months of access to tests, drills, and lessons

More information can be found on The Princeton Review's Web site at www.princetonreview.com.

Youel's™ Prep, Inc.

Youel's Prep, Inc., has specialized in medical board preparation for 30 years. The company provides DVDs, audiotapes, videotapes, a CD (PowerPrep Quick Study), books, live lectures, and tutorials for small groups as well as for individuals (TutorialPrep™). All DVDs, videotapes, audiotapes, live lectures, and tutorials are correlated with a three-book set of Prep Notes consisting of two textbooks, *Youel's Jewels I* and *Youel's Jewels II* (984 pages), and *Case Studies*, a question-and-answer book (1854 questions, answers, and explanations).

The Comprehensive DVD program consists of 56 hours of lectures by the systems with a three-book set: *Youel's Jewels I and II* and *Case Studies*. Integrated with these programs are pre-tests and post-tests.

All Youel's Prep courses are taught and written by physicians, reflecting the clinical slant of the boards. All programs are systems based. In addition, all programs are updated continuously. Accordingly, books are not printed until the order is received.

Delivery in the United States or overseas is usually within 1 week. Optional express delivery is also available. Youel's Prep Home Study Program™ allows students to own their materials and to use them for repetitive study in the convenience of their homes. Purchasers of any of Youel's Prep materials, programs, or services are enrolled as members of the Youel's Prep Family of Students™, which affords them access to free telephone tutoring at (800) 645-3985. Students may call 24/7. Youel's Prep live lectures are held at select medical schools at the invitation of the school and students.

Programs are custom-designed for content, number of hours, and scheduling to fit students' needs. First-year students are urged to call early to arrange live-lecture programs at their schools for next year.

For more information, contact:

Youel's Prep, Inc.
P.O. Box 31479
Palm Beach Gardens, FL 33420
Phone: (800) 645-3985
Fax: (561) 622-4858
Email: info@youelsprep.com
www.youelsprep.net

Publisher Contacts

ASM Press
P.O. Box 605
Herndon, VA 20172
(800) 546-2416
Books@asmusa.org
www.asmpress.org

CRC Press
Taylor & Francis Group
6000 Broken Sound Parkway, NW, Suite 300
Boca Raton, FL 33487
(800) 272-7737
Fax: (800) 374-3401
orders@crcpress.com
www.crcpress.com

Elsevier, Inc.
3251 Riverport Lane
Maryland Heights, MO 63043
(800) 401-9962
Fax: (800) 535-9935
www.us.elsevierhealth.com

Exam Master
100 Lake Drive, Suite 6
Newark, DE 19702
(800) 572-3627
Fax: (302) 283-1222
customerservice@exammaster.com
www.exammaster.com

Garland Science
711 Third Avenue, 8th Floor
New York, NY 10017
(203) 281-4487
Fax: (212) 947-3027
orders@taylorandfrancis.com
www.garlandscience.com

Gold Standard Board Prep
Apollo Audiobooks, LLC
2508 27th Street
Lubbock, TX 79410
(806) 773-3197
info@ApolloAudiobooks.com
www.boardprep.net

John Wiley & Sons
1 Wiley Drive
Somerset, NJ 08875-1272
(800) 225-5945
Fax: (732) 302-2300
custserv@wiley.com
www.wiley.com

Kaplan, Inc.
395 Hudson Street, 4th Floor
New York, NY 10014
(800) 527-8378
customer.care@kaplan.com

Lippincott Williams & Wilkins
16522 Hunters Green Parkway
Hagerstown, MD 21740
(800) 638-3030
Fax: (301) 223-2400
orders@lww.com
www.lww.com

McGraw-Hill Companies
Order Services
P.O. Box 182604
Columbus, OH 43272-3031
(888) 955-4600
Fax: (614) 759-3749
pbg.ecommerce_custserv@mcgraw-hill.com
www.mhprofessional.com

MedMaster, Inc.
P.O. Box 640028
Miami, FL 33164
(800) 335-3480
Fax: (954) 962-4508
mmbks@aol.com
www.medmaster.net

Princeton Review
2315 Broadway
New York, NY 10024
(888) 955-4600
www.princetonreview.com

Thieme Medical Publishers, Inc.
333 Seventh Avenue
New York, NY 10001
(800) 782-3488
Fax: (212) 947-0108
www.thieme.com
customerservice@thieme.com

▶ NOTES

SECTION IV

Abbreviations and Symbols

ABBREVIATION	MEANING
1°	primary
2°	secondary
3°	tertiary
A-a	alveolar-arterial [gradient]
AA	Alcoholics Anonymous, amyloid A
AAMC	Association of American Medical Colleges
Ab	antibody
ABP	androgen-binding protein
ACA	anterior cerebral artery
Acetyl-CoA	acetyl coenzyme A
ACD	anemia of chronic disease
ACE	angiotensin-converting enzyme
ACh	acetylcholine
AChE	acetylcholinesterase
ACL	anterior cruciate ligament
ACom	anterior communicating [artery]
ACTH	adrenocorticotropic hormone
ADA	adenosine deaminase, Americans with Disabilities Act
ADH	antidiuretic hormone
ADHD	attention-deficit hyperactivity disorder
ADP	adenosine diphosphate
ADPKD	autosomal-dominant polycystic kidney disease
AFP	α-fetoprotein
Ag	antigen, silver
AICA	anterior inferior cerebellar artery
AIDS	acquired immunodeficiency syndrome
AIHA	autoimmune hemolytic anemia
AL	amyloid light [chain]
ALA	aminolevulinic acid
ALL	acute lymphoblastic (lymphocytic) leukemia
ALP	alkaline phosphatase
α_1, α_2	sympathetic receptors
ALS	amyotrophic lateral sclerosis
ALT	alanine transaminase
AMA	American Medical Association, antimitochondrial antibody
AML	acute myelogenous (myeloid) leukemia
AMP	adenosine monophosphate
ANA	antinuclear antibody
ANCA	antineutrophil cytoplasmic antibody
ANOVA	analysis of variance
ANP	atrial natriuretic peptide
ANS	autonomic nervous system
anti-CPP	anti-cyclic citrullinated peptide

ABBREVIATION	MEANING
AO×3	alert and oriented to time, place, and person
AOA	American Osteopathic Association
AP	action potential, A & P [ribosomal binding sites]
A & P	ribosomal binding sites
APC	antigen-presenting cell, activated protein C
APP	amyloid precursor protein
APRT	adenine phosphoribosyltransferase
APSAC	anistreplase
aPTT	activated partial thromboplastin time
Apo	apolipoprotein
AR	attributable risk, autosomal recessive, aortic regurgitation
ara-C	arabinofuranosyl cytidine (cytarabine)
ARB	angiotensin receptor blocker
ARDS	acute respiratory distress syndrome
Arg	arginine
ARMD	age-related macular degeneration
ARPKD	autosomal-recessive polycystic kidney disease
AS	aortic stenosis
ASA	acetylsalicylic acid, anterior spinal artery
ASD	atrial septal defect
ASO	anti–streptolysin O
AST	aspartate transaminase
AT	angiotensin, antithrombin
ATCase	aspartate transcarbamoylase
ATN	acute tubular necrosis
ATP	adenosine triphosphate
ATPase	adenosine triphosphatase
AV	atrioventricular
AVM	arteriovenous malformation
AZT	azidothymidine
β_1, β_2	sympathetic receptors
BAL	British anti-Lewisite [dimercaprol]
BCG	bacille Calmette-Guérin
BIMS	Biometric Identity Management System
BM	basement membrane
BMI	body-mass index
BMR	basal metabolic rate
BP	bisphosphate, blood pressure
BPG	bisphosphoglycerate
BPH	benign prostatic hyperplasia
BT	bleeding time
BUN	blood urea nitrogen
Ca^{2+}	calcium ion
CAD	coronary artery disease

ABBREVIATION	MEANING
CAF	common application form
CALLA	common acute lymphoblastic leukemia antigen
cAMP	cyclic adenosine monophosphate
CBG	corticosteroid-binding globulin
Cbl	cobalamin
CBSSA	Comprehensive Basic Science Self-Assessment
CBT	computer-based test, cognitive behavioral therapy
CCK	cholecystokinin
CCS	computer-based case simulation
CCT	cortical collecting tubule
CD	cluster of differentiation
CDK	cyclin-dependent kinase
cDNA	complementary deoxyribonucleic acid
CEA	carcinoembryonic antigen
CETP	cholesterol-ester transfer protein
CF	cystic fibrosis
CFTR	cystic fibrosis transmembrane conductance regulator
CFX	circumflex [artery]
CGD	chronic granulomatous disease
cGMP	cyclic guanosine monophosphate
CGN	cis-Golgi network
CGRP	calcitonin gene–related peptide
C_H1–C_H3	constant regions, heavy chain [antibody]
ChAT	choline acetyltransferase
CHF	congestive heart failure
χ^2	chi-squared
CI	confidence interval
CIN	candidate identification number, carcinoma in situ, cervical intraepithelial neoplasia
CIS	Communication and Interpersonal Skills
CK	clinical knowledge, creatine kinase
CK-MB	creatine kinase, MB fraction
C_L	constant region, light chain [antibody]
CL	clearance
Cl⁻	chloride ion
CLL	chronic lymphocytic leukemia
CML	chronic myelogenous (myeloid) leukemia
CMV	cytomegalovirus
CN	cranial nerve
CN⁻	cyanide ion
CNS	central nervous system
CNV	copy number variation
CO	carbon monoxide, cardiac output
CO_2	carbon dioxide
CoA	coenzyme A
COMLEX-USA	Comprehensive Osteopathic Medical Licensing Examination
COMSAE	Comprehensive Osteopathic Medical Self-Assessment Examination
COMT	catechol-O-methyltransferase
COOH	carboxyl group
COP	coat protein
COPD	chronic obstructive pulmonary disease
CoQ	coenzyme Q
COX	cyclooxygenase

ABBREVIATION	MEANING
C_p	plasma concentration
CPAP	continuous positive airway pressure
CPK	creatine phosphokinase
CPR	cardiopulmonary resuscitation
Cr	creatinine
CRC	colorectal cancer
CREST	calcinosis, Raynaud phenomenon, esophageal dysfunction, sclerosis, and telangiectasias [syndrome]
CRH	corticotropin-releasing hormone
CRP	C-reactive protein
CS	clinical skills
C-section	cesarean section
CSF	cerebrospinal fluid
CT	computed tomography
CTL	cytotoxic T lymphocyte
CTP	cytidine triphosphate
CV	cardiovascular
CVA	cerebrovascular accident
CVID	common variable immunodeficiency
CXR	chest x-ray
Cys	cysteine
DAF	decay-accelerating factor
DAG	diacylglycerol
dATP	deoxyadenosine triphosphate
DCIS	ductal carcinoma in situ
DCT	distal convoluted tubule
ddC	dideoxycytidine [zalcitabine]
ddI	didanosine
DES	diethylstilbestrol
DHAP	dihydroxyacetone phosphate
DHB	dihydrobiopterin
DHEA	dehydroepiandrosterone
DHF	dihydrofolic acid
DHS	Department of Homeland Security
DHT	dihydrotestosterone
DI	diabetes insipidus
DIC	disseminated intravascular coagulation
DIP	distal interphalangeal [joint]
DKA	diabetic ketoacidosis
DM	diabetes mellitus
DNA	deoxyribonucleic acid
dNTP	deoxynucleotide triphosphate
DO	doctor of osteopathy
DPGN	diffuse proliferative glomerulonephritis
DPM	doctor of podiatric medicine
DPP-4	dipeptidyl peptidase-4
DS	double stranded
dsDNA	double-stranded deoxyribonucleic acid
dsRNA	double-stranded ribonucleic acid
d4T	didehydrodeoxythymidine [stavudine]
dTMP	deoxythymidine monophosphate
DTR	deep tendon reflex
DTs	delirium tremens
dUDP	deoxyuridine diphosphate

ABBREVIATION	MEANING
dUMP	deoxyuridine monophosphate
DVT	deep venous thrombosis
EBV	Epstein-Barr virus
EC	ejection click
ECF	extracellular fluid
ECFMG	Educational Commission for Foreign Medical Graduates
ECG	electrocardiogram
ECL	enterochromaffin-like [cell]
ECM	extracellular matrix
ECT	electroconvulsive therapy
ED_{50}	median effective dose
EDRF	endothelium-derived relaxing factor
EDTA	ethylenediamine tetra-acetic acid
EDV	end-diastolic volume
EEG	electroencephalogram
EF	ejection fraction
EGF	epidermal growth factor
EHEC	enterohemorrhagic *E. coli*
ELISA	enzyme-linked immunosorbent assay
EM	electron micrograph/microscopy
EMB	eosin–methylene blue
Epi	epinephrine
EPO	erythropoietin
EPS	extrapyramidal system
ER	endoplasmic reticulum, estrogen receptor
ERAS	Electronic Residency Application Service
ERCP	endoscopic retrograde cholangiopancreatography
ERP	effective refractory period
ERPF	effective renal plasma flow
ERT	estrogen replacement therapy
ERV	expiratory reserve volume
ESR	erythrocyte sedimentation rate
ESRD	end-stage renal disease
ESV	end-systolic volume
ETEC	enterotoxigenic *E. coli*
EtOH	ethyl alcohol
EV	esophageal vein
F	bioavailability
FA	fatty acid
Fab	fragment, antigen-binding
FAD	flavin adenine dinucleotide
FAD^+	oxidized flavin adenine dinucleotide
$FADH_2$	reduced flavin adenine dinucleotide
FAP	familial adenomatous polyposis
F1,6BP	fructose-1,6-bisphosphate
F2,6BP	fructose-2,6-bisphosphate
FBPase	fructose bisphosphatase
Fc	fragment, crystallizable
FcR	Fc receptor
5f-dUMP	5-fluorodeoxyuridine monophosphate
Fe^{2+}	ferrous ion
Fe^{3+}	ferric ion
Fe_{Na}	excreted fraction of filtered sodium
FEV_1	forced expiratory volume in 1 second

ABBREVIATION	MEANING
FF	filtration fraction
FFA	free fatty acid
FGF	fibroblast growth factor
FGFR	fibroblast growth factor receptor
FISH	fluorescence in situ hybridization
FKBP	FK506 binding protein
FLAIR	fluid-attenuated inversion recovery
f-met	formylmethionine
FMG	foreign medical graduate
FMN	flavin mononucleotide
FN	false negative
FNHTR	febrile nonhemolytic transfusion reaction
FP	false positive
F1P	fructose-1-phosphate
F6P	fructose-6-phosphate
FRC	functional residual capacity
FSH	follicle-stimulating hormone
FSMB	Federation of State Medical Boards
FTA-ABS	fluorescent treponemal antibody—absorbed
5-FU	5-fluorouracil
FVC	forced vital capacity
GABA	γ-aminobutyric acid
Gal	galactose
GBM	glomerular basement membrane
GC	glomerular capillary
G-CSF	granulocyte colony-stimulating factor
GERD	gastroesophageal reflux disease
GFAP	glial fibrillary acid protein
GFR	glomerular filtration rate
GGT	γ-glutamyl transpeptidase
GH	growth hormone
GHB	γ-hydroxybutyrate
GHRH	growth hormone–releasing hormone
G_I	G protein, I polypeptide
GI	gastrointestinal
GIP	gastric inhibitory peptide
GIST	gastrointestinal stromal tumor
GLUT	glucose transporter
GM	granulocyte macrophage
GM-CSF	granulocyte-macrophage colony stimulating factor
GMP	guanosine monophosphate
GnRH	gonadotropin-releasing hormone
GP	glycoprotein
G3P	glucose-3-phosphate
G6P	glucose-6-phosphate
G6PD	glucose-6-phospate dehydrogenase
GPe	globus pallidus externa
GPi	globus pallidus interna
GPI	glycosyl phosphatidylinositol
GRP	gastrin-releasing peptide
G_S	G protein, S polypeptide
GS	glycogen synthase
GSH	reduced glutathione
GSSG	oxidized glutathione

ABBREVIATION	MEANING
GTP	guanosine triphosphate
GTPase	guanosine triphosphatase
GU	genitourinary
H^+	hydrogen ion
H_1, H_2	histamine receptors
HAART	highly active antiretroviral therapy
HAV	hepatitis A virus
HAVAb	hepatitis A antibody
Hb	hemoglobin
Hb^+	oxidized hemoglobin
Hb^-	ionized hemoglobin
HBcAb	hepatitis B core antibody
HBcAg	hepatitis B core antigen
HBeAb	hepatitis B early antibody
HBeAg	hepatitis B early antigen
HBsAb	hepatitis B surface antibody
HBsAg	hepatitis B surface antigen
$HbCO_2$	carbaminohemoglobin
HBV	hepatitis B virus
HCC	hepatocellular carcinoma
hCG	human chorionic gonadotropin
HCO_3^-	bicarbonate
Hct	hematocrit
HCTZ	hydrochlorothiazide
HCV	hepatitis C virus
HDL	high-density lipoprotein
HDV	hepatitis D virus
H&E	hematoxylin and eosin
HEV	hepatitis E virus
Hfr	high-frequency recombination [cell]
HGPRT	hypoxanthine-guanine phosphoribosyltransferase
HHb	human hemoglobin
HHV	human herpesvirus
5-HIAA	5-hydroxyindoleacetic acid
HIE	hypoxic ischemic encephalopathy
His	histidine
HIT	heparin-induced thrombocytopenia
HIV	human immunodeficiency virus
HL	hepatic lipase
HLA	human leukocyte antigen
HMG-CoA	hydroxymethylglutaryl-coenzyme A
HMP	hexose monophosphate
HMSN	hereditary motor and sensory neuropathy
HMWK	high-molecular-weight kininogen
HNPCC	hereditary nonpolyposis colorectal cancer
hnRNA	heterogeneous nuclear ribonucleic acid
H_2O	water
H_2O_2	hydrogen peroxide
HPA	hypothalamic-pituitary-adrenal [axis]
HPO	hypothalamic-pituitary-ovarian [axis]
HPV	human papillomavirus
HR	heart rate
HRE	hormone receptor element
HRT	hormone replacement therapy

ABBREVIATION	MEANING
HSV	herpes simplex virus
5-HT	5-hydroxytryptamine (serotonin)
HTLV	human T-cell leukemia virus
HTN	hypertension
HTR	hemolytic transfusion reaction
HUS	hemolytic-uremic syndrome
HVA	homovanillic acid
HZV	herpes zoster virus
IBD	inflammatory bowel disease
IBS	irritable bowel syndrome
IC	inspiratory capacity, immune complex
I_{Ca}	calcium current [heart]
I_f	funny current [heart]
ICA	internal carotid artery
ICAM	intracellular adhesion molecule
ICD	implantable cardioverter defibrillator
ICE	Integrated Clinical Encounter
ICF	intracellular fluid
ID	identification
ID_{50}	dose at which pathogen produces infection in 50% of population
IDDM	insulin-dependent diabetes mellitus
IDL	intermediate-density lipoprotein
I/E	inspiratory/expiratory [ratio]
IF	immunofluorescence, initiation factor
IFN	interferon
Ig	immunoglobulin
IGF	insulin-like growth factor
I_K	potassium current [heart]
IL	interleukin
IM	intramuscular
IMA	inferior mesenteric artery
IMED	International Medical Education Directory
IMG	international medical graduate
IMP	inosine monophosphate
IMV	inferior mesenteric vein
I_{Na}	sodium current [heart]
INH	isonicotinic hydrazine [isoniazid]
INO	internuclear ophthalmoplegia
INR	International Normalized Ratio
IO	inferior orbital [muscle]
IOP	intraocular pressure
IP_3	inositol triphosphate
IPV	inactivated polio vaccine
IR	current × resistance [Ohm's law], inferior rectus [muscle]
IRV	inspiratory reserve volume
ITP	idiopathic thrombocytopenic purpura
IUD	intrauterine device
IUGR	intrauterine growth retardation
IV	intravenous
IVC	inferior vena cava
IVDU	intravenous drug use
JAK/STAT	Janus kinase/signal transducer and activator of transcription [pathway]

ABBREVIATION	MEANING
JGA	juxtaglomerular apparatus
JVD	jugular venous distention
JVP	jugular venous pulse
K^+	potassium ion
KatG	catalase-peroxidase produced by *M. tuberculosis*
K_e	elimination constant
K_f	filtration constant
KG	ketoglutarate
K_m	Michaelis-Menten constant
KOH	potassium hydroxide
L	left
LA	left atrial, left atrium
LAD	left anterior descending [artery]
LAF	left anterior fascicle
LCA	left coronary artery
LCAT	lecithin-cholesterol acyltransferase
LCFA	long-chain fatty acid
LCL	lateral collateral ligament
LCME	Liaison Committee on Medical Education
LCMV	lymphocytic choriomeningitis virus
LCX	left circumflex artery
LD	loading dose
LD_{50}	median lethal dose
LDH	lactate dehydrogenase
LDL	low-density lipoprotein
LES	lower esophageal sphincter
LFA	leukocyte function–associated antigen
LFT	liver function test
LGN	lateral geniculate nucleus
LGV	left gastric vein
LH	luteinizing hormone
LLQ	left lower quadrant
LM	light microscopy
LMN	lower motor neuron
LP	lumbar puncture
LPL	lipoprotein lipase
LPS	lipopolysaccharide
LR	lateral rectus [muscle]
LSE	Libman-Sacks endocarditis
LT	labile toxin leukotriene
LV	left ventricle, left ventricular
Lys	lysine
M_1-M_5	muscarinic (parasympathetic) ACh receptors
MAC	membrane attack complex, minimal alveolar concentration
MALT	mucosa-associated lymphoid tissue
MAO	monoamine oxidase
MAOI	monoamine oxidase inhibitor
MAP	mean arterial pressure, mitogen-activated protein
MASP	mannose-binding lectin–associated serine protease
MBL	mannose-binding lectin
MC	midsystolic click
MCA	middle cerebral artery
MCAT	Medical College Admissions Test
MCHC	mean corpuscular hemoglobin concentration

ABBREVIATION	MEANING
MCL	medial collateral ligament
MCP	metacarpophalangeal [joint]
MCV	mean corpuscular volume
MD	maintenance dose
MEN	multiple endocrine neoplasia
Mg^{2+}	magnesium ion
MGN	medial geniculate nucleus
$MgSO_4$	magnesium sulfate
MGUS	monoclonal gammopathy of undetermined significance
MHC	major histocompatibility complex
MI	myocardial infarction
MIF	müllerian inhibiting factor
MLCK	myosin light-chain kinase
MLF	medial longitudinal fasciculus
MMC	migrating motor complex
MMR	measles, mumps, rubella [vaccine]
MOPP	mechlorethamine-vincristine (Oncovin)-prednisone-procarbazine [chemotherapy]
6-MP	6-mercaptopurine
MPGN	membranoproliferative glomerulonephritis
MPO	myeloperoxidase
MPO-ANCA/ p-ANCA	perinuclear antineutrophil cytoplasmic antibody
MR	medial rectus [muscle], mitral regurgitation
MRI	magnetic resonance imaging
mRNA	messenger ribonucleic acid
MRSA	methicillin-resistant *S. aureus*
MS	mitral stenosis, multiple sclerosis
MSH	melanocyte-stimulating hormone
MSM	men who have sex with men
mtDNA	mitochondrial DNA
mtRNA	mitochondrial RNA
mTOR	mammalian target of rapamycin
MTP	metatarsophalangeal [joint]
MTX	methotrexate
MUA/P	Medically Underserved Area and Population
MVO_2	myocardial oxygen consumption
MVP	mitral valve prolapse
N/A	not applicable
Na^+	sodium ion
NAD	nicotinamide adenine dinucleotide
NAD^+	oxidized nicotinamide adenine dinucleotide
NADH	reduced nicotinamide adenine dinucleotide
$NADP^+$	oxidized nicotinamide adenine dinucleotide phosphate
NADPH	reduced nicotinamide adenine dinucleotide phosphate
NBME	National Board of Medical Examiners
NBOME	National Board of Osteopathic Medical Examiners
NBPME	National Board of Podiatric Medical Examiners
NC	no change
NE	norepinephrine
NF	neurofibromatosis
NFAT	nuclear factor of activated T-cell
NH_3	ammonia
NH_4^+	ammonium
NIDDM	non-insulin-dependent diabetes mellitus

ABBREVIATION	MEANING
NK	natural killer [cells]
N_M	muscarinic ACh receptor in neuromuscular junction
NMDA	N-methyl-D-aspartate
NMJ	neuromuscular junction
NMS	neuroleptic malignant syndrome
N_N	nicotinic ACh receptor in autonomic ganglia
NRMP	National Residency Matching Program
NNRTI	non-nucleoside reverse transcriptase inhibitor
NO	nitric oxide
N_2O	nitrous oxide
NPH	neutral protamine Hagedorn
NPV	negative predictive value
NRI	norepinephrine receptor inhibitor
NRTI	nucleoside reverse transcriptase inhibitor
NSAID	nonsteroidal anti-inflammatory drug
OAA	oxaloacetic acid
OCD	obsessive-compulsive disorder
OCP	oral contraceptive pill
OH	hydroxy
OH_2	dihydroxy
$1,25\text{-OH } D_3$	calcitriol (active form of vitamin D)
$25\text{-OH } D_3$	storage form of vitamin D
$3'$ OH	hydroxyl
OMT	osteopathic manipulative technique
OPV	oral polio vaccine
OR	odds ratio
OS	opening snap
OTC	ornithine transcarbamoylase
OVLT	organum vasculosum of the lamina terminalis
P-450	cytochrome P-450 family of enzymes
PA	posteroanterior
PABA	*para*-aminobenzoic acid
$Paco_2$	arterial Pco_2
$PAco_2$	alveolar Pco_2
PAH	*para*-aminohippuric acid
PAN	polyarteritis nodosa
Pao_2	partial pressure of oxygen in arterial blood
PAo_2	partial pressure of oxygen in alveolar blood
PAP	Papanicolaou [smear], prostatic acid phosphatase
PAS	periodic acid–Schiff
PBP	penicillin-binding protein
PC	plasma colloid osmotic pressure, platelet count, pyruvate carboxylase
PCA	posterior cerebral artery
PCL	posterior cruciate ligament
Pco_2	partial pressure of carbon dioxide
PCom	posterior communicating [artery]
PCOS	polycystic ovarian syndrome
PCP	phencyclidine hydrochloride, *Pneumocystis carinii* pneumonia
PCR	polymerase chain reaction
PCT	proximal convoluted tubule
PCWP	pulmonary capillary wedge pressure
PD	posterior descending [artery]
PDA	patent ductus arteriosus

ABBREVIATION	MEANING
PDC	pyruvate dehydrogenase complex
PDE	phosphodiesterase
PDGF	platelet-derived growth factor
PDH	pyruvate dehydrogenase
PE	pulmonary embolism
PECAM	platelet–endothelial cell adhesion molecule
$Peco_2$	expired air Pco_2
PEP	phosphoenolpyruvate
PF	platelet factor
PFK	phosphofructokinase
PFT	pulmonary function test
PG	phosphoglycerate, prostaglandin
P_i	plasma interstitial osmotic pressure, inorganic phosphate
PICA	posterior inferior cerebellar artery
PID	pelvic inflammatory disease
Pio_2	Po_2 in inspired air
PIP	proximal interphalangeal [joint]
PIP_2	phosphatidylinositol 4,5-bisphosphate
PKD	polycystic kidney disease
PKU	phenylketonuria
PLP	pyridoxal phosphate
PLS	Personalized Learning System
PML	progressive multifocal leukoencephalopathy
PMN	polymorphonuclear [leukocyte]
P_{net}	net filtration pressure
PNET	primitive neuroectodermal tumor
PNS	peripheral nervous system
Po_2	partial pressure of oxygen
PO_4	salt of phosphoric acid
PO_4^{3-}	phosphate
PPAR	peroxisome proliferator-activated receptor
PPD	purified protein derivative
PPI	proton pump inhibitor
PPV	positive predictive value
PR3-ANCA/ c-ANCA	cytoplasmic antineutrophil cytoplasmic antibody
PrP	prion protein
PRPP	phosphoribosylpyrophosphate
PSA	prostate-specific antigen
PSS	progressive systemic sclerosis
PT	prothrombin time
PTH	parathyroid hormone
PTHrP	parathyroid hormone–related protein
PTSD	post-traumatic stress disorder
PTT	partial thromboplastin time
PV	plasma volume, venous pressure
PVC	polyvinyl chloride
PVR	pulmonary vascular resistance
R	correlation coefficient, right, R variable [group]
R_3	Registration, Ranking, & Results [system]
RA	right atrium
RAAS	renin-angiotensin-aldosterone system
RANK-L	receptor activator of nuclear factor-κ B ligand
RAS	reticular activating system

ABBREVIATION	MEANING
RBC	red blood cell
RBF	renal blood flow
RCA	right coronary artery
REM	rapid eye movement
RER	rough endoplasmic reticulum
Rh	*rhesus* antigen
RLQ	right lower quadrant
RNA	ribonucleic acid
RNA$_i$	ribonucleic acid interference
RNP	ribonucleoprotein
ROS	reactive oxygen species
RPF	renal plasma flow
RPGN	rapidly progressive glomerulonephritis
RPR	rapid plasma reagin
RR	relative risk, respiratory rate
rRNA	ribosomal ribonucleic acid
RS	Reed-Sternberg [cells]
RSV	respiratory syncytial virus
RTA	renal tubular acidosis
RUQ	right upper quadrant
RV	residual volume, right ventricle, right ventricular
RVH	right ventricular hypertrophy
Rx	medical prescription
[S]	substrate concentration
SA	sinoatrial
SAA	serum amyloid–associated [protein]
SAM	S-adenosylmethionine
SARS	severe acute respiratory syndrome
SAT	Scholastic Aptitude Test
SC	subcutaneous
SCC	squamous cell carcinoma
SCID	severe combined immunodeficiency disease
SCJ	squamocolumnar junction
SCM	sternocleidomastoid muscle
SCN	suprachiasmatic nucleus
SD	standard deviation
SEM	standard error of the mean
SEP	Spoken English Proficiency
SER	smooth endoplasmic reticulum
SERM	selective estrogen receptor modulator
SHBG	sex hormone–binding globulin
SIADH	syndrome of inappropriate [secretion of] antidiuretic hormone
SLE	systemic lupus erythematosus
SLL	small lymphocytic lymphoma
SLT	Shiga-like toxin
SMA	superior mesenteric artery
SMX	sulfamethoxazole
SNc	substantia nigra pars compacta
SNP	single nucleotide polymorphism
SNr	substantia nigra pars reticulata
SNRI	serotonin and norepinephrine receptor inhibitor
snRNP	small nuclear ribonucleoprotein
SO	superior oblique [muscle]

ABBREVIATION	MEANING
SOAP	Supplemental Offer and Acceptance Program
spp.	species
SR	superior rectus [muscle]
SS	single stranded
ssDNA	single-stranded deoxyribonucleic acid
SSPE	subacute sclerosing panencephalitis
SSRI	selective serotonin reuptake inhibitor
ssRNA	single-stranded ribonucleic acid
SSSS	staphylococcal scalded-skin syndrome
ST	Shiga toxin
STD	sexually transmitted disease
STEMI	ST-segment elevation myocardial infarction
STN	subthalamic nucleus
SV	sinus venosus, splenic vein, stroke volume
SVC	superior vena cava
SVT	supraventricular tachycardia
$t_{1/2}$	half-life
T_3	triiodothyronine
T_4	thyroxine
TA	truncus arteriosus
TAPVR	total anomalous pulmonary venous return
TB	tuberculosis
TBG	thyroxine-binding globulin
3TC	dideoxythiacytidine [lamivudine]
TCA	tricarboxylic acid [cycle], tricyclic antidepressant
Tc cell	cytotoxic T cell
TCR	T-cell receptor
TDF	tenofovir disoproxil fumarate
TdT	terminal deoxynucleotidyl transferase
TFT	thyroid function test
TG	triglyceride
6-TG	6-thioguanine
TGA	*trans*-Golgi apparatus
TGF	transforming growth factor
TGN	*trans*-Golgi network
Th cell	helper T cell
THF	tetrahydrofolic acid
TI	therapeutic index
TIA	transient ischemic attack
TIBC	total iron-binding capacity
TIPS	transjugular intrahepatic portosystemic shunt
TLC	total lung capacity
T_m	maximum rate of transport
TMP	trimethoprim
TN	true negative
TNF	tumor necrosis factor
TNM	tumor, node, metastases [staging]
TOEFL	Test of English as a Foreign Language
ToRCHeS	*Toxoplasma gondii*, rubella, CMV, HIV, HSV-2, syphilis
TP	true positive
tPA	tissue plasminogen activator
TPP	thiamine pyrophosphate
TPR	total peripheral resistance
TR	tricuspid regurgitation

ABBREVIATION	MEANING
TRAP	tartrate-resistant acid phosphatase
TRH	thyrotropin-releasing hormone
tRNA	transfer ribonucleic acid
TSH	thyroid-stimulating hormone
TSI	thyroid-stimulating immunoglobulin
TSS	toxic shock syndrome
TSST	toxic shock syndrome toxin
TTP	thrombotic thrombocytopenic purpura
TTR	transthyretin
TV	tidal volume
Tx	translation [factor]
TXA_2	thromboxane A_2
UCV	Underground Clinical Vignettes
UDP	uridine diphosphate
UMN	upper motor neuron
UMP	uridine monophosphate
UPD	uniparental disomy
URI	upper respiratory infection
USMLE	United States Medical Licensing Examination
UTI	urinary tract infection
UTP	uridine triphosphate
UV	ultraviolet
V_1, V_2	Vasopressin receptors
VA	Veterans Affairs
VC	vital capacity
V_d	volume of distribution
VD	physiologic dead space
V(D)J	heavy-chain hypervariable region [antibody]

ABBREVIATION	MEANING
VDRL	Venereal Disease Research Laboratory
VEGF	vascular endothelial growth factor
V_H	variable region, heavy chain [antibody]
VHL	von Hippel-Lindau [disease]
VIP	vasoactive intestinal peptide
VIPoma	vasoactive intestinal polypeptide-secreting tumor
VJ	light-chain hypervariable region [antibody]
VL	ventral lateral [nucleus]; variable region, light chain [antibody]
VLDL	very low density lipoprotein
VMA	vanillylmandelic acid
V_{max}	maximum velocity
VPL	ventral posterior nucleus, lateral
VPM	ventral posterior nucleus, medial
VPN	vancomycin, polymyxin, nystatin [media]
V/Q	ventilation/perfusion [ratio]
VRE	vancomycin-resistant enterococcus
VSD	ventricular septal defect
V_T	tidal volume
vWF	von Willebrand factor
VZV	varicella-zoster virus
WHOML	"worst headache of my life"
WBC	white blood cell
XR	X-linked recessive
XX	normal complement of sex chromosomes for female
XY	normal complement of sex chromosomes for male
ZDV	zidovudine [formerly AZT]

Image Acknowledgments

In this edition, in collaboration with McGraw-Hill, MedIQ Learning, LLC, and a variety of other partners, we are pleased to have expanded the clinical images and diagrams for the benefit of integrative student learning.

℞ Portions of this book identified with the symbol ℞ are copyright © USMLE-Rx.com (MedIQ Learning, LLC).

RU Portions of this book identified with the symbol RU are copyright © Dr. Richard Usatine and are provided under license through MedIQ Learning, LLC.

✺ Portions of this book identified with the ✺ symbol are listed below by page number.

⊜ This symbol refers to the Creative Commons Attribution license, full text at: *http://creativecommons.org/licenses/by/3.0/legalcode.*

⊜ BY-SA This symbol refers to the Creative Commons Attribution-Share Alike license, full text at: *http://creativecommons.org/licenses/by-sa/3.0/us/legalcode.*

Biochemistry

78 **Cilia structure.** ⊜ Courtesy of Louise Howard and Michael Binder.

80 **Osteogenesis imperfecta: Image A (left).** Radiograph of child. This image is a derivative work, adapted from the following source, available under ⊜ BY-SA. Vanakker OM, Hemelsoet D, De Paepe. Hereditary connective tissue diseases in young adult stroke: a comprehensive synthesis. *Stroke Res Treat* 2011;712903. doi 10.4061/2011/712903. The image may have been modified by cropping, labeling, and/or captions. MedIQ Learning, LLC makes this image available under the ⊜ BY-SA.

80 **Osteogenesis imperfecta: Image A (right).** Radiograph of adult. Reproduced, with permission, from Dr. Frank Gaillard and *www.radiopaedia.org.*

80 **Osteogenesis imperfecta: Image B.** Blue sclera. This image is a derivative work, adapted from the following source, under ⊜. Fred H, van Dijk H. Images of memorable cases: cases 40, 41 & 42. Connexions Web site. December 3, 2008. Available at: *http://cnx.org/content/m15020/1.3/.*

89 **Muscular dystrophies.** Fibrofatty replacement of muscle. ⊜ Courtesy of the U.S. Department of Health and Human Services and Dr. Edwin P. Ewing, Jr. The image may have been modified by cropping, labeling, and/or captions. All rights to this adaptation by MedIQ Learning, LLC are reserved.

95 **Vitamin D.** Rickets. This image is a derivative work, adapted from the following source, under ⊜ BY-SA. Courtesy of Dr. Michael L. Richardson.

97 **Malnutrition.** Child with kwashiorkor. ⊜ Courtesy of the U.S. Department of Health and Human Services and Dr. Lyle Conrad.

114 **Lysosomal storage diseases: Image A.** Gaucher disease. This image is a derivative work, adapted from the following source, under ⊜. Sokołowska B, Skomra D, Czartoryska B, et al. Gaucher disease diagnosed after bone marrow trephine biopsy. A report of two cases. *Folia Histochemica et Cytobiologica* 2011;49:352-356. doi 10.5603/FHC.2011.0048. The image may have been modified by cropping, labeling, and/or captions. All rights to this adaptation by MedIQ Learning, LLC are reserved.

114 **Lysosomal storage disease: Image B.** Niemann-Pick disease. Reproduced, with permission, from Lichtman MA et al. *Lichtman's Atlas of Hematology.* New York: McGraw-Hill, 2007: Fig. V.H.18.

114 **Lysosomal storage diseases: Image C.** Tay-Sachs disease. This image is a derivative work, adapted from the following source, under ⊜. Courtesy of Dr. Jonathan Trobe.

Microbiology

120 **Bacterial structures.** Adapted, with permission, from Levinson W, Jawetz E. *Medical Microbiology and Immunology: Examination and Board Review,* 9th ed. New York: McGraw-Hill, 2006:7.

127 **Endotoxin.** Adapted, with permission, from Levinson W. *Review of Medical Microbiology and Immunology,* 12th ed. New York: McGraw-Hill, 2012: Fig. 7-4.

130 *Staphylococcus aureus.* ⊜ Courtesy of the U.S. Department of Health and Human Services and Dr. Richard Facklam.

132 *Corynebacterium diphtheriae.* This image is a derivative work, adapted from the following source, under ⊜ BY-SA. Wikimedia Commons. The image may have been modified by cropping, labeling, and/or captions. MedIQ Learning, LLC makes this image available under the ⊜ BY-SA.

133 **Anthrax: Image A (left).** Gram-positive rods. ⊜ Courtesy of the U.S. Department of Health and Human Services and John A. Jernigan, David S. Stephens, David A. Ashford, and others.

133 **Anthrax: Image A (right).** Ulcer. ⊜ Courtesy of the U.S. Department of Health and Human Services and James H. Steele.

134 *Actinomyces vs. Nocardia*: Image A. *Actinomyces.* This image is a derivative work, adapted from the following source, under ⊜. Nathan Reading.

134 *Actinomyces vs. Nocardia*: Image B. *Nocardia.* ⊜ Courtesy of the U.S. Department of Health and Human Services and Dr. Hardin. The image may have been modified by cropping, labeling, and/or captions. All rights to this adaptation by MedIQ Learning, LLC are reserved.

Pathology

226 **Granulomatous diseases.** [PUBLIC DOMAIN] Courtesy of Sanjay Mukhopadhyay.

227 **Amyloidosis: Image A.** Congo red stain. This image is a derivative work, adapted from the following source, under [CC BY-SA] Dr. Ed Uthman.

227 **Amyloidosis: Image A.** Congo red stain under polarized light. This image is a derivative work, adapted from the following source, under [CC BY-SA]. Dr. Ed Uthman.

228 **Lipofuscin.** This image is a derivative work, adapted from the following source, under [CC BY-SA]. Nephron. The image may have been modified by cropping, labeling, and/or captions. MedIQ Learning, LLC makes this image available under the [CC BY-SA].

235 **Psammoma bodies.** [PUBLIC DOMAIN] Courtesy of Armed Forces Institute of Pathology.

236 **Common metastases: Image A.** Metastases to brain. [PUBLIC DOMAIN] Courtesy of Armed Forces Institute of Pathology.

236 **Common metastases: Image B.** Metastases to liver, gross specimen. [PUBLIC DOMAIN]. Courtesy of J. Hayman.

236 **Common metastases: Image C.** Metastases to liver, CT. This image is a derivative work, adapted from the following source, under [CC BY-SA]. Dr. James Heilman.

236 **Common metastases: Image D.** Bone metastases, gross specimen. This image is a derivative work, adapted from the following source, under [CC BY-SA]. M. Emmanuel.

Pharmacology

240 **Elimination of drugs.** Adapted, with permission, from Katzung BG, Trevor AJ. *Pharmacology: Examination & Board Review*, 5th ed. Stamford, CT: Appleton & Lange, 1998:5.

242 **Receptor binding: Images A and B.** Adapted, with permission, from Trevor AJ et al: *Katzung & Trevor's Pharmacology: Examination & Board Review*, 8th ed. New York: McGraw-Hill, 2008:14.

242 **Receptor binding: Image C.** Adapted, with permission, from Katzung BG. *Basic and Clinical Pharmacology*, 7th ed. Stamford, CT: Appleton & Lange, 1997:13.

243 **Central and peripheral nervous system.** Adapted, with permission, from Katzung BG. *Basic and Clinical Pharmacology*, 10th ed. New York: McGraw-Hill, 2007:76.

249 **Norepinephrine vs. isoproterenol.** Adapted, with permission, from Katzung BG, Trevor AJ. *Pharmacology: Examination & Board Review*, 5th ed. Stamford, CT: Appleton & Lange, 1998:72.

250 **Alpha-blockers.** Adapted, with permission, from Katzung BG, Trevor AJ. *Pharmacology: Examination & Board Review*, 5th ed. Stamford, CT: Appleton & Lange, 1998:80.

Cardiovascular

284 **Hypertension: Image A.** Fibromuscular dysplasia. This image is a derivative work, adapted from the following source, under [CC 0]. Plouin PF, Perdu J, LaBatide-Alanore A, et al. Fibromuscular dysplasia. *Orphanet J Rare Dis* 2007;7:28. PMID 17555581. The image may have been modified by cropping, labeling, and/or captions. All rights to this adaptation by MedIQ Learning, LLC are reserved.

284 **Hypertension: Image B.** Hypertensive nephropathy. This image is a derivative work, adapted from the following source, under [CC BY-SA]. Nephron. The image may have been modified by cropping, labeling, and/or captions. MedIQ Learning, LLC makes this image available under the [CC BY-SA].

285 **Hyperlipidemia signs: Image C.** Tendinous xanthoma. This image is a derivative work, adapted from the following source, under [CC BY-SA] Min.neel. The image may have been modified by cropping, labeling, and/or captions. MedIQ Learning, LLC makes this image available under the [CC BY-SA].

285 **Arteriosclerosis: Image A.** Monckeberg medial calcific sclerosis. This image is a derivative work, adapted from the following source, under [CC BY-SA]. C.E. Couri, G.A. da Silva, J.A. Martinez, F.A. Pereira, and F. de Paula. The image may have been modified by cropping, labeling, and/or captions. MedIQ Learning, LLC makes this image available under the [CC BY-SA].

285 **Atherosclerosis: Image B.** Hyaline type. This image is a derivative work, adapted from the following source, under [CC BY-SA]. Nephron.

285 **Atherosclerosis: Image C.** Hyperplastic type. This image is a derivative work, adapted from the following source, under [CC BY-SA]. Paco Larosa.

286 **Atherosclerosis: Image B.** Carotid plaque. This image is a derivative work, adapted from the following source, under [CC BY-SA]. Dr. Ed Uthman. The image may have been modified by cropping, labeling, and/or captions. MedIQ Learning, LLC makes this image available under the [CC BY-SA].

286 **Aortic aneurysms: Image B.** Thoracic aortic aneurysm. Reproduced, with permission, from Dr. Frank Gaillard and *www.radiopaedia.org*.

287 **Aortic dissection.** This image is a derivative work, adapted from the following source, under [CC 0]. Apostolakis EE, Baikoussis NG, Katsanos K, et a. Postoperative peri-axillary seroma following axillary artery cannulation for surgical treatment of acute type A aortic dissection: case report. *J Cardiothor Surg* 2010;5:43. doi 0.1186/1749-8090-5-43. The image may have been modified by cropping, labeling, and/or captions. All rights to this adaptation by MedIQ Learning, LLC are reserved.

291 **CHF.** Pedal edema. This image is a derivative work, adapted from the following source, under [CC BY-SA]. Dr. James Heilman.

292 **Rheumatic fever.** Aschoff body and Anitschkow cells. This image is a derivative work, adapted from the following source, under [CC BY-SA]. Dr. Ed Uthman. The image may have been modified by cropping, labeling, and/or captions. MedIQ Learning, LLC makes this image available under the [CC BY-SA].

293 **Cardiac tamponade.** This image is a derivative work, adapted from the following source, under [CC 0]. Jana M, Gamanagatti SR, Kumar A. Case series: CT scan in cardiac arrest and imminent cardiogenic shock: case series. *Indian J Radiol Imaging* 2010;20:150?153. doi 10.4103/0971-3026.63037. The image may have been modified by cropping, labeling, and/or captions. All rights to this adaptation by MedIQ Learning, LLC are reserved.

294 **Raynaud phenomenon.** This image is a derivative work, adapted from the following source, under [CC BY-SA]. Jamclaassen.

297 **Vasculitis: Image A: Temporal arteritis histology.** This image is a derivative work, adapted from the following source, under [CC BY-SA]. Marvin.

297 **Vasculitis: Image B.** Takayasu arteritis angiography. ⌖ Courtesy of the U.S. Department of Health and Human Services and Justin Ly.

297 **Vasculitis: Image C.** Microaneurysms in polyarteritis nodosa. Reproduced, with permission, from Dr. Frank Gaillard and *www.radiopaedia.org.*

297 **Vasculitis: Image D.** Kawasaki disease and strawberry tongue. This image is a derivative work, adapted from the following source, under ⌖ BY-SA. Natr.

297 **Vasculitis: Image E.** Kawasaki disease and coronary artery aneurysm. This image is a derivative work, adapted from the following source, under ⌖ BY-SA, Wikimedia Commons. The image may have been modified by cropping, labeling, and/or captions. All rights to this adaptation by MedIQ Learning, LLC are reserved.

297 **Vasculitis: Image F.** Granulomatosis with polyangiitis (Wegener) and PR3-ANCA/c-ANCA. ⌖ Courtesy of M.A. Little.

297 **Vasculitis, Image G.** Microscopic polyangiitis and MPO-ANCA/p-ANCA. ⌖ Courtesy of M.A. Little.

297 **Vasculitis, Image H.** Churg-Strauss syndrome histology. This image is a derivative work, adapted from the following source, under ⌖ BY-SA. Nephron.

297 **Vasculitis, Image I.** Henoch-Schonlein purpura. ⌖ Courtesy of Okwikikim.

300 **Lipid-lowering agents.** Adapted, with permission, from Katzung BG, Trevor AJ. *USMLE Road Map: Pharmacology*, 1st ed. New York: McGraw-Hill, 2003:56.

Endocrine

306 **Thyroid development.** Thyroid duct cyst. Reproduced, with permission, from Dr. Frank Gaillard and *www.radiopaedia.org.*

314 **PTH.** Adapted, with permission, from Chandrosoma P et al. *Concise Pathology*, 3rd ed. Stamford, CT: Appleton & Lange, 1998.

317 **Cushing syndrome: Image A.** Coronal MRI in Cushing disease. This image is a derivative work, adapted from the following source, under ⌖ BY-SA. H. Elhateer, T. Muanza, Roberge D, et al. Fractionated stereotactic radiotherapy in the treatment of pituitary macroadenomas. *Curr Oncol* 2008;15:286-292. PMC2601024. The image may have been modified by cropping, labeling, and/or captions. All rights to this adaptation by MedIQ Learning, LLC are reserved.

318 **Addison disease.** ⌖ Courtesy of FlatOut. The image may have been modified by cropping, labeling, and/or captions. All rights to this adaptation by MedIQ Learning, LLC are reserved.

318 **Neuroblastoma: Image B.** MRI. Reproduced, with permission, from Dr. Frank Gaillard and *www.radiopaedia.org.*

319 **Pheochromocytoma: Image A.** CT. This image is a derivative work, adapted from the following source, under ⌖ BY-SA. Drahreg. The image may have been modified by cropping, labeling, and/or captions. MedIQ Learning, LLC makes this image available under the ⌖ BY-SA.

319 **Pheochromocytoma: Image B.** Pheochromocytoma involving adrenal medulla. This image is a derivative work, adapted from the following source, under ⌖ BY-SA. Dr. Michael Feldman.

319 **Pheochromocytoma: Image C.** Chromaffin cells. This image is a derivative work, adapted from the following source, available under ⌖ BY-SA. KGH. The image may have been modified by cropping, labeling, and/or captions. MedIQ Learning, LLC makes this image available under the ⌖ BY-SA.

320 **Hypothyroidism: Image B: Congenital hypothyroidism.** This image is a derivative work, adapted from the following source, under ⌖ BY-SA. Sadashiv Swain.

320 **Hypothyroidism: Image C.** Before and after treatment of congenital hypothyroidism. ⌖ Wikimedia Commons.

323 **Hyperparathyroidism: Image A.** Osteitis fibrosa cystica. Reproduced, with permission, from Dr. Frank Gaillard and *www.radiopaedia.org.*

324 **Pituitary adenoma.** Reproduced, with permission, from Dr. Frank Gaillard and *www.radiopaedia.org.*

327 **Diabetes mellitus.** Diabetic retinopathy. This image is a derivative work, adapted from the following source, under ⌖ BY. Yanagi Y. Role of peroxisome proliferator activator receptor on blood retinal barrier breakdown. *PPAR Res* 2008;2008:679237. doi 10.1155/2008/679237.

Gastrointestinal

348 **Peyer patches.** This image is a derivative work, adapted from the following source, under ⌖ BY-SA. Plain paper.

349 **Achalasia.** This image is a derivative work, adapted from the following source, under ⌖ BY-SA. Farnoosh Farrokhi and Michael F. Vaezi.

350 **Barrett esophagus.** This image is a derivative work, adapted from the following source, under ⌖ BY-SA. Nephron. The image may have been modified by cropping, labeling, and/or captions. MedIQ Learning, LLC makes this image available under the ⌖ BY-SA.

352 **Ulcer complications.** Reproduced, with permission, from Dr. Frank Gaillard and *www.radiopaedia.org.*

354 **Inflammatory bowel disease: Image A.** Crohn disease. This image is a derivative work, adapted from the following source, under ⌖ BY. Al-Mofarreh MA, Al Mofleh IA, Al-Teimi IN, et al. Crohn's disease in a Saudi outpatient population: is it still rare? *Saudi J Gastroenterol* 2009;15:111-116. doi 10.4103/1319-3767.45357. The image may have been modified by cropping, labeling, and/or captions. All rights to this adaptation by MedIQ Learning, LLC are reserved.

355 **Diverticula of the GI tract: Image B.** Diverticulitis. This image is a derivative work, adapted from the following source, under ⌖ BY-SA. Dr. James Heilman.

356 **Zenker diverticulum.** This image is a derivative work, adapted from the following source, under ⌖ BY-SA. Bernd Bragelmann.

360 **Cirrhosis and portal hypertension: Image A.** CT. This image is a derivative work, adapted from the following source, under ⌖ BY-SA. Inversitus. The image may have been modified by cropping, labeling, and/or captions. MedIQ Learning, LLC makes this image available under the ⌖ BY-SA.

360 **Cirrhosis and portal hypertension: Image B.** Histology. This image is a derivative work, adapted from the following source, under ⌖ BY-SA. Nephron.

362 **Hepatocellular carcinoma: Image A.** Gross specimen. Reproduced, with permission, from Jean-Christophe Fournet and *www.humpath.com*.

363 **Jaundice.** [PUBLIC DOMAIN] Courtesy of the U.S. Department of Health and Human Services and Dr. Thomas F. Sellers.

367 **Gallstones: Image A.** Gross specimen. This image is a derivative work, adapted from the following source, under [CC BY-SA]. M. Emmanuel.

367 **Gallstones: Image B.** Ultrasound. This image is a derivative work, adapted from the following source, under [CC BY-SA]. Dr. James Heilman.

368 **Porcelain gallbladder.** This image is a derivative work, adapted from the following source, under [CC 0]. Fred H, van Dijk H. Images of memorable cases: case 19. Connexions Web site. December 4, 2008. Available at: *http://cnx.org/content/ m14939/1.3/*. The image may have been modified by cropping, labeling, and/or captions. All rights to this adaptation by MedIQ Learning, LLC are reserved.

368 **Acute pancreatitis.** This image is a derivative work, adapted from the following source, under [CC BY-SA]. Hellerhoff. The image may have been modified by cropping, labeling, and/or captions. MedIQ Learning, LLC makes this image available under the [CC BY-SA].

368 **Chronic pancreatitis.** This image is a derivative work, adapted from the following source, under [CC BY-SA]. Hellerhoff. The image may have been modified by cropping, labeling, and/or captions. MedIQ Learning, LLC makes this image available under the [CC BY-SA].

369 **Pancreatic adenocarcinoma: Image A.** Histology. This image is a derivative work, adapted from the following source, under [CC BY-SA]. KGH. The image may have been modified by cropping, labeling, and/or captions. MedIQ Learning, LLC makes this image available under the [CC BY-SA].

369 **Pancreatic adenocarcinoma: Image B.** CT scan. [PUBLIC DOMAIN] Courtesy of MBq.

370 **GI therapy.** Adapted, with permission, from Katzung BG, Trevor AJ. *USMLE Road Map: Pharmacology*, 1st ed. New York: McGraw-Hill, 2003:159.

Hematology and Oncology

374 **Erythrocyte.** [PUBLIC DOMAIN] Courtesy of the U.S. Department of Health and Human Services and Drs. Noguchi, Rodgers, and Schechter.

374 **Platelet.** Reproduced, with permission, from Mescher AL. *Junqueira's Basic Histology: Text and Atlas*, 12th ed. New York: McGraw-Hill, 2010: Fig. 12-13A.

374 **Neutrophil.** [PUBLIC DOMAIN] Wikimedia Commons.

375 **Monocyte.** This image is a derivative work, adapted from the following source, under [CC BY-SA]. Graham. Colm.

375 **Macrophage.** Reproduced, with permission, from Lichtman MA et al. *Lichtman's Atlas of Hematology*. New York: McGraw-Hill, 2007: Fig. V.H.11.

375 **Eosinophil.** This image is a derivative work, adapted from the following source, under [CC BY-SA]. Dr. Ed Uthman.

375 **Basophil.** Reproduced, with permission, from Lichtman MA et al. *Lichtman's Atlas of Hematology*. New York: McGraw-Hill, 2007: Fig. 12-10A.

375 **Mast cell.** Reproduced, with permission, from Lichtman MA et al. *Lichtman's Atlas of Hematology*. New York: McGraw-Hill, 2007: Fig. 5-5A.

376 **Dendritic cell.** This image is a derivative work, adapted from the following source, under [CC 0]. Behnsen J, Narang P, Hasenberg M, et al. Environmental dimensionality controls the interaction of phagocytes with the pathogenic fungi *Aspergillus fumigatus* and *Candida albicans*. PLoS Pathogens 2007;3:e13. doi 10.1371/ journal.ppat.0030013.

376 **Lymphocyte.** This image is a derivative work, adapted from the following source, under [CC BY-SA]. Wikimedia Commons.

380 **Pathologic RBC forms: Image A.** Acanthocyte. This image is a derivative work, adapted from the following source, under [CC 0]. Courtesy of Dr. Ed Uthman.

380 **Pathologic RBC forms: Image B.** Basophilic stippling. Reproduced, with permission, from Lichtman MA et al. *Lichtman's Atlas of Hematology*. New York: McGraw-Hill, 2007: Fig. I.B.1.

380 **Pathologic RBC forms: Image C.** Bite cell. Reproduced, with permission, from Lichtman MA et al. *Lichtman's Atlas of Hematology*. New York: McGraw-Hill, 2007: Fig. I.C.33.

380 **Pathologic RBC forms: Image D.** Elliptocyte. Reproduced, with permission, from Lichtman MA et al. *Lichtman's Atlas of Hematology*. New York: McGraw-Hill, 2007: Fig. I.A.4.

380 **Pathologic RBC forms: Image E.** Macro-ovalocyte. Reproduced, with permission, from Lichtman MA et al. *Lichtman's Atlas of Hematology*. New York: McGraw-Hill, 2007: Fig. I.C.88.

380 **Pathologic RBC forms: Image F.** Ringed sideroblast. Reproduced, with permission, from Lichtman MA et al. *Lichtman's Atlas of Hematology*. New York: McGraw-Hill, 2007: Fig. V.G.12.

380 **Pathologic RBC forms: Image G.** Schistocyte. [PUBLIC DOMAIN] Dr. Ed Uthman. The image may have been modified by cropping, labeling, and/ or captions. All rights to this adaptation by MedIQ Learning, LLC are reserved.

381 **Pathologic RBC forms: Image J.** Teardrop cell. Reproduced, with permission, from Fauci AS et al. *Harrison's Principles of Internal Medicine*, 17th ed. New York: McGraw-Hill, 2008: Fig. 58-7.

381 **Other RBC pathologies: Image A.** Heinz bodies. Reproduced, with permission, from Lichtman MA et al. *Lichtman's Atlas of Hematology*. New York: McGraw-Hill, 2007: Fig. I.B.2.

381 **Other RBC pathologies: Image B.** Howell-Jolly bodies. Reproduced, with permission, from Lichtman MA et al. *Lichtman's Atlas of Hematology*. New York: McGraw-Hill, 2007: Fig. I.B.3.

383 **Microcytic, hypochromic anemia: Image D.** Lead poisoning. Reproduced, with permission, from Dr Abhijit Datir, Dr. Frank Gaillard, and *www.radiopaedia.org*.

383 **Microcytic, hypochromic anemia: Image E.** Sideroblastic anemia. This image is a derivative work, adapted from the following source, under [CC BY-SA]. Paulo Henrique Orlandi Moura.

384 **Macrocytic anemia.** This image is a derivative work, adapted from the following source, under [CC 0]. Dr. Ed Uthman.

393 **Multiple myeloma: Image B.** Peripheral blood smear. This image is a derivative work, adapted from the following source, under [cc 0]. Sharma A, Kaushal M, Chaturvedi NK, et al. Cytodiagnosis of multiple myeloma presenting as orbital involvement: a case report. *Cytojournal* 2006;3:19. doi 10.1186/1742-6413-3-19. The image may have been modified by cropping, labeling, and/or captions. All rights to this adaptation by MedIQ Learning, LLC are reserved.

396 **Langerhans cell histiocytosis: Image A.** Lytic lesions. Reproduced, with permission, from Dr. Frank Gaillard and *www.radiopaedia. org.*

396 **Langerhans cell histiocytosis: Image B.** Birbeck granules. Reproduced, with permission, from Lichtman MA et al. *Lichtman's Atlas of Hematology.* New York: McGraw-Hill, 2007: Fig. IV.C.2.

397 **Chronic myeloproliferative disorders: Image A.** Polycythemia vera. This image is a derivative work, adapted from the following source, under [cc 0]. Fred H, van Dijk H. Images of memorable cases: case 151. Connexions Web site. December 4, 2008. Available at: *http://cnx.org/content/m14932/1.3/.*

397 **Chronic myeloproliferative disorders: Image B.** Essential thrombocytosis. This image is a derivative work, adapted from the following source, under [cc BY-SA]. Simon Caulton. The image may have been modified by cropping, labeling, and/or captions. MedIQ Learning, LLC makes this image available under the [cc BY-SA].

397 **Chronic myeloproliferative disorders: Image C.** Myelofibrosis. This image is a derivative work, adapted from the following source, under [cc 0]. Dr. Ed Uthman. The image may have been modified by cropping, labeling, and/or captions. All rights to this adaptation by MedIQ Learning, LLC are reserved.

399 **Warfarin (Coumadin): Toxic effect.** This image is a derivative work, adapted from the following source, under [cc 0]. Fred H, van Dijk H. Images of memorable cases: cases 84 and 85. *Connexions Web site.* December 2, 2008. Available at: *http://cnx.org/content/ m14932/1.3/.*

401 **Cancer drugs—cell cycle.** Adapted, with permission, from Katzung BG, Trevor AJ. *USMLE Road Map: Pharmacology*, 1st ed. New York: McGraw-Hill, 2003:133.

Musculoskeletal, Skin, and Connective Tissue

412 **Wrist bones.** Adapted, with permission, from Brunicardi FC et al. *Schwartz' Principles of Surgery*, 9th ed. New York: McGraw-Hill, 2009: Fig. 44-2B.

414 **Upper extremity nerves.** Adapted, with permission, from White JS. *USMLE Road Map: Gross Anatomy*, 2nd ed. New York: McGraw-Hill, 2005:145-147.

420 **Osteopetrosis.** This image is a derivative work, adapted from the following source, under [cc 0]. V. Soultanis KC, Payatakes AH, Chouliaras VT, et al. Rare causes of scoliosis and spine deformity: experience and particular features. *Scoliosis* 2007;2:15. doi 10.1186/1748-7161-2-15.

420 **Paget disease of bone: Image A.** Histology. This image is a derivative work, adapted from the following source, under [cc BY-SA]. Nephron.

420 **Paget disease of bone: Image B.** Thickened calvarium. This image is a derivative work, adapted from the following source, under [cc 0]. Dawes L. Paget's disease. [Radiology Picture of the Day Website]. Published June 21, 2007. Available at *http://www. radpod.org/2007/06/21/pagets-disease/.*

422 **Primary bone tumors: Image A.** Giant cell tumor. Reproduced, with permission, from Dr. Frank Gaillard and *www.radiopaedia. org.*

422 **Primary bone tumors: Image B.** Radiograph of osteosarcoma. Reproduced, with permission, from Dr. Frank Gaillard and *www.radiopaedia.org.*

422 **Primary bone tumors: Image C.** MRI of osteosarcoma. Reproduced, with permission, from Dr. Frank Gaillard and *www.radiopaedia. org.*

425 **Gout: Image B.** Podagra. Reproduced, with permission, from LeBlond RF et al. *DeGowin's Diagnostic Examination*, 9th ed. New York: McGraw-Hill, 2009: Plate 30.

426 **Pseudogout.** [cc] Courtesy of the U.S. Department of Health and Human Services.

426 **Seronegative spondyloarthropathies: Image C (left).** Bamboo spine. This image is a derivative work, adapted from the following source, under [cc BY-SA]. Stevenfruitsmaak. The image may have been modified by cropping, labeling, and/or captions. MedIQ Learning, LLC makes this image available under the [cc BY-SA].

426 **Seronegative spondyloarthropathies: Image C (right).** Bamboo spine. This image is a derivative work, adapted from the following source, under [cc BY-SA]. Heather Hawker. The image may have been modified by cropping, labeling, and/or captions. All rights to this adaptation by MedIQ Learning, LLC are reserved.

428 **Sarcoidosis.** Reproduced, with permission, from Dr. Frank Gaillard and *www.radiopaedia.org.*

429 **Polymyositis/dermatomyositis: Image A.** Gottron papules. This image is a derivative work, adapted from the following source, under [cc 0]. Dhoble J, Puttarajappa C, Neiberg A. Dermatomyositis and supraventricular tachycardia. *Int Arch Med* 2008;1:25. doi 10.1186/1755-7682-1-25. The image may have been modified by cropping, labeling, and/or captions. All rights to this adaptation by MedIQ Learning, LLC are reserved.

429 **Myositis ossificans.** This image is a derivative work, adapted from the following source, under [cc BY-SA]. T. Dvorak. The image may have been modified by cropping, labeling, and/or captions. MedIQ Learning, LLC makes this image available under the [cc BY-SA].

432 **Common skin disorders: Image O.** Seborrheic keratosis. This image is a derivative work, adapted from the following source, under [cc BY-SA]. Dr. James Heilman.

434 **Blistering skin disorders: Image A.** Pemphigus vulgaris. Reproduced, with permission, from Hurwitz RM et al. *Pathology of the Skin: Atlas of Clinical-Pathological Correlation*, 2nd ed. Stamford, CT: Appleton & Lange, 1998.

434 **Blistering skin disorders: Image D.** Bullous pemphigoid. This image is a derivative work, adapted from the following source, under [cc 0]. Emmanuel M. The image may have been modified by cropping, labeling, and/or captions. All rights to this adaptation by MedIQ Learning, LLC are reserved.

434 **Blistering skin disorders: Image E.** Dermatitis herpetiformis. This image is a derivative work, adapted from the following source, under [BY-SA]. Dr. Thomas Habif.

439 **Arachidonic acid products.** Adapted, with permission, from Katzung BG, Trevor AJ. *Pharmacology: Examination & Board Review*, 5th ed. Stamford, CT: Appleton & Lange, 1998:150.

Neurology

446 **Syringomyelia.** Reproduced, with permission, from Dr. Yuranga Weerakkody, Dr. Frank Gaillard, and *www.radiopaedia.org*.

451 **Sleep stages.** Adapted, with permission, from Barrett KE et al. *Ganong's Review of Medical Physiology*, 23rd ed. New York: McGraw-Hill, 2010: Fig. 15-7.

457 **Central pontine myelinolysis.** Reproduced, with permission, from Dr. Frank Gaillard and *www.radiopaedia.org*.

461 **Aneurysms: Berry aneurysm.** This image is a derivative work, adapted from the following source, under [BY-SA]. Friedman JA, Kumar R. Intraoperative angiography should be standard in cerebral aneurysm surgery. *BMC Surg* 2009;9:7. doi 10.1186/1471-2482-9-7. The image may have been modified by cropping, labeling, and/or captions. MedIQ Learning, LLC makes this image available under the [BY-SA].

462 **Intracranial hemorrhage: Image A (left and right).** Epidural hematoma. This image is a derivative work, adapted from the following source, under [BY-SA]. Hellerhoff. The image may have been modified by cropping, labeling, and/or captions. MedIQ Learning, LLC makes this image available under the [BY-SA].

462 **Intracranial hemorrhage: Image B (left).** Subdural hematoma. Reproduced, with permission, from Chen MY et al. *Basic Radiology*, 1st ed. New York: McGraw-Hill, 2005: Fig. 12-32.

476 **Eye and retina.** Reproduced, with permission, from Mescher A. *Junqueira's Basic Histology: Text & Atlas*, 12th ed. New York: McGraw-Hill, 2010: Fig 23-1.

477 **Common eye conditions: Image A.** Uveitis. This image is a derivative work, adapted from the following source, under [BY]. Agrawal RV, Murthy S, Sangwan V, et al. Current approach in diagnosis and management of anterior uveitis. *Indian J Ophthalmol* 2010;58:11-19. doi 10.4103/0301-4738.58468. The image may have been modified by cropping, labeling, and/or captions. All rights to this adaptation by MedIQ Learning, LLC are reserved.

477 **Common eye conditions: Image B.** Retinitis. [PUBLIC DOMAIN] Courtesy of the U.S. Department of Health and Human Services.

478 **Aqueous humor pathway.** Adapted, with permission, from Riordan-Eva P, Whitcher JP. *Vaughan & Asbury's General Ophthalmology*, 17th ed. New York: McGraw-Hill, 2008.

478 **Cataract.** This image is a derivative work, adapted from the following source, under [BY-SA]. Rakesh Ahuja.

479 **Extraocular muscles and nerves.** Reproduced, with permission, from Morton D et al. *The Big Picture: Gross Anatomy*. New York: McGraw-Hill, 2011: Fig. 18-3C.

480 **Pupillary light reflex.** Adapted, with permission, from Simon RP, et al. *Clinical Neurology*, 7th ed. New York: McGraw-Hill, 2009: Fig. 4-12.

481 **Age-related macular degeneration.** [PUBLIC DOMAIN] Courtesy of the U.S. Department of Health and Human Services.

484 **Multiple sclerosis.** Reproduced, with permission, from Dr. Frank Gaillard and *www.radiopaedia.org*.

487 **Neurocutaneous disorders: Image A.** Sturge-Weber syndrome and port wine stain. This image is a derivative work, adapted from the following source, under [BY]. Prashant Babaji et al.

487 **Neurocutaneous disorders: Image B.** Sturge-Weber syndrome CT scan. Reproduced, with permission, from Dr. Frank Gaillard and *www.radiopaedia.org*.

487 **Neurocutaneous disorders: Image C.** Tuberous sclerosis. This image is a derivative work, adapted from the following source, under [BY]. Fred H, van Dijk H. Images of memorable cases: case 143. Connexions Web site. December 4, 2008. Available at: *http://cnx.org/content/m14923/1.3/*.

487 **Neurocutaneous disorders: Image D.** Tuberous sclerosis and renal angiomyolipoma. This image is a derivative work, adapted from the following source, under [BY-SA]. KGH.

487 **Neurocutaneous disorders: Image E.** Neurofibromatosis and cafe-au-lait spots. This image is a derivative work, adapted from the following source, under [BY-SA]. Wikimedia Commons.

487 **Neurocutaneous disorders: Image F.** Lisch nodules in neurofibromatosis. [PUBLIC DOMAIN] Courtesy of the U.S. Department of Health and Human Services. The image may have been modified by cropping, labeling, and/or captions. All rights to this adaptation by MedIQ Learning, LLC are reserved.

487 **Neurocutaneous disorders: Image G.** Von Hippel-Lindau disease histology. This image is a derivative work, adapted from the following source, under [BY-SA] Wikimedia Commons. The image may have been modified by cropping, labeling, and/or captions. MedIQ Learning, LLC makes this image available under the [BY-SA].

487 **Neurocutaneous disorders: Image H.** Von Hippel-Lindau disease and hemangioblastoma. This image is a derivative work, adapted from the following source, under [BY]. Park DM, Zhuang Z, Chen L, et al. von Hippel-Lindau disease-associated hemangioblastomas are derived from embryologic multipotent cells. *PLOS Medicine* Feb. 13, 2007. doi 10.1371/journal.pmed.0040060.

488 **Adult primary brain tumors: Image A.** Glioblastoma multiforme at autopsy. [PUBLIC DOMAIN] Courtesy of Armed Forces Institute of Pathology.

488 **Adult primary brain tumors: Image B.** Glioblastoma multiforme histology. This image is a derivative work, adapted from the following source, under [BY-SA]. Wikimedia Commons. The image may have been modified by cropping, labeling, and/or captions. MedIQ Learning, LLC makes this image available under the [BY-SA].

488 **Adult primary brain tumors: Image C.** Dural tail in meningioma. [PUBLIC DOMAIN] Courtesy of Armed Forces Institute of Pathology. The image may have been modified by cropping, labeling, and/or captions. All rights to this adaptation by MedIQ Learning, LLC are reserved.

488 **Adult primary brain tumors: Image D.** Meningioma histology. This image is a derivative work, adapted from the following source, under [BY-SA]. Nephron. The image may have been modified by cropping, labeling, and/or captions. MedIQ Learning, LLC makes this image available under the [BY-SA].

546   Diuretics: site of action. Adapted, with permission, from Katzung BG. Basic and Clinical Pharmacology, 7th ed. Stamford, CT: Appleton & Lange, 1997:243.

Reproductive

555   Twinning. Adapted, with permission, from Cunningham FG et al. *Williams Obstetrics*, 23rd ed. New York: McGraw-Hill, 2009: Fig. 39.2.

557   Umbilical cord: Image A. Cross-section. This image is a derivative work, adapted from the following source, under [cc BY-SA]. Dr. Ed Uthman.

562   Male/female homologs. Adapted, with permission, from Strong B et al. *Human Sexuality: Diversity in Contemporary America*, 5th ed. New York: McGraw-Hill, 2005: Fig. 3.1.

566   Seminiferous tubules: Image A. Histology. This image is a derivative work, adapted from the following source, under [cc BY-SA]. Dr. Anil K. Rao.

579   Pregnancy complications: Image A. Ectopic pregnancy. This image is a derivative work, adapted from the following source, under [cc BY-SA]. Dr. Ed Uthman.

580   Endometritis. This image is a derivative work, adapted from the following source, under [cc BY-SA]. Nephron.

581   Leiomyoma (fibroid). This image is a derivative work, adapted from the following source, under [cc BY-SA]. Hic et nunc. The image may have been modified by cropping, labeling, and/or captions. MedIQ Learning, LLC makes this image available under the [cc BY-SA].

581   Polycystic ovarian syndrome. This image is a derivative work, adapted from the following source, under [cc 0]. Raine-Fenning N, Fleischer A. Clarifying the role of three-dimensional transvaginal sonography in reproductive medicine: an evidenced-based appraisal. *J Exp Clin Assist Reprod* 2005;2:10. doi 10.1186/1743-1050-2-10.

582   Ovarian neoplasms: Image C. Mature cystic teratoma. This image is a derivative work, adapted from the following source, under [cc BY-SA]. Nephron.

583   Ovarian neoplasms: Image F. Yolk sac tumor. This image is a derivative work, adapted from the following source, under [cc BY-SA]. Jensflorian. The image may have been modified by cropping, labeling, and/or captions. MedIQ Learning, LLC makes this image available under the [cc BY-SA].

585   Malignant breast tumors: Image B. Comedocarcinoma. Reproduced, with permission, from Schroge JO et al. *Williams Gynecology*. New York: McGraw-Hill, 2008: Fig. 12-11.

585   Malignant breast tumors: Image C. Paget disease. This image is a derivative work, adapted from the following source, under [cc BY-SA]. Nephron. The image may have been modified by cropping, labeling, and/or captions. MedIQ Learning, LLC makes this image available under the [cc BY-SA].

587   Varicocele. Reproduced, with permission, from Dr. Frank Gaillard and *www.radiopaedia.org*.

589   Control of reproductive hormones: female. Adapted, with permission, from Katzung BG. *Basic And Clinical Pharmacology*, 10th ed. New York: McGraw-Hill, 2006: Fig. 40-5.

589   Control of reproductive hormones: male. Adapted, with permission, from Katzung BG. *Basic And Clinical Pharmacology*, 10th ed. New York: McGraw-Hill, 2006: Fig. 40-6.

Respiratory

602   Rhinosinusitis. This image is a derivative work, adapted from the following source, under [cc 0]. Smith KD, Edwards PC, Saini TS, et al. The prevalence of concha bullosa and nasal septal deviation and their relationship to maxillary sinusitis by volumetric tomography. *Int J Dent* 2010; 10:404982. doi 10.1155/2010/404982.

603   Pulmonary emboli: Image A. CT scan. Reproduced, with permission, from Dr. Frank Gaillard and *www.radiopaedia.org*.

604   Obstructive lung diseases: Image A. Emphysema histology. This image is a derivative work, adapted from the following source, under [cc BY-SA]. Nephron.

604   Obstructive lung disease: Image B. Centriacinar emphysema. [public domain] Courtesy of the U.S. Department of Health and Human Services and Dr. Edwin P. Ewing, Jr.

606   Pneumoconioses: Image A. CT scan of asbestosis. This image is a derivative work, adapted from the following source, under [cc 0]. Miles SE, Sandrini A, Johnson AR, et al. Clinical consequences of asbestos-related diffuse pleural thickening: a review. *J Occup Med Toxicol* 2008;3:20. doi 10.1186/1745-6673-3-20. The image may have been modified by cropping, labeling, and/or captions. All rights to this adaptation by MedIQ Learning, LLC are reserved.

606   Pneumoconioses: Image B. Ferruginous bodies in asbestosis. This image is a derivative work, adapted from the following source, under [cc BY-SA]. Nephron.

610   Pancoast tumor. Reproduced, with permission, from Dr. Frank Gaillard and *www.radiopaedia.org*.

611   Pneumonia: Image B (left). Bronchopneumonia. This image is a derivative work, adapted from the following source, under [cc BY-SA] Yale Rosen. The image may have been modified by cropping, labeling, and/or captions. MedIQ Learning, LLC makes this image available under the [cc BY-SA].

611   Pneumonia: Image B (right). Lobar pneumonia. This image is a derivative work, adapted from the following source, under [cc BY-SA]. Yale Rosen.

611   Pneumonia: Image C. Bronchopneumonia histology. This image is a derivative work, adapted from the following source, under [cc BY-SA]. Yale Rosen.

611   Lung abscess. Reproduced, with permission, from Dr. Frank Gaillard and *www.radiopaedia.org*.

Index